Emergency Neurology

This work will serve to increase the emergency physician's sense of confidence in the assessment and management of the acute neurologically impaired patient. Furthermore, it will provide the emergency physician a conceptual framework for the efficient assessment and management of the patient with a neurological emergency.

From the Foreword by John G. Wiegenstein, MD

This clinician's reference provides the necessary resources for emergency physicians to care for the patient presenting with a neurological emergency. Reflecting the central place of neurological evaluation and management in the daily practice of emergency medicine, it systematically reviews the main interventions in emergency neurology, at all levels of emergency care, from prehospital management, through the emergency department, to the final disposition of the patient. The book is divided into seven sections, each integrating neurological concepts with the practical realities and demands of emergency care:

- Neurological examination and neurodiagnostic testing
- Common neurological presentations
- Specific neurological conditions
- Neurological trauma and environmental emergencies
- Pediatric neurological emergencies
- Pregnancy-related neurological emergencies
- Neurotoxicology and brain resuscitation

Combining the expertise of emergency physicians, neurologists and other specialists this highly practical text provides a constant reference source for trainees and experienced clinicians alike. Generously illustrated with scans and line diagrams, it also features management algorithms for many conditions, and each chapter ends with a list of "pearls and pitfalls." It is a comprehensive survey of best practice guidelines for emergency physicians, neurologists, and house officers in emergency medicine, neurology, neurosurgery, and critical care.

Emergency Neurology

Principles and Practice

Edited by

SID M. SHAH
Michigan State University–
  College of Human Medicine
Ingham Regional Medical Center
Lansing, Michigan

KEVIN M. KELLY
MCP Hahnemann University School of Medicine
Pittsburgh, Pennsylvania

Foreword by JOHN G. WIEGENSTEIN

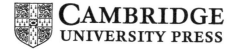

CAMBRIDGE
UNIVERSITY PRESS

CAMBRIDGE UNIVERSITY PRESS
Cambridge, New York, Melbourne, Madrid, Cape Town, Singapore, São Paulo

Cambridge University Press
The Edinburgh Building, Cambridge CB2 2RU, UK

Published in the United States of America by Cambridge University Press, New York

www.cambridge.org
Information on this title: www.cambridge.org/9780521496889

First published 1999
This digitally printed first paperback version 2006

A catalogue record for this publication is available from the British Library

Library of Congress Cataloguing in Publication data

Shah, Sid M.
    Emergency neurology : principles and practice / Sid M. Shah, Kevin
M. Kelly.
      p.   cm.
    ISBN 0-521-49688-8
    1. Neurologic emergencies.   I. Kelly, Kevin M.   II. Title.
    [DNLM: 1. Nervous System Diseases – diagnosis.   2. Neurologic
Examination.   3. Emergency Medicine.   WL 141 S525e 1999]
    RC350.7.S53   1999
    616.8'0425 – dc21
    DNLM/DLC
    for Library of Congress   98-19188
                                                                   CIP

ISBN-13 978-0-521-49688-9 hardback
ISBN-10 0-521-49688-8 hardback

ISBN-13 978-0-521-03428-9 paperback
ISBN-10 0-521-03428-0 paperback

To my wife Marsha Rappley
and our children
Maya and Neil.

SMS

To my wife Rosemary Cather Kelly
and our children
Aidan and Maura.

KMK

Contents

Part III. Specific Neurological Conditions

Preface

The past decade has brought a fundamental change in the way neurological emergencies are approached. The speciality of emergency medicine has been instrumental in this change by fostering a new awareness of the importance of providing early intervention for patients with neurological emergencies. Prior to this past decade, there was limited opportunity for therapeutic intervention for several neurological conditions. No longer simply a "triage center" for neurological emergencies, the emergency department has assumed a central role in the multifaceted evaluation and management of neurological conditions. *Emergency Neurology: Principles and Practice* is intended to enhance the awareness of important interventions in emergency neurology. It provides necessary resources for emergency department evaluation and management of patients with neurological emergencies.

Overviews of neurological emergencies are a part of most comprehensive books of emergency medicine and neurology. One of the two major themes of this book is to incorporate the principles of "emergency neurology" into the management of patients at all levels of emergency care, from the prehospital setting to the emergency department through final disposition. Prehospital care issues are reviewed, and appropriate intervention in the field is discussed. According to the patient's neurological condition, out-of-hospital evaluation and the demands of patient transport can direct and possibly change the initial diagnostic considerations and prehospital care. Emergency department evaluation is directed at rapid and focused general physical and neurological examinations. A review of key historical details guides examination, neuroanatomic localization, differential diagnosis, and intervention. Disposition of the patient from the emergency department details the principles of safe, prompt, and appropriate discharge and follow-up. Particular emphasis is placed on the various neurological entities that require patient transport to a tertiary care facility.

The other major theme of this book is the integration of neurological concepts with the practical realities and demands of emergency care. To accomplish this, we have divided the book into seven parts. Part I includes the basics of the neurological examination and neurodiagnostic testing. Chapters on lumbar puncture, electroencephalography, electronystagmography, and evoked potentials are included to familiarize the emergency physician with these neurodiagnostic tests. Although most of these tests are not components of evaluation in the emergency department, frequently they are the next step in the diagnostic process. Part II uses a symptom-oriented approach and includes a review of common neurological symptoms such as headache, weakness, and dizziness. Part III reviews specific neurological disorders. Subsequent sections are dedicated to topics of selected neurological emergencies that warrant separate review: neurological trauma, selected topics in emergency pediatric neurology, neurological complications of pregnancy, and neurotoxicology and brain resuscitation.

Some redundancy was difficult to avoid in the book, which involved the efforts of numerous authors. However, we believe that this work will find its place on the shelves of busy emergency departments where information can be retrieved easily. We thank all authors for their hard work and their patience in the final compilation of the book. The chief motivation for this effort was to provide an up-to-date resource for emergency physicians. We hope this book will be of value to neurologists, primary care physicians, and others involved in the daily care of patients with neurological emergencies.

Sid M. Shah
Kevin M. Kelly

Foreword

Full-time staffing of emergency departments by career emergency physicians began in the early 1960s, prompted by the increasing public demand for improved patient care. Prior to that time, the *least trained* members of the medical team typically staffed emergency departments. In 1968, the American College of Emergency Physicians (ACEP) was formally organized, and emergency medicine residency programs began to form. The formal approval of the specialty board followed eleven years later.

It has been interesting to watch the specialty mature during the past twenty years. Academic members of other specialties were *necessarily* called upon to author the early textbooks in emergency medicine. It has been most gratifying to observe graduates of emergency medicine residency programs assume academic positions. Certified emergency physicians, as authors, tend to focus more directly on the essential core of the specialty: the *time-dependent* process of initial recognition, evaluation, stabilization, treatment, and disposition of the emergency patient.

In the past ten years, the body of knowledge in emergency medicine has grown significantly. This has prompted academicians to more fully define certain sub-sections of the specialty and to produce textbooks relating to each sub-section or sub-specialty. Collaboration with other specialists is beneficial in this regard to assure that the work is accurate and comprehensive.

Such collaboration is evident in this excellent work on emergency neurology edited by Drs. Shah and Kelly. Dr. Shah is a residency-trained emergency physician, who graduated from the Michigan State University Emergency Medicine Residency Program where I was a faculty member. He is a valued member of the Department of Emergency Medicine at Ingham Regional Medical Center, and a respected teacher in the MSU Emergency Medicine Residency Program-Lansing.

Dr. Kelly is a neurologist and faculty member of Allegheny University of the Health Sciences. During his training and for a period of ten years he worked part-time in the busy emergency department at W. A. Foote Hospital, Jackson, Michigan. It was there that he met and worked with Dr. Shah. Their common experiences convinced them that a comprehensive text in emergency neurology, tailored to meet the special needs of the emergency physician, was needed.

If the 1980s can be labeled the "decade of the heart" in terms of emergency medicine making a difference in the outcome of patients with acute cardiac events, the 1990s can be truly labeled the "decade of the brain." Just as cardiologists have recognized the paramount importance of emergency medicine in caring for the patient with acute myocardial infarction, neurologists now recognize the essential role of the emergency physician in caring for the patient with acute stroke.

As the field of emergency medicine expands, the standard of care in the management of neurological emergencies is beginning to evolve rapidly. At the same time, there is an ever-increasing need for emergency physicians to understand and apply the basic and most advanced principles of neurology.

This work will serve to increase the emergency physician's sense of confidence in the assessment and management of the acute neurologically impaired patient. Furthermore, it will provide the emergency physician a conceptual framework for the efficient assessment and management of the patient with a neurological emergency.

John G. Wiegenstein, M.D.
Professor
Emergency Medicine
Michigan State University

Acknowledgments

A work of this magnitude is accomplished with extensive support from friends and colleagues. The editors wish to thank Ms. Teresa Hentosz, Ms. Carrie Tumpa, Ms. Karen Jury, and Ms. Anna Unglo for their monumental help with the manuscript. Teresa and Carrie committed themselves tirelessly during the final hand over of the manuscript. We thank Mr. Gregory Connor and Dr. Linda Neal for their illustrations. Ms. Shayne Davidson, a friend and a medical illustration and graphics artist, helped us enormously with her patience and the promptness with which she was able to work with deadlines. The editors thank our colleagues in Lansing, Ann Arbor, and Pittsburgh, not only for their contributions but also for their ready willingness to review manuscripts. Dr. Earl Reisdorff, a friend and scholar, provided strong support for our endeavors from the time this project was conceived. Dr. John Wiegenstein, the "father of emergency medicine," fostered Dr. Shah's interest in emergency medicine, mentored him over the years, and was gracious enough to write the foreword for this book. We also extend our gratitude to the staff of the Chi Memorial Library at Ingham Regional Medical Center under the direction of Ms. Judy Barnes.

Dr. Richard Barling, the executive editor of Cambridge, embodies our positive interactions with Cambridge University Press. Dr. Barling took personal interest in promoting this project and helped us at each step along the way. We extend our deepest gratitude to Ms. Camilla Knapp, the production editor for her efforts and patience. We also thank Ms. Nancy Brochin and Ms. Jo-Ann Strangis at Cambridge. Finally, the editors thank all the authors who give us the benefit of their knowledge, insight, and experience in bringing forth this publication.

Contributors

James W. Albers, M.D., Ph.D.
Director, Neuromuscular Program
University of Michigan Medical Center
Ann Arbor, Michigan

Roger L. Albin, M.D.
University of Michigan Medical Center
Ann Arbor, Michigan

A. Sinan Baran, M.D.
Medical Director of Sleep Disorders Center
University of Mississippi Medical Center
Jackson, Mississippi

Mark Baratz, M.D.
MCP Hahnemann University
School of Medicine
Allegheny General Hospital
Pittsburgh, Pennsylvania

Ahman Beydoun, M.D.
University of Michigan Medical Center
Ann Arbor, Michigan

Charles Bill, M.D., Ph.D.
Michigan State University
E. W. Sparrow Hospital
Lansing, Michigan

Paul Blackburn, D.O., FACEP
Division of Emergency Medicine
University of Arizona
Residency Director of Emergency Medicine
Maricopa Medical Center
Phoenix, Arizona

Amy Blasen, D.O., FACEP
Michigan State University Emergency Medicine
    Residency Program - Lansing
Department of Emergency Medicine
E. W. Sparrow Hospital
Lansing, Michigan

William J. Brady, M.D.
University of Virginia Health Systems
Charlottesville, Virginia

Jon Brillman, M.D. FRCPI
MCP Hahnemann University
School of Medicine
Chairman-Department of Neurology
Allegheny General Hospital
Pittsburgh, Pennsylvania

Lynn Brown, M.D., FACEP
Department of Emergency Medicine
St. Luke's Shawnee Mission Medical Center
Overland Park, Kansas

David Castle, EMT
Michigan State University
College of Osteopathic Medicine
East Lansing, Michigan

Marc Chimowitz, M.D.
Emory University
Atlanta, Georgia

Kathleen Cowling, D.O., FACEP
Michigan State University Emergency Medicine
    Residency Program - Saginaw
St. Joseph Hospital
Saginaw, Michigan

Ivo Drury, MB, Bch
Department of Neurology
Henry Ford Hospital
Detroit, Michigan

Eric Eggenberger, D.O.
College of Osteopathic Medicine
Michigan State University
East Lansing, Michigan

Janet Eng, D.O.
Michigan State University
  Emergency Medicine Residency
  Program - Lansing
Ingham Regional Medical Center
E. W. Sparrow Hospital
Lansing, Michigan

William D. Fales, M.D.
Department of Emergency Medicine
Michigan State University
East Lansing, Michigan

Greg Fermann, M.D.
Director of Clinical Operations
University of Cincinnati
Cincinnati, Ohio

Thomas J. Fix, M.D.
Palm Beach Gardens Imaging Center
Palm Beach Gardens, Florida

Norman L. Foster, M.D.
University of Michigan Medical Center
Ann Arbor, Michigan

Michael R. Frankel, M.D.
Emory University
Grady Memorial Hospital
Atlanta, Georgia

Brent Furbee, M.D.
Methodist Hospital of Indiana
Indiana University School of Medicine
Indianapolis, Indiana

Douglas J. Gelb, M.D., Ph.D.
University of Michigan Medical Center
Ann Arbor, Michigan

Kevin J. Gingrich, M.D.
Director of Neuroanesthesiology, Pharmacology
  and Physiology
University of Rochester Medical Center
Rochester, New York

Andrew L. Goldberg, M.D.
MCP Hahnemann University
School of Medicine
Allegheny General Hospital
Pittsburgh, Pennsylvania

Barbara Good, Ph.D.
National Surgical Adjuvant Bowel and Breast Project
Allegheny General Hospital
Pittsburgh, Pennsylvania

Stephen Guertin, M.D.
Michigan State University
Director of Pediatric Intensive Care Unit
Medical Director
E. W. Sparrow Regional Childrens Center
Lansing, Michigan

Rae R. Hanson, M.D.
Department of Emergency Medicine
Midelfort Clinic
Eau Claire, Wisconsin

Ashok Harwani, M.D.
Department of Emergency Medicine
Flower Hospital
Sylvania, Ohio

Oliver W. Hayes, D.O., FACEP
College of Osteopathic Medicine
Michigan State University Emergency Medicine
  Residency Program - Lansing
East Lansing, Michigan

Judith L. Heidebrink, M.D.
University of Michigan Medical Center
Ann Arbor, Michigan

Tim Hodge, D.O.
Department of Emergency Medicine
E. W. Sparrow Hospital
Lansing, Michigan

J. Stephen Huff, M.D., FACEP
University of Virginia Health Systems
Charlottesville, Virginia

Mary Hughes, D.O., FACEP
College of Osteopathic Medicine
Michigan State University
Osteopathic Program Director
Michigan State University Emergency Medicine
    Residency Program - Lansing
East Lansing, Michigan

Ron Jakubiak, M.D.
Michigan State University
E. W. Sparrow Hospital
Lansing, Michigan

Imad Jarjour, M.D.
MCP Hahnemann University
School of Medicine
Allegheny General Hospital
Pittsburgh, Pennsylvania

Robert G. Kaniecki, M.D.
MCP Hahnemann University
School of Medicine
Allegheny General Hospital
Pittsburgh, Pennsylvania

Kevin M. Kelly, M.D., Ph.D.
MCP Hahnemann University
School of Medicine
Allegheny General Hospital
Pittsburgh, Pennsylvania

Ario Keyarash, M.D.
Department of Orthopedic Surgery
Allegheny General Hospital
Pittsburgh, Pennsylvania

Henry R. Landsgaard, D.O.
Department of Emergency Medicine
Genesis Health Systems
Grand Blanc, Michigan

Patricia Lanter, M.D.
Department of Emergency Medicine
Cook County Hospital
Chicago, Illinois

Mary Beth Miller, D.O.
Assistant Director of Education
Michigan State University Emergency Medicine
    Residency Program - Lansing
Lansing, Michigan

Herbert Newton, M.D.
Director, Division of Neuro-Oncology
Ohio State University
Columbus, Ohio

David Overton, M.D., FACEP
Michigan State University
Michigan State University Emergency Medicine
    Residency Program - Kalamazoo
Kalamazoo, Michigan

Robert Prodinger, D.O.
Michigan State University Emergency Medicine
    Residency Program - Lansing
E.W. Sparrow Hospital
Department of Emergency Medicine
Lansing, Michigan

Marsha Rappley, M.D.
Department of Pediatrics and
    Human Development
College of Human Medicine
Michigan State University
East Lansing, Michigan

Danielle Ray, M.D.
Michigan State University Emergency Medicine
    Residency Program - Kalamazoo
Kalamazoo, Michigan

Earl J. Reisdorff, M.D., FACEP
Michigan State University
Michigan State University Emergency Medicine
    Residency Program - Lansing
Lansing, Michigan

David Rossi, M.D.
Department of Emergency Medicine
Burgess Medical Center
Kalamazoo, Michigan

Thomas F. Scott, M.D.
MCP Hahnemann University
School of Medicine
Allegheny General Hospital
Pittsburgh, Pennsylvania

L. R. Searls, D.O.
Michigan State University Emergency Medicine
    Residency Program - Lansing
Ingham Regional Medical Center
Lansing, Michigan

Sid M. Shah, M.D., FACEP
Michigan State University Emergency Medicine
    Residency Program - Lansing
Ingham Regional Medical Center
E.W. Sparrow Hospital
Lansing, Michigan

Neil T. Shepard, Ph.D.
Department of Otorhinolaryngology,
    Head and Neck Surgery
University of Pennsylvania Health System
Philadelphia, Pennsylvania

George A. Small, M.D.
MCP Hahnemann University
School of Medicine
Allegheny General Hospital
Pittsburgh, Pennsylvania

Jerald A. Solot, D.O., FACEP, FACOEP
University of Pittsburgh School of Medicine
Chairman of Emergency Medicine
UPMC Shadyside
Pittsburgh, Pennsylvania

Craig A. Taylor, M.D.
MCP Hahnemann University
School of Medicine
Allegheny General Hospital
Pittsburgh, Pennsylvania

Steven A. Tellan, M.D.
Department of Otorhinolaryngology
University of Michigan Medical Center
Ann Arbor, Michigan

Jane L. Turner, M.D.
Department of Pediatrics and Human Development
College of Human Medicine
Michigan State University
East Lansing, Michigan

James P. Valeriano, M.D.
MCP Hahnemann University
School of Medicine
Allegheny General Hospital
Pittsburgh, Pennsylvania

Navin K. Varma, M.D.
Ogden, Utah

John J. Wald, M.D.
Neuromuscular Program
University of Michigan Medical Center
Ann Arbor, Michigan

W. Lee Warren, M.D.
Department of Neurosurgery
Allegheny General Hospital
Pittsburgh, Pennsylvania

Mary Ellen Wermuth, M.D.
Methodist Hospital of Indiana
Indiana University School
    of Medicine
Indianapolis, Indiana

James E. Wilberger, Jr., M.D.
MCP Hahnemann University
School of Medicine
Department of Neurosurgery
Allegheny General Hospital
Pittsburgh, Pennsylvania

Brian Zink, M.D.
University of Michigan
Department of Emergency Medicine
University of Michigan Medical Center
Ann Arbor, Michigan

Scott R. Zittel, D.O.
Michigan State University
    Emergency Medicine Residency
    Program - Lansing
Lansing, Michigan

ONE Neurological Examination and Neurodiagnostic Testing

1 The Neurological Examination

THOMAS F. SCOTT

SUMMARY The neurological history and examination provide physicians with information to localize lesions of the nervous system. Neuroanatomical localization allows formulation of a focused differential diagnosis, diagnostic plan, and treatment plan. Although aspects of the neurological examination differ based on the clinical situation, the standard elements of the neurological examination remain the same. A review of the neurological examination as it applies to emergency department evaluation is provided.

Introduction

An adequate neurological examination can differ significantly among various clinical situations. An emergency physician caring for a patient with a gastrointestinal problem may limit the neurological examination to observance of speech and motor movements during the interview and the general medical examination, and document an abbreviated neurological examination. A patient who has symptoms that suggest a neurological or a musculoskeletal problem requires a detailed neurological examination. The purpose of this chapter is to review the elements of a focused neurological examination for use in a busy emergency department.

The neurological examination is primarily a bedside tool that allows clinicians to localize lesions in the nervous system. Typically, a combination of findings on the examination allows this localization. If an examination suggests multiple lesions in the nervous system, the implications of each lesion are considered individually and in combinations. Evidence of *systemic disease* (involving more than one organ system) is considered in the interpretation of the neurological findings. Thus the neurological examination is incorporated in the context of the patient's overall health history and general physical examination.[1,2]

A standard neurological examination begins with a brief assessment of the patient's mental status, followed by testing of cranial nerve function, motor function, deep tendon reflexes, sensory modalities, and pathological reflexes (i.e., snout, grasp, and Babinski reflex) generally presented in that order in documentation.[3] Time constraints in the emergency department frequently prevent a comprehensive neurological examination. However, an abbreviated and focused neurological examination is adequate for most patients presenting with a focal problem such as a typical migrainous headache, unilateral limb pain, or back pain. A focused neurological examination is directed at a specific clinical condition and includes site-specific components of neurological evaluation. Patients who are being admitted to the hospital for nonneurological conditions require a documented "abbreviated" evaluation that includes a brief mental status examination, testing of cranial nerves II to VII, motor function, and sensory function.

The goal of an emergency department neurological examination is the ability to answer confidently the following questions: Is there a neurological condition? Where is (are) the lesion(s) located? What are the possible causes? Can the patient be discharged safely from the emergency department or is hospitalization required?

Emergency Department Evaluation

Neurological History

A detailed neurological history allows the emergency physician to focus on important components of the neurological examination, thus saving time and resources. A specific and detailed history enhances the likelihood of making a definite diagnosis in the emergency department. About 75% of neurological diagnoses are made while obtaining the patient's history. One of the key elements in obtaining a neurological history in the emergency department is the *directed history*, which allows development of a relevant differential diagnosis. An account from family members and bystanders can be an important source of information in the emergency department. The history obtained from the patient can be considered a part of the mental status examination, providing information about the patient's affect, speech, memory, logical thought, and any psychiatric symptoms. Important historical elements to elicit are the time and mode of onset, temporal relationship of symptoms, progression of symptoms, associated symptoms, and exacerbating and alleviating factors. Symptoms that indicate involvement of a particular region of the nervous system are explored. A history of a similar event in the past is of singular historical importance. A history of medication use, illicit drug use, exposure to toxins, and head trauma is important.

Neurological Examination

Mental Status Examination. The mental status examination is performed and documented as the first part of the neurological examination because its findings have bearing on the reliability of the remainder of the examination. For example, patients with an abnormal affect may be more likely to show signs of functional (somatoform) illness, and demented or encephalopathic patients may not be able to cooperate fully during the examination. Due to time constraints of the emergency department, the reporting of mental

TABLE 1.1. Glasgow Coma Scale

Eye opening	
Opens eyes spontaneously	4
Opens eyes to verbal command	3
Opens eyes to pain	2
Does not open eyes	1
Verbal response	
Alert and oriented	5
Converses but disoriented	4
Speaking but nonsensical	3
Moans or makes unintelligible sounds	2
No response	1
Motor response	
Follows commands	6
Localizes pain	5
Movement or withdrawal from pain	4
Abnormal flexion (decorticate)	3
Abnormal extension (decerebrate)	2
No response	1
TOTAL	3–15

status is often abbreviated, sometimes being reduced to a single phrase such as "patient alert and a good historian." Such limited documentation can make changes in mental status difficult to assess during the course of a hospitalization. Ideally, the record adequately reflects the patient's baseline mental functioning prior to hospitalization.

Level of alertness is noted first, as either alert, confused, drowsy, stuporous (tending to drift into sleep during the examination, or arousable for only brief periods), or comatose (with or without spontaneous or purposeful movements). An assigned number on a coma scale is no substitute for a precise description of mental status. However, the Glasgow Coma Scale is often used as a method of briefly quantitating neurological dysfunction (see Table 1.1).[4] Coma with certain combinations of ocular findings and breathing patterns can indicate specific neuroanatomical substrates for the coma.[5] Bilateral pinpoint pupils in a comatose patient with apneustic or agonal respirations implies a pontine lesion with high morbidity and mortality, but these findings can also occur as a result of narcotics overdose. Loss of the oculocephalic reflex, or "doll's eyes," is rarely seen in drug overdose and implies brainstem injury (normally, eye movements are opposite to rotary movements of the head performed by the examiner). A unilateral dilated pupil in a comatose patient implies brainstem herniation, usually related to contralateral hemispheric mass effect. Bilateral dilated and fixed pupils and loss of all brainstem reflexes and respiratory drive occur in brain death. Paralytic agents can produce a similar clinical presentation, but typically pupils are not affected.

In alert patients, a comment regarding affect is made when noting the patient's behavior and insight during the interview and examination. Orientation is checked in four "spheres": person (self and others), place, time, and purpose. The remainder of the mental status examination varies among clinicians, but several of the following tests are performed at the bedside routinely: naming presidents, "serial sevens," registration of three objects and recalling them at five minutes, repeating digit span forward and backward, interpreting proverbs and similarities, complex figure drawing, spelling "world" forward and backward, and naming five cities. A standardized mini mental status examination such as the Folstein MMSE is used occasionally. Determination of probable mild to severe dementia is often made with only a brief neurological examination using these tests.

More specific bedside testing of higher cortical functions is often added to the mental status examination in patients with evidence of focal lesions. Delineation of aphasias can involve detailed testing but is usually limited to gross observation of speech output, conduction (ability to repeat), and comprehension. Bedside testing also includes object naming, awareness of right/left, and testing for visual and sensory neglect (especially important in parietal and thalamic lesions).

Cranial Nerve Examination. An abnormality on cranial nerve examination may relate to lesion(s) in the cortex, deep gray matter (for example, thalamus), brainstem (including nuclei), or along the course of a cranial nerve through soft and bony tissues. Certain patterns of cranial nerve dysfunction allow localization of lesions to these areas, and many such patterns are considered to be "classic" findings related to specific neuroanatomical substrates. It is often necessary to combine a cranial nerve finding with other neurological deficits in order to localize a lesion precisely (see Fig. 1.1).[6]

- *Cranial Nerve I.* Although the first cranial nerve is often omitted as part of the routine examination, a deficit of smell is often an important clue to a diagnosis. Lesions of the olfactory groove (typically, a meningioma) can have associated psychiatric symptoms related to frontal lobe injury, and loss of sense of smell due to compression of the olfactory nerves. Loss of sense of smell is also common after head trauma and is due to shearing of the branches of the olfactory nerves as they pass through the cribriform plate. Coffee grounds are often used to test sense of smell. Noxious smells such as isopropyl alcohol should be avoided because they stimulate cranial nerve V.

- *Cranial Nerve II.* Visual disturbances are listed as part of the cranial nerve examination regardless of the location of the lesion. A visual field disturbance related to hemispheric injury (e.g., a homonymous hemianopsia) is noted. Lesions limited to the optic nerve produce monocular visual disturbance. Typically, visual acuity is tested when the patient's complaints are primarily ocular. In patients with near blindness, the distance at which the patient can count fingers is sometimes noted. A funduscopic examination is done routinely and reported as negative when the retina, retinal vessels, and optic discs are free of lesions. Papilledema (swelling of the optic disc) is a classic finding of increased intracranial pressure due to tumor, hydrocephalus, or other causes. Visual field neglect, frequently associated with contralateral parietal lesions, is usually noted as part of the mental status examination or under the topic of "higher cortical functions." When intact, several optic nerve functions are commonly summarized by the abbreviation PERRLA (pupils equal, round, and reactive to light and accommodation). The swinging flashlight test may reveal a consensual response (contralateral pupillary constriction with stimulation) despite a relatively poor direct response ipsilaterally (afferent pupillary defect, also known as a Marcus Gunn pupil), due to an optic nerve lesion.

  Findings of the neurological examination that are listed under cranial nerve II include the following: a Hollenhorst plaque, a bright-appearing

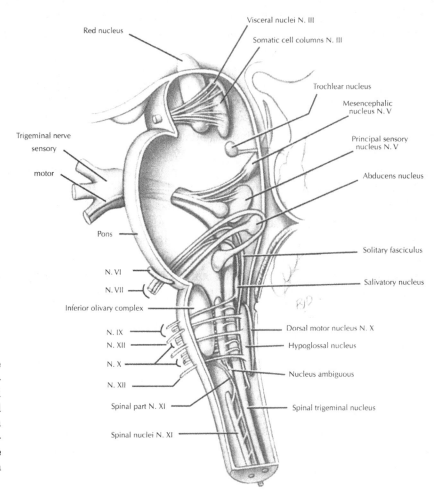

Red nucleus

Trigeminal nerve
sensory

motor

Pons

N. VI
N. VII
Inferior olivary complex
N. IX
N. XII
N. X
N. XII
Spinal part N. XI
Spinal nuclei N. XI

Visceral nuclei N. III
Somatic cell columns N. III
Trochlear nucleus
Mesencephalic
nucleus N. V
Principal sensory
nucleus N. V
Abducens nucleus
Solitary fasciculus
Salivatory nucleus
Dorsal motor nucleus N. X
Hypoglossal nucleus
Nucleus ambiguous
Spinal trigeminal nucleus

FIGURE 1.1. Sagittal view of the brainstem showing selected anatomical features to demonstrate cranial nerve nuclei, cranial nerves, and their anatomical relationships. An abnormality of cranial nerve function may localize a lesion to the brainstem when associated with other specific neurological deficits.

cholesterol or atheromatous embolus visualized by funduscopic examination of the retinal vessels, implying an embolic process. Visual field defects include: homonymous hemianopsia, a large hemispheric lesion or lesion of the lateral geniculate ganglion; bitemporal hemianopsia, a lesion of the pituitary area compressing the optic chiasm; central scotoma, a lesion of the optic nerve that typically occurs with optic neuritis, superior quadrantanopsia, a contralateral temporal lobe lesion.

- *Cranial Nerves III, IV, VI.* Cranial nerves that control eye movements are frequently described by the abbreviation EOMI (extraocular muscles intact). Dysfunction of these nerves can be localized by noting the direction of gaze, which causes or worsens a diplopia, and any loss of upgaze, downgaze, or horizontal movements in either eye. Diplopia that worsens on lateral gaze

(while the patient tracks a hand-held object or finger) suggests an ipsilateral palsy of cranial nerve VI or lateral rectus weakness. Cranial nerve III and sympathetic fibers are responsible for eye opening; consequently, ptosis, without or with a Horner's syndrome (ptosis, miosis, anhydrosis), is recorded as part of the extraocular muscle examination (although the pupil abnormalities associated with these syndromes can be recorded as part of the visual examination). A classic finding of abnormal ocular motility is referred to as an internuclear ophthalmoplegia (INO). Abnormal ipsilateral adduction with visual tracking of the eye is seen with lacunar infarcts of the medial longitudinal fasciculus (MLF) or with multiple sclerosis plaques in the MLF.

- *Cranial Nerve V.* Facial sensation is tested with light touch, pinprick, and temperature. A cooled tuning fork or ice bag can be used to test temperature. If an abnormality is found in only one or two divisions of V_1–V_3, the findings imply a lesion distal to the gasserian ganglion. Distinct splitting of sensory function at the midline face is unusual and can imply a functional disorder. Vibration is not tested for cranial nerve V function, but splitting of vibratory sensation across the forehead or skull is further evidence of a functional component in a patient's clinical presentation.

- *Cranial Nerve VII.* Seventh cranial nerve lesions are referred to as either central or peripheral. In central lesions, located proximal to the seventh nerve nucleus and contralateral to the resulting facial droop, the upper face (periorbital area and forehead) will be relatively spared. The palpebral fissure may be slightly larger ipsilateral to the facial droop. In peripheral lesions, weakness is ipsilateral to the lesion of the seventh cranial nerve nucleus or the nerve itself. Other brainstem signs are seen typically when a lesion involves the nerve nucleus; the term *Bell's palsy* commonly refers to lesions of the nerve distal to the nucleus. Eye closure may be lost in severe cases of peripheral seventh nerve lesions. Hyperacusis is due to loss of the seventh nerve's dampening influence on the stapes.

- *Cranial Nerve VIII.* The eighth cranial nerve consists of an auditory component and a vestibular component. Deafness rarely results from cortical lesions, which more often cause difficulty with sound localization. Common bedside testing involves comparison for gross symmetry with a high-pitched tuning fork (512 or 256 Hz) or by finger rubbing near the ear, and the Weber and Rinne tests (for air conduction compared to bone conduction of sound). Lesions of the vestibular nuclei and the vestibular portion of the eighth cranial nerve can product vertigo, nausea, vomiting, and nystagmus.

- *Cranial Nerves IX and X.* The examiner records symmetry of palatal elevation and the gag reflex, functions subserved by these cranial nerves. Hoarseness and dysphagia can be seen with unilateral or bilateral injury to cranial nerve X (vagus); however, lesions of cranial nerve IX may be undetectable clinically.

- *Cranial Nerve XI.* Strength of the sternocleidomastoid and trapezius muscles is tested with resistance to head turning and shoulder shrug, respectively. The loss of strength is often greater with nuclear or peripheral lesions as opposed to a supranuclear injury.

- *Cranial Nerve XII.* On protrusion, a unilateral weak tongue deviates toward the side of weakness in lesions of the nucleus and peripheral nerve injury, but away from supranuclear lesions. Nuclear and peripheral lesions are associated with atrophy when chronic.

The Motor System. *Tone and Power.* Normal muscle tone refers to the slight tension present in muscles at rest. Muscle tone can be increased in both pyramidal and extrapyramidal disturbances. Muscle tone is evaluated at bedside by passive movements of joints through a range of motion at varying velocities. In slowly evolving extrapyramidal disorders such as Parkinson's disease, rigidity occurs.

Tremor plus rigidity yields "cogwheel" rigidity. Acute central nervous system (CNS) lesions involving the pyramidal tracts often produce hypotonia. This finding evolves over days, producing hyperreflexia and hypertonicity, referred to as spasticity. Spasticity is a velocity-dependent increase in tone, waxing and waning through the range of motion. Hypertonicity can occur acutely in brainstem lesions (decorticate or decerebrate posturing). Hypotonicity may be present chronically in neuromuscular disease.

After resistance to passive manipulation is tested manually, individual muscle group power is graded on a scale of 0–5 as follows: 0 equals no muscle contraction, 1 equals muscle contraction without joint movement, 2 equals partial movement with gravity eliminated, 3 equals movement against gravity, 4 equals resistance given, 5 equals normal strength. For detection of mild weakness, the examiner assesses for pronator drift (the patient with arms extended and supinated tends to pronate and lower the whole arm with flexion at the elbow) and observes the gait (including heel and toe walking).

The neurological history and examination usually can localize weakness to upper motor neuron dysfunction, lower motor neuron dysfunction, or the neuromuscular junction or muscle (see Table 1.2).[7] Predominant proximal muscle weakness or atrophy, when symmetrical, usually suggests a myopathic

TABLE 1.2. Changes in Motor Function

	Loss of Power	Tone	Atrophy	Fasciculations	Ataxia
Spinomuscular lesion					
a. Anterior horn cell	Focal	Flaccid	Present	Present	Absent
b. Nerve root, plexus, peripheral nerve	Focal or segmental	Flaccid	Present	Occasionally present	Absent
c. Neuromuscular junction	Diffuse	Usually normal	Usually normal	Absent	Absent
d. Muscle	Diffuse	Flaccid	Present but later than a. and b.	Absent	Absent
Extrapyramidal lesion	None or mild	Rigid	Absent	Absent	Absent
Corticospinal tract lesion	Generalized Incomplete	Spastic	Absent	Absent	Absent
Cerebellar lesion	None; ataxia may simulate loss of power	Hypotonic (ataxia)	Absent	Absent	Absent
Psychogenic disorder	Bizarre No true loss of power May simulate any type	Normal or variable Often	Absent	Absent	Absent (may simulate ataxia)

Source: From Haerer AF. 5th ed. *DeJong's The Neurologic Examination.* Philadelphia, Pa: JB Lippincott Co; 1992. Courtesy of and with permission from publisher, Lippincott-Raven.

condition. Flabby or flaccid weak muscles, often atrophic, are seen in lower motor neuron disorders and are associated with a decrease in deep tendon reflexes (e.g., peripheral neuropathy, spinal muscle atrophy). Upper motor neuron disorders are distinguished by spasticity, increased tone, and increased deep tendon reflexes. In some neurological disorders (e.g., amyotrophic lateral sclerosis, vitamin B_{12} deficiency) a mixture of upper motor neuron and lower motor neuron dysfunction evolves over time.

Coordination. Equilibrium refers to the coordination and balance of the whole body; when equilibrium is impaired, it is referred to as truncal ataxia. This is tested at bedside by observing sitting, balance when standing, and gait (classically "wide-based" in cases of mild to moderate ataxia). The examination is refined with testing of tandem gait (placing one heel directly in front of the opposite toes), and by testing for the Romberg sign (swaying and truncal movements) when the eyes are closed after the feet are placed together with the arms at the sides.

Limb ataxia (appendicular ataxia) can be present in a single extremity (usually an arm) but is more often seen in an ipsilateral arm and leg pattern, with the patient exhibiting a tendency to fall to that side. When limb ataxia is combined with weakness, the tem *ataxic hemiparesis* applies (classic for an internal capsule or pontine lacunar stroke when present-

TABLE 1.2. Changes in Motor Function (cont.)

Reflexes	Abnormal Movements	Pathologic Associated Movements
Decreased or absent	None except for fasciculations	Absent
Decreased or absent	None except for rare fasciculations	Absent
Usually normal	None	Absent
Decreased	None	Absent
Muscle stretch reflexes normal or variable Superficial reflexes normal or slightly increased No corticospinal tract responses	Present	Absent
Muscle stretch reflexes hyperactive Superficial reflexes diminished to absent Corticospinal tract responses	None	Absent
Muscle stretch reflexes diminished or pendular Superficial reflexes normal No corticospinal tract responses	May be present (intention tremor and ataxia)	Absent
Muscle stretch reflexes normal or increased (range) Superficial reflexes normal or increased No corticospinal tract responses	May be present	Absent

ing as a pure motor stroke syndrome). Limb ataxia is demonstrated by testing finger-to-nose and heel-to-shin movements. Although limb ataxia can be seen in sensory disorders (pseudoathetosis), it is a classic indicator of lesions of the cerebellar system, producing intention tremor (see below) and dysdiadochokinesia (impairment of rapid alternating movements). Limb ataxia in the absence of weakness suggests a lesion of the cerebellar hemispheres and their projections, whereas truncal ataxia in isolation suggests a lesion of midline cerebellar structures and their projections.

Abnormal Movements. Essential or physiological tremor (commonly 8–11 Hz) can be a normal finding. Essential tremor is assessed by having the patient forcibly extend the arms and digits; tremor is demonstrated distally. The term *benign essential tremor* denotes a pathological idiopathic high-frequency tremor that is often familial. Essential tremor can be accentuated or attenuated by drugs and disease states. Tremulousness generally refers to transient high-frequency tremor associated with acute illness or anxiety. In severe metabolic disturbances, tremor can coexist with other abnormal movements such as myoclonus (rapid and tense contractions of large muscle groups) and asterixis (intermittent lapses of tone-interrupting voluntary movements).

Intention tremor refers to to-and-fro motions that increase in amplitude as the patient's finger approaches a target. This tremor is usually demonstrated on finger-to-nose testing in patients with lesions of cerebellar hemispheres and their projections into the brainstem and ventral posterolateral thalami.

Parkinsonian tremor is typically at a lower frequency than essential tremor and is often described as a "pill-rolling" tremor. Unlike the "action" tremors described above, tremor in Parkinson's disease is present at rest (at least intermittently), is variably affected by changes in position, and is associated with stiffness (hence cogwheel rigidity) and bradykinesia.

Bradykinesia, Akinesia, and Dyskinesia:

Bradykinesia is a reduction of normal spontaneous or unconscious semipurposeful movements such as blinking, shifting movements, and facial expressions. A classic symptom of Parkinson's disease, bradykinesia also occurs in other neurodegenerative syndromes, multi-infarct state, and depression.

Akinetic mutism is a condition of extreme lack of movement and interaction, verbal and nonverbal, that occurs in patients with brainstem lesions or bilateral hemispheric or deep gray matter lesions. It also occurs in patients with end-stage neurodegenerative disorders. Catatonic mutism refers to a similar condition – regarded as a manifestation of severe psychiatric disturbance, not structural lesions – and generally is associated with waxy flexibility (maintaining an unusual posture positioned passively) or rigidity.

Dyskinesia is a nonspecific term for complex irregular involuntary movements involving multiple muscle groups. Most patients with dyskinesia have medication-induced side effects of neuroleptics and antiparkinsonian drugs containing L-dopa. Tardive dyskinesia refers to the late-developing, neuroleptic-induced choreoathetoid movements primarily of the face, head, shoulders, and upper trunk.

Rapid dyskinetic movements are often referred to as *choreiform.* This term accurately describes many patients with tardive dyskinesia, Huntington's disease, and Sydenham chorea. Dystonic movements are slower and associated with increased tone or rigidity (for example, dystonia musculorum deformans) and can occur in patients with Parkinson's disease and as acute reactions to neuroleptics. Athetoid movements are intermittent in speed between chorea and dystonia, and have a writhing or more rhythmic quality.

Other miscellaneous abnormal movements include ballismus, tics, and akathisia:

- Ballismus refers to an abrupt flailing movement of an extremity that can occur following stroke involving the subthalamic nucleus.
- Tics refer to rapid movements that are stereotyped and repetitive. Tics are classic in Tourette's syndrome but can occur with mental retardation.
- Akathisia can be thought of as the opposite of bradykinesia. Normal spontaneous movements increase in the waking state. Patients with akathisia may be "fidgety" and often pace.

Deep Tendon Reflexes, Cutaneous Reflexes, and Miscellaneous Signs. Deep tendon reflexes are elicited by percussion over tendon insertions that produces a rapid muscle stretch. These reflexes are mediated by reflex arcs originating in intramuscular organs that are sensitive to stretching; they transmit impulses to alpha motor neurons within the spinal cord, which produces a contraction of the percussed muscle. When deep tendon reflexes are increased or hyperactive, reflex "spread" occurs in other local muscles, resulting in an increased intensity of muscle contraction. Deep tendon reflexes are generally graded on a 0–4 basis: 0 indicates that a reflex is not elicited; 1 indicates a hypoactive reflex or one that is present only with reinforcing maneuvers; 2 indicates a normal reflex; 3 indicates reflexes that appear to be hyperactive but may not necessarily be pathological; 4 indicates clonic reflexes that may or may not be pathological.

Cutaneous reflexes consist of the abdominal reflex (abdominal wall muscle contraction), elicited by stimulation of the skin over the four quadrants of the abdomen, the cremasteric reflex (testicular elevation), elicited by stimulation of the skin over the scrotal area, and the anal wink reflex (anal contraction with stimulation).

Pathological reflexes can be associated with the following signs:

- Frontal release signs consist of glabellar, snout, suck, root, grasp, and palmomental reflexes. These signs usually indicate bilateral frontal lobe disease.

- Hoffmann's sign indicates hyperreflexia in the upper extremities, elicited by brisk tapping of the distal digits in the hand and observing for flexion of the thumb.
- Babinski sign occurs when plantar stimulation of the foot with a blunt object produces extension of the great toe and fanning of the other toes. This reflex is synonymous with an extensor plantar response and is a sign of upper motor neuron dysfunction. Other methods of eliciting an "upgoing toe" involve stimulation of the lateral foot (Chaddock's sign) or pinprick over the dorsum of the foot (Bing's sign).

Psychogenic disorders can be associated with the following findings:

- Splitting the tuning fork test is administered to patients with psychogenic sensory disturbance. These patients typically have a sharply demarcated loss of sensation to the midface and may complain of a lack of vibratory sensation when tested on the affected side of the forehead, with intact vibratory sensation on the unaffected side.
- The hand–face drop test is used in patients with psychogenic coma who appear flaccid. When the patient's hand is held over the face and dropped, the patient in psychogenic coma typically avoids letting the hand hit the face with subtle movements to the side.
- Hoover's sign (of psychogenic neurological dysfunction): The examiner places one hand under each heel with the patient in the supine position. The patient is asked to raise one leg, and the examiner feels downward pressure of the opposite leg when voluntary effort is intact. Absence of pressure suggests lack of effort and possible contralateral functional weakness.
- Astasia – abasia is a lurching, unusual gait symptomatic of psychogenic ataxia.

Sensory Examination. Similar to the rest of the neurological examination, the sensory examination is an organized assessment of neuroanatomical structures and systems. It is usually performed last because findings related to cognition and higher cortical functions have bearing on its interpretation. Testing of light touch and pinprick sensation assesses the integrity of the peripheral nervous system and spinal cord sensory tracts, and it can also be used to assess the presence of a cortical lesion (e.g., "extinction" in parietal lobe lesions occurs when bilateral stimuli are presented and the sensory stimulus is neglected contralateral to the lesion).

The sensory examination is routinely documented as a response to five modalities: pinprick, light touch, vibration, position, and temperature. The tools used for these tests include a safety pin or other sharp object, a cotton swab, a 128-Hz tuning fork, an ice bag or metal object such as a tuning fork placed over a cooling vent or in ice water, and calipers to test two-point discrimination. Perception of temperature or pain requires integrity of unmyelinated peripheral nerves (which originate as bipolar neurons in the dorsal root ganglia), the spinothalamic tracts of the spinal cord and brainstem, the ventral posterolateral and ventral posteromedial thalami, and thalamic projections to the parietal lobes. Sensation of light touch is transmitted similarly, but is also likely transmitted through the posterior columns. Sensory loss to light touch and pinprick can occur in the distribution of a single nerve, nerve root, plexus pattern, hemicord pattern, transverse cord pattern, or crossed brainstem pattern (see below), or somatotopically, corresponding to lesions above the brainstem (for example, contralateral face-arm-leg). A lesion is localized to the brainstem when sensory loss occurs on one side of the face and contralateral body. A "stocking-glove" pattern is usually seen in patients with polyneuropathy, often due to diabetes. Perception of vibratory and position sense requires integrity of myelinated nerve fibers (originating as bipolar neurons in the dorsal root ganglion), the posterior columns, the medial lemniscus, ventral posterolateral nucleus of the thalamus, and cortex. Lesions of the posterior columns are demonstrated by loss of vibratory and position sense disproportionate to the loss of other modalities (e.g., B_{12} deficiency). Vibratory sensation is best tested with a 128-Hz tuning fork, and position sense is tested by small excursions of the distal digits.

Sample Examinations

The following two examinations are examples of neurological examinations as they might appear in a hospital chart in typed, dictated, or handwritten form. Handwritten examinations tend to include several commonly used abbreviations.

EXAMINATION:

Mental status: 0 × 4, alert, appropriate, digits 6# $\leftrightarrows$ presidents✓, 3/3 5 min. memory, proverbs✓, serial 7s ✓

Cranial nerves: II - XII intact (PERRLA, EOMI, face-gag-palatal symmetrical, V_i–V_3 ✓) fundi ⊙

Motor: Strength 5/5, normal tone/bulk, ∅ drift, F→N✓, gait heel/toe/tandem✓, H→S

Sensory:

Vibration✓
Position✓
Light touch✓
Pinprick✓
Temp✓

DTRs:

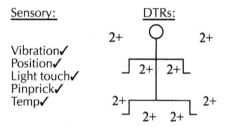

Imp: Right upper extremity parasthesias of uncertain etiology (normal exam)

FIGURE 1.2. A representative chart note of a normal neurological examination: 0 × 4 denotes orientation in four spheres, digits 6# $\leftrightarrows$ denotes digit span, PERRLA denotes pupils, equal, round, and reactive to light and accommodation, EOMI denotes extraocular muscles intact, V_1–V_3 denotes intact fifth nerve, ∅ drift denotes no pronator drift, F→N denotes finger-to-nose testing, H→S denotes heel-to-shin testing, stick figure denotes basic deep tendon reflexes. For example: 2+ over knee means that the knee is normal, whereas 1+ means trace reflexes and ∅ denotes loss of reflexes.

Sample Examination #1
A normal neurological examination (see Fig. 1.2):
Mental status: Patient is alert and oriented times four. Affect appropriate. Names presidents back to Carter easily, registers 3 out of 3 complex objects and recalls them at 5 minutes. Proverbs and serial 7's intact. Digit span 6 or 7 numbers forward and backward. On cranial nerve examination, fundi are benign. Pupils equal, round, and reactive to light and accommodation. Extraocular muscles intact. Face, gag, and palate elevation symmetrical. Facial sensation intact in all divisions of cranial nerve V. On motor examination, strength is 5/5 with normal tone and bulk. No pronator drift. Finger-to-nose testing and fine finger movements normal. Gait testing including heel, toe, and tandem walk intact. Heel-to-knee-to-shin intact. Deep tendon reflexes

are 2+ throughout and symmetrical with downgoing toes. No pathological reflexes. Sensory examination is intact to vibration, position, light touch, pinprick, and temperature.

Sample Examination #2
The following neurologic examination could be recorded in a patient with an acute right middle cerebral artery distribution infarct and moderate idiopathic Parkinson's disease:
Mental status: Patient is slightly drowsy. Patient is oriented to place, year, season but not month, or day of the week, or time of day. Patient does not know how long he has been in the hospital or the reason for hospitalization. Patient refuses to consider the possibility that he might have left-sided weakness due to a stroke (anosognosia or denial). Patient seems to neglect the left visual field. Patient can name only one recent president. Patient knows his address and phone number but has trouble naming his four children. He is unable to register three complex objects. He is unable to perform simple calculations. On cranial nerve examination, the patient has a left central seventh nerve palsy and some mild tongue deviation on tongue protrusion. Sensory examination of V_1 through V_3 is not reliable. Patient does not cross the midline with conjugate gaze. Gag intact. Patient is noted to have a snout and glabellar tap reflex. On motor examination, the patient has increased tone and cogwheel rigidity on the right, and his left upper extremity is flaccid. The left lower extremity is remarkable for trace proximal movements to command, and proximal and distal withdrawal movements to deep pain. Bilateral Babinskis are present, and deep tendon reflexes are symmetrical and 2+. All sensory modalities are decreased on the left versus neglect on the left. Patient distinguishes different sensory modalities on the right but reliability is questionable.

PEARLS AND PITFALLS

- Examination findings for patients with neurological disease can be mistaken for hysteria.
- Abnormal findings on neurological examination can result from one or more disease processes. Findings are considered in isolation and in combination.

- An age-associated loss of upgaze and vibratory sensation is normal in elderly patients.
- A detailed neurological examination evaluating the entire neuroaxis is not practical in the emergency department setting; therefore, the examination is tailored to the patient's specific complaints to localize lesions.
- An abnormal gait can be the only sign of serious neurological disease.

REFERENCES

1. Adams RD, Victor M. 3rd ed. *Principles of Neurology.* New York, NY: McGraw-Hill Book Co.; 1985.

2. Rowland LP. 9th ed. *Merritt's Textbook of Neurology.* Baltimore, Md: Williams & Wilkins; 1995.

3. Mancall E. 2nd ed. *Alpers and Mancall's Essentials of the Neurologic Examination.* Philadelphia, Pa: FA Davis Co; 1981.

4. Henry GL. Coma and altered states of consciousness. In: Tintinalli JE, Ruiz E, Krome RL, eds. *Emergency Medicine: A Comprehensive Study Guide.* 4th ed. New York, NY: McGraw-Hill Book Co; 1996:227.

5. Plum F, Posner JB. 3rd ed. *The Diagnosis of Stupor and Coma.* Philadelphia, Pa: FA Davis Co; 1982.

6. Carpenter MB. 3rd ed. *Core Text of Neuroanatomy.* Baltimore, Md: Williams & Wilkins; 1985.

7. Haerer AF. 5th ed. *DeJong's The Neurologic Examination.* Philadelphia, Pa: JB Lippincott Co; 1992.

2 Neuroradiology

ANDREW L. GOLDBERG AND THOMAS J. FIX

SUMMARY This chapter delineates the role of neuroradiology in the emergency department evaluation of a patient with a neurological emergency. Appropriate selection of diagnostic imaging techniques is discussed, with an emphasis on computerized tomography (CT) and magnetic resonance imaging (MRI). Important safety considerations unique to MRI are stressed. The imaging appearances of neurological emergencies such as acute intracranial injury, subarachnoid hemorrhage, and occlusive vascular disease are presented. The complementary roles of CT and MRI in the evaluation of acute spinal trauma are emphasized. Other entities such as degenerative disease of the spine and inflammatory and neoplastic disorders of the brain are described. Finally, the imaging appearances of numerous congenital anomalies and normal variants found in the general population are reviewed.

Introduction

The development of modern imaging technologies has expanded the physician's ability to diagnose neurologic disorders accurately. Computerized tomography (CT) and magnetic resonance imaging (MRI) are paramount among the tools that are available in the modern hospital for this purpose. In years past, patients without life-threatening conditions would frequently be admitted to the hospital for diagnostic evaluation. Contemporary trends emphasize the importance of a definitive diagnosis and treatment plan prior to hospitalization. A sophisticated familiarity with neuroradiological imaging procedures is essential for the emergency physician to diagnose and treat neurological problems accurately. To this end, broad categories of neurological disease are presented with emphasis on how the clinical presentation directs the choice of diagnostic procedure, usually CT or MRI. Myelography is utilized primarily for patients with symptoms of myelopathy or radiculopathy, in whom MRI is contraindicated. Contraindications for MRI include pacemakers and virtually all cerebral aneurysm clips. A comprehensive discussion of MRI-

related safety issues has been published by the Safety Committee of the International Society of Magnetic Resonance in Medicine.[1,2] A number of patients will also not be able to undergo MRI due to obesity or claustrophobia. A trend has developed toward establishing open-configuration MRI units in proximity to emergency departments. However, the ultimate role of this design is unsettled.[3] Cerebral angiography is an important, but no longer primary, neuroradiological procedure. It is performed frequently on an emergency basis, after CT or MRI, to evaluate the possibility of ruptured aneurysm or arteriovenous malformation, or to exclude acute intracranial arterial occlusion ("brain attack").

Computerized Tomography versus Magnetic Resonance Imaging

CT is sensitive to acute hemorrhage and is the procedure of choice for acute trauma. CT can clearly depict skull base, facial, and calvarial fractures, and it is usually in close proximity to the emergency department. CT is readily adaptable to patients requiring life sup-

Sid M. Shah and Kevin M. Kelly, eds., *Emergency Neurology: Principles and Practice.* Copyright © 1999 Cambridge University Press. All rights reserved.

port equipment. MRI can identify acute hemorrhage, particularly within the brain parenchyma, but it is typically unreliable in the diagnosis of subarachnoid hemorrhage.[4,5] MRI can create a confined environment for the patient, which may increase heart rate and blood pressure, an added hazard for the patient with a ruptured intracranial aneurysm.

For patients with subacute or chronic symptoms, the choice between CT and MRI is less clear. MRI is favored frequently because its multiplanar capability and superb soft tissue contrast sensitivity provide an excellent means to diagnose both intra- and extra-axial mass lesions, especially when supplemented by intravenous contrast. Hemorrhagic brain lesions have a characteristic appearance with MRI, and chronic subdural collections are more easily distinguished from adjacent bone with MRI than with CT.[6] Magnetic resonance angiography (MRA) can image flowing blood without intravenous contrast, thus evaluating arterial or venous pathology.

A multispecialty consortium (societies of neurology, neurosurgery, neuroradiology, and emergency medicine) has issued a practice parameter statement, for use in neuroimaging for new-onset seizures and chronic seizure disorders.[7] Emergency scanning is recommended if the patient presents with new focal deficits, persistent altered mental status, fever, recent trauma, intractable headache, history of cancer, history of anticoagulation, or suspicion of AIDS. An increased likelihood of a structural lesion is also present in patients over the age of 40 and in those presenting with partial-onset seizure.

Vascular Disease

The diagnosis and treatment of acute occlusive vascular disease (stroke) is one of the most challenging and rapidly evolving areas of emergency neurology. Ready access to CT and its accurate interpretation is essential for the patient presenting with a new ischemic neurological deficit. Acute hemorrhage or hemorrhagic infarction must be excluded prior to initiating anticoagulant therapy. Thrombolytic intervention has increased in use and requires sophisticated analysis of the CT examination. The "hyperdense middle cerebral artery sign" is insensitive but has strongly positive predictive value for the onset of major hemispheric infarction (Fig. 2.1)[8,9] and suggests a

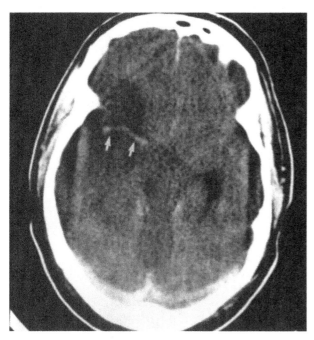

FIGURE 2.1A. CT scan showing a linear hyperdensity (arrows) corresponding to thrombus in the M1 segment of the right middle cerebral artery. Surrounding edema indicates the incipient infarction in this vascular territory.

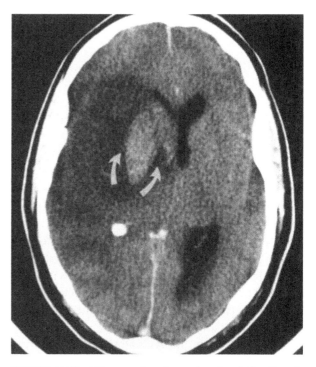

FIGURE 2.1B. CT scan showing extensive infarction in the right middle cerebral artery territory. There is a hemorrhagic component in the basal ganglia (curved arrows). There is mass effect on the ventricular system, and midline structures are shifted from right to left.

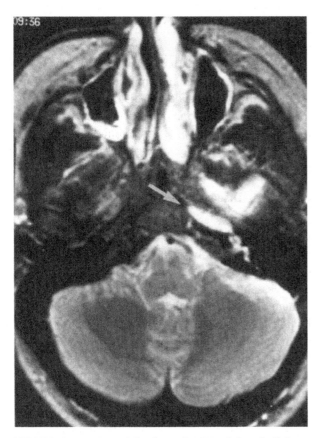

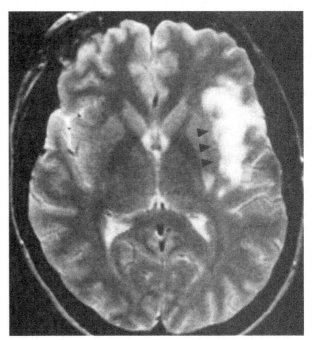

FIGURE 2.2B. T2-weighted axial MRI showing hyperintensity in the left insular cortex (arrowheads) indicating ischemic infarction in the left middle cerebral artery territory.

FIGURE 2.2A. T2-weighted axial MRI of the skull base showing asymmetrical hyperintensity in the petrous portion of the left internal carotid artery (arrow) suggestive of thrombosis. By contrast, flow-void is seen in the basilar artery.

poor prognosis. When this sign is absent and the CT shows abnormal hypodensity involving less than one-third of the affected hemisphere, cerebral angiography and possible thrombolysis are considered. MRA and CT angiography allow further noninvasive evaluation, but their use may be limited by the need for timely thrombolytic therapy.

Transcatheter angiography may be needed for definitive diagnosis of internal carotid artery dissection, although the diagnosis can be made with MRI and MRA. This entity can be an unexpected cause of stroke, particularly after apparent minor trauma (Fig. 2.2).

MRA is useful in the evaluation of the posterior circulation in patients with vertebrobasilar transient ischemic attacks (TIAs). Typically, these are elderly patients for whom selective catheterization of the vertebral arteries presents a relatively high risk. MRA can support the clinical impression of

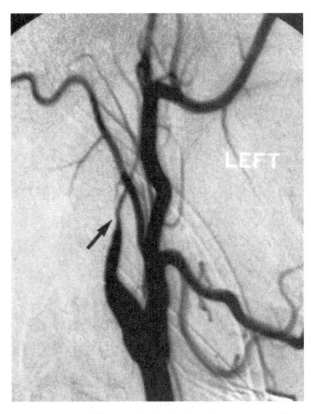

FIGURE 2.2C. Selective angiography showing tapered occlusion of the left internal carotid artery (arrow) characteristics of intimal dissection.

posterior circulation TIA by revealing vertebrobasilar stenoses and/or occlusions (Fig. 2.3). In a cooperative patient, the carotid bifurcations can be evaluated at the same time.

Cerebral venoocclusive disease (dural sinus thrombosis) is an important entity that can present with misleading or nonspecific symptoms and signs. Oral contraceptives, connective tissue diseases, systemic neoplasia, parameningeal inflammation (e.g., otomastoiditis), and trauma are predisposing factors. A CT scan can be obtained for symptoms that range from persistent headache to coma. The results can be normal or show subtle postcontrast abnormalities such as the "delta" sign.[10,11] This consists of a triangular hypodensity representing thrombus, surrounded by the enhancing wall of the superior sagittal (or other dural) sinus. Intracerebral hemorrhage occurs in many cases. MRI with mag-

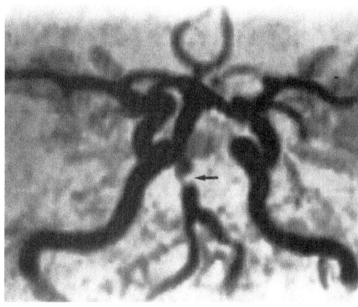

A

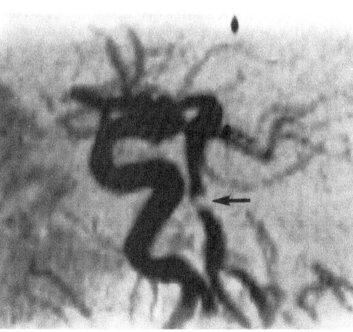

B

FIGURE 2.3. Three-dimensional time-of-flight MRA, in both (A) frontal and (B) lateral projections. There is focal stenosis (arrow) in the proximal basilar artery.

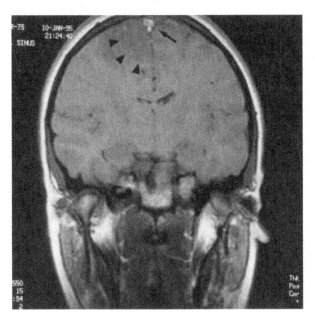

FIGURE 2.4A. Coronal T1-weighted MRI. There is focal hyperintensity in the superior sagittal sinus (arrow). It is difficult to distinguish thrombus from artifact (flow-related enhancement); however, surrounding edema (arrowheads) strongly favors thrombus.

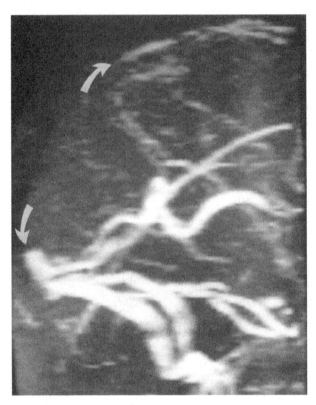

FIGURE 2.4B. Magnetic resonance venography using two-dimensional time-of-flight technique and arterial presaturation. Absence of flow (arrows) in the mid and distal superior sagittal sinus is demonstrated.

netic resonance venography facilitates accurate diagnosis of dural sinus thrombosis.[12,13] Thromboses can occur either in the superior sagittal sinus (Fig. 2.4) or in the lateral and sigmoid sinuses. Invasive angiography is an adjunct to transvenous thrombolysis in most cases.

Subarachnoid and Intracerebral Hemorrhage

Emergency CT scanning is used in the evaluation of sudden headache. Acute subarachnoid hemorrhage is readily diagnosed when blood is abundant; however, a CT scan is also crucial to detect smaller traces of hemorrhage, as many of these patients are intact neurologically and will realize maximal benefit from early angiography and surgical clipping (or endovascular coil occlusion). The sylvian fissures and interpeduncular cistern are scrutinized for any hyperdensity (Fig. 2.5). Dilatation of the temporal horns of the lateral ventricles often indicates impending hydrocephalus.

The current standard of care requires evaluation of acute subarachnoid hemorrhage by emergent transarterial angiography, despite impressive ad-

vances in MRA.[14,15,16] MRA is used more frequently to detect unruptured aneurysms after CT scanning has demonstrated an abnormality or in patients being screened for higher than average risk of subarachnoid hemorrhage, for example, polycystic kidney disease.

Rupture of arteriovenous malformations can result in subarachnoid, intracerebral, and/or intraventricular hemorrhage. CT scanning, especially following administration of intravenous contrast, often suggests the diagnosis of subarachnoid hemorrhage, which requires angiographic confirmation. Cavernous angioma is a specific vascular malformation that is imaged particularly well by MRI. Gradient echo sequences are sensitive to the magnetic susceptibility effect of hemosiderin deposition, and often reveal multiple lesions (Fig. 2.6). These lesions can be associated with anomalous venous drainage (venous angiomas).[17]

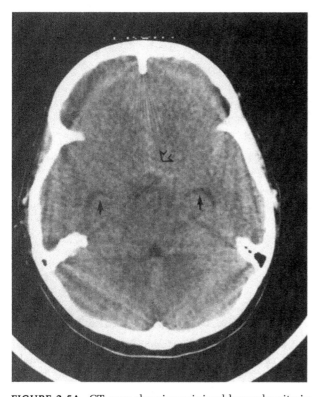

FIGURE 2.5A. CT scan showing minimal hyperdensity in the anterior aspect of the suprasellar cistern extending into the interhemispheric fissure (open arrow). There is associated moderate enlargement of the temporal horns of the lateral ventricles for a young patient (closed arrows). These findings are consistent with a "sentinel" subarachnoid hemorrhage with early hydrocephalus.

Spontaneous intracerebral hemorrhage can occur as a result of coagulopathy, toxins, hypertensive vasculopathy, or amyloid angiopathy, or with primary or metastatic tumors (Fig. 2.7). It is difficult to exclude the possibility of an underlying tumor with CT findings of acute intracerebral hemorrhage, particularly if the density and margins of the hematoma are irregular. MRI without and with contrast can be helpful when there is an enhancing component distinct from the intensity changes due to hemorrhagic breakdown products. In metastatic disease, additional lesions can exist that are remote from the hematoma. A repeat examination after six weeks or more may be necessary for a definitive diagnosis. Edema and mass effect resolve in cases of nonneoplastic hematoma.

Craniospinal Trauma

Availability of cross-sectional imaging for acute intracranial injury is an essential and potentially lifesaving component of evaluation in the emergency department. Expeditious diagnosis of acute epidural and subdural hematomas is critical. Epidural hematomas are often associated with fractures, which should be evaluated with CT bone settings and the accompanying lateral digital radiograph. In epidural hematomas, the brain is less likely to be injured than in trauma that results in subdural hematoma. The

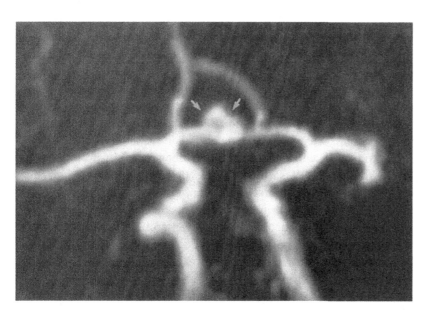

FIGURE 2.5B. Three-dimensional time-of-flight MRA centered on the circle of Willis. There is a saccular aneurysm (arrows) arising from the anterior communicating artery.

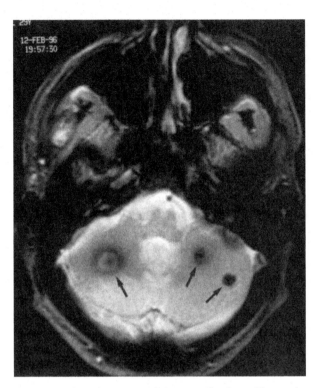

FIGURE 2.6. MRI susceptibility-weighted gradient echo image shows well-demarcated hypointense lesions (arrows) without surrounding edema in the cerebellum. There are multiple additional lesions (not shown) in the supratentorial region. These findings are characteristic of cavernous angiomata.

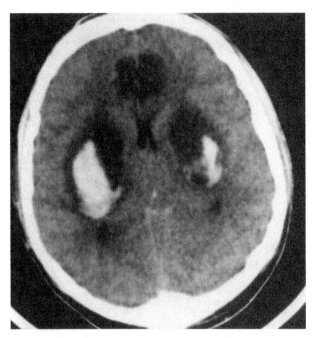

FIGURE 2.7. CT scan showing hemorrhagic infarction in the putamina of a young patient who ingested methanol. There is nonhemorrhagic infarction in the medial frontal lobes.

prognosis associated with epidural hematoma is favorable once mass effect is alleviated (Fig. 2.8). A subacute subdural hematoma can be imaged as isodense on CT. MRI is particularly sensitive in demonstrating subacute subdural hematomas because of its inherent soft tissue contrast characteristics and its multiplanar capability. Free dilute methemoglobin creates panhyperintensity in these collections on all MRI sequences (Fig. 2.9).[18,19]

Traumatic brain injury can result from shearing forces. Treatment is based on control of hyperemic brain swelling. This form of brain injury is known as *diffuse axonal injury* and can be better visualized on MRI than on CT. T2-weighted spin echo, T2*-weighted gradient echo, or fluid-attenuated inversion recovery (FLAIR) images show multiple small tissue tear hemorrhages (Fig. 2.10).[20]

Intracranial trauma can also precipitate cerebral infarction. For example, uncontrolled intracranial hypertension can lead to caudal herniation with compression of the posterior cerebral arteries. Trans-

falcine herniation can compromise the anterior cerebral arteries.[21] These herniation syndromes result in infarction in the involved vascular territories.

Evaluation of acute spinal trauma begins with plain radiographs. CT and MRI allow the neuroradiologist to refine diagnostic accuracy. MRI has elucidated the spectrum of spinal cord injury, including cord contusions, hemorrhage, and transection in severe cases.[22] The sagittal and parasagittal images generated by MRI are useful in evaluating alignment abnormalities. Unilateral facet lock (Fig. 2.11) can be difficult to discern on plain radiographs.

It is well known that sprain due to cervical hyperextension can result in serious neurological deficits, which may not be evident on plain radiographs.[23] MRI shows anterior ligamentous disruption, discovertebral separation, extrinsic cord compression, and intrinsic cord contusion (Fig. 2.12). In contrast, flexion injuries cause anterolisthesis and posterior longitudinal ligament disruption (Fig. 2.13).

At the craniocervical junction, a combination of CT and MRI is useful to assess fractures (Fig. 2.14). MRI is superior in defining nonosseous compressive lesions such as epidural hematoma and herniated

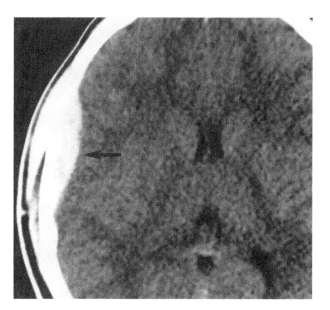

FIGURE 2.8A. CT scan showing the typical lentiform hyperdensity of a right convexity epidural hematoma (arrow).

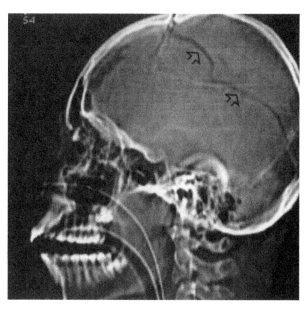

FIGURE 2.8B. Lateral digital radiograph shows the associated fracture extending from the coronal to the lambdoidal suture (open arrows). The fracture's parallel orientation to the plane of section made its identification difficult with CT scanning that included bone windows (not shown).

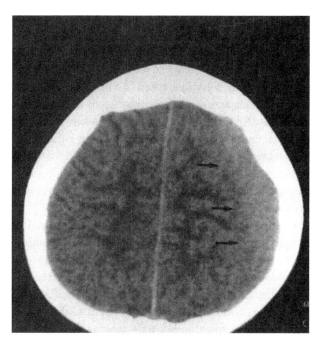

FIGURE 2.9A. CT scan showing a left convexity subdural hematoma (arrows) that is virtually isodense to the underlying brain.

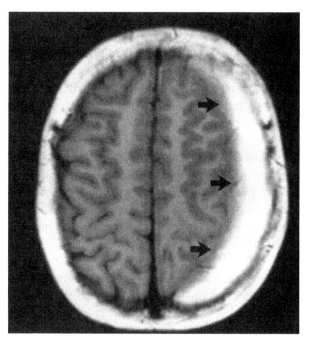

FIGURE 2.9B. T1-weighted MRI shows a hyperintense hematoma (arrows) due to the paramagnetic effect of free-dilute methemoglobin.

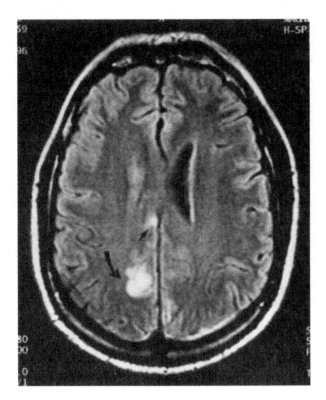 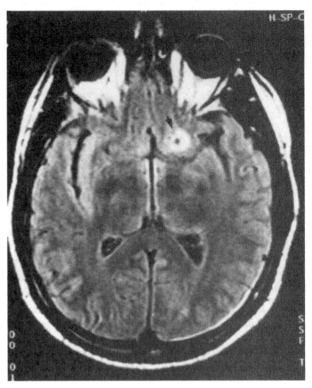

FIGURE 2.10A, B. Fluid-attenuated inversion recovery (FLAIR) axial MRIs following head trauma showing hyperintense foci of shearing injury that were not visible on preceding CT scan (not shown). The most prominent high signal abnormality is in the right medial occipital lobe (curved arrow). Additional sites of diffuse axonal injury are noted in the splenium of the corpus callosum and the left inferior frontal lobe (small arrows).

disc, and it can demonstrate horizontally oriented fracture lines that are parallel to the CT plane of section. CT more clearly depicts bony disruption of the neural arch. Similarly, these two techniques are complementary in the evaluation of burst fractures and flexion-distraction injuries (Chance or seat belt–type fractures) at the thoracolumbar junction (Fig. 2.15). MRI can elucidate pathologic fractures associated with abnormal marrow infiltration by metastases, myeloma, lymphoma, or leukemia that result from relatively minor trauma. Appropriate use of noninvasive cross-sectional imaging markedly reduces the need for myelography in evaluating acute trauma.

Degenerative Disease of the Spine

Radiologic evaluation of lumbar and/or cervical radiculopathy frequently begins with plain radiographs, which expose the patient to ionizing radiation and result in little diagnostic information, unlike the clinical setting of acute trauma, where plain radiographs are important. In many cases, no imaging is necessary for radicular symptoms, which are often self-limited or respond to conservative measures. When indicated, cross-sectional imaging can demonstrate abnormalities such as disc herniation and spinal stenosis. CT scanning may be adequate for the lumbar region, particularly when there is sufficient epidural fat, which acts as a natural contrast agent between the extruded disc and the thecal sac. However, MRI has superior contrast resolution, multiplanar capability, improving technique, and declining cost.[24] For these reasons, MRI is preferred, especially in imaging the cervical spine, where little epidural fat results in relatively ineffective noncontrast CT scanning.

Disc herniation is a common cause of radicular symptoms, and often presents acutely in middle-aged adults. The typical finding of an extradural compressive mass that is contiguous with the parent intervertebral disc is readily seen by MRI. Variants include far lateral herniations, which are important to detect on cross-sectional imaging because they are inapparent on myelography. Herniated fragments can migrate cranially and caudally but rarely cross the midline due to a median septum in the epidural space.[25] Very

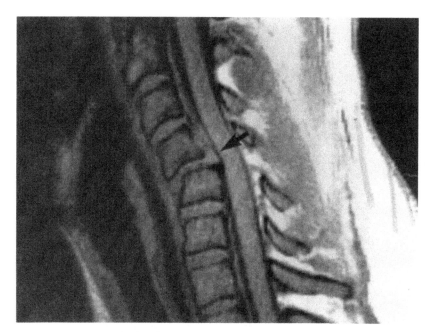

FIGURE 2.11A. Midsagittal T1-weighted MRI showing anterolisthesis of C-4 on C-5 with an associated disc herniation that impinges on the spinal cord (arrow).

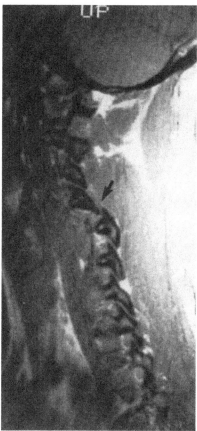

FIGURE 2.11B. Parasagittal T1-weighted MRI identifies a locked facet (arrow). Cranial and caudal levels show normal imbrication of the facets. The opposite side (not shown) was normal. (Reprinted with permission from: *Imaging of Vertebral Trauma*, R. H. Daffner. 2nd ed. Philadelphia, PA: Lippincott-Raven, 1996.)

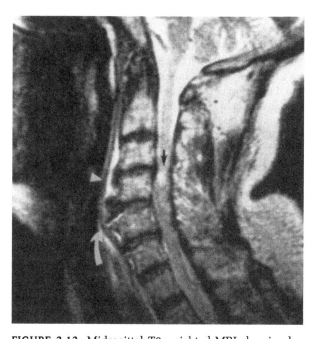

FIGURE 2.12. Midsagittal T2-weighted MRI showing hyperextension sprain. There is a hyperintensity consistent with a prevertebral hematoma in the high cervical region (arrowhead). There is disruption of the anterior longitudinal ligament at the C4–5 level (curved arrow). The anterior aspect of the disc space is widened abnormally. A linear hyperintensity that reflects blood and/or edema defines the superior endplate of C-5. A focal intramedullary hyperintensity represents spinal cord contusion (small arrow).

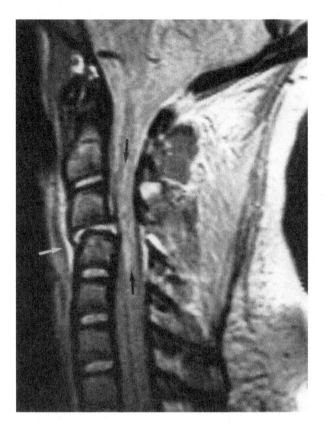

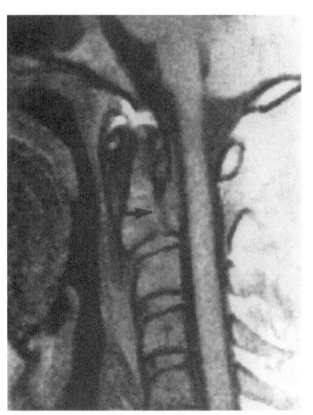

FIGURE 2.13. Proton-density-weighted MRI showing findings associated with hyperflexion sprain. The posterior aspect of the C3–4 interspace is widened with associated disruption of the posterior longitudinal ligament and anterolisthesis of C-3 on C-4. There is a small prevertebral hematoma (white arrow). There are intramedullary hyperintensities consistent with spinal cord contusion (black arrows). (Reprinted with permission from: *Imaging of Vertebral Trauma,* R. H. Daffner. 2nd ed. Philadelphia, PA: Lippincott-Raven, 1996.)

FIGURE 2.14A. A fracture extending vertically from the dens through the body of C-2 is noted on this midsagittal T1-weighted MRI (arrow). There is prevertebral hematoma. There is no cord compression.

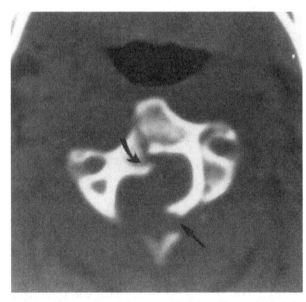

FIGURE 2.14B. Axial CT scan showing disruption of the neural arch (straight arrow) and the vertebral body fracture (curved arrow). (Reprinted with permission from: *Imaging of Vertebral Trauma,* R. H. Daffner. 2nd ed. Philadelphia, PA: Lippincott-Raven, 1996.)

large disc herniations can suggest the possibility of tumor. Intravenous contrast produces rim enhancement that is characteristic of the inflammatory reaction surrounding the herniated disc (Fig. 2.16); a neoplasm typically enhances homogeneously.[26,27]

Degenerative spinal stenosis is a common cause of age-related morbidity. Attention is focused on the compression of the thecal sac, visible on CT or MRI. Moderate disc bulging flattens the thecal sac, which becomes more deformed with facet degeneration. Myelography provides weight-bearing views that elucidate the severity of multilevel stenosis. Blockage of the caudal flow of contrast occurs in advanced cases.

Synovial cyst is a degenerative compressive lesion that is identified with cross-sectional imaging.[28] These cysts are usually of water density or in-

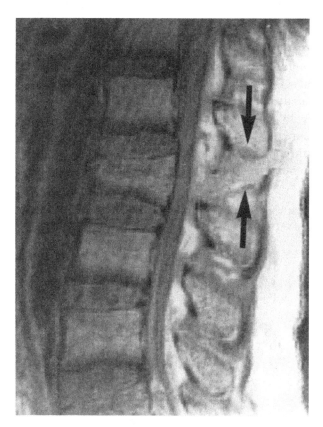

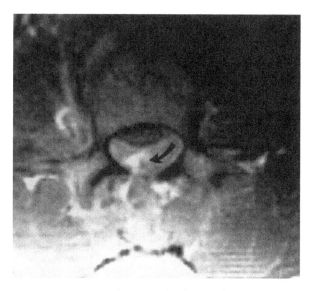

FIGURE 2.15B. Axial T1-weighted MRI showing the thecal sac displaced anteriorly by an epidural hematoma. Conversion to methemoglobin resulted in a focal hyperintensity (curved arrow).

FIGURE 2.15A. Midsagittal T1-weighted MRI showing a compression deformity of the L-2 vertebral body and disruption of the interspinous ligament (black arrows) consistent with a flexion distraction (seat belt–type) injury.

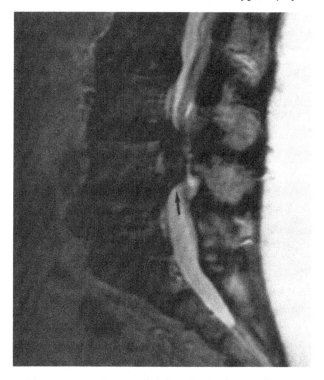

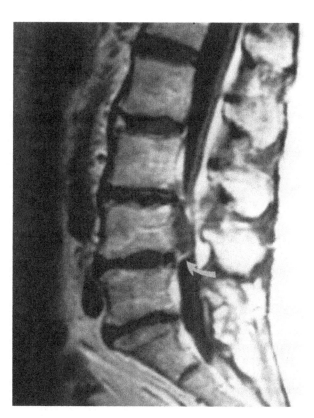

FIGURE 2.16A. T-2 weighted midsagittal MRI showing a mass (arrow) that fills much of the epidural space between the L3–4 and L4–5 interspaces.

FIGURE 2.16B. T1-weighted midsagittal MRI following intravenous contrast administered to exclude a neoplastic lesion. The image shows rim enhancement of the herniated disc (curved arrow). A cleavage plane is seen between the disc material and the L4–5 interspace, further suggesting an L3–4 disc herniation with caudal migration.

tensity, and can contain air or rim calcification. They are commonly seen at L4–5 and are usually closely apposed to the medial aspect of an adjacent degenerated facet joint (Fig. 2.17).

Spondylolisthesis usually results from a stress phenomenon that causes spondylolysis of the pars interarticularis, typically at the L5 level (Fig. 2.18).

Spondylolisthesis can be seen on plain radiographs, but CT or MRI are useful in assessing possible associated disc herniation at the involved or adjacent level. When anterolisthesis is seen at a level other than L5–S1, it is usually due to degenerative facet arthropathy rather than spondylolysis, and is frequently associated with canal stenosis.

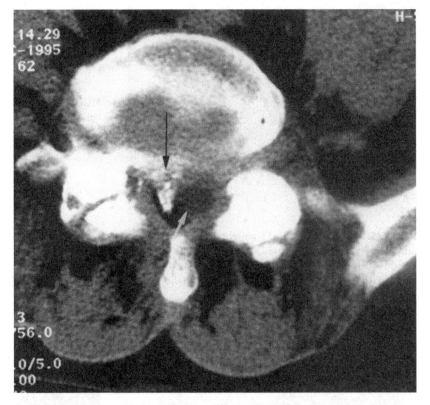

FIGURE 2.17A. Postmyelographic CT scan of an epidural mass at the L4–5 level (white arrow) that is intermediate in density between fat and the intervertebral disc. The contrast-filled thecal sac (black arrow) is displaced to the right. The findings are consistent with synovial cyst.

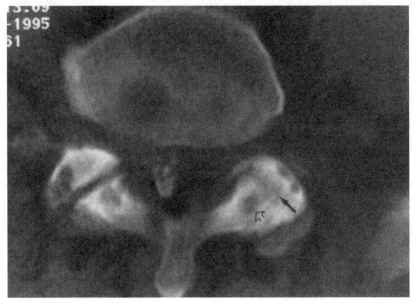

FIGURE 2.17B. Postmyelographic CT scan with bone window settings of the previous image showing marked facet degeneration with joint space narrowing (long black arrow) and subchondral cyst formation (open arrow).

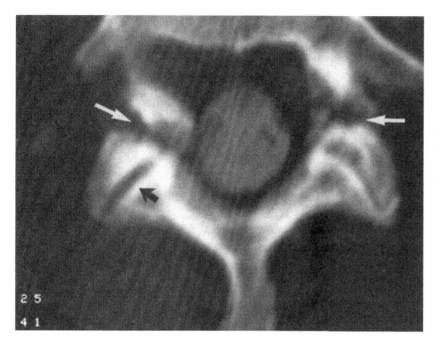

FIGURE 2.18. Axial postmyelographic CT scan showing bilateral isthmic defects of the pars interarticularis (spondylolysis). The irregular nonsclerotic appearance of the pars defects (white arrows) is seen in contrast to the smooth sclerotic articulation of the adjacent facet joint (black arrow).

Inflammatory Disease of the Central Nervous System

Diagnostic imaging is an important component of a comprehensive evaluation of possible inflammatory disease of the central nervous system (CNS). Detection and analysis of extra-axial and parenchymal lesions are valuable in establishing a presumptive diagnosis. Imaging performed for suspected bacterial meningitis is typically normal and excludes hydrocephalus or a focal mass lesion prior to lumbar puncture. CT scanning, and especially MRI, can reveal infarction, cerebritis, or subdural empyema in complicated cases (Fig. 2.19). Cerebritis can result in

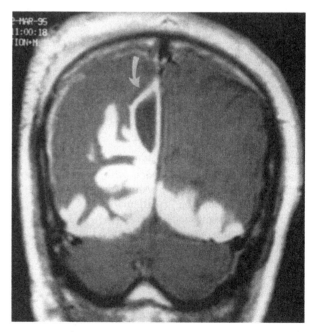

FIGURE 2.19A. Coronal CT scan showing asymmetrical soft tissue density consistent with right maxilloethmoid sinusitis.

FIGURE 2.19B. Coronal postcontrast T1-weighted MRI showing gyriform enhancement associated with cerebritis. The rim-enhancing extra-axial collection in the interhemispheric fissure (curved arrow) is a subdural empyema.

a brain abscess, which can occur following penetrating trauma, tuberculosis, or fungal disease. These entities have been observed with increased frequency because of acquired immunodeficiency syndrome (AIDS), but can be seen in immunologically normal patients, especially in parts of the world where these infections are endemic (Fig. 2.20).

Herpes simplex encephalitis is an acute viral inflammatory process that has specific imaging abnormalities affecting the temporal lobes, insular cortex, and orbitofrontal region.[29] The putamen is spared. MRI has shown greater evidence of bilateral involvement (areas of T2 hyperintensity) than has CT. Contrast enhancement is variable, but a gyriform pattern is typical (Fig. 2.21).

Human immunodeficiency virus (HIV) infection is associated with brain imaging abnormalities due to a variety of opportunistic infections. Imaging is often not helpful in arriving at a specific diagnosis, and is generally normal in asymptomatic patients.[30] HIV can result in an encephalitis that affects deep gray matter and periventricular white matter and is seen as hyperintensity on T2-weighted images and as low density on CT images. HIV is associated with cytomegalovirus, toxoplasmosis, progressive multifocal leukoencephalopathy, and primary CNS lymphoma. A mass lesion suggests toxoplasmosis or lymphoma. Differentiating these two entities can be difficult clinically, but certain imaging features are helpful. Lymphoma has higher density on noncontrast CT and lower signal intensity on T2-weighted MRI than does toxoplasmosis, which is usually hyperintense (Fig. 2.22). For a patient with AIDS, neither lesion multiplicity nor enhancement pattern (ring versus solid) is particularly helpful in differentiating the two entities. Subependymal spread of the lesion favors lymphoma, but the two lesions can coexist.[31]

There are several CNS inflammatory processes for which a causative agent has not yet been identified. Multiple sclerosis (MS) is the most significant clinically. MRI has reduced diagnostic uncertainty because of characteristic findings, especially in young patients. Proton density, T2-weighted, and FLAIR images show deep white matter hyperintensities that tend to have a periventricular orientation in the periventricular region (*ovoid lesions*) (Fig. 2.23). Contrast enhancement provides a measure of lesion activity by demonstrating blood–brain barrier disruption. An MS plaque will present occasionally as a ring-enhancing tumefactive lesion that simulates a neoplasm. Little mass effect relative to the

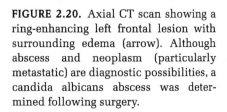

FIGURE 2.20. Axial CT scan showing a ring-enhancing left frontal lesion with surrounding edema (arrow). Although abscess and neoplasm (particularly metastatic) are diagnostic possibilities, a candida albicans abscess was determined following surgery.

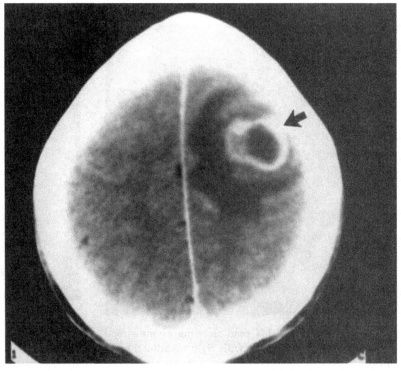

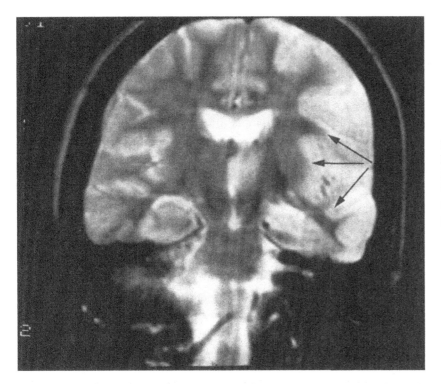

FIGURE 2.21A. Coronal T2-weighted MRI showing gyral swelling of the left frontotemporal region with constriction of the normal ramifying subcortical white matter tracts (arrows) compared to the right side.

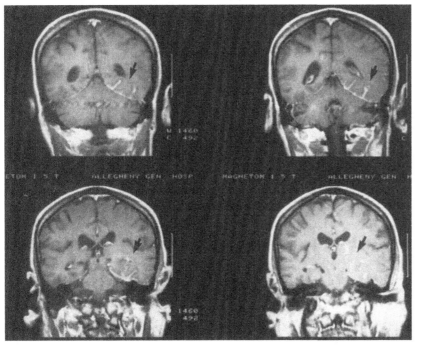

FIGURE 2.21B. Contiguous coronal T1-weighted postcontrast MRIs extending from the parieto-occipital region through the frontotemporal area showing a pattern of gyriform enhancement that extends to the tentorial surface. The findings are consistent with blood–brain barrier breakdown due to the inflammatory process.

size of the lesion suggests a demyelinating process. Acute disseminated encephalomyelitis is an infrequent monophasic illness that occurs after a viral illness or vaccination and results in neurological deficits. Multiple ring-enhancing or solidly enhancing lesions are seen on brain MRI.[32]

Vertebral discitis/osteomyelitis can occur following surgery for lumbar disc disease and in septicemia. On MRI, findings of T1 hypointensity in adjacent vertebral bodies, T2 hyperintensity in the intervening disc space, and irregularity of the end plates are diagnostic (Fig. 2.24). Following adminis-

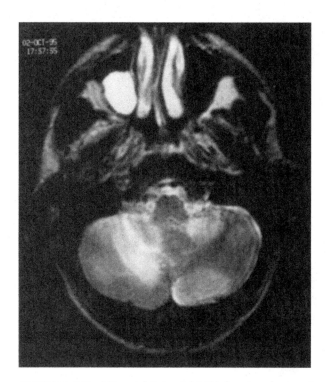

FIGURE 2.22A. T2-weighted axial MRI showing abnormal hyperintensity in the cerebellar hemispheres in a nonvascular distribution. Right maxillary sinusitis is present in this HIV-positive patient.

tration of intravenous contrast, patchy enhancement is seen in the disc space and spreads into the vertebral bodies. This finding is different from the normal uniform linear enhancement seen postoperatively.

Other entities that can simulate the MRI findings of infection include neuropathic joint, ankylosing spondylitis complicated by discovertebral destruction, dialysis-associated spondyloarthropathy, and gout. In contrast, tuberculous spondylitis involves longer segments of the spine, is less destructive of the disc spaces, and is associated with prominent prevertebral or paraspinal masses. These findings are similar to those of metastatic disease.

Brain Tumors

The brain and meninges are sites of benign and malignant neoplasia. Neuroimaging is obtained in the emergency department in the evaluation of intractable headaches or neurological deficits associated with these lesions. Benign lesions, such as meningioma, are frequent incidental findings of neuroimaging obtained for patients for other reasons.

FIGURE 2.22B. Postcontrast T1-weighted coronal MRI showing enhancement of the lesions, with edema noted surrounding a large right cerebellar mass (arrow), and a smaller vermian mass – in this case, of cerebellar toxoplasmosis.

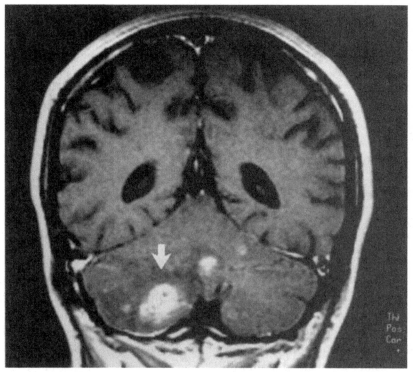

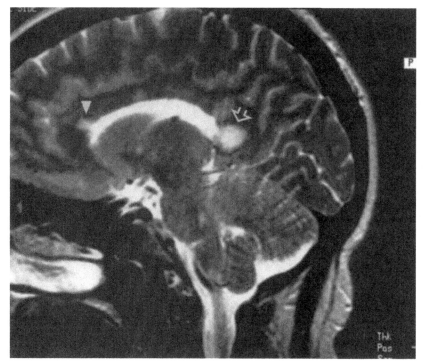

FIGURE 2.23A. Midsagittal T2-weighted MRI showing abnormal hyperintensity involving the corpus callosum at multiple foci along the callosal septal interface including the rostrum (arrowhead) and the splenium (open arrow).

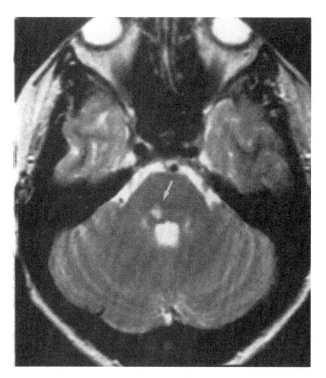

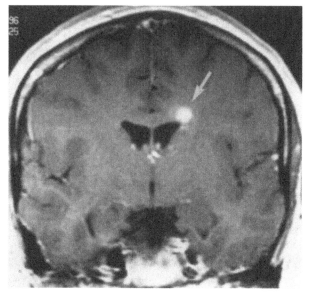

FIGURE 2.23C. Coronal postcontrast MRI showing asymmetrical enhancement involving the left forceps minor (arrow) indicating active blood–brain barrier breakdown in a plaque of MS.

FIGURE 2.23B. Midsagittal T2-weighted MRI showing a focal lesion in the pontine tegmentum (arrow) probably involving the medial longitudinal fasciculus.

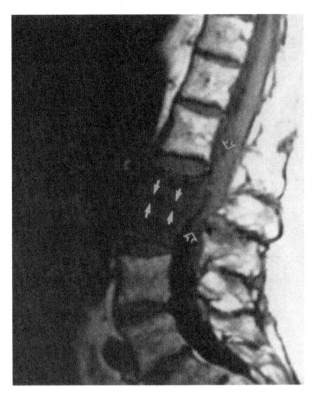

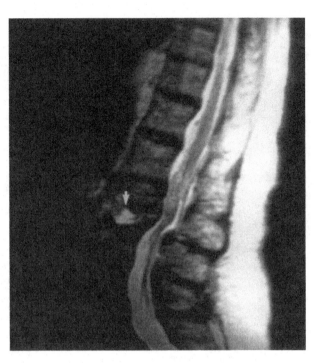

FIGURE 2.24A. Midsagittal T1-weighted MRI showing marked hypointensity in the L2 and L3 vertebral bodies and obliteration of the intervertebral disc (solid arrows). Extension of abnormal signal (intermediate between spinal cord substance and CSF) into the spinal canal is seen (open arrows).

FIGURE 2.24B. T2-weighted midsagittal MRI showing marked hyperintensity in the L2–3 interspace. Findings on T1- and T2-weighted MRIs are characteristic of discitis-osteomyelitis. The proximal cauda equina is obscured by amorphous soft tissue intensity consistent with abscess or phlegmon.

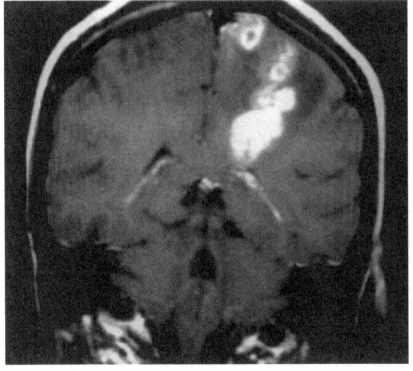

FIGURE 2.25. Coronal postcontrast MRI showing a multinodular enhancing lesion due to metastatic melanoma extending in a radial pattern from the ventricular surface to the parietal cortex.

Primary gliomas are common and generally easy to diagnose by CT or MRI. The prognosis for middle-aged or elderly adults is poor. Glioblastoma multiforme is observed as a mass of heterogeneous density or intensity associated with contrast enhancement and surrounding edema. A solitary metastatic lesion can appear identical when the pattern of glioma growth is more globoid than infiltrative (Fig. 2.25). When the process involves the corpus callosum, the differential diagnosis is limited; primary lymphoma can grow in a similar fashion but is characterized by more uniform enhancement.

Meningiomas have a favorable prognosis, although those that arise from the skull base tend to grow in an en plaque fashion and create surgical difficulties. Multiplanar evaluation with contrast-enhanced MRI is the most helpful diagnostic approach. Small meningiomas without significant edema can be similar in intensity to brain parenchyma on noncontrast T1- and T2-weighted images.[33] Large meningiomas arising from the high cerebral convexity or skull base can be embolized preoperatively. Evaluation of the patency of the superior sagittal sinus is important (Fig. 2.26). CT scanning depicts the typical hyperostotic calvarial reaction very well.

Acoustic schwannoma is a benign extra-axial lesion that can cause sensorineural hearing loss in an adult. Newer three-dimensional sequences of MRI with thin sections through the internal auditory canals provide excellent anatomical detail. Intracanalicular lesions can be diagnosed without administration of intravenous contrast.[34] However, gadolinium use is common because of the intense enhancement of these lesions. Bilateral acoustic schwannomas are diagnostic of neurofibromatosis type II (Fig. 2.27).

Intra-axial posterior fossa masses occur most frequently in young patients and can be associated with nausea and vomiting. A choroid plexus papilloma is shown in Figure 2.28. These lesions can cause hydrocephalus due to intraventricular obstruction, overproduction of cerebrospinal fluid (CSF), and/or the coagulative effect of tumor hemorrhage.

The sella turcica and parasellar region constitute a small area but are associated with a broad variety of pathology. Pituitary macroadenomas are sometimes detected as incidental findings on CT scans

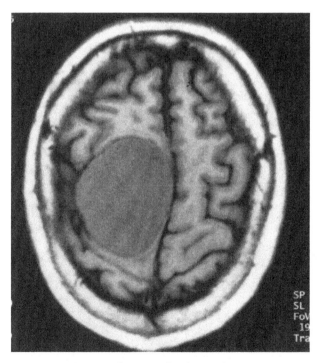

FIGURE 2.26A. Axial T1-weighted MRI showing a globoid mass that is slightly hypointense to the adjacent brain. The falx cerebri is displaced focally from right to left.

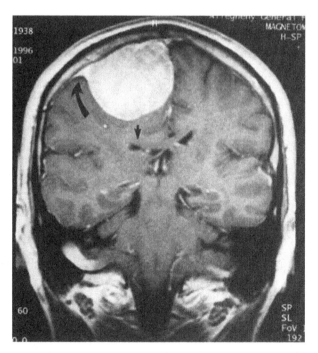

FIGURE 2.26B. Axial T1-weighted MRI following infusion of intravenous contrast showing homogeneous enhancement of the same mass consistent with a meningioma. An enhancing dural tail is present (curved arrow), indicating origin from the high right cerebral hemispheric convexity with secondary displacement of the falx. Mass effect is noted on the right lateral ventricle (arrow).

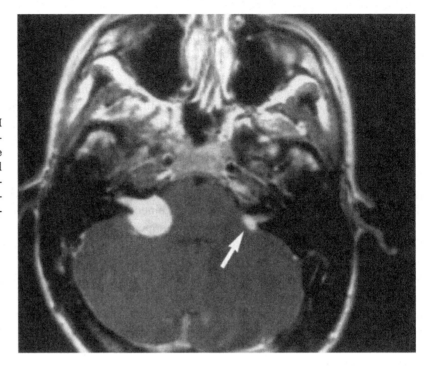

FIGURE 2.27. Axial postcontrast MRI showing a globoid, uniformly enhancing lesion in the right cerebellopontine angle extending into the right internal auditory canal. A smaller second lesion is seen on the left (arrow). Bilateral acoustic schwannomas are diagnostic of neurofibromatosis type II.

obtained in the emergency department. Aneurysms must be excluded when parasellar or suprasellar abnormalities are present. Suprasellar neoplasms include gliomas, metastases, germ cell tumors, lymphomas, and cranipharyngiomas (Fig. 2.29).

The spinal cord and vertebral column are sites for a variety of tumors. Histopathology can be identical to that of intracranial tumors, although the biological behavior can differ. A slow, insidious onset of neurological deficit delays diagnosis of intrinsic

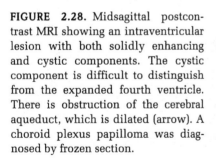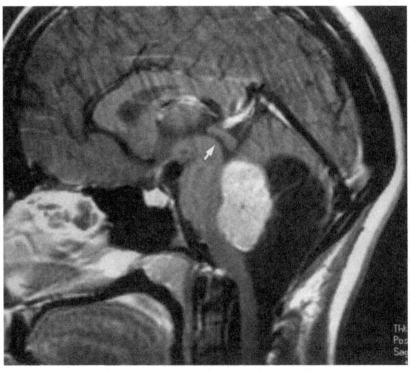

FIGURE 2.28. Midsagittal postcontrast MRI showing an intraventricular lesion with both solidly enhancing and cystic components. The cystic component is difficult to distinguish from the expanded fourth ventricle. There is obstruction of the cerebral aqueduct, which is dilated (arrow). A choroid plexus papilloma was diagnosed by frozen section.

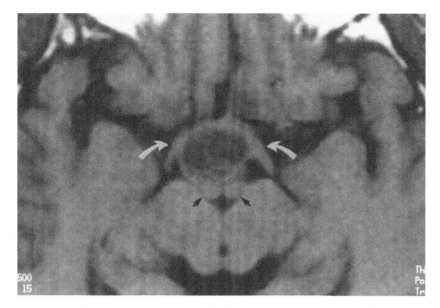

FIGURE 2.29A. Axial T1-weighted MRI showing a septated cystic lesion that occupies the suprasellar cistern. The mass occurs between a compressed and displaced anteriorly optic chiasm (curved white arrows) and the mammillary bodies posteriorly (small black arrows).

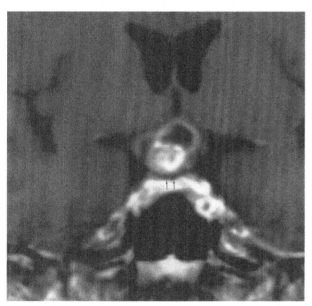

FIGURE 2.29B. Coronal T1-weighted MRI following administration of intravenous contrast showing enhancement of a more inferior solid component of the lesion. The mass, a craniopharyngioma, is separated by a cleavage plane from the superior aspect of the normally enhancing anterior pituitary gland (small black arrows).

spinal cord neoplasms such as ependymoma or astrocytoma. Ependymoma is generally an encapsulated mass that allows surgical enucleation (Fig. 2.30); astrocytoma is usually more infiltrative. Other spinal cord tumors are hemangioblastomas and intramedullary metastases. These lesions, especially hemangioblastomas, can be associated with

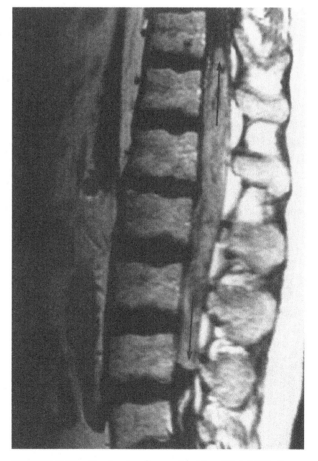

FIGURE 2.30. Contrast-enhanced midsagittal MRI showing an elongated, expansile mass obscuring the normal distinction between the conus medullaris and the cauda equina (arrows). The lesion spans five vertebral bodies, but the relatively sharp demarcation of its borders is typical of an ependymoma.

nonneoplastic syrinx cavities, which need to be distinguished from intratumoral cysts. Spinal cord tumors generally show greater contrast enhancement on MRI compared with inflammatory lesions such as demyelinating plaques.[35]

Spinal schwannomas and meningiomas are commonly multiple in neurofibromatosis type II, but they can also occur as solitary, intradural/extramedullary lesions. In females, spinal meningiomas occur with greater frequency than do intracranial meningiomas.

Vertebral metastases which compress the spinal canal and/or spinal cord occur more frequently than intrinsic cord lesions. The noncontrast T1-weighted MRI best demonstrates these lesions (Fig. 2.31). Phased array surface coil technology has facilitated metastatic survey of the entire spinal axis; sensitivity is similar to radionuclide bone scanning, and specificity is superior.[36]

Congenital Abnormalities

Congenital abnormalities that are observed on images of the brain and spine may be unrelated to presenting symptoms in the emergency department; others have etiologic significance. Ventricular size and configuration are assessed on every CT and MRI examination. Hydrocephalus, regardless of its cause, is a treatable neurosurgical condition. Ventriculomegaly due to certain congenital malformations, such as holoprosencephaly, Chiari II malformation, and hydranencephaly, generally presents in infancy or early childhood. In other conditions, such as aqueductal stenosis or Dandy-Walker malformation, the age of

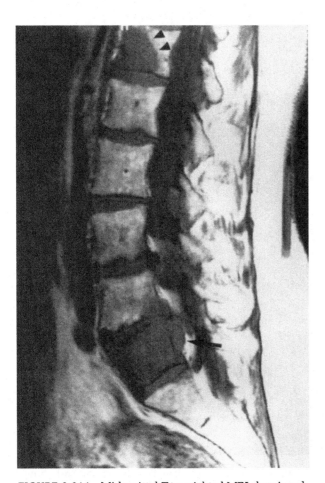

FIGURE 2.31A. Midsagittal T1-weighted MRI showing abnormal hypointensity consistent with marrow infiltration by metastatic carcinoma in the L5 and T12 (arrowheads) vertebral bodies. Canal encroachment by an epidural mass is seen at the L5 level (arrow).

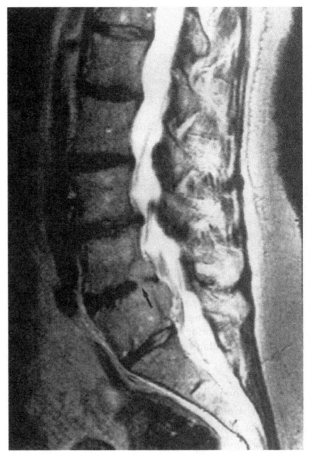

FIGURE 2.31B. T2-weighted midsagittal MRI showing a lesion at L5 that has the unusual feature of disc space invasion (arrow).

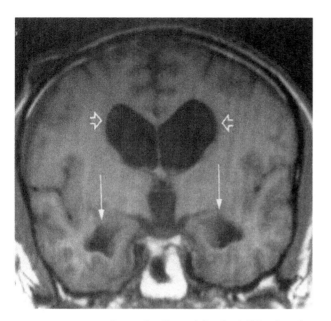

FIGURE 2.32A. Coronal T1-weighted MRI showing rounding of the frontal horns (open arrows) and dilatation of the temporal horns (solid arrows).

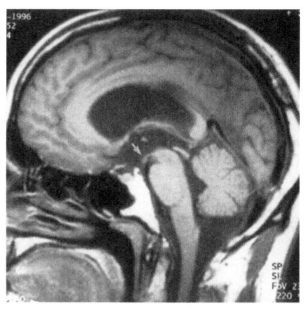

FIGURE 2.32B. Midsagittal T1-weighted MRI showing dilatation of the recesses of the third ventricle with diminution of the mammillopontine distance (arrow). This finding and those shown in Figure 2.32A likely indicate obstructive hydrocephalus.

presentation varies (Fig. 2.32). Obstructive hydrocephalus results in a characteristic alteration of ventricular configuration that distinguishes it from the increased ventricular volume associated with cerebral atrophy. The frontal horns become rounded, and they have less distinct margins due to transependymal resorption of CSF. The temporal horns enlarge disproportionately, the third ventricle enlarges and assumes an ovoid rather than a rectangular shape as the anterior recesses dilate, and the mamillopontine distance diminishes.[37] Sagittal MRI demonstrates these findings particularly well. Enlargement of the fourth ventricle suggests communicating (extraventricular obstructive) hydrocephalus, which can occur with a normal-sized fourth ventricle. Absence of the septum pellucidum indicates an abnormality of development, such as septo-optic dysplasia, associated with an attenuated optic chiasm that can be demonstrated by MRI (Fig. 2.33). Distinction is made between an absent septum pellucidum and a normal variant involving separation of its leaves (cavum septi pellucidi).

MRI has also enabled diagnosis of various neuronal migration disorders, which are typically obscure on CT. These entities include schizencephaly (Fig. 2.34), heterotopias, pachygyria, polymicrogyria, hemimegalencephaly, and the most severe

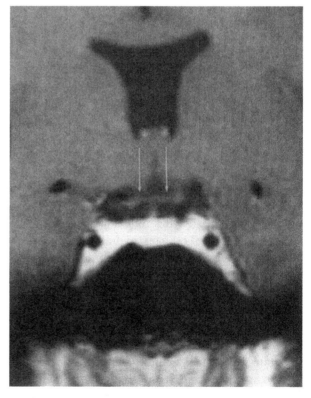

FIGURE 2.33. Coronal postcontrast T1-weighted MRI through the suprasellar region showing an abnormally attenuated optic chiasm (arrows). This finding and an absent septum pellucidum is diagnostic of septo-optic dysplasia.

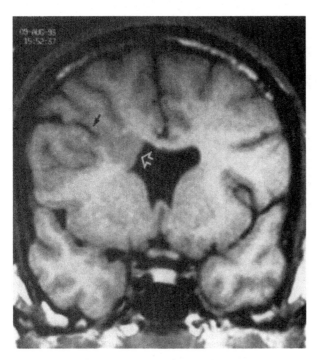

FIGUR 2.34. Coronal T1-weighted MRI showing an asymmetrical cleft (closed arrow) and a radially oriented gray matter isointensity mass that deforms the right frontal horn (open arrow). The findings are consistent with schizencephaly, closed-lip type.

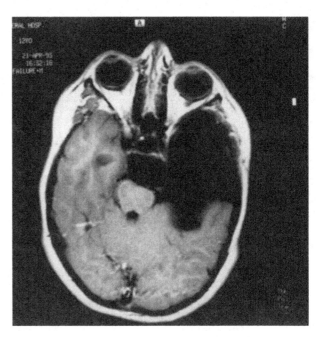

FIGURE 2.35. Postcontrast T1-weighted axial MRI showing a CSF isointensity mass that expands the left temporal fossa, and extends into the prepontine cistern. The findings are characteristic of a large arachnoid cyst.

form, lissencephaly.[38,39] Seizures are a frequent presenting symptom.

Benign cysts (usually arachnoid) are a common and typically incidental finding on brain imaging. They usually occur in the middle cranial fossa (Fig. 2.35). Posterior fossa cysts can be congenital or due to remote infection or hemorrhage.

Colloid cysts typically occur in the anterior third ventricle. These cysts are usually incidental findings, but they can obstruct the foramina of Monro and cause symptomatic or fatal hydrocephalus. These cysts can vary in density on CT and in intensity on MRI. They are not likely to enhance significantly. Colloid cysts have high protein content and/or paramagnetic substances and are often hyperintense on T1-weighted MR images. This hyperintensity can simulate an aneurysm on time-of-flight MRA (Fig. 2.36).

Commonly, spinal malformations are not evaluated on an emergency basis. Occult dysraphism can present in late life when symptoms are exacerbated by superimposed degenerative change. Tethering of the spinal cord by a bony spur in a case of diastematomyelia is shown in Figure 2.37.

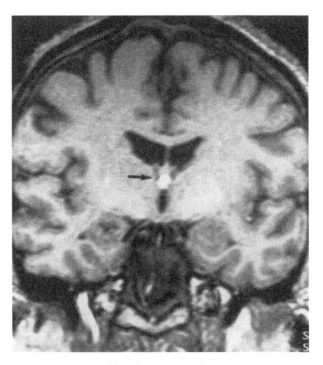

FIGURE 2.36A. Coronal noncontrast T1-weighted MRI showing a hyperintense lesion (arrow) bridging the superior third ventricle and the foramina of Munro, consistent with a colloid cyst.

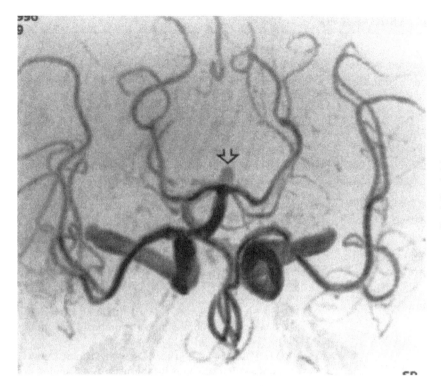

FIGURE 2.36B. Projection reconstruction of a time-of-flight MRA image showing how the T1 hyperintensity of the cyst can simulate a basilar tip aneurysm (open arrow).

Conclusion

Modern neuroimaging has made a significant impact on the evaluation of neurological problems in the emergency setting. Consultation with a neuroradiologist for the appropriate choice of procedure and expert interpretation of neuroimaging examina-

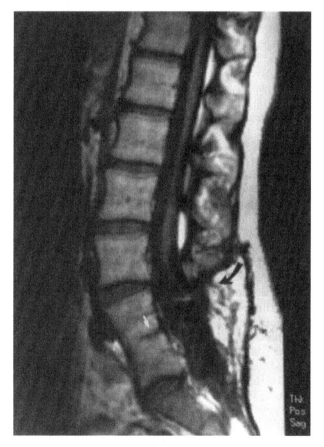

FIGURE 2.37A. Midsagittal T1-weighted MRI showing abnormal caudal and dorsal termination of the spinal cord consistent with tethering (curved black arrow). The vertebral bodies of L4 and L5 represent a congenital block vertebra with a rudimentary interspace (small white arrow).

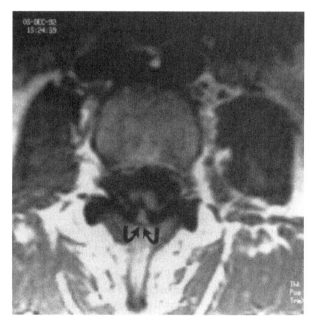

FIGURE 2.37B. Axial T1-weighted MRI showing tethering of the spinal cord by a bony spur (curved arrows). A short segment of rostral spinal cord was cleft, i.e., diastematomyelic (not shown).

tions is important. When not in the hospital, a neuroradiologist can review imaging studies by modern digital communication technology.

PEARLS AND PITFALLS

- CT, not MRI, is essential in the diagnosis of sudden headache because CT is sensitive to subarachnoid hemorrhage.
- The "dense middle cerebral artery sign" can indicate an impending hemispheric infarction.
- Cavernous angiomas appear as "black holes" without surrounding edema on gradient echo MRI.
- Isodense subdural hematomas on CT are hypointense of all MRI sequences.
- Hyperextension sprain without associated fracture can result in spinal cord contusion, which is demonstrated on MRI.
- Lateral disc herniations are diagnosed by CT or MRI; these herniations are inapparent on myelography.
- MRI demonstrates that herpes simplex encephalitis frequently involves both cerebral hemispheres.
- Colloid cysts vary in size, CT density, and MRI signal intensity but are enhanced significantly with contrast agents.

REFERENCES

1. Kanal E, Shellock FG, Talagala L. Safety considerations in MR imaging. *Radiology.* 1990;176:593–606.
2. Shellock FG, Kanal E. Policies, guidelines, and recommendations for MR imaging safety and patient management. *J Magn Reson Imaging.* 1991;1:97–101.
3. Doezema D, King JN, Tandberg D, et al. Magnetic resonance imaging in minor head trauma. *Ann Emerg Med.* 1991;20:1281–5.
4. Gomori JM, Grossman RI, Goldberg HI, et al. Intracranial hematomas. Imaging by high field MR. *Radiology.* 1985;157:87–93.
5. Grossman RI, Kemp SS, Ip CY, et al. Importance of oxygenation in the appearance of acute subarachnoid hemorrhage on high field magnetic resonance imaging. *Acta Radiol.* 1986;369(suppl):56–8.
6. Kelly AB, Zimmerman RD, Snow RB, et al. Head trauma: comparison of MR and CT – experience in 100 patients. *AJNR.* 1988;9:699–708.
7. Greenberg MK, Barsan WG, Starkman S. Neuroimaging in the emergency patient presenting with seizure. *Neurology.* 1996;47:26–32.
8. Tomsick T, Brott T, Barsan W, et al. Prognostic value of the hyperdense middle cerebral artery sign and stroke scale score before ultraearly thrombolytic therapy. *AJNR.* 1996;17:79–85.
9. Von Kummer R, Meyding-lamade' U, Forstung M, et al. Sensitivity and prognostic value of early CT in occlusion of the middle cerebral artery trunk. *AJNR.* 1994;15:9–15.
10. Goldberg AL, Rosenbaum AE, Wang E, et al. Computed tomography of dural sinus thrombosis. *J Comput Assist Tomogr.* 1986;10:16–20.
11. Kim KS, Walczak TS. Computed tomography of deep venous thrombosis. *J Comput Assist Tomogr.* 1986;10(3):386–90.
12. Macchi PJ, Grossman RI, Gomori JM, et al. High field MR imaging of cerebral venous thrombosis. *J Comput Assist Tomogr.* 1986;10:10–15.
13. Rippe DJ, Boyko OB, Spritzer CE, et al. Demonstration of dural sinus occlusion by the use of MR angiography. *AJNR.* 1990;11:199–201.
14. Gouliamos A, Gotsis E, Vlanos L, et al. Magnetic resonance angiography compared to digital subtraction arteriography in patients with subarachnoid hemorrhage. *Neuroradiology.* 1992;35:46–9.
15. Litt AW. MR angiography of intracranial aneurysms: proceed, but with caution. *AJNR.* 1994;15:1615–16.
16. Ross JS, Masaryk TJ, Modic MT, et al. Intracranial aneurysms: evaluation by MR angiography. *AJNR.* 1990;11:449–56.
17. Wilms G, Bleus P, Demaerel G, et al. Simultaneous occurrence of developmental venous anomalies and cavernous angiomas. *AJNR.* 1994;15:1247–54.
18. Gomori JM, Grossman RI. Mechanisms responsible for the MR appearance of evolution of intracranial hemorrhage. *RadioGraphics.* 1988;8:427–40.
19. Grossman RI, Gomori JM, Goldberg HI, et al. MR imaging of hemorrhagic conditions of the head and neck. *RadioGraphics.* 1988;8:441–54.
20. Rydberg JN, Hammond CA, Grimm RC, et al. Initial clinical experience in MR imaging of the brain with a fast fluid-attenuation inversion recovery pulse sequence. *Radiology.* 1994;193:173–80.
21. Rothfus WE, Goldberg AL, Tabas JH, et al. Callosomarginal infarction secondary to transfalcial herniation. *AJNR.* 1987;8:1073–6.
22. Silberstein M, Tress BM, Hennessy O. Prediction of neurologic outcome in acute spinal cord injury: the role of CT and MR. *AJNR.* 1992;13:1597–608.
23. Burke DC. Hyperextension injuries of the spine. *J Bone Joint Surg Br.* 1971;53B:3–12.
24. Robertson WD, Jarvik JG, Tsuruda JS, et al. The comparison of a rapid screening MR protocol with a conventional MR protocol for lumbar spondylosis. *AJR.* 1996;166:909–16.

25. Schellinger D, Manz HJ, Vidic B, et al. Disk fragment migration. *Radiology.* 1990;175:831–6.
26. Modic MT, Masaryk TJ, Ross JS, et al. Imaging of degenerative disk disease. *Radiology.* 1988;168:177–86.
27. Valk J. Gd-DTPA in MR of spinal lesions. *AJNR.* 1988;9:345–50.
28. Silbergleit R, Gebarski SS, Brunberg JA, et al. Lumbar synovial cysts: correlation of myelographic, CT, MR, and pathologic findings. *AJNR.* 1990;11:777–9.
29. Demaerel PH, Wilms G, Robberecht W, et al. MRI of herpes simplex encephalitis. *Neuroradiology.* 1992;34:490–3.
30. Raininko R, Elovaara I, Virta A, et al. Radiological study of the brain at various stages of human immuno-deficiency virus infection: early development of brain atrophy. *Neuroradiology.* 1992;34:190–6.
31. Chang L, Cornford ME, Chiang FL, et al. Radiologic-pathologic correlation: cerebral toxoplasmosis and lymphoma in AIDS. *AJNR.* 1995;16:1653–63.
32. Caldemeyer KS, Harris TM, Smith RR, et al. Gadolinium enhancement in acute disseminated encephalomyelitis. *J Comput Assist Tomogr.* 1991;15:673–5.
33. Zimmerman RD, Fleming CA, Saint-Louis LA, et al. Magnetic resonance imaging of meningiomas. *AJNR.* 1985;6:149–57.
34. Casselman W, Kuhweide R, Deimling M, et al. Constructive interference in steady state-3DFT MR imaging of the inner ear and cerebellopontine angle. *AJNR.* 1993;14:47–57.
35. Sze G, Krol G, Zimmerman RD, et al. Intramedullary disease of the spine: diagnosis using gadolinium-DTPA-enhanced MR imaging. *AJNR.* 1988;9:847–58.
36. Avrahami E, Tadmor R, Dally O, et al. Early MR demonstration of spinal metastasis in patients with normal radiographs and CT and radionuclide bone scans. *J Comput Assist Tomogr.* 1989;13:598–602.
37. El Gammal T, Allen MB Jr, Brooks BS, et al. MR evaluation of hydrocephalus. *AJNR.* 1987;8:591–7.
38. Barkovich AJ, Gressens P, Evrard P. Formation, maturation, and disorders of brain neocortex. *AJNR.* 1992;13:423–46.
39. Byrd SE, Bohan TP, Osborn RE, et al. The CT and MR evaluation of lissencephaly. *AJNR.* 1988;9:923–7.
40. Daffner RH. *Imaging of Vertebral Trauma.* 2nd ed. Philadelphia, Pa: Lippincott-Raven, 1966.

3 Electroencephalography

IVO DRURY AND AHMAD BEYDOUN

SUMMARY This chapter reviews the methods used to obtain electroencephalograms (EEGs), the major features of the normal EEG, and abnormal EEG features seen in patients with seizure disorders and various encephalopathies. It concludes with the value of EEG in several clinical circumstances where patients may present to an emergency department.

Introduction

The electroencephalogram (EEG) measures temporal changes in summated postsynaptic potentials from the superficial layers of the cerebral cortex. In the past, the EEG was used widely as a diagnostic test in clinical neurology. Today, use of the EEG has evolved to two major areas of clinical practice: the investigation of (1) patients with seizure disorders, and (2) patients with altered states of consciousness. Both conditions can result in patients presenting to an emergency department. Although patients requiring emergency EEGs are likely to be under the care of a neurologist or a neurosurgeon, it is important that the emergency physician be knowledgeable about the utility and limitation of the EEG in these clinical states.

Methods

EEGs are made by a technologist and interpreted by a physician. This interpretation is usually performed after completion of the study, but in emergency situations the physician should view the EEG on site while it is being recorded. A series of electrodes is placed in symmetric locations over the patient's scalp and connected to a specialized recording device. Typically, a routine EEG takes 30 minutes to record. While the EEG is being recorded, the technolo-gist documents the patient's behavioral state (awake, drowsy, stuporous, etc.), asks the patient to perform certain tasks in order to judge level of alertness, has the patient open and close his or her eyes, and performs activation procedures such as hyperventilation and photic stimulation. The technologist observes the patient closely and indicates on the record any alteration in responsiveness, seizure-like activity, or responses to noxious or auditory stimuli. In certain clinical circumstances, such as status epilepticus (SE), the physician may administer antiepileptic drugs (AEDs) intravenously during the study.

The Normal Electroencephalogram

The appearance of the normal EEG changes significantly from birth through the teenage years, then remains relatively unchanged until at least age 80. Unlike most imaging studies of the brain, the EEG also changes markedly depending on the behavioral state of the patient. Physicians interpreting EEG studies need to be familiar with changes that may be explained by age and state. EEG rhythms are divided into four normal frequency bands: delta (0.1–3.9 Hz), theta (4–7.9 Hz), alpha (8–12.9 Hz), and beta (13 Hz or greater). In the normal awake adult whose eyes are closed, the background rhythms consist of sinusoidal activity of 9–10 Hz over the parieto-occipital region, which attenuates when the eyes are open. A mixture of faster and slower frequencies over the more anterior head regions is relatively unaffected by eye opening or closure. In younger children, the rhythms are somewhat slower and less organized. In very advanced age (>80 years), there is some slowing of this dominant posterior rhythm and a greater amount of intermittent, more focal slowing.

Hyperventilation provokes physiological slowing of the background rhythm and further intermittent slowing in many normal subjects. These changes are most pronounced in young children. Intermittent photic stimulation may evoke a repetitive, time-locked occipital rhythm at the frequency or a harmonic of the frequency of the photic stimulus in normal subjects. Drowsiness and sleep result in characteristic changes in the EEG background, including increasing amounts of slower frequencies. There are characteristic EEG features to drowsiness, each stage of nonrapid eye movement sleep, and rapid eye movement (REM) sleep itself. In many pa-

tients with seizures, it is of particular value to record the EEG during or after sleep deprivation because abnormal waveforms may be seen more commonly in these recording conditions.

The Abnormal Electroencephalogram

There are numerous ways in which the EEG may be abnormal, but they can be reduced to two fundamental types: (1) changes seen in patients with seizure disorders and (2) various types of slow-wave abnormality. EEG findings in certain clinical conditions are summarized in Table 3.1.

Electroencephalogram Changes in the Epilepsies

Nearly every epileptic syndrome can be defined according to the following four categories: generalized or partial, that is, due to a diffuse brain abnormality or a more focal brain abnormality, respectively; and idiopathic or symptomatic, that is, usually

TABLE 3.1. EEG Findings in Major Neurological Conditions

Diagnosis	EEG Findings
Metabolic encephalopathies (e.g., renal or hepatic)	Generalized background slowing; intermittent rhythmic delta, triphasic waves; severity of slowing correlates with depression of mental status
Focal brain lesions (e.g., stroke, tumor, inflammatory)	Focal slowing; PLEDs if acute
Encephalitis	PLEDs or Bi-PLEDs; generalized or multifocal slowing
Anoxic brain injury: Mild to moderate	Slowing with or without reactivity
Severe	Alpha coma; burst suppression; periodic generalized sharp waves
Brain death	Isoelectric EEG
History of seizures: Focal epilepsy	Focal slowing; focal epileptiform discharges
Idiopathic generalized epilepsy	Normal background; generalized epileptiform discharges
Symptomatic generalized epilepsy	Slowing of background; generalized epileptiform discharges
Status epilepticus: Nonconvulsive	Recurrent focal seizures (complex partial SE) Generalized spike-wave activity (nonconvulsive generalized SE)
Convulsive	Generalized spike-wave activity with periods of voltage attenuation
Syncope	Normal EEG; EKG abnormalities
Psychogenic unresponsiveness	Normal background
Pseudostatus epilepticus	Normal background; muscle and movement artifacts

benign and commonly occurring on a heredofamilial basis, or when due to some underlying insult, respectively. Thus, the prototypical patient with an idiopathic generalized epilepsy might have generalized tonic-clonic convulsions but a normal neurological examination, whereas a patient with a symptomatic generalized epilepsy might also have generalized tonic-clonic convulsions but probably would have abnormal findings on the neurological examination. EEG findings in these four major categories of epilepsies parallel the clinical features. Patients with idiopathic epilepsies have normal background; patients with symptomatic epilepsies have an abnormal background. Epileptiform discharges seen in patients with generalized epilepsies are generalized; those in patients with focal (partial) epilepsies are focal.

EEG analysis begins with an assessment of the background activity. If the EEG is normal for age and behavioral state, the patient probably has an idiopathic epilepsy. Epileptiform abnormalities on the EEG may be either interictal (i.e., occurring between seizures), or ictal (i.e., the EEG rhythm seen during the course of a clinical seizure). Interictal epileptiform discharges are spikes, sharp waves, or spike-wave complexes. Their morphology, topography, frequency, and appearance in different states of behavior and in response to different activation procedures will vary depending on the patient's underlying epileptic syndrome. Acute cortical insults may lead to periodic lateralized epileptiform discharges (PLEDs), which are high-amplitude, regularly recurring sharp waves on a markedly attenuated background (Fig. 3.1). PLEDs are most commonly seen in patients with stroke or encephalitis. Ictal EEG discharges are more prolonged than interictal activity and, especially in the partial epilepsies, show an evolution in frequency, morphology, and topography during a clinical seizure.

Slow-Wave Abnormalities

EEG abnormalities that are slower than expected for the age and behavioral state of the patient are referred to as slow-wave abnormalities. These may be generalized or focal, and intermittent or persistent, the latter defined as present for greater than 80% of an EEG. Slow-wave abnormalities can be seen in patients with epilepsy; however, when they occur without other associated abnormalities, they are always nonspecific in nature. Focal slow-wave abnormalities imply a local disturbance of cortical and sometimes adjacent subcortical structures in the focal epilepsies; they can also occur in other conditions such as severe migraine or after head trauma where there is a localized injury. Generalized intermittent slowing occurs most commonly in diverse encephalopathies. The frequency of the slowing and the percent to which it is present in the EEG correlate with the severity of the encephalopathy. A stu-

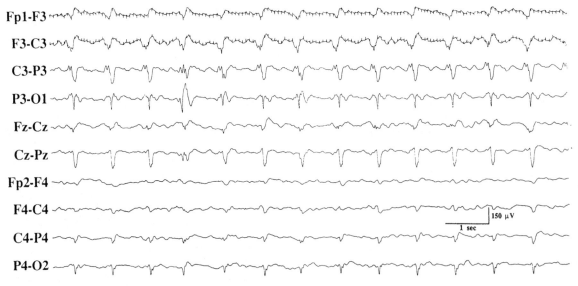

FIGURE 3.1. PLEDs arising from the posterior regions of the left hemisphere in a patient after a large left hemisphere stroke.

porous patient will show a moderate degree of slowing of background rhythms and brief trains of even slower waveforms intermittently. Stimulation of the patient will cause an acceleration of background frequency. A comatose patient will show a more marked and persistent degree of slowing that typically will not change with stimulation.

Special Clinical Circumstances

Status Epilepticus

Status epilepticus (SE) is defined as a continuous seizure lasting 30 minutes or more, or the occurrence of two or more seizures without full recovery of the baseline level of consciousness. Although a variety of classifications exists, a simple and practical one describes SE as either convulsive or nonconvulsive. The nonconvulsive types may be either complex partial SE or nonconvulsive generalized SE, the latter type may be referred to as absence status or spike-wave stupor.

Convulsive SE is a major medical emergency associated with significant morbidity and mortality and is discussed in Chapter 12, "Seizures." EEG recordings are of immense value in the pharmacological management of patients with convulsive SE. An EEG should be obtained as quickly as possible, but treatment is never delayed while awaiting an EEG recording. EEG can confirm SE and exclude the rare patient who has pseudo-SE. It also monitors the response to treatment given acutely[1] and can document the presence of subclinical (electrographic) seizures when overt seizure activity may not be apparent, indicating an incomplete response to the AEDs administered. In patients with refractory convulsive SE, the EEG is essential to ensure the adequacy of burst suppression intervals in pentobarbital-induced coma.

Nonconvulsive SE can occur in patients with a known history of epilepsy, or it may be the de novo manifestation of a seizure disorder. This diagnosis is always considered in patients who demonstrate a relatively acute onset of mental status changes and have no medical, psychiatric, or toxic/metabolic explanation for their illness.[2] On occasion, such patients will present with purely psychiatric symptoms. A diagnosis of nonconvulsive SE is always considered in patients with an unexpectedly prolonged postictal state. A conclusive diagnosis of either complex partial SE or absence SE can be made only by concurrent EEG recording. Psychogenic causes of unresponsiveness can be determined with certainty by a normal EEG. A neurologist should review the EEG during the recording period. If a diagnosis of nonconvulsive SE is established, the electrographic and clinical responses to intravenous administration of benzodiazepines (Fig. 3.2) and more long-acting AEDs such as phenytoin or phenobarbital are assessed.

First Seizure

Although there are many different types of seizures, the typical presentation of a first seizure in the emergency department is a generalized tonic-clonic (grand mal) event. Unless the underlying cause of the seizure is certain (e.g., alcohol withdrawal), all patients experiencing their first tonic-clonic seizure should be evaluated with an EEG. The results of the EEG in conjunction with the history, physical examination, and results of an imaging study are crucial in determining whether the patient is in need of ongoing treatment and, when indicated, which AED to use. There is a significantly increased likelihood of subsequent seizures when a patient's EEG is abnormal.[3] It is not essential that the EEG is performed at the time of the visit to the emergency department, but ideally it should be accomplished within a short interval after the first seizure.

The Patient with Altered Mental Status

EEGs can be of value in diagnosing patients with altered mental status not due to nonconvulsive SE. Occasionally, EEG findings in a comatose patient strongly suggest a particular etiology. A combination of unreactive delta range slowing with superimposed, widespread beta rhythms is likely to lead to a suspicion of overdose with barbiturates or benzodiazepines. In the heavily sedated patient or the patient who has been paralyzed with neuromuscular blocking agents, the EEG can be an extremely useful bedside measure of the integrity of brain function. The EEG is one of the confirmatory tests that can be useful in establishing a diagnosis of brain death; it should be used as such only when the patient has met all clinical criteria for the absence of any brain or brainstem function due to a known and irreversible cause. The EEG provides a measure of the function of the neocortex only. It is crucial that the patient's blood pressure and temper-

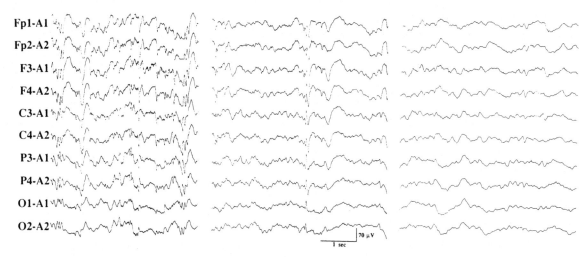

FIGURE 3.2. Three discontinuous samples of EEG from a 65-year-old woman in nonconvulsive generalized SE. The patient experienced repeated episodes of intermittent stupor, some associated with generalized tonic-clonic seizures, since age 50. The first EEG sample occurred after several hours of a confusional state and showed generalized irregular polyspike-and-wave activity. The next two samples were obtained 90s and 115s, respectively, after intravenous administration of 7.5 mg diazepam and showed prompt resolution of the epileptiform activity. (Reprinted with permission from Drury and Henry. Ictal patterns in generalized epilepsy. *J Clin Neurophysiol*. 1993;10:268–280, Raven Press, New York.

ature is normal or close to normal at the time the study is performed and that the patient is on no central nervous system depressant agents.

In patients with well-defined focal brain lesions such as tumors or stroke, there is no indication for the routine use of EEG. Certain focal brain lesions may present with a more global alteration in neurological function, most commonly in patients with encephalitis. It can also occur in patients with lesions such as tumors or strokes who develop an extensive region of epileptogenic tissue in the area adjacent to the lesion associated with a marked alteration in consciousness with or without subtle focal seizure activity. PLEDs typically occur in the cerebral hemisphere affected by an acute cortical lesion such as stroke or encephalitis; in encephalitis, these discharges may also appear independently over both hemispheres and are referred to as Bi-PLEDs.

PEARLS AND PITFALLS

■ EEG is used in the evaluation of patients with seizure disorders and patients with altered states of consciousness.

■ Interictal epileptiform discharges occur between seizures and consist of spikes, sharp waves, or spike-wave complexes.

■ PLEDs are most commonly observed in patients with acute stroke or encephalitis.

■ EEG slowing in a comatose patient is marked and persistent and typically does not change with stimulation of the patient.

■ EEG can provide evidence of subclinical seizures indicating an incomplete response to AEDs administered in the treatment of SE.

■ Psychogenic causes of unresponsiveness can be determined by a normal EEG.

REFERENCES

1. Privitera MD, Strawsburg RH. Electroencephalographic monitoring in the emergency department. *Emerg Med Clin North Am*. 1994;12:1089–100.
2. Lee SI. Nonconvulsive status epilepticus. Ictal confusion in later life. *Arch Neurol*. 1985;42:778–81.
3. Hauser WA, Anderson VE, Loewenson RB, McRoberts SM. Seizure occurrence after a first unprovoked seizure. *N Engl J Med*. 1982;307:522–8.
4. Drury I, Henry TR. Ictal patterns in generalized epilepsy. *J Clin Neurophysiol*. 1993;10:268–80.

4 Lumbar Puncture

JAMES P. VALERIANO AND DOUGLAS J. GELB

SUMMARY Lumbar puncture (LP) for the analysis of cerebrospinal fluid is the most frequently performed invasive diagnostic procedure in neurology. The two most common indications for performing LP in the emergency department are suspected meningitis and subarachnoid hemorrhage. Infection at the site of puncture is the only absolute contraindication for LP. A potential asymmetrical rise of intracranial pressure (ICP) that can lead to brain herniation is a relative contraindication for LP. In cases where the rise of ICP is more diffuse, as in meningitis, LP is reasonably safe; clinical deterioration and death occur only rarely.

Introduction

Lumbar puncture (LP) is indicated in the emergency department when an acute meningeal process such as meningitis or subarachnoid hemorrhage (SAH) is suspected. Characteristic symptoms and signs occur with any irritative process involving the meninges. Typical symptoms include neck and back pain, which can be diffuse, or radicular when individual nerve roots are involved. Photophobia and phonophobia are common. Classic meningeal signs, or stiff neck are common but not always present. Systemic signs include fever, diaphoresis, tachycardia, and tachypnea, and are often accompanied by mild agitation or irritability.

Neurological signs of meningeal irritation include Brudzinski's sign, an involuntary flexion of the hips and knees when the patient's neck is flexed by the examiner, and Kernig's sign, which is pain in the back or neck when the hip is flexed and the knee is extended. These signs are essentially flexor protective reflexes elicited by stretching of inflamed meninges. Elicitation of these signs requires a cooperative patient. Focal neurological signs can occur, and reflect involvement of particular cranial nerves or nerve roots. More generalized neurological signs include a decreased level of consciousness. Poor clinical outcome is suggested when deterioration of mental status occurs rapidly with signs of a meningeal process such as rapidly progressive bacterial meningitis or SAH. Any impairment of the level of consciousness with findings of meningeal involvement requires an emergency examination of the cerebrospinal fluid (CSF).

Performing Lumbar Puncture

The LP procedure, along with its risks (complications) and benefits, is explained to the patient and documented. A written consent for the procedure is obtained at most institutions in the United States.

There are relatively few contraindications for an LP. LP is contraindicated when infection exists at or near the site of the puncture (cellulitis, furuncle), and it is relatively contraindicated when there may be increased intracranial pressure (ICP) due to a space-occupying lesion. An asymmetric rise in ICP can precipitate brain herniation (discussed later in this section). LP is performed in hypocoagulable states, when the benefit of CSF analysis outweighs the potential risk of hemorrhage. Platelets can be infused prior to the procedure with severe thrombocytopenia.

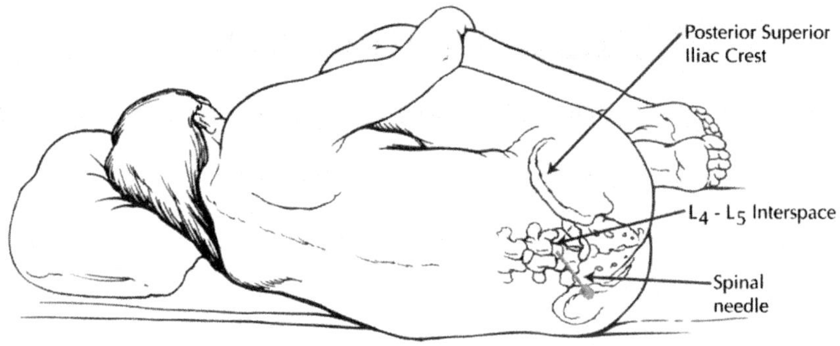

FIGURE 4.1. Lumbar puncture in an adult – left lateral decubitus fetal position.

LP is usually performed at the L3–4 or the L4–5 intervertebral space with the patient in the left lateral decubitus position (right-handed examiner) (Fig. 4.1). The patient's knees are pulled toward the chest and the head is flexed slightly. The spine is aligned as straight as possible. The shoulders and hips are positioned perpendicular to the examining table or bed. A firm table allows the best positioning of the patient. The patient's lower back is arched out toward the examiner. Marked flexion of the neck does not help the physician to position the patient and causes discomfort. Alternatively, LP can be performed with the patient sitting and bending forward (Fig. 4.2). This body position can allow better visual inspection of the patient's back, and better palpation

and digital localization of landmarks in some patients. Restraints are used for agitated and delirious patients. Conscious sedation of the patient may be required in order to perform LP in the emergency department, especially in young patients.

Following positioning of the patient, a sterile field is established. The patient's skin is prepared by vigorously rubbing an iodine-based solution. The skin and the deeper subcutaneous tissues are infiltrated with a 1% lidocaine solution for local anesthesia. A 20-gauge 3.5-inch spinal needle with stylet is used in adult patients. The spinal needle is inserted in the midline at an appropriate vertebral space with the bevel parallel to the long axis of the body so that it separates, rather than cuts through,

FIGURE 4.2. Lumbar puncture in an adult – sitting.

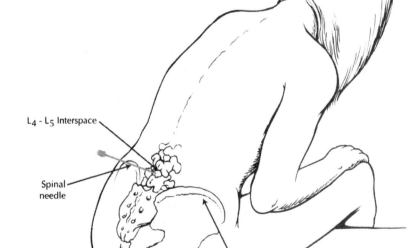

48

the fibers of the ligamentum flavum, which covers the interlaminary space between the vertebrae and offers resistance to the needle. The needle is directed toward the umbilicus, and a "pop" is felt when the needle tip punctures the ligament and the underlying dural sheath. If no "pop" is felt and the needle encounters bone, the needle is withdrawn to the subcutaneous tissue and redirected. The ligament can be calcified in the older patient, making a midline LP difficult. A slightly lateral approach can be used in this case. It is better to have someone else perform the LP after two or three unsuccessful attempts. When the needle enters the subarachnoid space, the stylet is removed slowly and CSF is allowed to flow one drop at a time. After the position of the needle is confirmed, the stylet is replaced, and the patient is asked to relax and extend the head and legs. The stylet is removed and the manometer is attached to the spinal needle to record the opening pressure of CSF. The normal CSF pressure is less than 200 mm CSF (water). After CSF is collected, the needle is removed and the site is covered with an adhesive bandage. The patient is asked to remain supine for at least 30 min. Traumatic LPs can be avoided by properly positioning the patient and by precisely introducing and directing the spinal needle. A hemorrhagic CSF sample is obtained when the spinal needle is advanced too far ventrally or directed laterally. The L4 vertebral spinous process lies approximately at the level of the highest point of the iliac crest. The adjacent interspace above or below can be used depending on the width of the space on palpation. In the adult, the spinal cord extends to the caudal end of the L1 vertebral body or just below it. Therefore, LP in adults or older children is performed below the L2 verte-

bral body. The spinal cord extends to the level of the L3 vertebra at birth. Therefore, in infants and young children, LP is performed at L4–5 or L5–S1 vertebral level (Fig. 4.3).

The major complication of LP is brain herniation, which occurs rarely. Herniation syndromes are reviewed in Chapter 26 ("Increased Intracranial Pressure"). Spinal epidural hematoma can occur in patients receiving anticoagulants or in patients with bleeding disorders. Spinal subdural hematomas following LP are rare. Meningitis can develop when LP is performed in a bacteremic patient. One series reported that meningitis developed in 7 out of 46 bacteremic children following an initial LP that had normal CSF results.[1] "LP-induced" meningitis occurred in children less than 1 year of age who did not receive antimicrobial therapy at the time of the initial cultures of CSF.[2,3] However, bacteremia is not a contraindication for LP because the benefits of CSF analysis outweigh the risks of iatrogenic meningitis.

Minor backache is a common complaint after LP. Disc herniation is a rare complication of LP, it occurs when the needle passes beyond the subarachnoid space and into the annulus fibrosis. Transient sensory symptoms due to nerve root irritation of the cauda equina are common. Complaints of motor weakness, sensory loss, or incontinence following LP require thorough investigation.

Performing Lumbar Puncture Prior to Computerized Topography Scanning

Two clinical conditions, suspected meningitis and SAH, account for most of the LPs performed in the emergency department. A definitive diagnosis of

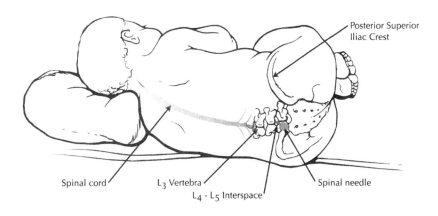

Posterior Superior
Iliac Crest

Spinal cord

L₃ Vertebra

L₄ - L₅ Interspace

Spinal needle

FIGURE 4.3. Lumbar puncture in an infant – left lateral decubitus fetal position.

meningitis is based on the examination of CSF. SAH can be identified on CT scanning in about 90–95% of cases. When SAH is suspected and it is not demonstrated on a CT scan, an examination of CSF to detect blood is necessary. The traditional premise of obtaining a CT scan of the brain prior to performing LP is based on the possible LP-induced rapid decompression of the central nervous system (CNS) in patients with increased ICP. This is of special concern in patients with a potential for an asymmetrical increase in ICP caused by mass lesions such as tumors, abscesses, and intra- or extra-axial hematomas. Asymmetrical ICP can cause a shift of intracranial contents when suddenly relieved from below. This can result in herniation syndromes, including transtentorial herniation, transfalcial herniation, or herniation of the cerebellar tonsils through the foramen magnum. When the rise in ICP is more diffuse or symmetrical, as in meningitis, LP is considered a relatively safe procedure, although clinical deterioration and death can occur.[4]

Most patients with either meningitis or SAH do not have intracranial mass lesions. Unless physical examination provides strong evidence of an intracranial mass lesion – specifically: a consistent asymmetry in sensory, motor, or reflex findings; papilledema, or a lesion of the third cranial nerve – LP can be performed before CT scanning is obtained. It is reasonable to obtain a CT scan when it can be performed quickly because it can potentially identify SAH noninvasively. Prudent clinical judgment is required when deciding to proceed with LP before obtaining a CT scan of the brain.

Papilledema on funduscopic examination is an accessible bedside finding of increased ICP. Papilledema depends on the chronicity and absolute increase of ICP, so it can be present with only modest elevations of ICP that have been present for a long period of time. Papilledema is not an absolute contraindication for LP. Therapeutic LPs are performed in certain conditions of diffuse increased ICP, such as pseudotumor cerebri (idiopathic intracranial hypertension) (see Chapter 27, "Idiopathic Intracranial Hypertension"). However, the finding of papilledema requires further investigation with CT scanning or magnetic resonance imaging (MRI) to assess for an intracranial lesion(s) that could result in an asymmetrical increase in ICP. Venous pulsations of the optic disk are not found on funduscopic examination of all normal individuals; however, when present, they reliably indicate a pressure of less than 200 mm CSF.

Interpretation of Lumbar Puncture Results

Following LP, the initial appearance of the CSF is described, the opening pressure is measured and recorded, and any difficulty performing the procedure is noted. Specimens are sent to the laboratory for determination of glucose, protein, cell count, and bacterial culture. Assays of bacterial antigens are done when indicated. In some clinical settings, it may be appropriate to send samples for fungal cultures or cytology. A small amount of CSF is retained for Gram stain and determination of xanthochromia (a yellow appearance resulting from the breakdown of red blood cells (RBCs)). In addition, a sample of CSF is saved in the emergency department or laboratory in the event that CSF results suggest the need for additional tests.

Cellular Content

CSF is normally acellular, so the presence of blood cells suggests an abnormality. However, a few white blood cells (WBCs), fewer than 5 cells/ml, can be a normal finding when they are primarily lymphocytes and there is no other evidence of pathology.[5] The presence of polymorphonuclear leukocytes (PMNs) is generally considered a sign of infection. The most frequent cause of a few RBCs in the CSF is a traumatic LP.

Glucose

Glucose enters the CSF by a carrier-mediated transport system,[6] and the usual ratio of CSF glucose to serum glucose is 0.6. A concomitant measurement of serum glucose can help to determine an expected range of CSF glucose. Because entrance of glucose into the CSF is a transport-mediated process, the carrier system can become saturated. At serum glucose levels greater than 250 mg/dl, the ratio of CSF glucose to serum glucose tends to decline. CSF glucose is reduced in conditions such as fungal or bacterial infections, and in carcinomatous meningitis. This decrease is likely caused by two mechanisms: (1) the decreased transport of glucose into the CSF, caused by pathological inflammation and/or injury to the meninges; and (2) increased utilization of glucose by polymorphonuclear cells. In

TABLE 4.1. Cerebrospinal Fluid Findings in Different Pathological Conditions

	Protein mg/dl	Glucose mg/dl	Cell Count/mm³ WBCs
Viral meningitis	Mild ↑	↔	10–200 Mainly lymphocytes
Bacterial meningitis	↑-↑↑	↓-↓↓	1,000–10,000 Mainly PMNs
Fungal meningitis	↑-↑↑	↓	100–1,000 Mainly lymphocytes
Tuberculosis meningitis	↑-↑↑	↓-↓↓	100–5,000 Mainly lymphocytes
Acute subarachnoid hemorrhage	↑	↔-↓	Markedly ↑ RBCs; often > 100,000; ↑ WBCs with PMN predominance

severe infections, CSF glucose can fall to very low levels (<5 mg/dl). Very low levels of CSF glucose are usually associated with poor clinical outcome. Glucose levels for various conditions are outlined in Table 4.1.

Protein

Most proteins found in the CSF are derived from the serum – with some notable exceptions (e.g., myelin basic protein). Protein enters the CSF by a pinocytotic process involving capillary endothelial cells,[7] and reflects serum concentration of the specific protein. Disruption of the blood–brain barrier by a pathological process, such as tumor, inflammation, or infection, disrupts the endothelial cell "tight junctions"[4] and causes increased permeability of serum protein, thus increasing total CSF protein content.

A normal CSF protein level is approximately 45 mg/dl. In conditions that affect reabsorption of CSF protein (e.g., meningitis, cancer, brain tumors), levels as high as 3.5 g/dl can occur. In general, elevated levels of CSF protein can be interpreted as a nonspecific response to a disease state that has disrupted the blood–brain barrier. Very high levels of CSF protein (750–1000 mg/dl) can be observed in spinal block (Froin's syndrome). Mild to moderate elevation of CSF protein is common in Guillain-Barré syndrome, diabetes, polyneuropathy, CNS in-

fections, and certain brain tumors. In multiple sclerosis (MS), the CSF protein elevation is seldom greater than 80–100 mg/dl.[8,9]

CSF Opening Pressure

CSF opening pressure is measured before CSF samples are obtained. The patient's legs are extended, because flexion at the knees and hips can elevate venous pressure and indirectly increase CSF pressure. The manometer is held upright perpendicular to the patient, and the CSF is allowed to rise freely. The opening pressure is reached when the meniscus of the CSF varies with respiration: decreasing with inspiration (due to lowered intrathoracic pressure and decreased venous pressure), and increasing with expiration or with Valsalva's maneuver. Normal CSF pressure is less than 200 mm CSF, and values above this represent increased ICP. Increased ICP is a nonspecific finding that can occur in processes such as tumor, abscess, hemorrhage, or infection. Very high pressures can be recorded with pseudotumor cerebri, at times in the range of 600 mm CSF.

Low opening pressure of CSF suggests obstruction of the needle by the meninges. Spinal block can also cause a low pressure reading. Other rare causes of low pressure conditions include barbiturate intoxication, following neurosurgical proce-

TABLE 4.2. Timing of CSF Changes after Subarachnoid Hemorrhage

	RBCs	Xanthochromia
First appearance (range)	≤30 minutes	2–24 hours
Present in all patients	0–12 hours	12 hours–2 weeks
Disappearance by (range)	1–24 days	2–7 weeks
	(Avg.: 3–9 days)	(Avg.: 3–4 weeks)

dures, and secondary to subdural hematomas in the elderly.

Identifying Traumatic Lumbar Puncture

SAH can result in RBCs in the CSF, xanthochromia or both, depending on the timing of the LP relative to the SAH. A general guideline is provided by the "rules of halves": half an hour after the event, RBCs appear in the CSF; at half a day, xanthochromia appears; at half a week, the RBCs disappear; and at half a month, the xanthochromia resolves. More precise time ranges are listed in Table 4.2.[10–14]

There is often uncertainty about whether RBCs were introduced to the CSF at the time of LP (a "traumatic tap"). This is a particular concern when the procedure is technically difficult, requiring several passes with the needle. The most reliable way to resolve this issue is to centrifuge the sample immediately and examine the supernatant for xanthochromia.[13–15] Xanthochromia results from the release of pigments as RBCs degenerate in the CSF. These pigments include oxyhemoglobin, causing a red color, bilirubin causing a yellow color, and methemoglobin, causing a brown color. Oxyhemoglobin pigment remains in suspension after cells are spun to the bottom of the tube, and is viewed as xanthochromia. RBCs that enter the CSF because of the procedure (a traumatic tap) do not have sufficient time to degenerate and therefore are associated with a clear supernatant. The most reliable way to detect xanthochromia is with a spectrophotometer,[13,14] but this instrument is not generally available. Direct visual inspection is the usual method of determining xanthochromia, but it is relatively unreliable. Discriminating xanthochromia is improved when the sample of spun CSF is compared directly to an equal volume of water, holding both against a white background in bright light. If there is any discernible difference in hue, the fluid is considered xanthochromic. Because of the critical implications of this determination, emergency physicians should perform this test themselves rather than relying on laboratory personnel.

The presence of bilirubin in the CSF involves the conversion of oxyhemoglobin by the enzyme heme-oxygenase. This enzyme is found in the choroid plexus, the arachnoid granulations, and the meninges. Enzyme activity appears approximately 12 hours after hemorrhage. Bilirubin can persist in CSF for 2–4 weeks. Bilirubin in CSF caused by hepatic or hemolytic disease does not appear until a serum level of 10–15 mg/dl total bilirubin is reached, unless there is an underlying disease associated with high CSF protein. Methemoglobin is a reduction product of oxyhemoglobin, and is typically found in encapsulated subdural hematomas or in old intracerebral hematomas.

Other methods for distinguishing preexisting SAH from traumatic LP are less reliable. One common practice is to perform a cell count on the first and last tubes of CSF collected, because blood introduced at the time of the procedure is usually most prominent in the first tube and clears rapidly. However, there are no guidelines for determining whether the rate of "clearing" is consistent with traumatic blood. Additionally, patients with SAH can undergo traumatic LP, which introduces additional blood into the first samples of CSF collected. In this situation, significant clearing of blood can occur in subsequent samples. Unless the blood in the CSF clears to an insignificant number of RBCs in the final tube, it is not possible to exclude the possibility of SAH.[15] Thus the absolute RBC count in the final tube is the most important finding, not the degree of RBC clearing.

Another less accurate method to determine whether blood in the CSF is due to traumatic LP is by observing the presence of clots in the CSF. Clotting of blood in the CSF indicates RBC counts of 200,000 cells/ml, counts usually indicative of traumatic LP.[16] However, high RBC counts do not exclude SAH. At one time, crenated RBCs were thought to differentiate SAH from traumatic LP. However, it is now known that crenated RBCs can occur in both circumstances.[10]

When LP is performed at least 24 hours after the onset of symptoms, a significantly elevated WBC count provides evidence of SAH. Leukocytosis occurs with traumatic LP, but the expected WBC count can be readily calculated:[17]

$$\text{Expected CSF WBC count} = \frac{(\text{CSF RBCs}) \times (\text{peripheral WBCs})}{(\text{peripheral RBCs})}$$

Typical peripheral RBC counts are $4\text{--}6 \times 10^6$ cells/ml, whereas normal peripheral WBC counts are $4\text{--}11 \times 10^3$ cells/ml. According to the formula above, approximately one WBC can be expected in the CSF for every 500–1000 RBCs introduced by a traumatic LP. When the CSF WBC count is substantially higher than predicted on this basis, the results cannot be explained simply by traumatic LP. Similarly, an increase in CSF protein of about 1 mg/dl can be expected for every 1000 RBCs present in the CSF;[16] CSF protein elevation greater than that expected from this estimate indicates an abnormality that cannot be attributed to a traumatic LP.

Distinguishing Bacterial Meningitis from Viral Meningitis

The CSF WBC count is the most important test in diagnosing meningitis. Any count greater than 5 cells/ml is abnormal,[17] but WBC counts for bacterial meningitis typically range from 1000–10,000 cells/ml.[17-20] WBC counts in viral meningitis are usually lower and typically range from 5–1000 cells/ml.[17-20] Therefore, bacterial meningitis is unlikely with WBC counts of less than 100 cells/ml,

and WBC counts greater than 1000 cells/ml make viral meningitis unlikely. No single clinical or laboratory parameter reliably distinguishes between viral and bacterial infections in the intermediate range of 100–1000 cells/ml. The differential cell count is an unreliable measure in this range. In general, a mononuclear predominance is typical of viral meningitis and a polymorphonuclear predominance is the rule in bacterial meningitis, but 15% of patients with acute bacterial meningitis have a lymphocytic predominance.[19] Additionally, lymphocytic predominance is common in patients with low total CSF WBC counts, the subgroup of patients in whom the diagnosis is most uncertain.[18,21] In a series of patients with culture-proven bacterial meningitis, 41% of patients with total CSF WBC counts of less than 100 cells/ml had a lymphocytic predominance (as opposed to 1% of patients whose total WBC counts exceeded 100 cells/ml).[21] Furthermore, polymorphonuclear granulocytes can predominate in viral meningitis, especially in the first 72 hours.[19]

The CSF glucose content is usually reduced in bacterial meningitis and is characteristically normal in viral meningitis, but there are exceptions to both of these general rules. The ratio of CSF glucose to serum glucose is more sensitive than the absolute CSF glucose level for detecting meningitis, because the serum glucose is often elevated in this condition.[19,21] However, some patients with bacterial meningitis have a normal ratio of CSF glucose to serum glucose. Alternatively, a ratio value of less than 0.25 almost never occurs in viral meningitis.[19] The CSF protein is typically elevated in both viral and bacterial meningitis. Protein levels tend to be higher in bacterial meningitis than in viral meningitis, but this finding is not sufficiently reliable to aid significantly in determining the diagnosis. CSF opening pressure is also elevated in both conditions. A positive CSF Gram stain permits diagnosis of bacterial meningitis, but a negative Gram stain does not exclude the diagnosis. Similarly, assays of specific bacterial antigens can help to identify the pathogen, but false-negative results can occur.

A reliable differentiation between viral meningitis and bacterial meningitis is not possible on the basis of a single CSF parameter. A combination of several independent parameters (variables) can have greater predictive power than any of the variables individually. High diagnostic accuracy is achieved using a formula derived from four parame-

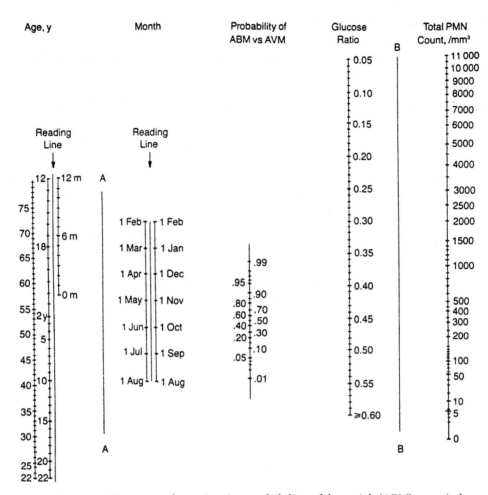

FIGURE 4.4. Nomogram for estimating probability of bacterial (ABM) vs. viral (AVM) meningitis. Step 1, place ruler on reading lines for patient's age and month of presentation and mark intersection with line A; step 2, place ruler on values for glucose ratio and total polymorphonuclear leukocyte (PMN) count in cerebrospinal fluid and mark intersection with line B; step 3, use ruler to join marks on lines A and B, then read off the probability of ABM vs. AVM.

ters: (1) the total CSF polymorphonuclear leukocyte count; (2) the ratio of CSF glucose to blood glucose; (3) the month of presentation; and (4) the age of the patient.[19] A nomogram summarizing that formula is shown in Figure 4.4. Because two of the four parameters used in this calculation (month of presentation and age) are epidemiological, the formula needs to be confirmed in other geographic and demographic circumstances to determine its widespread applicability. Until such verification occurs, patients with negative CSF Gram stain and CSF WBC counts in the range of 100–1000 cells/ml are treated empirically for bacterial meningitis because

the complications of treatment are far less dangerous than the failure to treat. Treatment continues until blood and CSF cultures are negative for 48 hours. Empirical treatment with acyclovir is appropriate when the clinical course is consistent with Herpes simplex meningoencephalitis.

Because prompt treatment of SAH and bacterial meningitis can potentially prevent catastrophic consequences, a sense of urgency attends the evaluation until these diagnoses have been either excluded or treated. One common management error is the failure to administer antibiotics promptly while awaiting CT scanning and LP results.[22] Although there is justifiable concern that CSF culture results can be obscured when antibiotics are given prior to LP, this concern is weighted against the risk of overwhelming bacterial infection when antibiotics are given too late. When LP is performed and CSF collected within 2 hours of intravenous antibiotic administration (especially if antibiotic inhibitors are added to the culture medium), it is possible to achieve a high rate of positive culture results. Several human studies have demonstrated a 20–40% positive rate of CSF cultures up to 24 hours after administration of intravenous antibiotics, with higher rates of culture positivity when the interval from antibiotic administration to LP is shorter.[22] Moreover, CSF cultures are not the only means available for identifying the bacterial etiology of meningitis. Roughly 50% of patients with bacterial meningitis have positive blood cultures, and bacterial antigen studies are nearly as sensitive as CSF Gram stains.[17,22]

The following approach to empirical antibiotic therapy is reasonable. Patients who are hemodynamically compromised or appear gravely ill should have blood cultures obtained, followed immediately by intravenous antibiotics and LP. Patients with papilledema or prominent focal abnormalities on neurological examination are more likely to have an intracranial mass lesion. In these patients, blood cultures should be obtained followed by a noncontrast CT scan of the brain. LP is performed following a normal CT scan. A single dose of antibiotics is given immediately after obtaining the CSF (and before results are available), unless the suspicion of bacterial meningitis is very low, that is, the patient is afebrile and CSF is clear on gross inspection.

PEARLS AND PITFALLS

- The site of LP in infants and young children is *lower* (L4–L5 or L5–S1 vertebral level) than in adults (L3–4 or L4–5 vertebral level).
- In patients suspected of having SAH, LP and examination of CSF are necessary when CT scanning of the brain fails to demonstrate SAH.
- The traditional practice of obtaining a CT scan of the brain prior to performing LP is tempered with

clinical reasoning and a comprehensive neurological examination.

- Papilledema observed on funduscopic examination is a readily accessible bedside finding of increased ICP. Papilledema is not an absolute contraindication for an LP.
- Papilledema depends on the absolute increase in ICP and the chronicity of ICP elevation.
- There is no ideal test to distinguish traumatic from nontraumatic LP. Although direct visual inspection can be unreliable, it is the usual method of determining xanthochromia.
- There is no single clinical or laboratory parameter that can reliably distinguish between viral and bacterial infections when the CSF WBC count is in the intermediate range of 100–1000 cells/ml.

REFERENCES

1. Teele DW, Dashefsky B, Rakusan T, Klein JO. Meningitis after lumbar puncture in children with bacteremia. *N Engl J Med.* 305:1079–981.
2. Krishra V, Liu V, Singleton AF. Should lumbar puncture be routinely performed in patients with suspected bacteremia? *J Nat Med Assoc.* 1983;75:1153.
3. Fedor HM, Adelman AM, Pugno PA, Dallman J. Meningitis following normal lumbar puncture. *J Fam Pract.* 1985;20:437.
4. Swartz MN, Dodge PR. Bacterial meningitis – a review of selected aspects, I: general clinical features, special problems and unusual meningial reactions mimicking bacterial meningitis. *N Engl J Med.* 1965;272:725–31, 779–87, 842–8, 898–902.
5. Ford DH. Blood-brain barrier: a regulatory mechanism. *Rev Neurosci.* 1976;2:1–42.
6. Fishman RA. Carrier transport of glucose between blood and cerebrospinal fluid. *Am J Physiol.* 1964;206:836–44.
7. Brightman MW, Klatzo I, Olsosan Y, Reese TS. The blood-brain barrier to proteins under normal and pathological conditions. *J Neurol Sci.* 1970;10:215–39.
8. Shenkin HA, Finneson BE. Clinical significance of low cerebral spinal fluid pressure. *Neurology* 1958;8:157.
9. Bell WE, Joynt RJ, Sahs A: Low spinal fluid pressure syndromes. *Neurology* 1060;10:512.
10. Matthews WF, Frommeyer WB. The in vitro behavior of erythrocytes in human cerebrospinal fluid. *J Lab Clin Med.* 1955;45:508–15.
11. Sengupta RP, McAllister VL, Gates P. Differential diagnosis. In: Sengupta RD, McAllister VL, eds. *Suberachnoid Haemorrhage.* Berlin: Springer-Verlag, 1986:79–92.
12. Maurice-Williams RS. *Subarachnoid Hemorrhage: Aneurysms and Vascular Malformations of the Central*

Nervous System. Bristol, England: Wright; 1987: 83–100.

13. Vermeulen M, Hasan D, Blijenberg BG, Hijdra A, van Gijn J. Xanthochromia after subarachnoid haemorrhage needs no revision. *J Neurol Neurosurg Psychiatry* 1989;52:826–8.

14. Weir B. Headaches from aneurysms. *Cephalalgia* 1994; 14:79–87.

15. Vermeulen M, van Gijn J. The diagnosis of subarachnoid haemorrhage. *J Neurol Neurosurg Psychiatry* 1990;53:365–72.

16. McMenemey WH. The significance of subarachnoid bleeding. *Proc Roy Soc Med.* 1954;47:701–4.

17. Fishman RA. 2nd ed. *Cerebrospinal Fluid in Diseases of the Nervous System.* Philadelphia, Pa: WB Saunders; 1992.

18. Overturf GD. Pyogenic bacterial infections of the CNS. *Neurol Clin.* 1986;4:69–90.

19. Spanos A, Harrell FE, Durack DT. Differential diagnosis of acute meningitis. An analysis of the predictive value of initial observations. *JAMA* 1989;262: 2700–7.

20. Durand ML, Calderwood SB, Weber DJ, et al. Acute bacterial meningitis in adults. A review of 493 episodes. *N Engl J Med.* 1993;328:21–8.

21. Powers WJ. Cerebrospinal fluid lymphocytosis in acute bacterial meningitis. *Am J Med.* 1985;79: 216–20.

22. Talan DA, Guterman JJ, Overturf GD, Singer C, Hoffman JR, Lambert B. Analysis of emergency department management of suspected bacterial meningitis. *Ann Emerg Med.* 1989;18:856–62.

5 Electromyography

JAMES W. ALBERS AND JOHN J. WALD

SUMMARY There are few indications for emergency electromyography testing. However, it is important that the emergency department physician is familiar with those indications and has a basic understanding of the electrophysiological changes associated with acute peripheral nervous system lesions. Familiarity with the temporal changes that occur in electrodiagnostic measures facilitates scheduling decisions, both for differentiating acute from preexisting lesions and for providing appropriate test results to subsequent treating physicians. A basic understanding of the electromyography report also permits proper use of existing electrodiagnostic information in making emergency clinical decisions.

Introduction

Nerve conduction studies and needle electromyography are commonly referred to as electromyogram (EMG) testing. These tests consist of sensitive, objective measures used in the diagnosis of peripheral nervous system disorders. For several reasons, the emergency department physician rarely uses the results of an EMG in making emergency decisions. First, when indicated in an emergency setting, the neuromuscular problem is typically limb- or life-threatening, resulting in immediate surgical intervention or admission of the patient. In this setting, EMG studies may be ordered by the admitting physician to identify nerve continuity in a paralyzed limb after acute trauma or defective neuromuscular transmission or diffuse motor neuron disease in the presence of weakness and respiratory failure. Second, some EMG findings do not appear immediately after onset of a peripheral disorder, but become apparent only after days to weeks. For example, the finding of fibrillation potentials, a sensitive indicator of denervation, does not occur for days to weeks after an acute nerve lesion. However,

other abnormalities appear immediately, some of which are useful in establishing prognosis. In addition, identification of a preexisting lesion often is important in establishing the cause of a problem, and the best documentation of the timing of a lesion is derived from serial evaluations. EMG studies are scheduled occasionally by the emergency department physician so that results will be available at follow-up evaluations. An understanding of the indications and timing of electrodiagnostic studies is useful in making scheduling decisions, and a familiarity with the EMG report allows interpretation of available electrodiagnostic information in making emergency clinical decisions.

Description of Electromyography

The EMG evaluation includes nerve conduction studies (motor and sensory) and the needle examination of muscle. The studies are based on sound neurophysiological principles, and they provide sensitive, objective measures of nerve and muscle functions. A thorough EMG evaluation establishes the distribution, severity, pathophysiology, and temporal profile of a peripheral disorder. Even when the results do not establish a specific diagnosis, the information is useful in accurately localizing the disorder, thereby directing the subsequent evaluation.

Technical Considerations

Nerve conduction techniques are standardized, with minor differences existing from laboratory to laboratory.[1,2] Many results are age-dependent, and some vary according to certain physical dimensions of the patient.[3,4] Normal values exist for a variety of techniques, and the EMG report should include appropriate normal values. The most important technical consideration is limb temperature, a significant source of variability.[5,6] Cooling decreases the rate at which ionic channels open, producing decreased conduction velocity. The prolonged opening of ionic channels when the limb is cool also produces an increased response amplitude, particularly in sensory nerves. The combination of increased amplitude and reduced conduction velocity is atypical for any pathological process. Standard practice requires the electromyographer to monitor and record limb temperature, warming when necessary to approximately 31–36°C.

Nerve Conduction Studies

Nerve conduction studies evaluate propagation of nerve action potentials along motor or sensory nerves. These responses are produced by depolarizing peripheral nerves with a percutaneous electrical stimulus. Techniques also exist to evaluate reflex pathways, conduction along proximal portions of the motor nerve root, and neuromuscular transmission. Nerve conduction studies evaluate a variety of peripheral disorders, including neuropathy, plexopathy, myopathy, defective neuromuscular transmission, and motor neuron disease. An important characteristic of nerve conduction studies is their ability to distinguish peripheral from central abnormalities.

Motor and Sensory Nerve Conduction. Motor or sensory nerve action potentials are recorded using surface electrodes placed on the skin (Figs. 5.1 and 5.2). Motor responses are biphasic when recorded directly over the endplate region. Sensory responses usually are triphasic, reflecting the signal as it approaches, passes beneath, and then travels away from the recording electrode, although the initial positivity is not always apparent. Motor or sensory amplitudes are important measures, as they essentially reflect the number and size of functioning nerve or muscle fibers.[7,8] Motor amplitudes are expressed in millivolts (mV), and sensory amplitudes are expressed in microvolts (μV). Lesions involving loss of peripheral axons from any cause produce reduced amplitude.[2]

Conduction velocity (M/s) of the fastest fibers is calculated by stimulating the nerve at two sites,

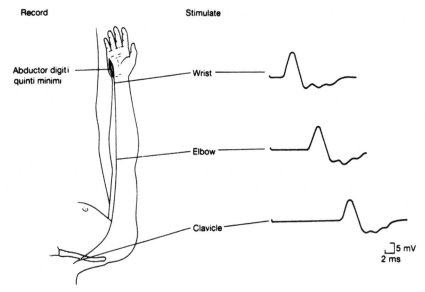

FIGURE 5.1. Representative motor nerve conduction study. Motor responses recorded following stimulation of the ulnar nerve at the wrist, elbow, and clavicle, recorded from the hypothenar muscles. Calibration: 2 ms and 5 mV. Reprinted with permission from Albers, J.W., Leonard, J.A. Jr. 1992. Nerve conduction studies and electromyography. In *Neurosurgery, The Scientific Basis of Clinical Practice,* 2nd ed. vol 2, eds. A. Crockard, R. Hayward, J.T. Hoff, pp. 735–757. Boston: Blackwell Scientific Publications.

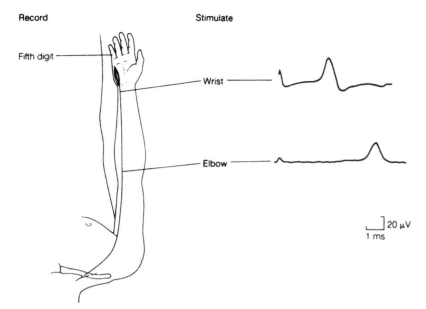

Record   Stimulate

Fifth digit

Wrist

Elbow

]20 μV
1 ms

FIGURE 5.2. Representative sensory nerve conduction study. Sensory responses recorded following supramaximal percutaneous stimulation of the ulnar nerve at the wrist and elbow, recorded from the fifth digit. Calibration: 1 ms and 20 μV. Reprinted with permission from Albers, J.W., Leonard, J.A. Jr. 1992. Nerve conduction studies and electromyography. In *Neurosurgery, The Scientific Basis of Clinical Practice,* 2nd ed. vol 2, eds. A. Crockard, R. Hayward, J.T. Hoff, pp. 735–757. Boston: Blackwell Scientific Publications.

measuring the stimulus to response onset latencies, and dividing the distance between the two sites by the latency difference. Distal latency (ms) is another measure of the rate of conduction, expressed as the elapsed time from the stimulus to response onset at a fixed distance from the end of the nerve. Conduction speed reflects many physiological and technical components of peripheral nerve function, including nerve size, amount and integrity of myelin, nodal and internodal lengths, axonal resistance, nerve temperature, and age.[2]

F Wave Latency. The F wave is a small motor response produced by one or more motor units (Fig. 5.3). The F wave occurs after antidromic stimulation of a motor nerve (e.g., toward the spinal cord, away from muscle), resulting in activation of some anterior horn cells and transmission of an action potential back down the same nerve. The stimulation to response latency can be measured, representing a transmission time of the signal along and then back the entire nerve (stimulation site to spinal cord to muscle). The F wave evaluates transmission over the entire motor nerve, including the proximal motor nerve, a portion not evaluated by standard conduction studies.

H Reflex Latency. The H reflex is a monosynaptic reflex analogous to the Achilles reflex, differing only in the method of activation. For the Achilles reflex, muscle stretch activates intrafusal muscle receptors, whereas for the H reflex, sensory afferents in the tibial nerve are activated by a percutaneous electrical stimulus at the knee, not muscle stretch. The resultant action potentials depolarize the same spinal cord motor neuron pool, however. The H reflex has limited use, but it does study conduction along the entire S1 reflex arc.

Repetitive Motor Nerve Stimulation. The most common technique available to evaluate neuromuscular transmission utilizes repetitive motor nerve stimulation.[2] Neuromuscular transmission failure is identified as a decrement in the motor amplitude with repeated depolarization, whereas the normal response shows no amplitude variation. Neuromuscular transmission depends on many factors, including availability and release of acetylcholine (ACh), inactivation of ACh in the synaptic cleft, and the presence of functional ACh receptors on muscle; abnormality of any of these may result in impaired neuromuscular transmission. The optimal stimulus rate for demonstrating defective neuromuscular transmission in disorders such as myasthenia gravis or anticholinesterase intoxication is 2–5 Hz. The effects of calcium-dependent facilitation are studied by volitional exercise or high-rate stimulation (50 Hz) to demonstrate abnormal facilitation in the Lambert-Eaton myasthenic syndrome or botulism intoxication.

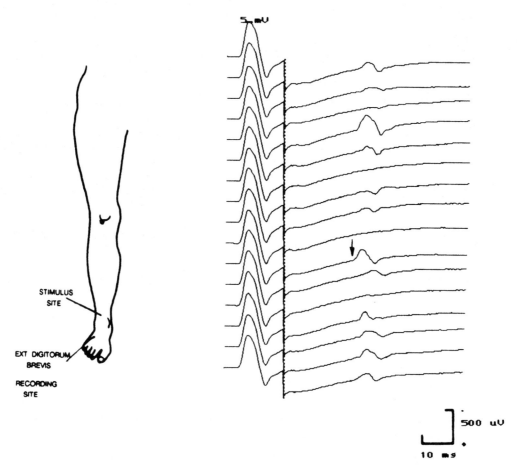

FIGURE 5.3. Representative F wave following percutaneous antidromic stimulation of the peroneal nerve at the ankle. The resultant F wave is shown at the right of the recording, with the motor response on the left. Calibration: 20 ms and 1 mV (the 5 mV legend refers to the calibration of the direct motor response.) Reprinted with permission from Albers, J.W., Leonard, J.A. Jr. 1992. Nerve conduction studies and electromyography. In *Neurosurgery, The Scientific Basis of Clinical Practice,* 2nd ed. vol 2, eds. A. Crockard, R. Hayward, J.T. Hoff, pp. 735–757. Boston: Blackwell Scientific Publications.

Needle Electromyogram

Electrical signals from muscle are recorded using a sterile needle electrode inserted through the skin into muscle, and displayed on an oscilloscope and heard through a loudspeaker.[2,9,10] These signals are recorded in the patient at rest (insertional activity) and in response to voluntary activation of the muscle. The needle EMG is used to evaluate many disorders also studied by nerve conduction techniques; however, it has the advantage of access to muscles, such as the paraspinal muscles, that cannot be otherwise studied. Its greatest utility is as a sensitive indicator of ongoing or previous motor nerve or muscle fiber degeneration. The needle EMG exami-

nation is very sensitive and frequently detects abnormalities that are neither clinically apparent nor symptomatic.

Insertional Activity. The response to electrode insertion and the presence or absence of spontaneous electrical activity are two characteristics of the EMG signal. Normal muscle is electrically silent when recording away from the endplate region. With electrode movement, a brief discharge is a normal finding (normal insertional activity). Examples of abnormal spontaneous activity include positive waves and fibrillation potentials. Each represents involuntary muscle fiber discharges by reflecting muscle fiber hypersensitivity to ACh following separation of the muscle fiber from nerve, regardless of cause. They are easily recognized, are not easily confused with other EMG signals, and are not present in normal muscle. These potentials are shown in Figure 5.4. The amplitude of positive waves and fibrillation potentials diminishes over months, corresponding to muscle fiber atrophy, thereby providing an approximation of lesion onset.

Motor Units. Activated muscle fibers generate and transmit a muscle fiber action potential (MFAP) analogous to the nerve action potential. The needle electrode records electrical activity from individual motor units consisting of muscle fibers originating from a single lower motor neuron. The resulting signal is called a motor unit action potential, or motor unit, and represents a compound action potential that consists of a summation of all the individual MFAPs of a given anterior horn cell. The motor unit interference pattern is recorded during voluntary activation of a muscle, and consists of as few as one to many motor units. Examination of the interference pattern includes evaluation of motor unit size,

configuration (amplitude, duration, and number of phases), and activation pattern.[11]

Because the motor unit is a summation of individual MFAPs, an increase in muscle fiber density produces an increased amplitude, and a decrease in density produces a decreased amplitude. The activation pattern refers to the sequential introduction (recruitment) of motor units into the interference pattern as force is voluntarily increased. Those motor units activated initially discharge at 5–15 Hz. As force is increased, the discharge rate increases until a second motor unit is activated, the pattern repeating with increasing force. Decreased recruitment results from loss of individual motor units, whereas increased recruitment reflects decreased force generation by individual motor units. A recruitment pattern that is irregular or occurs in bursts is characteristic of patients with upper motor neuron disorders, poor cooperation, or pain inhibition. Representative recruitment patterns are shown in Figure 5.5.

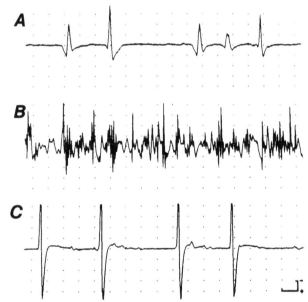

FIGURE 5.5. Motor unit interference pattern demonstrating recruitment at low levels of muscle force. (A) Normal recruitment with 3 motor units present, as demonstrated by the different amplitude responses. (B) Increased recruitment with many short-duration polyphasic motor units despite low level of force, as seen in myositis. (C) Decreased recruitment with only one motor unit firing rapidly, as seen in partial denervation. Calibration: 10 ms and 200 μV. Modified with permission from Bromberg, M.B., Albers, J. W. 1988. Electromyography in idiopathic myositis. *Mt Sinai J Med.* 55:459–464.

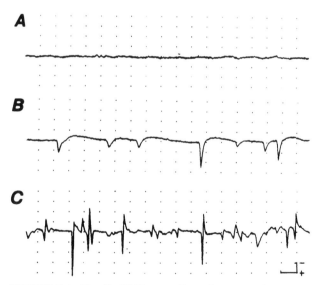

FIGURE 5.4. Needle EMG recordings from muscle at rest. (A) Normal muscle with no evidence of abnormal spontaneous activity. (B) Abnormal spontaneous activity consisting of positive waves. (C) Abnormal spontaneous activity consisting of fibrillation potentials and occasional positive waves. Calibration: 10 ms and 50 μV. Modified with permission from Bromberg, M.B., Albers, J. W. 1988. Electromyography in idiopathic myositis. *Mt Sinai J Med.* 55:459–464.

Expected Findings Following an Acute Axonal Lesion

EMG findings associated with acute neuromuscular disorders are important to the emergency physician, and problems may be overlooked if the temporal changes that occur in the EMG evaluation are not understood. These changes are best demonstrated by considering what happens after acute nerve transection. It is well known that immediately after transection, stimulation of the transected nerve distal to the transection produces a normal muscle contraction.[12] Furthermore, this response persists for several days but then diminishes and disappears in about one week. Nerve conduction studies demonstrate similar findings. Immediately after transection, nerve stimulation produces normal motor and sensory responses in the distal portion of the transected nerve. Of course, responses cannot be produced by stimulation proximal to the lesion. The needle examination initially demonstrates normal insertional and rest activity, but motor units cannot be activated, as voluntary activity cannot be transmitted across the lesion.

Within several days, motor and sensory amplitudes decrease and ultimately disappear in about one week. Before they disappear, conduction velocities and distal latencies remain essentially normal, becoming slightly abnormal only when amplitude is substantially diminished. Depending upon the proximity of the muscle to the lesion, needle examination abnormalities suggestive of denervation appear within one to three weeks. The initial abnormality is prolonged insertional activity, usually consisting of unsustained positive waves, followed by sustained positive wave and fibrillation potentials.

The first sign of reinnervation is the appearance of small-amplitude, long-duration, polyphasic motor units, usually in association with a decrease in abnormal spontaneous activity. These changes develop prior to clinical evidence of recovery. As reinnervation progresses, individual motor units capture more muscle fibers through collateral sprouting and the motor unit amplitude increases. Nevertheless, recruitment remains decreased as long as the total number of motor units is decreased. Eventually, small sensory and motor responses appear, and serial studies

TABLE 5.1. EMG Changes After Nerve Transection

	Immediate	1–3 Days	3–7 Days	7–10 Days	1–2 Weeks	2–4 Weeks	>4 Weeks
Conduction studies							
Motor and sensory responses following stimulation							
Proximal to lesion	NR	NR	NR	NR	NR	NR	NR
Distal to lesion:							
Amplitude	N	Slight ↓	Marked ↓	NR	NR	NR	NR
Conduction velocity	N	N	Slight ↓	NR	NR	NR	NR
Distal latency	N	N	Slight ↑	NR	NR	NR	NR
F wave latency	NR	NR	NR	NR	NR	NR	NR
Needle examination							
Insertional activity	N	N	N	N	Slight ↑ (near lesion)	↑	↑
Fibrillation potentials	0	0	0	0	0 to +	+ to ++	+++ to ++++
Motor units	None	None	None	None	None	None	None

N = normal.
NR = no response.

demonstrate progressive increases in amplitude. Residual deficits may persist, but most motor abnormalities eventually resolve. Table 5.1 summarizes the sequential EMG changes after nerve transection.

Selected Examples of Electromyogram Findings

It is beyond the scope of this chapter to describe EMG findings for all disorders encountered in the emergency department, and descriptions exist in standard texts. The examples that follow highlight important considerations in the EMG evaluation and interpretation process. For each example, information regarding the temporal changes described above are included when relevant, but they are not reported in detail for each disorder. It is understood that the differential diagnosis for each example includes a variety of peripheral disorders, and that each would be addressed as part of the EMG evaluation.

Mononeuropathy

A suspected mononeuropathy may vary in severity from mild focal compression to complete transection. The expectation is that the electromyographer will determine if the problem can be localized to a single nerve, performing sufficient evaluation to exclude involvement of other nerves or nerve roots. With focal compression, conduction slowing across the compression is the earliest abnormality, preferentially involving large sensory fibers because they are the most vulnerable to compression.[13,14,15] Mild nerve conduction abnormalities should be confirmed by evaluating adjacent nerves, as well as contralateral recordings. Mild slowing may or may not be important, and segmental slowing (e.g., ulnar conduction across the elbow compared to the forearm) of less than 20% should be interpreted cautiously.[2] Any substantial compression produces axonal damage, and any axonal lesion at or distal to the dorsal root ganglia (DRG) produces a reduced sensory amplitude. Failure to demonstrate a reduced or absent sensory response in the presence of clinical sensory loss argues against the presence of a lesion distal to the DRG. In nerves containing sensory and motor fibers, decreased motor and sensory amplitudes correspond to the amount of axon loss, assuming the lesion is at least one week old. Not all

nerves are readily assessable for nerve conduction evaluation. A list of readily assessable nerves commonly evaluated is shown in Table 5.2. Some nerves are assessable at multiple points along their length, facilitating evaluation across common points of entrapment or injury.

The ability to localize a lesion on the needle examination depends upon the presence or absence of axonal damage. In addition, the number and location of nerve branches facilitate location of the lesion by demonstrating normal needle examination findings in muscles innervated by branches of the nerve above the lesion and abnormalities in muscles innervated by branches below the lesion. For some nerves, such as the radial nerve, testing precision is high. By definition, examination of muscles innervated by other nerves would be normal in a mononeuropathy. When nerve transection is a consideration, the most important information is the presence of volitional motor units. The presence of even a single motor unit indicates partial anatomic continuity of the nerve, assuming that considerations regarding anomalous innervation are addressed. Because the absence of volitional motor units occurs in complete conduction block, nerve conduction studies alone are insufficient to exclude transection. Nevertheless, a persistent response with stimulation distal to the lesion excludes complete axonal degeneration.

Plexopathy

The EMG findings in plexopathy usually differ from those of an isolated mononeuropathy or radiculopathy.[16] In compressive plexus lesions, sensory axons are almost always involved, and sensory responses are abnormal because the lesion is distal to the DRG. Because sensory and motor fibers often follow different routes through the plexus, the combination of motor and sensory conduction abnormalities is useful in localizing the lesion within the brachial plexus.[17] For example, a lower trunk brachial plexopathy is characterized by abnormality of the ulnar motor and sensory responses and median motor responses in the involved hand. Other conduction studies, including the median sensory response, are normal because those fibers do not transverse the lower trunk of the brachial plexus.

The distribution of abnormalities on needle examination is of great importance in localizing a

TABLE 5.2. Commonly Performed Nerve Conduction Studies

Nerve	Record	Stimulate	Typical Reason for Evaluation
Facial M	Orbicularis oculi	Angel of jaw	Bell's palsy
Median M	Thenar	Palm to clavicle	Carpal tunnel syndrome, plexopathy
Median S	Digits 2, 4		
Ulnar M	Hypothenar	Palm to clavicle	Cubital tunnel syndrome, plexopathy
Ulnar S	Digits 4, 5		
Radial M	Extensor indices	Forearm to axilla	Wrist drop (spiral groove of radius)
Radial S	Digit 1, wrist		
Femoral M	Quadriceps	Inguinal ligament	Amyotrophy, femoral neuropathy
Peroneal M	EDB, foot extensors	Ankle to knee	Foot drop, neuropathy, radiculopathy
Peroneal S	Dorsum of foot		
Tibial M	Abductor hallucis	Ankle to knee	Neuropathy, radiculopathy
Sural S	Ankle	Calf	Neuropathy, radiculopathy, tarsal tunnel

M = motor.
S = sensory.

plexus lesion. The examination will show only decreased recruitment if the lesion is acute or consists only of conduction block (neurapraxic). If axonal loss is present and the lesion is greater than one to three weeks old, increased insertional activity, positive waves, fibrillation potentials, and appropriate motor unit changes also will be present. Needle examination abnormalities are limited to the anterior myotomes and generally are distributed among more than one nerve root or peripheral nerve. The paraspinal muscles, innervated by the posterior primary divisions that branch off the spinal nerves before the brachial plexus, are normal. The combination of abnormal sensory responses and a normal paraspinal examination are important findings that help distinguish a plexopathy from a radiculopathy.

Radiculopathy

Nerve conduction studies are of limited importance in the evaluation of radiculopathy, and their primary role is in excluding other problems, particularly those localized distal to the DRG. Because most muscles are innervated by more than one nerve root, even transection of a nerve root rarely causes substantial reduction of a motor response, and sensory response remains normal in radicu-

lopathy. The needle examination is used to demonstrate findings in anterior *and* posterior myotome muscles, localizing the problem to the spinal nerve before it separates into its anterior and posterior primary divisions.[16] This localization also accounts for the normal sensory conduction studies despite decreased sensation on clinical examination, because a lesion proximal to the DRG spares the sensory nerve cell bodies and distal axons. With chronic radiculopathy, reinnervation of proximal before distal muscles may obscure paraspinal muscle abnormalities.

Unlike the precise localization possible in some mononeuropathies, localization in the evaluation of radiculopathy is imprecise, and even localization to a single nerve root does not identify the site of abnormality along that root. Specifically, electrodiagnostic studies alone are unable to distinguish whether the nerve root lesion is extradural, intradural-extramedullary, or intramedullary, and involvement of the spinal nerve root proximal to the DRG up to and including the anterior horn cell resembles a radiculopathy on EMG studies.[18] Similar to any peripheral lesion, EMG changes develop sequentially after an acute lesion. These changes are summarized for radiculopathy in Table 5.3, and the distribution of

TABLE 5.3. EMG Changes in Radiculopathy

	<1 Week	1–6 Weeks	6 Weeks–3 Months	>3 Months
Conduction studies				
Motor amplitude	N	↓	↓	Slight ↓ or N
Motor conduction velocity	N	Slight ↓	Slight ↓	N
Motor distal latency	N	Slight ↑	Slight ↑	N
F wave and H reflex	N, prolonged, or NR	N, prolonged, or NR	N, prolonged, or NR	N, prolonged, or NR
Sensory response	N	N	N	N
Needle examination				
Fibrillation potentials	None	First proximal, then distal	+ to +++ (proximal and distal	+ to ++ distal, small amplitude
Motor units	↓ Recruitment, otherwise N	↓ recruitment and ↑ % polyphasic	↑duration, amplitude and % polyphasic	↑duration and amplitude (especially distal)

N = normal.
NR = no response.

abnormality in an acute right L5 radiculopathy (1–2 weeks' duration) is shown in Table 5.4.

Polyneuropathy

Acute Guillain-Barré syndrome (GBS) is an acute demyelinating polyneuropathy commonly encountered by the emergency physician. EMG evaluation in suspected GBS is similar to the evaluation of any polyneuropathy.[19] This evaluation includes motor and sensory nerve conduction studies in upper and lower extremities to determine the type and distribution of findings. Nerve conduction studies, when combined with F wave measurements, establish predominant involvement of sensory or motor fibers and determine whether the pathophysiology is primarily axonal loss or demyelination.[8] Proximal stimulation of motor nerves and F wave studies can be performed to measure proximal conduction along motor nerves, and absent F waves are frequently the earliest indication of abnormality.

Multifocal demyelination is the hallmark of all acquired demyelinating polyneuropathies, and marked slowing of conduction velocity is suggestive of demyelination.[20,21] Unfortunately, substantial slowing also can be seen in primary axonal disorders with severe axonal loss, so reduced conduction velocity must be interpreted in relation to other information, including motor amplitudes and disease duration. It is also important that localized compressive or entrapment neuropathies are not interpreted to represent diffuse or multifocal disease.

Abnormal dispersion of motor responses and partial conduction block with increasing conduction distance are useful indicators of acquired demyelination. The degree of abnormal temporal dispersion or partial conduction block in motor nerves can be approximated by calculating the ratio of motor amplitudes following proximal and distal stimulation.[8] Ratios of less than 70% cannot be attributed to axonal loss lesions, and reductions of greater than 50% almost always require at least some degree of conduction block. Duration measurements of the motor response are useful in determining the contribution of abnormal temporal dispersion. Duration increases of greater than 15% over short segments and less than 20% over longer segments are

TABLE 5.4. Distribution of EMG Changes in a Right L5 Radiculopathy of 1–2 Weeks' Duration

Muscle	Insertional Activity			Voluntary Motor Units		
	Insertion	Fibrillation or Positive Waves	Recruitment	Amplitude	Duration	Polyphasia
R anterior tibialis (L4, <u>L5</u>)	N	0	↓	N	N	N
R medial gastrocnemius (L5, <u>S1</u>, S2)	N	0	↓	N	N	N
R lateral gastrocnemius (<u>S1</u>, S2)	N	0	N	N	N	N
R internal hamstring (L4, <u>L5</u>, S1)	N	0	↓	N	N	N
R vastus lateralis (L2, L3, L4)	N	0	N	N	N	N
R posterior tibialis (<u>L5</u>, S1)	N	0	N	N	N	N
R abductor hallucis (S1, S2)	N	0	N	N	N	N
R gluteus medius (L4, <u>L5</u>, S1)	↑	+	↓	N	N	N
R paraspinal (midlumbar)	N	0				
R paraspinal (low lumbar)	↑	+				
R paraspinal (high sacral)	N	0				
L paraspinal (low lumbar)	N	0				

Note: The root innervation is indicated by parentheses and underlined if it is the primary innervation.
N = normal.

abnormal and consistent with increased temporal dispersion. Fortunately, it is not necessary to determine the contribution from either abnormal temporal dispersion or partial conduction block because both indicate demyelination (Fig. 5.6). Normal nerve conduction studies early in the course of the illness do not exclude the diagnosis of GBS.

The role of the needle examination in the evaluation of GBS is secondary. Early in the course of the disease when the diagnosis is in question, the only abnormality is decreased recruitment in proportion to the degree of clinical weakness. Evidence of profuse fibrillation potentials or chronic motor unit changes early in the course of the disease suggests a chronic or preexisting process.

Defective Neuromuscular Transmission

Patients with progressive weakness attributed to defective neuromuscular transmission occasionally are evaluated in the emergency department.[22] Examples include patients with myasthenia gravis, anticholinesterase toxicity, Lambert-Eaton myasthenic syndrome, and botulism. Impaired neuromuscular transmission is easily documented in the EMG laboratory.[2] Repetitive motor nerve stimulation at low rates (e.g., 3 Hz) is the most common technique used to demonstrate a decremental response.[23] In disorders such as myasthenia gravis, the first response is normal, but there is a subsequent decrease in the motor amplitude until about the third or fourth response, after which the amplitude stabilizes. This early decrement is related to physiological depletion of ACh and the resultant failure of some fibers to discharge because of their decreased transmission safety factor. The stabilization with continued stimulation relates to ACh mobilization, a normal physiological event. A true myasthenic decrement can be repaired (completely or partially) immediately after brief exercise (postactivation facilitation). Characteristic responses for a patient with moderately severe generalized myasthenia gravis are shown in Figure 5.7.

In the Lambert-Eaton myasthenic syndrome, the defect of neuromuscular transmission differs from

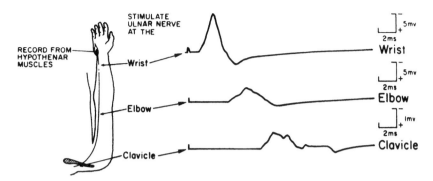

FIGURE 5.6. Motor responses recorded from hypothenar muscles following stimulation of ulnar nerve at distal and proximal sites. Abnormal responses obtained from a patient with Guillain-Barré syndrome demonstrating abnormal temporal dispersion with partial conduction block, increased motor response duration with proximal stimulation, and decreased conduction velocity. (Modified with permission from Albers, J.W. and Kelly, J.J. Jr. 1989. Acquired inflammatory demyelinating polyneuropathies; clinical and electrodiagnostic features. *Muscle Nerve* 12:435–451.

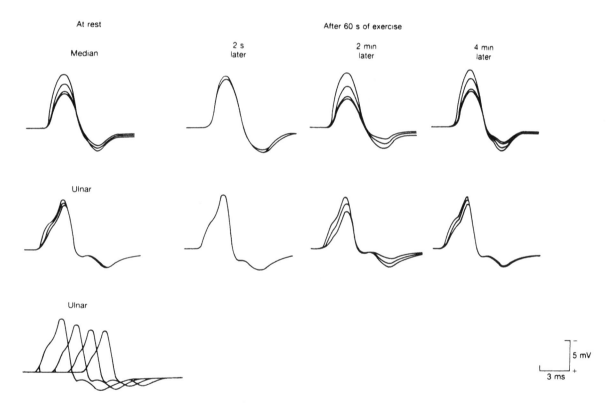

FIGURE 5.7. Motor responses following repetitive stimulation of the median and ulnar nerves at 3 Hz, recorded from thenar and hypothenar muscles, respectively, in a patient with myasthenia gravis. Four superimposed responses are shown at rest, and after 60 s of exercise (recording 2 s, 2 min, and 4 min later). The repair of the decrement immediately after exercise reflects postactivation facilitation. The increased decrement 2 min later reflects postactivation exhaustion. The ulnar responses at the bottom of the figure are shifted in time to demonstrate the changing decrement with sequential stimulations. Calibration: 3 ms and 5 mV. Reprinted with permission from Albers, J.W., Sanders, D.B. 1989. Repetitive stimulation. *American Academy of Neurology Annual Course No. 350.* American Academy of Neurology, Minneapolis, pp. 13–29.

that of myasthenia gravis and is associated with impaired release of ACh.[24] Motor conduction studies show reduced response amplitude. As in myasthenia gravis, in the Lambert-Eaton myasthenic syndrome repetitive motor nerve stimulation at low rates produces a small decrement. However, in the latter syndrome, the effect of postactivation facilitation in response to brief exercise is a dramatic increase (>200%) in the motor amplitude (Fig. 5.8). Similar findings are sometimes demonstrated in botulism toxicity.

Myopathy

Acute weakness is occasionally attributable to primary disease of muscle, as seen in fulminant polymyositis or dermatomyositis. However, certain EMG features are common to most myopathies, regardless of etiology.[25] For example, sensory studies remain normal, as do distal motor conduction studies and tests of neuromuscular transmission. However, motor recordings from weak proximal muscles may show reduced amplitude. The characteristic EMG abnormalities associated with inflammatory myopathy are seen on needle examination. These include increased insertional activity, positive waves and fibrillation potentials, complex repetitive discharges, and small-amplitude, short-duration poly-

phasic motor units with increased recruitment. These abnormalities are recorded from involved weak muscles in most patients, and they are most prominent in paraspinal muscles in inflammatory myopathy. A normal needle examination makes a diagnosis of inflammatory myopathy very unlikely.

Motor Neuron Disease

Patients with motor neuron disease are rarely seen in the emergency department for primary diagnostic purposes. Instead, respiratory distress or aspiration prompts emergency evaluation. Occasionally, patients in whom the diagnosis has not been suspected or established are evaluated when they are in acute distress. In these situations, EMG studies likely will not be obtained in the emergency department. Nevertheless, understanding the diagnostic criteria may be important in confirming the diagnosis or making emergency decisions. Because most forms of motor neuron disease such as amyotrophic lateral sclerosis are multifocal disorders, it is important that the EMG abnormalities cannot be explained by a single lesion.[26] For this reason, the needle examination must demonstrate evidence of chronic partial denervation and reinnervation in a multifocal distribution, involving at least three limbs (the head and thoracic paraspinal muscles are

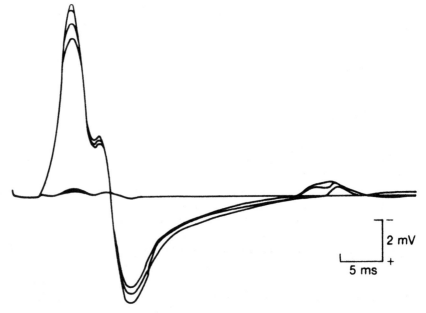

FIGURE 5.8. Motor responses following repetitive supramaximal ulnar motor nerve stimulation at 3 Hz, recorded from hypothenar muscle in a patient with Lambert-Eaton myasthenic syndrome. The smaller responses close to the baseline represent the markedly reduced compound muscle action potential (CMAP) amplitude with a small decrement in rested muscle. Upper tracing recorded immediately after 10 s of maximal voluntary contraction, representing marked postexercise facilitation. Calibration: 5 ms and 2 mV. Reprinted with permission from Albers, J.W., Sanders, D.B. 1989. Repetitive stimulation. *American Academy of Neurology Annual,* Minneapolis, pp. 13–29.

considered as "limbs"). Adherence to this rule requires documentation of widespread disease. Unfortunately, the EMG abnormalities in motor neuron disease cannot be distinguished from a multifocal polyradiculopathy, because paraspinal and extremity muscles are abnormal and sensory studies are normal in both disorders.

PEARLS AND PITFALLS

- A thorough EMG evaluation establishes the distribution, severity, temporal profile, and pathophysiology of a peripheral disorder.

- Substantial nerve compression produces axonal damage, and axonal lesions at or distal to the DRG produce a reduced sensory amplitude; normal sensory responses in the presence of clinical sensory loss argue against the presence of a lesion distal to the DRG.

- Following nerve transection, motor and sensory responses in the portion of the nerve distal to transection remain normal for several days before ultimately disappearing in about one week.

- Because motor units may be absent in complete conduction block, the absence of volitional activation on needle examination is insufficient to demonstrate nerve transection.

- In excluding nerve transection, the most important EMG information is the presence of volitional motor units; a single voluntary motor unit indicates partial anatomical continuity of the nerve, assuming that considerations regarding anomalous innervation are addressed.

- Abnormal sensory responses and a normal paraspinal needle examination are important findings that help distinguish a plexopathy or mononeuropathy from radiculopathy.

- Fibrillation potentials are sensitive indicators of denervation, but they do not appear for days to weeks after the occurrence of an acute nerve lesion. Nevertheless, EMG studies should not necessarily be delayed; other abnormalities appear immediately, and early evaluation permits documentation of preexisting lesions.

- In some acute disorders such as Guillain-Barré syndrome, normal nerve conduction studies performed early in the course of the illness do not exclude a peripheral disorder.

REFERENCES

1. Daube JR. Nerve conduction studies. In: Aminoff MJ, ed. *Electrodiagnosis in Clinical Neurology*. New York, NY: Churchill Livingstone; 1980:229–64.
2. Kimura J. *Electrodiagnosis in Disease of Nerve and Muscle: Principles and Practice*. 2nd ed. Philadelphia, Pa: FA Davis Co., 1989.
3. Bolton CF, Carter KM. Human sensory nerve compound action potential amplitudes: variation with sex and finger circumference. *JNNP.* 1980;43:925–8.
4. Rivner MH, Swift TR, Crout BO, Rhodes KP. Toward more rational nerve conduction interpretations: the effect of height. *Muscle Nerve.* 1990;13:232–9.
5. Denys EH. The influence of temperature in clinical electrophysiology. *Muscle Nerve.* 1991;14:795–811.
6. Nelson KR, Rivner MH. Electromyography and nerve conduction laboratory in clinical neurologic practice. *Semin Neurol.* 1990;10:131–40.
7. Gilliatt RW. Sensory conduction studies in the early recognition of nerve disorders. *Muscle Nerve.* 1978; 1:352–9.
8. Albers JW. Clinical neurophysiology of generalized polyneuropathy. *J Clin Neurophysiol.* 1993;10: 149–66.
9. Aminoff MJ. Electromyography. In: Aminoff MJ, ed. *Electrodiagnosis in Clinical Neurology*. New York, NY: Churchill Livingstone, 1980:197–228.
10. Daube JR. AAEM minimonograph #11: Needle examination in clinical electromyography. *Muscle Nerve* 1991;14:685–700.
11. Daube JR. The description of motor unit potentials in electromyography. *Neurology.* 1978;28:623–5.
12. Landau WM. The duration of neuromuscular function after nerve section in man. *J Neurosurg.* 1953;10:64–8.
13. Ochoa J, Marotte L. Nature of the nerve lesion underlying chronic entrapment. *J Neurol Sci.* 1973;19: 491–5.
14. Ochoa J, Fowler TJ, Gilliatt RW. Anatomical changes in peripheral nerves compressed by a pneumatic tourniquet. *J Anat.* 1972;113:433–55.
15. Rydevik B, Nordborg C. Changes in nerve function and nerve fibre structure induced by acute, graded compression. *J Neurol Neurosurg Psychiatry.* 1980;43: 1070–82.
16. Eisen AA. Radiculopathies and plexopathies. In: Brown WF, Bolton CF, eds. *Clinical Electromyography*. Boston, Mass: Butterworth Publishers; 1987: 51–73.
17. Wilbourn AJ. Brachial plexus disorders. In: Dyck PJ, Thomas PK, Griffin JW, Low PA, Podulso JF, eds. *Pe-*

ripheral Neuropathy. 3rd ed. Philadelphia, Pa: WB Saunders; 1993:911–50.

18. McGonagle TK, Levine SR, Donofrio PD, Albers JW. Spectrum of patients with EMG features of polyradiculopathy without neuropathy. *Muscle Nerve.* 1990;13:63–9.

19. Lisak RP, Brown MJ. Acquired demyelinating polyneuropathies. *Semin Neurol.* 1987;7:40–8.

20. Brown WF, Feasby TE. Conduction block and denervation in Guillain-Barré polyneuropathy. *Brain.* 1984; 107:219–39.

21. Albers JW, Kelly JJ Jr. Acquired inflammatory demyelinating polyneuropathies; clinical and electrodiagnostic features. *Muscle Nerve.* 1989;12:435–51.

22. Mendell J. Neuromuscular junction disorders: a guide to diagnosis and treatment. *Adv Neuroimmunol.* 1994; 1:9–16.

23. Litchy WJ, Albers JW. *Repetitive Stimulation. An AAEE Workshop.* Rochester, NY: American Association of Electromyography and Electrodiagnosis; 1984:1–18.

24. Lambert EH, Rooke DE, Eaton LM. Myasthenic syndrome occasionally associated with bronchial neoplasm. In: Viets HR, ed. *Myasthenia Gravis.* Springfield, Ill: Charles C Thomas Publisher, 1961:362–410.

25. Wilbourn AJ. The electrodiagnostic examination with myopathies. *J Clin Neurophysiol.* 1993;10:132–48.

26. Daube JR. Electrophysiologic studies in the diagnosis and prognosis of motor neuron diseases. *Neurol Clin.* 1985;3:473–93.

27. Albers JW, Leonard JA Jr. Nerve conduction studies and electromyography. In: Crockard R, Hayward R, Hoff JT, eds. *Neurosurgery. The Scientific Basis of Clinical Practice.* 2nd ed. Boston, Mass: Blackwell Scientific Publications; 1992;2:735–57.

28. Bromberg MB, Albers JW. Electromyography in idiopathic myositis. *Mt. Sinai J Med.* 1988;55:459–64.

29. Albers JW, Kelly JJ Jr. Acquired inflammatory demyelinating polyneuropathies; clinical and electrodiagnostic features. *Muscle Nerve.* 1989;12:435–51.

30. Albers JW, Sanders DB. Repetitive stimulation. *American Academy of Neurology Annual Course No. 350.* Minneapolis, Minn: American Academy of Neurology; 1989:13–29.

6 Electronystagmography

NEIL T. SHEPARD

SUMMARY The electronystagmogram (ENG) consists of a series of subtests designed to investigate aspects of the peripheral and central vestibular system. The primary purpose of the ENG is to help in determining site-of-lesion concerns for patients with complaints involving vertigo, lightheadedness, and/or unsteadiness. The constellation of subtests in ENG evaluates only a portion of the overall balance system, but it is a reasonable first step in the investigation of the vestibular system. When performed in a thorough manner, the ocular motor section of the ENG indicates possible brainstem or cerebellar system involvement. Indications for peripheral system involvement are suggestive of possible localization to the labyrinthine, eighth cranial nerve, or vestibular nucleus level of the brainstem. More specific site-of-lesion definition requires the use of auditory symptoms and signs together with ocular motor results. ENG is not a test that can be used while a patient is in the emergency department. Indications for specialty referral and guidelines for ordering ENG evaluation are discussed.

Introduction

The majority of patients who have an acute balance or dizziness disorder recover spontaneously with only symptomatic treatment.[1,2] For reasons that are poorly understood, some of these patients develop chronic balance system problems requiring significant care from a variety of medical and surgical specialists to evaluate and manage their disorder.

Vertigo and balance disorders constitute a significant public health problem. Estimates of the number of persons in the United States who seek medical care for disequilibrium or vertigo range as high as 7 million per year. Approximately 30% of the U.S. population has experienced episodes of dizziness by age 65.[3] There are no indications that the problem of balance disorders is diminishing, particularly as the population ages.[4,5] One of the purposes of balance function studies, and the most traditional purpose, is site-of-lesion localization. This localization can determine sensory input elements, motor output elements, or neural pathways that may be responsible for the reported symptoms. Such testing may also help estimate the extent of the lesion. Localizing the lesion site (e.g., peripheral versus central vestibular pathology, dysfunction in motor output systems) is important in making medical or surgical referrals that may be necessary for the continued evaluation and management of the patient. Extent- and site-of-lesion studies may also help confirm the suspected diagnosis, and, in cases of bilateral peripheral vestibular system paresis, they directly influence the patient's rehabilitative management program. It is critical to realize that the extent of a peripheral, central, or mixed lesion does not always correlate directly to the extent of functional disability experienced by the patient (Beynon G, Shepard NT, unpublished data).[6] The major reason for this finding relates to the ability of central nervous system (CNS) to undergo a compensation process, reducing symptoms from peripheral or limited central vestibular system injury.

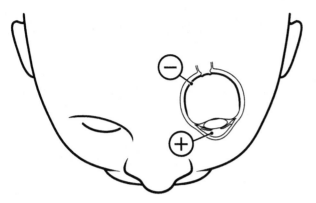

FIGURE 6.1. Shown schematically is the corneal-retinal potential that forms the basis for electro-oculography as an indirect recording technique for eye movement position as a function of time. Electrodes placed around the eyes (see Fig. 6.2) detect changes in electric field potential as the eyes move.

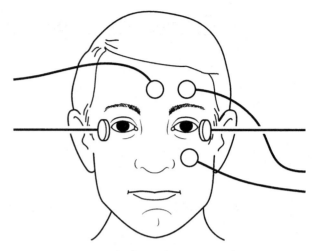

FIGURE 6.2. Typical electrode montage for monitoring eye position as a function of time in both the lateral and vertical dimensions. Note that given the dipole nature of the eyes shown in Figure 6.1, and the use of electrodes lateral and vertical to the anterior-posterior axis of the eye, this type of configuration is not responsive to torsional movements of the eyes. The torsional movements have as their axis of rotation the central anterior-posterior axis.

Traditional ENG, using electro-oculography for eye movement recordings, is a process that estimates eye movements indirectly. The estimates are reliable whether recorded with the patient's eyes open or closed, and in a darkened or well-lighted environment. Changes in eye position are indicated by the polarity of the corneal-retinal potential dipole relative to each electrode placed near the eye (Fig. 6.1). Typically, these electrodes are placed at each lateral canthus and above and below at least one eye, with a common electrode on the forehead (Fig. 6.2). Because the vestibular apparatus contributes significantly to the control of eye movements, the movements of the eyes may be used to examine the activity of the peripheral vestibular end organs and their central vestibulo-ocular pathways. Historically, ENG has become synonymous with vestibular function evaluation, and now it is viewed as only a portion of a more complete test battery. ENG typically consists of a series of subtests performed with eye movement recordings to assess the function of the vestibular end organs, the central vestibulo-ocular pathways, and ocular motor processes.

Neuroanatomy and Physiology

There is no single structure that subserves balance function. The balance system consists of multiple sensory inputs from the vestibular end organs, the visual system, and the somatosensory/propriocep-

tive systems. Input information is integrated in the brainstem and cerebellum with significant influence from the cerebral cortex, including the frontal, parietal, and occipital lobes. The integrated input information results in various motor and perceptual outputs. A brief overview of the major elements of the input and output structures and their basic physiological functioning is provided here.

The membranous labyrinth structure is housed within the bony labyrinth in the petrous portion of the temporal bone of the skull. The membranous labyrinth is secured by connective tissue and is bathed in perilymph. Endolymph is contained within the membranous structure, where specialized sensory neuroepithelium for hearing and balance is located. The vestibular apparatus consists of two groups of specialized sensory receptors: (1) the three semicircular canals – lateral (or horizontal), posterior, and superior – each of which originates from the utricle and terminates in a dilated end (ampulla) that also attaches to the utricle; and (2) the two otolithic organs – the utricular macula and the saccular macula (Fig. 6.3). The semicircular canals are oriented in orthogonal planes approximate to the other ipsilateral canals. While the two horizontal canals are in parallel planes, the two superior

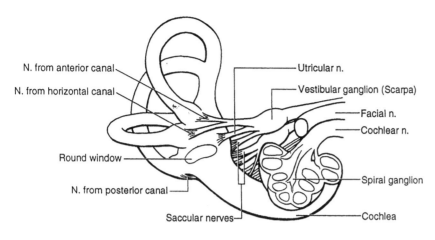

FIGURE 6.3. A schematic illustration of the membranous labyrinth of the otic capsule showing the relative positions of the semicircular canals, cochlea, and the neural innervation. (Reprinted with permission from: *Practical Management of the Balance Disorder Patient,* Shepard and Telian, 1996, Singular Publishing Group, San Diego.)

and the two posterior are in planes approximately orthogonal to each other. The canals are organized into functional pairs. The two members of each pair are in parallel planes of orientation. The three functional pairs are: (1) the two horizontal canals; (2) the superior canal and the contralateral posterior canal; and (3) the posterior canal and the contralateral superior canal. The semicircular canals are sensitive only to angular acceleration and deceleration forces. The three paired arrangements allow for angular acceleration and deceleration sensitivity in all planes of movements. The otolithic organs also function in a paired format, with the two utricular maculae in approximately the horizontal plane and the two saccular maculae in the nonparallel vertical plane.[5]

Contained within each semicircular canal ampulla and otolithic organ is an arrangement of hair cells that constitute the neuroepithelial transduction mechanism for the vestibular end organs. These hair cells are situated on a mound of supporting cells in the ampulla called the crista ampullaris, and within the maculae of the otolithic organ. Covering the hair cell projections (stereocilia and kinocilium) within the ampulla is a gelatinous membrane, the cupula. The cupula, having the same specific gravity as the endolymph, is not responsive to static position changes of the head in the gravitational field. The gelatinous covering over the hair cells of the otolithic maculae has calcium carbonate crystals called otoconia imbedded in its fibrous network. The presence of the otoconia increases the specific gravity significantly above that of endolymph. Thus the maculae are responsive to linear acceleration, including the force of gravity as the head is placed in different positions.

The axons of the vestibular portion of the cochleovestibular nerve each display the property of a spontaneous tonic firing rate that is generated intrinsically. In both the semicircular canals and the otolithic organs, the activated hair cells modulate the firing rate of the corresponding vestibular nerve fibers. If the stereocilia are bent in one direction, an increase (excitation) in the spontaneous neural firing rate results. A decrease (inhibition) in spontaneous firing rate results from shearing action in the opposite direction. Therefore, stimulation of any of the three functional pairs by angular acceleration in their plane of orientation causes an increase in the neural firing rate on one side and a decrease on the contralateral side. This same paired action scheme occurs in the otolithic organs; however, the morphological arrangement of the hair cells is significantly more complicated, allowing for sensitivity to linear acceleration in any direction.

The asymmetrical neural input from the vestibular nerves is interpreted by the CNS as either angular or linear acceleration. In addition, the asymmetry resulting from action of the semicircular canals causes a compensatory reflex eye movement in the plane of the canals being stimulated, known as the first of Ewald's three laws.[7,8] This compensatory reflex movement of the eye is produced by the vestibulo-ocular reflex, and is opposite to the direction of acceleration. To a lesser extent, this reflex also occurs for linear acceleration, mediated by the otolithic organs. The primary system utilized for evaluating patients with balance disorders is the vestibulo-ocular reflex from the horizontal semicircular canals, which is described in detail and illustrated in Figure 6.4. For example, consider a subject

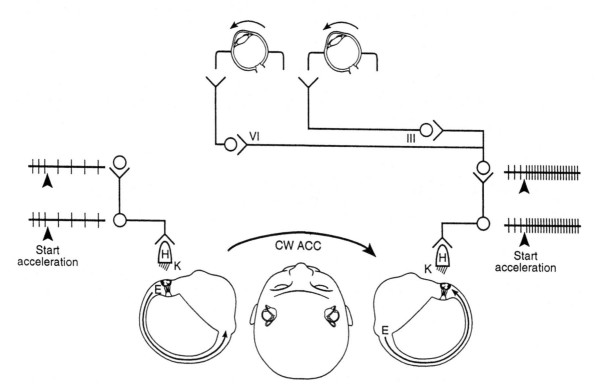

FIGURE 6.4. The orientation of the semicircular canals in the human skull. To each side of the head are enlargements of the horizontal canals illustrating the relative flow of endolymph (E) in each for a clockwise acceleration (CW ACC) of the head. The relative shearing of the stereocilia of the hair cells (H) to the position of the kinocilium (K) is shown. The neural firing rate from each side on the vestibular portion of the eighth cranial nerve is shown, marked with "start acceleration." For the right side the neural connections from the hair cells to the ocular motor nuclei (nuclei of cranial nerve III) and the nuclei of the abducens nerve (cranial nerve VI) are shown. The vestibulo-ocular reflex compensatory movement of the eyes in response to the acceleration is illustrated. (Reprinted with permission from: *Practical Management of the Balance Disorder Patient,* Shepard and Telian, 1996, Singular Publishing Group, San Diego.)

seated in a normal upright position and accelerated to the right rotating about the long axis of the body. Because the membranous horizontal canals are connected to the bony labyrinth within the petrous portion of the temporal bone, they also accelerate to the right. The endolymph, however, does not move immediately to the right but lags behind the membranous canal because of viscoelastic and inertial forces created by the capillary fluid mechanics of the canal. This effectively produces a relative flow of endolymph in the direction opposite that of the acceleration. Thus the cupula in the right canal is deflected toward the utricle, while that in the left is deflected away from the utricle. This action results in an excitation of the neural firing rate on the right

and an inhibition on the left. The individual perceives rotation to the right and, assuming no visual input (darkness or eyes closed), a reflexive eye movement to the left (mediated by the vestibulo-ocular reflex) is produced. This movement is interrupted by fast movements (saccades) of the eyes back in the direction of the acceleration. This fast saccadic eye movement is not part of the vestibulo-ocular reflex; it is a resetting reflex stimulated by the position of the eye within the orbit. If the acceleration continues, the vestibulo-ocular reflex again produces the slow component eye movement opposite the direction of acceleration. An individual viewing the eyes of the subject or recording their movement notes a repeated jerking motion to the right and a slower motion to the left. This eye movement is called jerk nystagmus, named for the direction of the fast (saccadic) component. In this example, the nystagmus would be right-beating. This reflex is significantly influenced by specific areas of the brainstem and the nodulus of the cerebellum.[9–10]

The horizontal canal-produced vestibulo-ocular reflex is mediated by a simple three-neuron arc involving the vestibular nuclei, and cranial nerves III and VI. Stimulation of the vertical canal pairs also produces a vestibulo-ocular reflex along analogous brainstem pathways. Oblique (or rotatory) nystagmus can be seen with stimulation of the horizontal canals and one of the vertical pairs. The CNS pathways from the vestibular nuclei to the extraocular muscles involve cranial nerves III, IV, and VI, the medial longitudinal fasciculus, and collateral neural inputs from the reticular formation in the brainstem.

The principal function of the vestibulo-ocular reflex is the control of eye position during transient head movements to maintain a stable visual image. In addition to this dynamic control system, several other neural pathways that are independent of head movement contribute to eye movement control. Control of smooth pursuit, saccadic, and optokinetic eye movements assists in maintaining clear visual images and contributes to the perception of speed and direction of body motion. The smooth pursuit system permits tracking of a visual target with a smooth, continuous movement of the eye. This mechanism provides for stable image projection to the fovea of the retina. The vestibulocerebellum (flocculus, nodulus, and posterior vermis) plays a dominant role in smooth pursuit; the remainder of the cerebellum, portions of the brainstem, and cortical areas also participate under certain conditions.[12]

The saccadic system of eye movement control provides the fast component during the production of jerk nystagmus. The primary functional goal of the saccadic movements is to reposition a visual target of interest onto the fovea with a single rapid eye motion.[12,13] In addition to the cortical activity, both the pontine reticular formation and the vestibulocerebellum participate in modulating the parameters of movement such as saccade latency, velocity, and accuracy.[14–16] When a target of interest is mov-

ing outside the operating parameters of the smooth pursuit system, the saccade system facilitates the tracking ability by superimposing jerk movements onto the smooth movements.

The optokinetic response is a combination of smooth pursuit and saccade mechanisms. This response can be produced by repeated movements of a visual target(s) across a stationary subject's visual field and/or by moving the subject in a stationary visual field. Evidence from research suggests that the optokinetic system is more than a simple superimposition of smooth pursuit and saccade systems.[12] The optokinetic response is a perception of movement and produces optokinetic jerk nystagmus (OKN) (nystagmus produced by the movement of objects in the visual field), similar in character to that of the vestibulo-ocular reflex. Right-beating OKN results from objects crossing from right to left in a subject's visual field. While there is some indication of a separate "optokinetic control system," eye movement experts generally agree that the smooth pursuit and saccade control centers in the brainstem and cerebellar pathways mentioned above are the predominant control mechanisms.[17–20] The main purpose of the optokinetic system is to provide for clear visual images during sustained head movements (constant velocity, no acceleration or deceleration) to which the peripheral vestibular system does not respond. The perception of motion that can be generated with optokinetic stimulation is so powerful that the vegetative symptoms of motion sickness (e.g., nausea and vomiting) can be produced without actual movement of the subject. This response is exploited commercially in amusement park attractions that simulate motion. The production of nystagmus and the perceptions of motion may suggest some direct interaction between the vestibular system and the optokinetic system. It has been demonstrated that this does not occur at the level of the periphery, but at the level of the vestibular nuclei and vestibulocerebellum.[21–23]

Another system of ocular motor control is visual fixation. This is the active process of maintaining a fixed line of gaze on a target of interest. Although this system shares a neurological substrate with the smooth pursuit system, evidence suggests that it is a separate control system.[12] When gaze is directed laterally or vertically, the initial movement and placement of the target on the fovea is a property of the saccade system; however, the maintenance of gaze for a prolonged period involves the visual fixation system together with mechanisms referred to as the saccade system for eccentric gaze. The integration of the vestibulo-ocular reflex and the ocular control systems are used to provide individuals with the ability to maintain a clear visual image of the seen world when the head is in motion and/or when visual targets are moving. It is through this integration of systems that accurate perceptions of orientation in space and direction of movement are derived.

Significant additions to the above systems for eye movement control are needed to subserve the functions of postural control. This involves volitional movements for learned, complex activities as well as maintaining quiet stance. Also involved is the ability to respond rapidly to unexpected perturbations in the position of one's center of mass (gravity). ENG testing does not assess this aspect of the balance system. Means for assessing the postural control system are part of a more complex laboratory and/or direct clinical evaluation.

Components of the Electronystagmogram

The ENG is potentially useful for all patients with chronic dizziness and balance disorders. The test consists of the following groups of subtests: ocular motor evaluation, typically with smooth pursuit tracking, saccade analysis, gaze fixation, and optokinetic stimulation; spontaneous nystagmus; rapid positioning; positional nystagmus; and caloric irrigations. The slow-component eye velocity of the nystagmus is the measurement of interest, as it reflects the portion of the nystagmus that is generated by the vestibulo-ocular reflex. Rapid positioning is analyzed by direct examination and does not require quantification or recording. The ocular motor tests are quantified according to the eye movements generated during the task. Each of these components will be considered in brief detail.

Ocular Motor Tests

Just as the eyes serve as the window for investigating the function of the peripheral vestibular system, they provide a means to investigate the ocular motor pathways in the brainstem and cerebellum that are required for the function of the vestibulo-ocular reflex.

A variety of testing paradigms are available to assist in identifying abnormalities in the central ocular motor control systems. Smooth pursuit is the most sensitive of the ocular motor tests, but it provides poor site-of-lesion localization within the multiple pathways involved in pursuit generation. Abnormalities with pursuit are typically taken as an indication of possible vestibulo-cerebellar region involvement. When tested with different paradigms, saccade testing (although not as sensitive as smooth pursuit testing) can provide information to differentiate brainstem from posterior vermis involvement. Suggestions for possible frontal or parietal lobe involvement can also be obtained from saccade testing. Gaze fixation provides general suggestions of brainstem/cerebellar involvement in most instances of abnormal results. Specific abnormalities of fixation of gaze can be indicative of specific cerebellar degenerative disorders. Optokinetic stimulation is the least sensitive, probably because the combination of both smooth pursuit and saccade systems allows the optokinetic nystagmus to be generated by a combination of foveal and retinal stimulation. At present, optokinetic stimulation best serves as a cross check with significant abnormalities seen during pursuit or saccade testing. Figures 6.5 and 6.6 are typical recordings and analyses of smooth pursuit and reactionary saccade testing.

Spontaneous Nystagmus

This test is performed with the patient sitting with head straight and eyes closed. The purpose is to record eye movements when visual fixation is removed, without any provocative head movements or positions. Jerk nystagmus is the principal abnormality of interest in most situations. Other forms of abnormal eye movements, such as pendular nystagmus, may be seen.

Clinically significant, direction-fixed nystagmus is interpreted to indicate pathology within the peripheral vestibular system when the ocular motor evaluation is normal (Fig. 6.7).

Hallpike Maneuver

This is a well-known outpatient procedure used to elicit evidence for benign paroxysmal positional ver-

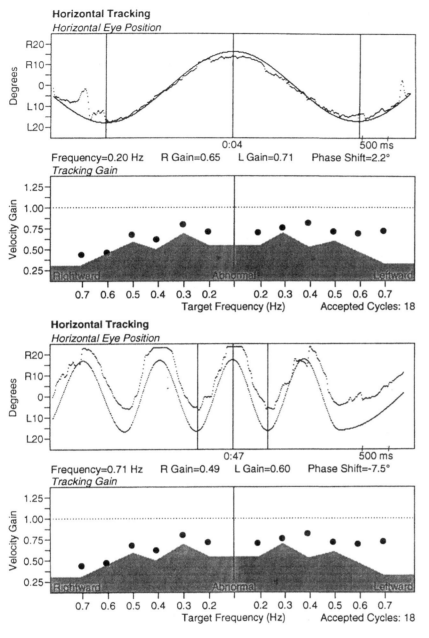

FIGURE 6.5. An example of smooth pursuit eye movement recording with the target at two of the multiple frequencies tested. Shown in both top and bottom panel sets is a plot of horizontal eye position as a function of time (500 ms time mark shown) for sinusoidal tracking (dotted trace). In the same plot (smooth line) the target position in degrees as a function of time is given. The panel below the eye and target position plots gives the value of velocity gain as a function of frequency of target movement. The shaded region represents abnormal performance. The top panel set is for a target frequency of 0.2 Hz, and the bottom panel set is for 0.71 Hz. (Reprinted with permission from: *Practical Management of the Balance Disorder Patient,* Shepard and Telian, 1996, Singular Publishing Group, San Diego.)

tigo (BPPV). The nystagmus produced by BPPV is the most common positive result induced by this maneuver; however, it is not the only one.

This maneuver (Figure 6.8) is also typically part of the standard electronystagmography protocol. However, the test is administered identically in both settings. Classically, positive Hallpike responses produce a torsional nystagmus with the fast phase directed toward the dependent ear (clockwise torsional for left ear down, and counterclockwise

for right ear down), as viewed by the examiner, not as recorded with standard surface electrode recordings.

Positional Nystagmus

The patient is moved slowly into stationary positions. The eye movements are monitored with a spontaneous nystagmus test, and the patient's eyes should be closed (Fig. 6.7). The more common positions include: sitting, with the head turned right;

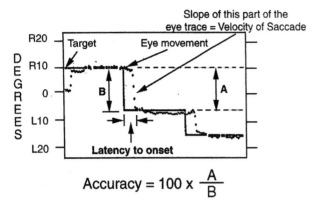

$$\text{Accuracy} = 100 \times \frac{A}{B}$$

FIGURE 6.6. Schematic of eye and target position in degrees, as a function of time demonstrating the calculations of velocity, latency, and accuracy of the saccade eye movement for analysis. The three parameters of velocity, latency, and accuracy are then used to characterize the patient's performance. (Reprinted with permission from: *Practical Management of the Balance Disorder Patient,* Shepard and Telian, 1996, Singular Publishing Group, San Diego.)

sitting, with the head turned left; supine; supine, with the head turned left; supine, with the head turned right; right decubitus (right side); left decubitus (left side); and preirrigation position (head and shoulders elevated by 30 degrees up from the horizontal plane). When there is no evidence of cervical region injury or active pathology, use of head hanging (neck hyperextended) straight, right, and left is safe and adds three positions for testing prior to placement of the patient in the preirrigation position. The purpose of this subtest is to investigate the effect of different head positions within the gravitational field. Positional nystagmus is typically classified by the direction of the fast component of the nystagmus. It may be either direction-fixed (always right-beating or always left-beating when present) or direction-changing (both right- and left-beating nystagmus observed during the examination). Direction-changing nystagmus may be subclassified, when appropriate, into geotropic (toward the pull of gravity, toward the underneath ear) or ageotropic

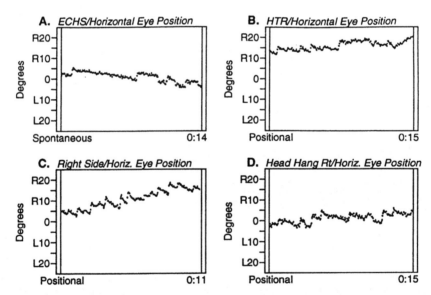

FIGURE 6.7. A–D plot horizontal eye position in degrees as a function of time, each showing right-beating nystagmus. The time in the lower right corner of each panel is the total elapsed time in seconds for that recording, not the total time shown. Each panel represents 7 s of tracing. (A) ECHS – eyes closed, head straight. (B) HTR – eyes closed, head turned right, sitting position. (C) Eyes closed, lying on the right side (right decubitus position). (D) Eyes closed, hyperextension of the neck (by approximately 30 degrees) with the head turned to the right. These are 4 of a total of 11 positions tested on this patient. (Reprinted with permission from: *Practical Management of the Balance Disorder Patient,* Shepard and Telian, 1996, Singular Publishing Group, San Diego.)

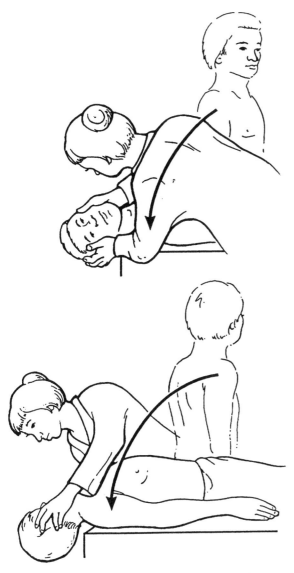

FIGURE 6.8. Illustrations of the technique for the Hallpike maneuver, for right side (top) and left side (bottom). Note the patient's eyes are open and fixated on the examiner. (Reprinted with permission from: *Practical Management of the Balance Disorder Patient,* Shepard and Telian, 1996, Singular Publishing Group, San Diego.)

(away from the pull of gravity, away from the underneath ear). The clinical interpretation of direction-changing nystagmus proceeds in the same manner as that for direction-fixed nystagmus. The exception is when the direction-changing nystagmus is observed while the patient remains in one head position, that is, without a change in gravitational orientation. This is typically interpreted as strongly indicative of central pathway involvement, independent of the ocular motor results, unless an alternative explanation is apparent.

Caloric Irrigations

The caloric test is the study that is most likely to lateralize a peripheral lesion with objective, repeatable eye movement data. The stimulus employed is nonphysiological compared to the normal function of the system during head motion, where one side is stimulated and the other is simultaneously inhibited. Nevertheless, the caloric test is the only portion of the test battery that measures unilateral labyrinthine function.

The three primary delivery methods for caloric irrigations are (Fig. 6.9): closed-loop water (water circulates in a thin latex balloon that expands in the external auditory canal); open-loop water (water runs into the external auditory canal and drains out); or airflow. In any of these methods, the fluid or air is set at temperatures above or below that of the body; typically, 44°C for warm and 30°C for cool are used for the closed-loop systems. All three methods are reasonably reliable when the tympanic membrane is intact. When a tympanic perforation or short ventilation tubes are present, the closed-loop water irrigation method is preferable. Studies in both terrestrial and weightless environments show that there appear to be at least two mechanisms operating to produce the caloric vestibulo-ocular reflex response to the temperature changes. The one that seems to predominate in routine testing involves gravity and the density changes that occur in the endolymph when it is heated or cooled (density decreased or increased, respectively). The patient's head is positioned so that the horizontal canal is oriented parallel to the gravitational vector, with the nose upward and the head tilted 30 degrees upward from the horizontal plane. During a warm irrigation, the less dense fluid attempts to rise. This produces a deviation of the cupula toward the utricle due to the pressure differential across the cupula, causing stimulation of the eighth cranial nerve. The reverse action occurs for the more dense area of cooled fluid, causing inhibition. This results in the well-known mnemonic "COWS," which refers to the direction of nystagmus: "cold opposite, warm same" (relative to the side of irrigation).[8,24–26]

Open-Loop Water   Closed-Loop Water   Air

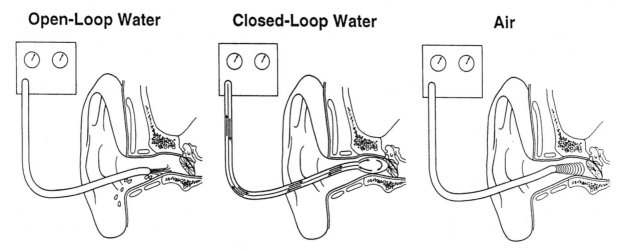

FIGURE 6.9. Three techniques for caloric irrigations are shown. (Reprinted with permission from: *Practical Management of the Balance Disorder Patient,* Shepard and Telian, 1996, Singular Publishing Group, San Diego.)

The traditional interpretation of caloric stimulation uses a relative comparison of maximum, average slow-component eye velocity on the right versus the left. These values are used to provide a percentage comparison of response magnitude (unilateral weakness) and direction bias of eye movement (directional preponderance) (Fig. 6.10).

Indications for Specialty Referral and Electronystagmography

The average patient with a self-limited vertigo syndrome can be managed successfully by the primary care physician who is familiar with common vestibular disorders. The otolaryngologist is commonly consulted when there is a hearing loss, when the primary care physician is uncertain about the diagnosis, or when symptoms persist. Together, these physicians should be able to evaluate and manage the vast majority of patients and dizziness. The otolaryngologist can prevent unnecessary and costly testing by carefully selecting the appropriate diagnostic evaluation. An otolaryngologist with special training or experience in neurotology can provide help with the differential diagnosis in difficult cases and provide surgical management when indicated. Therefore, referral for otolaryngology consultation should not necessarily include a request for an ENG, unless (1) this has been a long-standing problem for the patient; (2) abnormalities of smooth pursuit or

saccades, evaluated in the direct examination, are noted with no clear explanation; or (3) the symptom onset involved concomitant auditory loss of sensitivity perceived by the patient. An ENG is not necessary for the patient with first-time onset of symptoms and no auditory complaints or abnormalities in ocular motor direct examination. These patients should be managed initially by their primary physician and referral decisions developed as needed.

PEARLS AND PITFALLS

- The ENG, while providing information about the extent and site of lesions, represents an evaluation of only a limited part of the overall balance system but provides for a comprehensive evaluation of the ocular motor system regarding brainstem and cerebellar involvement.
- A normal ENG helps to rule out specific central ocular motor involvement, but it cannot be used to exclude completely peripheral system involvement of labyrinthine or eighth cranial nerve origin.
- Care is taken in assuming the actual site of lesion with peripheral indications from the ENG without considering the full neurotologic history and hearing evaluation.
- ENG results do not correspond closely to the patient's functional disability.

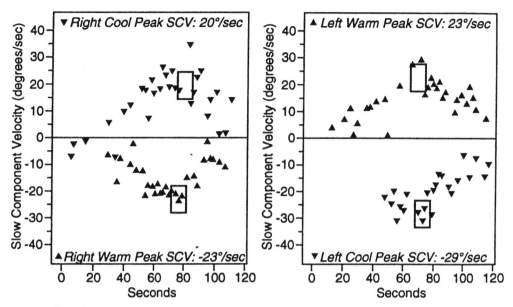

Caloric Weakness: 9% in the right ear
Directional Preponderance: 9% to the right

FIGURE 6.10. Plots of slow-component eye velocity (SCV) from nystagmus provoked by open-loop water irrigations as a function of time. Each triangle represents one slow-component velocity movement of the eye from the nystagmus trace. Responses for the right ear are shown on the left, those for the left ear on the right. The orientation of the triangles represents either cool (30°C), ▼, or warm (44°C), ▲, irrigations. The plots are arranged so that right-beating nystagmus SCVs are on the bottom (right warm, left cool) and left-beating nystagmus SCVs are on the top (right cool, left warm). The velocity values given in top or bottom of each plot represent the average maximum SCV calculated for the nystagmus beats within the rectangle shown on each plot. These maximum, average SCV values were used to calculate the caloric weakness and directional preponderance values shown at the bottom of the figure. Nine percent in the right ear means a 9% weaker response on the right compared to the left. Nine percent to the right means a 9% greater response for right-beating nystagmus compared to left-beating nystagmus. For purposes of calculations, rightward SCVs are assigned a negative number, leftward are assigned a positive number. (Reprinted with permission from: *Practical Management of the Balance Disorder Patient,* Shepard and Telian, 1996, Singular Publishing Group, San Diego.)

REFERENCES

1. Igarashi M. Vestibular compensation: an overview. *Acta Otolaryngol (Stockh).* 1984;406(suppl):78–82.
2. Pfaltz CR. Vestibular compensation: physiological and clinical aspects. *Acta Otolaryngol.* 1983;95: 402–6.
3. Roydhouse N. Vertigo and its treatment. *Drugs.* 1974;7:297–309.
4. Kroenke K, Mangelsdorff AG. Common symptoms in ambulatory care: incidence, evaluation, therapy and outcome. *Am J Med.* 1989;86:262–6.
5. Herdman SJ. Preface. In: Herdman SJ, ed. *Vestibular Rehabilitation.* Philadelphia, Pa: FA Davis Co; 1994:ix–x.

6. Gavie S, Shepard NT, Goldner N, Nihem C. Graded mobility tests: an assessment tool for balance disorders resulting from vestibular lesions. In: Abstracts of the 17th midwinter research meeting. St. Petersburg, Fla: Association for Research in Otolaryngology; 1994.
7. Ewald R. *Physiologishc Untersuch hber das Endorgan des Nervous Octavus.* Wiesbaden, Germany: Bergmann; 1892.
8. Baloh R, Honrubia V. *Clinical Neurophysiology of the Vestibular System.* 2nd ed. Philadelphia, Pa: FA Davis Co; 1990.
9. Raphan T, Matsuo V, Cohen B. Velocity storage in the vestibulo-ocular reflex arc (VOR). *Exp Brain Res.* 1979;35:229–48.

10. Cohen B, Henn V, Raphan T, Dennett D. Velocity storage, nystagmus, and visual-vestibular interactions in humans. *Ann NY Acad Sci.* 1981;374:421–33.

11. Waespe W, Cohen B, Raphan T. Dynamic modification of the vestibulo-ocular reflex by the nodulus and uvula. *Science.* 1985;228:199–202.

12. Leigh RJ, Zee DS. *The Neurology of Eye Movements.* 2nd ed. Philadelphia, Pa: FA Davis Co; 1991.

13. Leigh RJ, Zee DS. The diagnostic value of abnormal eye movements: a pathophysiological approach. *Johns Hopkins Med.* 1982;151:122–35.

14. Zee DS, Robinson DA. A hypothetical explanation of saccadic oscillations. *Ann Neurol.* 1978;5:405–14.

15. Cohen B, Buttner-Ennever JA. Projections from the superior colliculus to a region of the central mesencephalic reticular formation (cMRF) associated with horizontal saccadic eye movements. *Exp Brain Res.* 1984;57:167–76.

16. Cohen B, Henn V, Raphan T, Dennett D. Velocity storage, nystagmus, and visual-vestibular interactions in humans. *Ann NY Acad Sci.* 1981;374:421–33.

17. Zasorin NL, Baloh RW, Yee RD, Honrubia V. Influence of vestibulo-ocular reflex gain on human optokinetic responses. *Exp Brain Res.* 1983;51:271–4.

18. Rahko T. Optokinetic nystagmus. *Acta Ophthalmol Suppl.* 1984;161:153–8.

19. Ventre J. Cortical control of oculomotor functions, I: optokinetic nystagmus. *Behav Brain Res.* 1985;15:211–26.

20. Honrubia V, Baloh RW, Khalili R. Subjective and oculomotor responses during interaction of smooth pursuit with optokinetic and vestibular stimuli. In: Abstracts of the 12th midwinter research meeting. St. Petersburg, Fla: Association for Research in Otolaryngology; 1989.

21. Kubo T, Igarashi M, Wright W. Eye-head coordination and lateral canal block in squirrel monkeys. *Ann Otol Rhinol Laryngol.* 1981;90:154–7.

22. Zee DS, Yamazaki A, Butler P, Gucer G. Effects of ablation of flocculus and paraflocculus on eye movements in primate. *J Neurophysiol.* 1981;46:878–99.

23. Waespe W, Cohen B, Raphan T. Role of the flocculus and paraflocculus in optokinetic nystagmus and visual-vestibular interactions: effects of lesions. *Exp Brain Res.* 1983;50:9–33.

24. Barany R. Untersuchungen uber den vom vestibularapparat des ohres reflectorisch ausgelosten rhytmischen nystagmus und seine begleiterscheinungen. *Monatsschr Ohrenheilkd Laryngorhinol.* 1906;40:193–297.

25. Barany R, Witmaack K. Funktionelle prufung des vestibularapparates verhandl. *Dtsch Otolog Gesllsch.* 1911;20:37–184.

26. Jacobson GP, Newman CW, Kartush JM, eds. *Handbook of Balance Function Testing.* St. Louis, Mo: Mosby–Year Book, Inc; 1993.

27. Shepard NT, Telian SA. *Practical Management of the Balance Disorder Patient.* San Diego, Calif: Singular Publishing Group, 1996.

7 Evoked Potentials

NAVIN K. VARMA

SUMMARY This chapter reviews basic concepts of evoked potentials (EPs), which are rarely used in the emergency department. EPs are used to assess neurological function of certain neural pathways in routine neurological, neurosurgical, audiological, and orthopedic settings. Visual EPs assess pathways from the eye to the visual cortex. Brainstem auditory EPs assess pathways from the ear to the inferior colliculus. Somatosensory EPs assess pathways from a stimulated peripheral nerve through the dorsal columns and to the cerebral cortex. The interpretation of EPs relies on an understanding of the anatomical structures underlying the responses and is used as an extension of the neurological examination.[1,2]

Introduction

Evoked potentials (EPs) are time-locked electrophysiological responses obtained with stimulation of the nervous system that reflect changes in neurally generated electrical fields. EPs allow objective measures of deficits in neural pathways that subserve the stimulated modality and can give evidence of abnormality in clinically and radiographically normal systems. Routine use of EPs decreased considerably following the availability of magnetic resonance imaging (MRI), especially in evaluation of multiple sclerosis, the most common clinical setting in the past. EPs are now also used for operative monitoring and in the determination of neurological function in the comatose patient. EPs are used rarely in the emergency department. However, familiarity with the tests can assist in evaluating some patients.

Methods

In general, a stimulus results in a volley of electrophysiological information that is transmitted through a series of neuronal axons (nerves and tracts) and neuronal cell bodies (ganglia and nuclei) to the cerebral cortex. As this volley propagates across these structures, the electrical potential shifts generate electrical fields with varying spatial and temporal qualities. The spatial properties define the best location to measure the electrical field. Both spatial and temporal properties generate wave morphology. These waveforms are normally very low in amplitude and need to be elicited multiple times and averaged to reduce the interference of electrical noise (electroencephalogram, electrocardiogram, line frequency). The relationship of the amplitude of the EP to that of electrical noise determines the number of trials needed to produce a reproducible response. This is often in the range of 100–2000 responses. Cortically generated responses tend to have higher amplitude than subcortically generated responses and are therefore easier to identify.

Commonly used EPs involve stimulation of the visual, auditory, and somatosensory pathways. Other studies stimulate motor, pain, and endogenous (psychophysiological) pathways. The stimulus used is modality-specific but can vary from one laboratory to another. Patient and environmental factors can alter the results of EP testing. This requires standardization of techniques within each labora-

Sid M. Shah and Kevin M. Kelly, eds., *Emergency Neurology: Principles and Practice.* Copyright © 1999 Cambridge University Press. All rights reserved.

tory and the demonstration of reproducible results using the technique with control data of normal volunteers tested in the same laboratory. Reproducibility of the EP for an individual patient is documented by viewing multiple averaged waveforms of the response. Once representative waveforms are identified, they are reviewed by the neurophysiologist for two types of abnormality: (1) prolongation of propagation, and (2) disturbance in wave morphology or amplitude. Propagation time is statistically the most consistent feature of an EP and normally has a Gaussian distribution. Increased propagation time typically occurs with demyelination. Amplitude is highly variable normally and requires mathematical manipulation before statistical limits of significance can be identified. Waveform and amplitude typically reflect axonal physiology. Localization of the neuroanatomical site responsible for an abnormal waveform or prolonged latency is performed by correlating the known neural pathways (generators) and the corresponding portion of the EP.

Naming of EPs is not standard. Usually, a surface polarity is identified by capital letters followed by a sequence identifier. The latter can be a count or an average latency of the potential. For example, P100 identifies the cortical visual evoked potential (VEP) that is surface positive with an average latency of 100 ms; N1 is the first negativity in long latency endogenous EPs. Brainstem responses are designated by Roman numerals.

Visual Evoked Potential

VEPs are used to evaluate patency of visual pathways, typically in patients with suspected multiple sclerosis. VEPs are also used to monitor these pathways during surgical procedures such as pallidotomies, thalamotomies, and pineal resections. Many types of VEP stimuli have been used to improve the quality of the study and to localize various associative cortical regions. Most frequently, a black-and-white checkerboard pattern is used with reversal of the black and white checks as the stimulus. Full-field monocular stimulation of each eye is used, although some laboratories perform hemifield stimulation. Reliability of the VEP is highly dependent on certain patient factors; reliability is reduced by visual acuity less than 20/200, ocular opacity (corneal abrasions, cataracts), poor attention, and poor fixa-

tion. A noncooperative patient may have reliable testing only with specialized equipment. In certain laboratories, stroboscopic stimulation is used to assess visual pathways. Standard pattern reversal and stroboscopic stimulation do not assess vision; they test the patency of pathways from the stimulus to the primary visual cortex.[1,3]

Normal VEP

The normal VEP appears deceptively simple (Fig. 7.1). A low-amplitude N75 is followed by a high-amplitude P100 and a medium-amplitude broad N145. Clinically, the most important wave is the P100. Despite its simple appearance, it is one of the most complex electrical fields recorded. It is generated by at least six major dipoles from hemifields, parafoveal fibers, and foveal projections. These result in a single high-amplitude and backward-directed dipole that is normally easy to measure. The waveform should be a single negativity. Normal latency (+3 standard deviations) can be as high as 114 ms, but the results are dependent on the particular laboratory and the technique and should be compared to control data.

Abnormal VEP

VEP latency is abnormal in three basic ways: (1) it is prolonged in pathways anterior to the optic chiasm. This is observed when stimulation of one eye demonstrates a prolonged latency and the other demonstrates normal latency. Such a delay can be due to ocular conditions and is not specific to optic nerve function. (2) It is prolonged in pathways from both eyes with abnormalities that cannot be further localized. These delays can be anterior or posterior to the optic chiasm but must involve at least two lesions or a destruction of the chiasm itself. (3) It demonstrates a significant left versus right difference with or without prolonged absolute latencies. This indicates a delay anterior to the chiasm on the prolonged side.

VEP waveform abnormalities are difficult to interpret. Low-amplitude or wide waves are not necessarily abnormal. The single classic abnormality is the bifid or "w" waveform, which can indicate hemifield damage or scotomas. However, a bifid wave can also be interpreted as a variant of normal. This can be differentiated by specialized stimulation or recording paradigms.

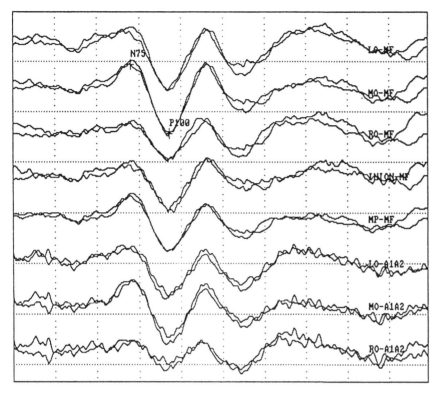

FIGURE 7.1. Normal VEPs obtained in a 31-year-old woman following left eye stimulation with a checkerboard pattern reversal stimulus. The multiple channels graph input from differential amplifiers between pairs of electrodes. This assists in identifying the waveform by its topography. The N75 and P100 waveforms are identified. The N145 is the negativity, upward deflected waveform, after the P100 waveform. Channel labels identify electrode sites: L = left, M = mid, R = right, O = occiput, P = parietal, F = frontal, A1 = left ear, A2 = right ear. For example: LO–MF is the channel graphing the electrical potential between the left occiput to the midfrontal region.

Brainstem Auditory Evoked Potential

Brainstem auditory evoked potentials (BAEPs) are used commonly to assess the patency of hearing pathways in neonates and to monitor the auditory nerve during surgery. BAEPs are extremely sensitive to auditory nerve damage and can give evidence of acoustic neuromas that are very small. The most common stimulus is a "click" that is composed of multiple frequencies and is presented to each ear individually. A stimulus with specific tones can be helpful in some instances. The BAEP is highly reproducible and can be measured while the patient is under general anesthesia. The extremely low amplitude of the BAEP requires 1000–2000 stimuli for a reproducible average response. Analogous to the VEPs, this test does not assess hearing, but rather the patency of neuroanatomical pathways within or caudal to the brainstem subserving hearing.[1,4]

Normal BAEP

The BAEP is marked by five waves that are the most important clinically and later waves that are normally variable in their presence (Fig. 7.2). The generators for these five waves are: I – cochlear nerve (CN) at the cochlea; II – CN at the internal au-

ditory meatus; III – CN at the cochlear nucleus and the cochlear nucleus itself; IV – superior olive and the lateral lemniscus; V – the lateral lemniscus and the inferior colliculus. These generators are within close proximity, therefore, the BAEP is a very detailed assessment of the brainstem. Wave V is the most reproducible. Waves I, III, and V are necessary to assess the pathways thoroughly. The most important properties are the absolute latencies of the waves, the interpeak latencies from waves I–III, III–V, and I–V, and the ratio (often a visual assessment) of wave V/I amplitude. The relationship of wave V absolute latency and stimulation intensity is charted in the evaluation of hearing.

Abnormal BAEP

Abnormalities of absolute or interpeak latency can be observed with any of the waves. Prolonged interpeak latency indicates a lesion within the pathway between the two generators. A prolonged absolute latency without interpeak latency changes is more difficult to localize, except with wave I (peripheral or at the cochlea). Wave I changes can be due to acoustic problems alone (e.g., scarred tympanic membrane) and may not reflect neurological injury.

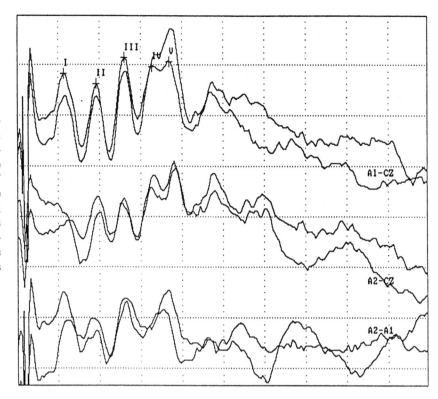

FIGURE 7.2. Normal BAEPs obtained in the same patient described in Figure 7.1 following left ear stimulation with clicks. Waves I–V are identified. Note that waves IV and V make up a complex waveform. The characteristics of the individual waves in the other two channels help to identify the waves in difficult cases. A1 and A2 are electrodes at the ears as in VEPs. CZ records from the vertex.

Amplitude abnormalities are observed with a reversal of the wave V/I ratio or with the absence of wave I, III, or V. This indicates a conduction defect at or peripheral to the generator of that waveform. The latency–intensity curve of wave V can distinguish conductive hearing loss from sensorineural hearing loss.

Somatosensory Evoked Potential

Somatosensory evoked potentials (SSEPs) are used to test large fiber, non–pain-mediating, sensory pathways of the upper or lower extremities. An electrical stimulus is applied to a peripheral nerve at a level of intensity sufficient to result in contraction of the associated muscle. In some patients, even maximum stimulation is insufficient to result in muscle movement. In this situation, absent waveforms require guarded interpretation because this finding may indicate insufficient stimulus intensity rather than abnormality. Stimulation is sometimes painful, and a study will be limited by muscle artifact when the patient becomes tense. Mild sedation can help these patients complete testing. The cortical components of the SSEP are sensitive to deep anesthesia; subcortical responses are well-sustained. The SSEP is relatively independent of patient factors.

SSEPs are most often used to monitor the state of the spinal cord during surgery because they test the patency of the sensory tracts, implying patency of the nearby motor pathways. SSEPs are used as a prognostic tool in the intensive care unit to establish function of the somatosensory cortex in comatose patients. At some centers, the SSEP is used to identify the somatosensory cortex intraoperatively during cortical resection.[2,5]

Normal SSEP

Upper limb: The median nerve is usually stimulated at the wrist (Fig. 7.3). Potentials commonly identified are measured at the bend of the shoulder (P9), brachial plexus (EP), dorsal root entry zone (P11), ipsilateral spinal cord (N13), medial lemniscus (P13, labeled by some as P14), perithalamic region (N18), and cortex (N20). The most important waveforms are the EP, N18, and N20, and a fused waveform, N/P13.

Lower limb: The posterior tibial nerve is usually stimulated at the ankle (Fig. 7.4). Potentials commonly identified are measured at the popliteal

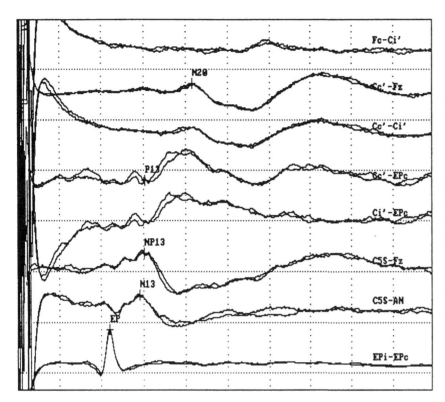

FIGURE 7.3. Normal SSEPs in a 37-year-old man following left median nerve stimulation at the wrist. The lowest channel identifies the EP at Erb's point. The next channel identifies the N13 waveform at the spinal cord. The third channel is a composite waveform of the N/P13 waveforms. The fourth and fifth channels identify the N18 waveform; this is the upward deflected waveform that follows the P13 waveform identified in the fifth channel. The uppermost three channels identify the cortical potential.

fossa (PF), spinal cord entry zone (LP), perithalamic region (N34), and the cerebral cortex (P37). The most important waveforms are the lumbar and cortical potentials (LP, P37) for routine studies and the subcortical potential (N34) for intraoperative monitoring.

Absolute and interpeak latencies are measured, along with amplitude. Absent waveforms or marked side-to-side differences are noted. Commonly, subcortical responses are not seen in routine studies following lower limb stimulation. Intraoperatively, the cortical response can be reduced in amplitude and the subcortical response can be more easily recognized, perhaps secondary to sedation. In this setting, subcortical responses have greater importance.

Abnormal SSEP

Prolonged interpeak latency identifies lesions between the generators as in BAEPs. Prolonged absolute latency without prolonged interpeak latency is not specific except in the most peripheral potential. In intraoperative monitoring, a greater than 50% decrease in amplitude or a greater than 10% prolongation of latency is considered significant and requires evaluation for potential causes.

Other Evoked Potentials

Other types of evoked potentials have different applications. Their utility in routine clinical practice is undetermined. Motor evoked potentials stimulate either the cerebral cortex or the spinal cord while measuring responses peripherally. Dermatomal stimulation of pain fibers tests the anterior spinothalamic and thalamocortical tracts to obtain an objective measure of pain. Endogenous responses test attention and the effect of various psychophysiological conditions.[1,2]

Case Histories

Case 1:

A 57-year-old woman arrives at the emergency department with subacute left arm paresis. She experienced a visual phenomenon six months prior to presentation but cannot describe it. She has 4/5 power in the left arm. The remainder of her neurological examination is normal. Differential diagnosis includes new stroke with a history of amaurosis fugax, an exacerbation of multiple sclerosis with a history of optic neuritis, or cervical disease. MRI and magnetic resonance angiography reveal no lesions. Lumbar puncture reveals a mild elevation of

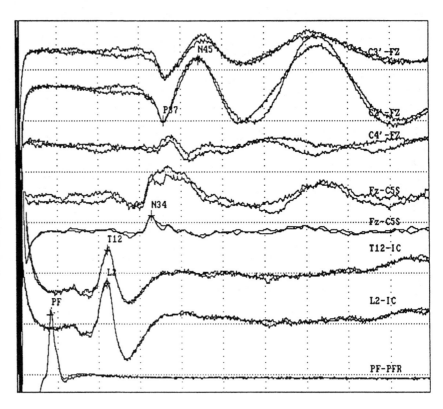

FIGURE 7.4. Normal SSEPs in a 31-year-old woman following left posterior tibial nerve stimulation at the ankle. The lowest channel identifies the response of the peripheral nerve at the popliteal fossa, the next two identify the lumbar potentials at L2 and T12 spinal levels, respectively. The middle two channels identify the subcortical perithalamic potential. The upper three channels identify the cortical potential.

protein. VEPs show a prolonged P100 waveform with left eye stimulation and normal responses to right eye stimulation. SSEPs show a delay between the EP and N18 with left arm stimulation and a delay between the LP waveform and P37 waveform bilaterally. BAEPs are normal. The results indicate abnormalities in the visual pathways subserving the left eye anterior to the optic chiasm, between the branchial plexus and the perithalamic region subserving the left arm, and of the somatosensory pathways subserving both legs. A diagnosis of multiple sclerosis was made and appropriate therapy begun.

Case 2:

A 16-year-old boy is brought to the emergency department after having hit a tree while driving a snowmobile. He has multiple left pelvic girdle fractures with internal hemorrhage. He is taken to the operating room with SSEP monitoring. During closure, the N34 waveform following left posterior tibial nerve stimulation is lost. Repeat testing confirms absence of the waveform. Loss of the N34 waveform suggests injury to the sciatic nerve, most likely within the surgical field. The wound is reopened and a bone chip is found compressing the sciatic nerve anteriorly. The bone chip is removed and the

N34 waveform returns with normal latency and amplitude over the next 15 minutes. The incision is closed without further abnormality in the SSEP. The manual search and removal of the chip likely resulted in saving the nerve from postoperative complications.

Case 3:

An 8-year-old girl is comatose after a motor vehicle accident but has spontaneous eye opening. The parents want to know if she can see. Stroboscopic stimulation of the eyes evokes a normal response. This result indicates functional visual pathways, but it cannot determine whether the child sees or will see following recovery from the coma.

PEARLS AND PITFALLS

EPs

■ EPs provide objective evidence of neurological pathway patency.
■ EPs do not study the complete pathways, and they should not be used to "confirm" full function of a modality.

■ EPs do provide an excellent method to monitor changes in pathways.

VEPs

■ VEPs assess visual pathways from the eye to the primary visual cortex.

■ VEPs are sensitive to patient and laboratory factors and require particular attention to local control data.

■ VEPs do not assess vision.

■ Ocular abnormalities can affect VEPs, and interpretation should include an assessment of these.

BAEPs

■ BAEPs assess auditory pathways from the ear to the inferior colliculus, and thus provide an evaluation of the brainstem from the cochlear nucleus to the inferior colliculus.

■ BAEPs can differentiate between conductive and sensorineural hearing loss.

■ BAEPs do not assess hearing.

SSEPs

■ SSEPs assess the large fiber somatosensory pathways from the site of stimulation to the cerebral cortex.

■ SSEPs can monitor changes in individual nerve or nerve tract function during an operation. Because of the proximity of the posterior columns and the corticospinal tracts, the SSEP provides a presumptive (not direct) measure of motor function during surgery.

■ The absence of SSEPs can be the result of multiple factors including insufficient stimulation, for example, in an obese patient. Therefore absence of SSEPs may not indicate an abnormality.

REFERENCES

1. Chiappa KH, ed. *Evoked Potentials in Clinical Medicine.* 3rd ed. Philadelphia, Pa: Lippincott-Raven; 1997.

2. Pedley TA, Emerson RG. Electroencephalography and evoked potentials. In: Bradley WG, Daroff RB, Fenichel GM, Marsden CD, eds. *Neurology in Clinical Practice.* Boston, Mass: Butterworth-Heinemann; 1991.

3. Celesia G. Visual evoked potentials in clinical neurology. In: Aminoff MJ, ed. *Electrodiagnosis in Clinical Neurology.* 3rd ed. New York, NY: Churchill Livingstone; 1980.

4. Stockord JJ, Pope-Stockard JE, Sharbrough F. Brainstem auditory evoked potentials in neurology: methodology, interpretation, and clinical application. In Aminoff MJ, ed. *Electrodiagnosis in Clinical Neurology.* 3rd ed. New York, NY: Churchill Livingstone; 1980.

5. Aminoff MJ, Eisen A. Somatosensory evoked potentials. In: Aminoff MJ, ed. *Electrodiagnosis in Clinical Neurology.* 3rd ed. New York, NY: Churchill Livingstone; 1980.

TWO Common Neurological Presentations

8 Altered Level of Consciousness

J. STEPHEN HUFF AND WILLIAM J. BRADY

SUMMARY Neurological symptoms are traditionally divided into negative symptoms, or loss of function, and positive symptoms, with excessive or abnormal sensory or motor phenomena. Altered mental status can be characterized similarly. Decreased level of consciousness, a loss of function, has coma as an end point. Agitated or hyperactive altered mental status, an excess of function, has delirium as an end point. Both these conditions represent central nervous system (CNS) dysfunction caused by primary problems of the CNS or secondary to other medical conditions. A methodical evaluation of patients with an altered level of consciousness in the emergency department includes a description of their behavior or their response to stimulation. In many cases of patients with an altered level of consciousness, a definitive diagnosis is made in the emergency department.

Introduction

Evaluation of a patient with altered mental status in the emergency department can be difficult because the patient's baseline mental functioning may not be known (e.g., the geriatric patient with mild dementia). In other patients, a change in the level of consciousness may be obvious but its cause is unknown (e.g., a previously normal individual who becomes comatose suddenly). Time constraints in the emergency department may not allow a thorough assessment of the patient's behavioral functioning. When the patient's clinical condition worsens in the emergency department, appropriate intervention is undertaken; typically, admission to the hospital is necessary.

Coma can be defined as an eyes-closed, unresponsive state. Jennett and Teasdale described coma as a state of "not obeying commands, not uttering words, and not opening the eyes".[1] They attempted to quantify it with their Glasgow Coma Scale (Table 8.1), the most widely used of a number of rating scales for level of consciousness. A brief description of the patient's appearance and the response to stimulation provides the most useful patient information. A variety of terms are used to describe unresponsive states: *obtundation* is a blunting of consciousness. *Stupor* is a sleep-like condition from which the patient may be aroused to full alertness with vigorous stimulation; when left alone, the patient returns to the sleep-like state.[2-4] Because these terms are commonly misused, clinical description of the individual patient is encouraged.

Despite the broad differential diagnosis of coma and altered mental status, certain factors are encountered commonly in the emergency department. In a study from Boston City Hospital in the 1930s, alcohol was the predominant cause of coma, accounting for nearly 60% of cases. In this study, trauma accounted for 13% of cases, cerebrovascular events accounted for 10% of cases, and poisoning, epilepsy, diabetes, meningitis, pneumonia, and cardiac failure accounted for less than 10% but more than 1% of cases.[5]

Modern prehospital emergency department medical services have changed the relative frequency of the different causes of coma on presentation of patients in the emergency department. In a recent

TABLE 8.1. Glasgow Coma Scale

Coma score (E + M + V = 3 to 15)	
Eye opening	E
Spontaneous	4
To speech	3
To pain	2
None	1
Best motor response	M
Obeys	6
Localizes	5
Withdraws	4
Abnormal flexion	3
Extensor response	2
None	1
Best verbal response	V
Oriented	5
Confused conversation	4
Inappropriate words	3
Incomprehensible sounds	2
None	1

study of comatose patients with spontaneous circulation presenting to an emergency department, 16% experienced multiple trauma and 9% had isolated cranial trauma.[6] Nontraumatic intracranial masses, primarily spontaneous intracerebral hemorrhages, accounted for 21%; other neurological disorders, primarily seizures, accounted for 16%. Patients with medical conditions, primarily resuscitated cardiac patients and patients with sepsis, accounted for 13% and 12%, respectively. Toxicological causes were encountered in 6% of patients, and psychiatric causes in 3%. No conclusive cause of coma was determined in 3% at time of death.[6] Toxic causes of coma may be represented with greater frequency at other facilities, and the relative numbers of various causes of coma vary from urban to rural hospitals, from one region of the country to another, and possibly from season to season.

Modern laboratory procedures, rapid neuroimaging, and supportive care allow for determination of the cause of coma in almost all patients in the emergency department. Reversible causes of coma such as hypoglycemia, seizures with postictal behavior, and many intoxications can be expected to improve or resolve in the emergency department. Patients with persistent coma are admitted to the hospital by the appropriate specialty services: for example, patients with serious intoxications and sepsis are referred to internists; those with tumors and intracranial hemorrhages are referred to neurosurgeons; and those experiencing ischemic strokes and seizures are referred to neurologists. In most cases, the emergency physician makes these decisions based on patient history and physical examination and the results of neuroimaging.

A variety of coma-like conditions can be observed in the emergency department. A vegetative state refers to a condition of chronic unresponsiveness in which the patient has no meaningful cognitive awareness; there is no voluntary motor activity, and sleep–wake cycles may be present. A patient in a "locked-in" state is awake and alert but has lost all motor outflow to the body except purposeful vertical extraocular movements. Destructive pontine lesions are the usual cause. These states usually are diagnosed by extended observation.[2,3]

At the other end of the behavioral spectrum is the patient with delirium who demonstrates excessive and abnormal motor and verbal activity. As with coma, reversible causes of delirium are identified and treated appropriately.

Prehospital Management

Prehospital care providers responding to a patient with altered mental status can distinguish between a diminished level of consciousness and excessive behavior. Witnesses may be present but not helpful. Typically, useful information is obtained when family members are present.

Immediate attention is given to the patient's airway, ventilation, and circulation. When the patient is conscious, breathing and circulation are present. When the patient is unconscious, a primary survey follows. Most of the initial neurological examination is performed in the primary survey. This includes assessment of the patient's level of consciousness, motor functions, and sensory functions. Out-of-hospital examination is necessarily brief. When the patient is not alert, stimulation is applied until there is a response. When this is ineffective, more forceful stimulation is used until the patient is deemed unresponsive. When the patient is alert, speech is assessed, as is orientation to time, person, and place. Observation for movement of all extremities and response to commands completes the evaluation.

For the patient who remains unresponsive despite stimulation, further assessment follows the primary survey. The patient is assessed for response to painful stimulation: Is the response purposeful, and do the patient's left and right sides move equally? The mnemonic "AVPU" has been recommended to describe the patient's mental state: A indicates alert, V indicates responses to voice commands, P indicates response to painful stimulation, and U indicates unresponsive.[7] Other examinations need not be detailed. A search for traumatic injuries occurs as part of the primary survey. Examination of the cranial nerves can be confined to the pupils, noting symmetry and size. A variety of medical, traumatic, and neurological conditions can cause a patient to be restless or confused. Quick and simple evaluation includes determining whether the patient speaks spontaneously and coherently, and responds meaningfully to questions. When the patient is alert but without meaningful speech, the possibility of a disturbance of language or an aphasia is considered.

Traditionally, out-of-hospital administration of a "coma cocktail," consisting of dextrose, naloxone, and thiamine, has been advocated for patients with altered mental status. This practice has recently been critically reviewed.[8] The use of rapid reagent tests may aid in identifying patients with hypoglycemia, but these tests are not without error. The administration of hypertonic dextrose is recommended for patients with nonfocal neurological examinations and low or borderline low glucose levels on reagent strips. When rapid testing is unavailable, dextrose is empirically administered to patients with no evidence of focal central nervous system (CNS) injury (primarily hemiparesis) on neurological examination. Oral administration of glucose and glucagon is not recommended, except when intravenous access cannot be obtained, because of the increased possibility of fluid aspiration by the patient with an altered mental status.[8] Patients with hypoglycemia can present with aphasia or other neurological findings. Clinical evidence suggests that stroke may worsen in the presence of hyperglycemia;[9,10] in patients with focal deficits, use of reagent strips to confirm hypoglycemia is recommended prior to administration of dextrose.[8] When rapid testing is not available, dextrose administra-tion is recommended for patients with focal CNS deficits to correct potential hypoglycemia; the risk of hypoglycemic encephalopathy from uncorrected hypoglycemia outweighs the risk of aggravating an ischemic stroke.[8]

As part of the "coma cocktail," thiamine is routinely recommended for the comatose patient, despite lack of proof of its efficacy.[8] The opiate antagonist, naloxone, is commonly recommended because of its efficacy in reversing narcotic overdose; however, some experts feel that its use should be based on a strong suspicion of opiate abuse or clinical signs of respiratory depression. In one study, a respiratory rate of 12 breaths per minute or less predicted response to naloxone.[11] Naloxone administration is not a substitute for definitive airway management. The risk of precipitating symptoms of narcotic withdrawal in opiate-addicted patients is significant. A typical initial dose of naloxone is 0.4–0.8 mg.

Any response to emergency medical services intervention is noted. Glasgow Coma Scale scores are frequently used and are probably most valuable as quick indicators of patient deterioration or progress (Table 8.1).[1] Contact with the emergency department's medical control is essential for decisions concerning other management issues.

Emergency Department Evaluation and Differential Diagnoses

The emergency department and treatment of patients with altered mental status proceed simultaneously. The approach to the comatose patient is best organized by initial assessment, immediate resuscitation, secondary survey (with emphasis on the neurological examination), and definitive care.[4,12] The following sections summarize the procedures involving initial assessment, patient history, and physical examination.

Initial Assessment

Airway, breathing, and circulation are assessed immediately after patient arrival in the emergency department. Administration of dextrose, thiamine, and naloxone is considered when not already given. Assessment of serum glucose is of paramount importance because hypoglycemia is common and readily reversed with the intravenous administration of dextrose. When hypoglycemia is unrecognized and untreated, CNS injury may continue to occur.

Patient History

In the evaluation of the patient with altered mental status, the most important information is contained in the history, which the patient may not be able to provide. When no history is obtainable including the patient's name, a condition sometimes called John Doe syndrome, there is high patient morbidity.[13,14] Emergency medical services personnel typically provide information regarding the patient's out-of-hospital setting. The presence of alcohol or drugs of abuse is noted. In this process, medications are often noticed and transported along with the patient. These medications often provide information not only about the patient's medical condition but also about the identity of the health care provider, who may be contacted for additional information. Less commonly, environmental toxins such as carbon monoxide or other inhaled toxins may be suspected. Caregivers and any witnesses to the circumstances are contacted.

Medical records are a source of additional patient information and are obtained when available. The presence of any underlying medical conditions is important to note. For example, the history of a seizure disorder can suggest a postictal state or ongoing seizures; a history of cancer can suggest a worsening of that condition from either CNS injury or a paraneoplastic condition; an abrupt severe headache prior to losing consciousness may be associated with an intracranial hemorrhage; a history of diabetes suggests possible severe hyperglycemia or hypoglycemia. Particularly for medical conditions, many other diagnostic possibilities exist. Hepatic encephalopathy is often a recurrent condition, as is respiratory failure. Patients with end-stage renal disease may present with cardiac decompensation, electrolyte abnormalities, or sepsis.

In many cases, the timing of the patient's illness suggests an etiology. Abrupt onset of altered mental status suggests stroke or seizure-related activity. Cardiac problems are another frequent cause of abrupt loss of consciousness. A more gradual onset of symptoms occurring over hours to days may suggest a more slowly progressive CNS lesion such as a subdural hematoma or tumor. Metabolic causes of encephalopathy such as hyperglycemia typically develop over several days.

Physical Examination

Initial Assessment. Initial assessment includes verifying airway integrity, defining the level of consciousness, assessing ventilation, and evaluating cardiovascular function. When the patient can be aroused to an eyes-open, responsive condition, ventilation and circulation are present. For the patient who is not arousable with vigorous verbal stimulation, progressive tactile and noxious stimuli are applied. When stimulation does not arouse the patient, immediate reassessment of airway, ventilation, and cardiovascular status occurs. Initial resuscitative measures take place simultaneously. A rapid head-to-toe survey notes any signs of trauma. Palpation of the head can reveal a boggy hematoma when no trauma was suspected. The cervical spine is protected when trauma is even remotely suspected. The chest wall is evaluated for any instability. A distended abdomen or a pulsatile mass is sought out. Extremities are evaluated for intactness and spontaneous movements or a patterned response to stimulation. This initial assessment takes approximately one minute to perform.

Secondary Assessment with Emphasis on Neurological Examination. Following initial assessment, additional data are gathered through the secondary assessment. Hypothermia is rarely a primary cause of coma[15] but suggests that thermal regulation has been deranged for at least a few hours. Hypothermia is common with hypoglycemia, sepsis, and intoxications. Elevated body temperature in patients suggests fever from sepsis or heat stress. More uncommon causes are endocrine emergencies such as thyroid storm or rare events such as neuroleptic malignant syndrome. Tachycardia may represent a stress response, hypovolemia, fever, hypoxia, or, rarely, a primary cardiac problem. Bradycardia may represent a primary cardiac problem or increased intracranial pressure (ICP). Deep, rapid respirations may represent attempted respiratory compensation for metabolic acidosis, or hyperventilation secondary to a CNS lesion.[2,16] Extreme hypertension with diastolic blood pressures of 120 mm Hg or more is often observed in patients with intraparenchymal hemorrhage and other stroke syndromes. Less commonly, uncontrolled hypertension may cause unresponsiveness with hypertensive encephalopathy. (Distinctive constellations of vital signs or toxidromes are observed in many toxic exposures; see Chapter 40, "Neurotoxicology.")

Oxygen saturation is commonly known as the "fifth vital sign." The advantage of early patient assessment is in the detection of hypoxia, which directs the resuscitation phase. Additionally, when hypoxia fails to correct after oxygen administration and ventilatory management, a systemic cause of hypoxia becomes more likely, such as low cardiac output or ventilation–perfusion mismatches.

The secondary assessment includes examination for cardiac murmurs, possibly suggesting acute cardiac dysfunction from complications of myocardial infarction or other problems such as endocarditis. Auscultation of the lungs may reveal signs of congestive heart failure, chronic obstructive pulmonary disease, or pneumonia. Examination of the skin and extremities is directed to the detection of any rashes suggesting systemic infection. Funduscopic examination may reveal hemorrhages suggestive of increased ICP; however, the absence of hemorrhages does not exclude intracranial hemorrhage.[17] The presence of spontaneous venous pulsations is an indication that ICP is not increased at the time.[18]

Neurological examination includes focused testing of cranial nerves, sensation, motor response, reflexes, and responsiveness. The general examination and history should indicate whether or not coma has resulted from global CNS dysfunction caused by systemic problems such as sepsis, shock of various etiologies, and hypoxia. Coma can be caused by primary CNS problems such as unilateral cerebral injury with secondary brainstem dysfunction, bilateral hemispheric dysfunction, and brainstem dysfunction.[2–4,12] Unilateral hemispheric dysfunction does not cause coma. When a unilateral destructive lesion is suggested by evaluation and the patient is comatose, then the other hemisphere is also dysfunctional, possibly due to a systemic cause, or concurrent brainstem dysfunction is present.

Global Central Nervous System Dysfunction

In the patient presenting with global CNS dysfunction, neurological examination does not reveal focal findings unless present from a preexisting condition. In "light" coma, the patient's pupils react to light symmetrically; spontaneous, conjugate eye movements may be present; and motor responses to pain may be purposeful or semipurposeful. Cranial reflexes are brisk and symmetrical. The presence of coherent speech excludes coma by definition; however, the utterance of brief groans or single words with a quick return to the unresponsive state is consistent with coma and useful in excluding dominant hemisphere lesions.[16] For example, when a painful stimulus is applied to the sternum, the patient's hand may reach up and grab. Simple flexion is purposeful movement but is more likely a component of a reflex flexion posture or decorticate posture. The only clearly purposeful response is the limb crossing the midline in order to ward off the stimulus; this implies a nonreflexive, cortical response.[2,16]

In the spectrum of global CNS dysfunction, an intermediate stage is represented by the patient with dysconjugate or skew gaze. In this patient, response to pain is inconsistent. Respiratory effort is variable and may be depressed. Pupils are symmetrically small and reactive, at times requiring magnification to appreciate. Extreme global CNS dysfunction is characterized by absence of response to painful stimulation, spontaneous respirations, provoked eye movements, and pupillary reaction.

Bilateral Hemisphere Dysfunction

Bilateral hemispheric dysfunction as a cause of acute coma can be confused with global CNS dysfunction. Bilateral hemispheric dysfunction interferes with cognitive abilities and the content of consciousness (as outlined in the following section). Brainstem functions such as pupillary response, corneal responses, and reflex eye movements are present. With cold water irrigation, the eyes move conjugately to the side of cold caloric irrigation. Nystagmus is absent.

Unilateral Hemisphere Dysfunction with Brainstem Compression

A unilateral hemispheric injury with symptoms such as headache or speech difficulty can be observed to progress to coma with signs of brainstem injury. For example, a patient suspected of having a large stroke progressively becomes drowsy and then has no meaningful motor response. The eyes are observed to deviate to the side of the lesion conjugately, then dysconjugately. One pupil may become sluggish in reaction to light, then become large without clear reaction to light. Respirations may become irregular. This condition can be caused by an enlarging hemispheric mass that secondarily compresses the brainstem, causing worsening of symptoms. Early treatment may be beneficial before irreversible brainstem damage occurs.

Brainstem Dysfunction

Primary brainstem dysfunction produces distinct clinical syndromes. For example, a pontine lesion may cause abrupt coma associated with pinpoint pupils that are reactive to light. Magnification is useful in determining pupil reactivity. Depending on the location of the brainstem injury, other brainstem reflexes may be asymmetrical or absent.

Pseudocoma

Psychogenic coma, or pseudocoma, implies that there is no neurological cause of coma. The patient is capable of interaction but either chooses not to interact or is psychologically incapable of making a meaningful response. In order to evaluate the patient, a physiologically intact cortex must be demonstrated. Various maneuvers can be performed, such as hand-dropping, to see if any avoidance occurs. "Geotropic eyes" is a term coined to describe eyes that seemingly deviate toward the ground no matter how the head is turned; that is, when the head is turned to the left, the eyes conjugately deviate to the left. When the head is turned to the right, the eyes both conjugately deviate to the right. This conjugate eye deviation dependent on head position is inconsistent with seizure activity or structural CNS pathology.[19] Active resistance to eye-opening is another useful sign.[20] Cold caloric stimulation is useful when there is any question of physiological impairment; when nystagmus is elicited, this is further evidence of physiological alertness.[16] A summary of causes of coma is presented in Table 8.2.

Delirium

The hyperactive or agitated patient with delirium presents differently from the patient with a de-

TABLE 8.2. Differential Diagnoses of Coma

Coma from causes affecting the brain diffusely
  Encephalopathies
    Hypoxic (includes respiratory failure, congestive heart failure, severe anemia, shock of different etiologies)
    Metabolic
      Hypoglycemia
      Diabetic ketoacidosis
      Hyperosmolar state
      Other electrolyte abnormalities
        Hyponatremia
        Hypercalcemia
      Organ system failure
        Hepatic encephalopathy
        Uremia/renal failure
        Endocrine
          myxedema coma
    Hypertensive encephalopathy
  Toxins and drug reactions
    CNS sedatives
    Alcohols
    Carbon monoxide, other inhalants
    Neuroleptic malignant syndrome
  Environmental causes
    Heat stroke
    Hypothermia
  Deficiency state
    Wernicke's encephalopathy
Coma from primary CNS disease or trauma
  Direct CNS trauma
    Diffuse axonal injury
    subdural hematoma
    epidural hematoma
    traumatic brain contusion or laceration
  Vascular disease
    Intraparenchymal hemorrhage
      Hemispheric
      Basal ganglia
      Brainstem
      Cerebellar
    Infarction
      Hemispheric
      Brainstem
    Subarachnoid hemorrhage
  CNS infections
  Neoplasms
    Metastatic
    Primary CNS
  Seizures
    Nonconvulsive status epilepticus
    Postictal state

pressed level of consciousness, although many of the causes are the same. The patient may not be coherent or may not provide accurate information. Histories elicited from family members or caregivers are therefore valuable. Quiet or hypoactive delirium is thought to be more common than delirium characterized by an agitated, confused state.

Delirium is defined as an acute reversible state of confusion; "acute confusional state" is synonymous. "Acute" in this setting means development over hours to days. Attention deficit is a key component; performing simple tests such as repetition of digits or short-term memory as tested by recall over a few minutes is impaired. Patients are easily distractable; attention cannot be focused or sustained. Behavior may fluctuate over hours; reversal of sleep–wake cycles is common. New focal cerebral signs are absent with rare exceptions.[21,22]

Detection of delirium can be difficult. Delirium often goes unrecognized in many elderly patients in the emergency department.[23,24] An organized approach with a standard test battery is useful in detecting cognitive changes associated with delirium.[25] A list of differential diagnoses of delirium is provided in Table 8.3.

The mini mental status examination has been studied for several years and is thought to be sensitive in detecting cognitive impairment. Key items include: specific orientation, three-item digit repetition and recall, attention and calculation (serial sevens for five answers or spelling the word "world" backward), simple language tests, and copying problems. A recent summary of this test provides specifics.[26]

Medication withdrawal, intoxication, or side effects are common precipitants of delirium; however, almost any medical condition can precipitate a change in mental status. Common causes are sepsis and electrolyte abnormalities; other causes include myocardial infarction and stroke. Information from caregivers and medical records is extremely important.

Patients with depression may present with agitation or psychomotor retardation. Other major depressive syndromes include loss of pleasure, fatigue, concentration problems, feelings of helplessness, hypersomnia or insomnia, or new delusional thinking; these symptoms tend to be common in all ages. Most often, these symptoms are of insidious onset and have been present for weeks to months.[27]

TABLE 8.3. Differential Diagnoses of Delirium*

Hypoxia/diffuse cerebral ischemia
Respiratory failure
Congestive heart failure
Severe anemia
Systemic diseases
Electrolyte & fluid disturbance
Endocrine disease
Thyroid
Adrenal
Hepatic failure
Nutrition/Wernicke's disease
Sepsis, infection
Intoxications and withdrawal
CNS sedatives
Ethanol
Corticosteroids
Other medications
CNS disease
Trauma
Infections
Stroke
Epilepsy
Neoplasm

*Causes are myriad; this is a partial list.

Relevant Neuroanatomy and Pathophysiology

At the cellular level, the neuron is the functional element of the nervous system. The substrates of glucose and oxygen must be supplied continuously for normal neuronal function. When hypoxia occurs, neuronal function is impaired. Other intracellular events such as accumulation of lactate and calcium, and oxidant generation may result in an irreversible cycle of cellular dysfunction leading to cellular death.

Adequate perfusion of blood to the brain is necessary to supply sufficient oxygen and glucose. Cerebral perfusion pressure is dependent on the variables of ICP and mean arterial pressure (MAP). Simply stated, when ICP is increased above MAP, cerebral perfusion stops and ischemic injury to the CNS follows shortly thereafter (see Chapter 26).

Complex interneuronal activity is also necessary for normal functioning of the CNS. Interference with synaptic transmission or the presence of false neurotransmitters has been proposed as a cause of some encephalopathies. Inhibitory and excitatory neuronal systems summate for simple reflex movements; complexities of neuronal activity for conscious behavior remain largely speculative.

Operationally, consciousness may be thought of as having two components. The first is the arousal state, which may be thought of as being generated in the brainstem. The other element of consciousness is the meaningful content of consciousness; the individual not only regards an object but also makes appropriate associations and responses. Meaningful content is generated by the cerebral hemispheres. A useful model in evaluating patients with disorders of consciousness is to determine whether the disorder is caused by a brainstem problem or a hemispheric problem – either bilateral or unilateral with secondary brainstem compression, or a diffuse dysfunction of the neurons throughout the CNS.[2] Although this model is inexact, it is clinically useful.

As part of normal wakefulness, eyes are open spontaneously or with appropriate stimulation; the individual regards the environment by tracking objects or responding to sounds or other stimulation. This alerting function is thought to reside in the ascending reticular activating system (ARAS), which is a collection of neurons located throughout the midbrain and pons; the anatomical organization of the ARAS is not fully elucidated. Isolated injury to the brainstem that contains the ARAS may result in an eyes-closed disorder of consciousness where the alerting response is absent.

The content of consciousness may be thought of as residing in the cerebral hemispheres, specifically in the cerebral cortex. Most individuals have dominant left hemispheres; that is, language function resides in the left hemisphere and the individuals are right-handed. An injury to the dominant hemisphere can be expected to cause a problem with language or motor function of the contralateral extremities (for example, dominant-hemisphere stroke) but should not in itself cause a disorder of arousal. When coma is present, the hemispheric lesion has caused secondary compression of the contralateral hemisphere or brainstem, or there is more diffuse

CNS dysfunction. Diffuse impairment of the CNS occurs with toxic or metabolic disorders.

Brain herniation syndromes described by Plum and Posner are useful models of progressive brain failure.[2] The syndrome of uncal herniation – pupillary dilation on the side of an expanding mass lesion resulting from pressure of the shifting temporal lobe on the ipsilateral oculomotor nerve against the tentorium – has been challenged. The fact that the pupillary dilation is at times reversed by hyperosmolar agents argues against pathological injury of the nerve; microvascular compromise of the blood supply to the nerve is speculated to be contributory. Instead of an orderly rostral to caudal pathological deterioration, complex interactions of ischemia, increased ICP, and hemorrhage are thought to contribute to progressive midbrain compression.[28,29]

Delirium represents another response to diffuse cerebral dysfunction. Reduced cerebral metabolism and reduction of synthesis of neurotransmitters have been proposed as pathophysiological mechanisms of delirium. The reduced synthesis of a neurotransmitter, such as acetylcholine (ACh), may lead to an imbalance of cholinergic and adrenergic neurotransmitters.[21] Patients with acute focal CNS lesions, such as stroke, can present with an acute confusional state, which complicates the diagnosis of delirium.[30]

Emergency Department Management and Disposition

Evaluation and management proceed simultaneously for the comatose patient. The patient without protective airway reflexes is at increased risk for aspiration of gastric contents. However, laryngoscopy and endotracheal intubation are associated with increases in ICP. For the patient with increased ICP, further increases may prove deleterious. Administration of intravenous lidocaine may attenuate the rise in ICP associated with intubation and is recommended at a dose of 1.5 mg/kg three minutes prior to intubation.[31] Other issues concerning airway management, including rapid sequence intubation, incorporate several aspects of the overall clinical condition.

A recent recommendation for use of naloxone in potentially narcotic-dependent patients is a low-dose regimen, giving a small initial dose of 0.1–0.2

mg. This approach is thought to increase patient arousal and respiratory effort without precipitating withdrawal symptoms. Doubling of the dose up to a total of 10-mg depends on clinical response. When no response is elicited by 10 mg, then isolated opioid intoxication is unlikely.[8] Flumazenil, a benzodiazepine antagonist, is not used in the management of suspected toxic coma or coma of unknown etiology. Malignant arrhythmias or seizures can result when it is administered in cases involving tricyclic antidepressants or benzodiazepine withdrawal.[8]

Aggressive supportive care with vigilant patient monitoring is necessary in the management of comatose patients. Administration of high-flow oxygen is indicated for all patients until they are stabilized. Continuous monitoring of vital signs, cardiac rhythm, and oxygen saturation is required. Laboratory work is guided by history, physical examination, and response to interventions. For patients who remain unresponsive after administration of dextrose, thiamine, and naloxone, basic laboratory work including complete blood cell count, serum chemistries, urinalysis, and arterial blood gas analysis is standard. Additional laboratory tests in selected patients include coagulation studies, antiepileptic drug levels, specific toxin assays, and special endocrine studies. Lumbar puncture (LP) is indicated when CNS infection is suspected. Cerebrospinal fluid analysis may be useful in providing alternative diagnoses; for example, subarachnoid hemorrhage may be suspected clinically but CSF may show meningitis. LP is commonly deferred when there is only a remote possibility of an intracranial lesion. When LP is delayed for computerized tomography (CT) scanning, prompt antibiotic administration is vital when bacterial meningitis is a possibility.

Rapid imaging of the brain, usually by CT scan, has become standard for patients with altered mental status. CT scanning is often used to exclude low-probability but important causes of coma such as occult subdural hematoma. Results of CT scanning aid in the ability of the emergency physician to refer patients to appropriate specialty services and hospital units.

An evolving responsibility of the emergency physician in the care of patients with altered mental status is to convey the likelihood of a poor prognosis and the diagnosis of brain death to family members and friends. Families may request that life-sustaining measures be withheld or withdrawn when the cause of coma is clearly determined during the course of emergency department evaluation, and the examination is compatible with brain death or severe disability with low likelihood of recovery. Alternatively, when a terminal illness or advanced dementia is present, family members may request supportive care only. Increasingly, brain death or severe impairment is diagnosed and support systems withheld or terminated in the emergency department; often this occurs in consultation with another physician. Local practices and policies vary substantially.

Traditionally, the diagnosis of brain death implies that no clinically detectable cortical and brainstem function is present. This diagnosis implies no motor response of any type to stimulation. Pupillary reaction to light is absent. There is no oculocephalic response to caloric irrigation. When the diagnosis of brain death is considered, a test for apnea can be performed. Oxygen (15 l/min) is supplied by a cannula inserted in the endotracheal tube during the assessment for respiratory activity, or hypoxia may result.[32] A positive apnea test consists of 10 minutes of observation without respiratory activity. The rationale of the apnea test is that increasing carbon dioxide levels will drive an intact respiratory center to activity. Controversy remains about the definition of brain death and the need to make the diagnosis of brain death prior to terminating life support measures. Practice guidelines exist for permitting termination of treatment of severely brain-injured patients.[33,34]

The hyperactive patient with delirium presents with symptoms very different from those indicating a depressed level of consciousness, despite the fact that both conditions can have common causes. Treatment typically is directed at the underlying medical cause. History suggests whether medication side effects or drug withdrawal is a problem. After infectious causes, electrolyte abnormalities, and cardiac causes are excluded, many delirious patients will not have a specific diagnosis.

Frequently, the emergency physician is asked to provide "medical clearance" for a patient with suspected psychiatric disturbance. Local practices vary. Causation is urged in using the term "medically cleared," and it is suggested that the results of the history and physical examination, including mental status testing, neurological examination, and laboratory testing, are documented carefully.[35]

Selected Clinical Conditions Presenting as Altered Mental Status

Subtle Status Epilepticus

An underappreciated cause of unresponsiveness in patients is continuing seizure activity. Postictal behavior varies greatly, but patients usually show some improvement in the level of consciousness 20–30 minutes after seizure activity has stopped. Careful observation of patients is necessary to ensure that seizure activity has halted; ongoing nystagmoid movements of the eyes or facial twitching may indicate continued seizure activity, perhaps best termed *subtle status epilepticus,* and the need for intervention.[16] Although used infrequently in the emergency department, electroencephalography (EEG) should be considered in selected cases. Uncommonly, electrical status epilepticus may be present without any appreciable abnormal motor activity, termed *nonconvulsive status epilepticus;* this is observed in patients following cardiac arrest and in patients with complex partial or absence seizures. Treatment with antiepileptic drugs is individualized; patients with epilepsy respond the best. Outcome usually reflects the severity of the underlying medical condition and any associated cortical injury. Correct diagnosis is possible only with EEG, which is not readily available in most emergency departments.

Cerebellar Hemorrhage

A cerebellar hemorrhage may progress in a manner similar to unilateral cerebral hemispheric dysfunction and cause secondary brainstem dysfunction. However, an expanding mass in the posterior fossa may cause abrupt brainstem compression and respiratory arrest. Particularly with cerebellar hemispheric hemorrhage or ischemic stroke, good clinical outcome is possible after evacuation of the injured cerebellar hemisphere. Symptoms of abrupt headache, nausea or emesis, and gait dysfunction, with progression to altered mental status, suggest this possibility. Prompt CT scanning expedites detection of this neurological emergency. Good recovery has been reported even with deeply comatose patients.[36]

Unusual Motor Responses (see Chapter 17)

Although unusual, abnormal flexor and extensor postures can simulate seizures particularly when they are fragmentary and brief and repeat rapidly.[37] These postures may occur in the setting of acute, severe CNS injury (subarachnoid hemorrhage, basilar artery thrombosis). Antiepileptic drugs have no effect on this type of abnormal motor activity.

Global CNS Dysfunction

Extensor posturing ("decerebrate") and flexor posturing ("decorticate") have been reported with drug overdoses and other metabolic causes of coma. Likewise, ophthalmoplegia in response to caloric testing (pupils "fixed and dilated") has been reported in "toxic" coma, resulting from an overdose of tricyclic antidepressants and carbamazepine.[39,40] These abnormal findings do not necessarily indicate a specific neuro-anatomic lesion.[2,38]

Hypoxic encephalopathy is a common sequela of the patient with cardiac arrest. Prognosis is often grave. A recent study has shown that early diagnostic findings such as impaired brainstem and abnormal motor responses correlate with death or disability but are best assessed at two to three days postarrest.[41] Early, accurate prognosis in cases of hypoxic encephalopathy is not possible in the emergency department.

Disorders of consciousness are sometimes incorrectly diagnosed as being psychiatric in origin. When the physician evaluates a patient with bizarre behavior, the typical initial response is that a psychiatric disorder is likely. The potential inaccuracy of "medical clearance" has been reported repeatedly.[35,42,43] In determining medical causes of altered mental status or behavior, abnormal vital signs and an attention deficit are important findings. Especially important is recognizing that certain illnesses, such as meningitis, may be fatal when undiagnosed and untreated.

Psychogenic Coma

Psychogenic disorders of consciousness do exist, e.g., psychogenic coma. An adequate history and brief confirmatory maneuvers for psychogenic unresponsiveness are urged before beginning treatment.[44]

Aphasias

Detection of patients with fluent aphasias can be difficult. Frequently, caregivers label these patients as having a psychiatric disturbance. In the absence of hemiparesis or knowledge of a language problem, the patient may indeed appear to be "talking crazy." In extreme cases, the patient will apparently answer questions and have some sentence structure in a fluent, articulated stream of completely incomprehensible noises. The rapidity of onset of symptoms, risk factors for cerebrovascular disease, and the lack of previous psychiatric problems suggests the possibility of a stroke. The presence of apraxia often helps to make the diagnosis of fluent aphasia. That is, a patient is asked to perform one task but instead performs a different but similar one, thinking the request has been carried out. For example, a patient asked to clinch his fist in a threatening manner instead waves goodbye. When consistently demonstrated, this type of parapraxic movement suggests that an aphasia may be present.[45]

PEARLS AND PITFALLS

- An impaired level of consciousness is caused by dysfunction of bilateral cerebral hemispheres or the brainstem.
- A patient with coma of unknown cause can be treated initially with dextrose, thiamine, and naloxone.
- The Glasgow Coma Scale score is an objective measure of neurological functioning and can be used serially to monitor changes in a patient's neurological condition.
- Psychogenic unresponsiveness resembles coma but has no underlying physiological cause.
- A patient with delirium can be hyperactive or agitated, or quiet.
- Medications are frequently the cause of coma and delirium.
- Brain death means that there is no detectable function of the cerebrum and brainstem.
- Termination of care of the severely brain-injured patient does not require a diagnosis of brain death.

REFERENCES

1. Jennett B, Teasdale G. Assessment of impaired consciousness. In: Jennett B, Teasdale G, eds. *Management of Head Injuries*. Philadelphia, Pa: FA Davis Co; 1981.
2. Plum F, Posner JB. The pathologic physiology of signs and symptoms of coma. In: Plum F, Posner JB, eds. *The Diagnosis of Stupor and Coma*. Philadelphia, Pa: FA Davis Co; 1980:1–86.
3. Samuels MA. The evaluation of comatose patients. *Hosp Pract*. 1993;28:165–182.
4. Huff JS. Coma. In: Rosen P, Baker FJ, Barkin RM, Braen GR, Dailey RH, Levy RC, eds. *Emergency Medicine, Concepts and Clinical Practice*. St. Louis, Mo: CV Mosby; 1984:249–69.
5. Solomon P, Aring CD. The causes of coma in patients entering a general hospital. *Am J Med Sci*. 1934; 188:805–11.
6. Huff JS. Contemporary etiology of coma presenting to academic medical center [abstract]. *Ann Neurol*. 1997; 42;3:471.
7. Hafen BQ, Karren KJ. Patient assessment. In: Hafen BQ, Karren KJ, eds. *Prehospital Emergency Care and Crisis Intervention*. Englewood Cliffs, NJ: Prentice-Hall, Inc; 1992:47–69.
8. Hoffman RS, Goldfrank LR. The poisoned patient with altered consciousness. Controversies in the use of a 'coma cocktail.' *JAMA*. 1994;274:562–9.
9. Pulsinelli WA, Levy DE, Sigsbee B, Scherer P, Plum F. Increased damage after ischemic stroke in patients with hyperglycemia with or without established diabetes mellitus. *Am J Med*. 1983;74:540–4.
10. Woo E, Chan YW, Yu YL, Huang CY. Admission glucose levels in relation to mortality and morbidity outcome in 252 stroke patients. *Stroke*. 1988;19:185–91.
11. Hoffman JR, Schriger DL, Luo JS. The empiric use of naloxone in patients with altered mental status. *Ann Emerg Med*. 1991;20:246–52.
12. Claps PJ, Berk WA. The John Doe syndrome. *Am J Emerg Med*. 1992;10:217–18.
13. Kothari M, Bazil C, Jafri S, Weinreb H. Patients of unknown identity: a neurodiagnostic challenge. *Am J Emerg Med*. 1994;12:510–11.
14. Aldrich E, Biniek R. How to approach an unconscious patient. In: Hacke W, Hanley DF, Einhaupl KM, Bleck TP, Diringer MN, eds. *NeuroCritical Care*. New York, NY: Springer-Verlag; 1994:23–85.
15. Fishbeck KH, Simon RP. Neurological manifestations of accidental hypothermia. *Ann Neurol*. 1981;10:384–5.
16. Fisher CM. The neurological evaluation of the comatose patient. *Acta Neurol Scand*. 1969;45:1–56.
17. Keane JR. Retinal hemorrhages: its significance in 100 patients with encephalopathy of unknown cause. *Arch Neurol*. 1979;36:691–4.
18. Levin BE. The clinical significance of spontaneous pulsations of the retinal vein. *Arch Neurol*. 1978;35:37–40.
19. Rosenberg ML. Geotropic eye movements and pseudoseizures. *Arch Neurol*. 1986;43:544.

20. Cain DL. A useful eye sign in the apparently unconscious patient. *Ann R Coll Surg Engl.* 1983;65:265.
21. Lipowski ZJ. Delirium (acute confusional states). *JAMA.* 1987;258:1789–92.
22. Rummans TA, Evans JM, Krahn LE, Fleming KC. Delirium in elderly patients: evaluation and management. *Mayo Clin Proc.* 1995;70:989–98.
23. Naughton BJ, Moran MB, Kadah H, Heman-Ackah Y, Longano J. Delirium and other cognitive impairment in older adults in an emergency department. *Ann Emerg Med.* 1995;25:751–5.
24. Lewis LM, Miller DK, Morley JE, Nork MJ, Lasater LC. Unrecognized delirium in ED geriatric patients. *Am J Emerg Med.* 1995;13:142–5.
25. Cummings JL. Mini-mental state examination: norms, normals, and numbers. *JAMA.* 1993;269:2420–1.
26. Crum RM, Anthony JC, Bassett SS, Folstein MF. Population-based norms for the mini-mental state examination by age and educational level. *JAMA.* 1993;269:2386–91.
27. Martin LM, Fleming KC, Evans JM. Recognition and management of anxiety and depression in elderly patients. *Mayo Clin Proc.* 1995;70:999–1006.
28. Fisher CM. Acute brain herniation: a revised concept. *Semin Neurol.* 1984;4:417–21.
29. Fisher CM. Observations concerning brain herniation. *Ann Neurol.* 1983;14:110.
30. Benbadis SR, Sila CA, Cristea RL. Mental status and stroke. *J Gen Intern Med.* 1994;9:485–7.
31. Murphy MF. Increased intracranial pressure. In: Dailey RH, Simon B, Young GP, Stewart RD, eds. *The Airway: Emergency Management.* St. Louis, Mo: Mosby–Year Book, Inc; 1992:271–81.
32. Marks SJ, Zisfein J. Apneic oxygenation in apnea tests for brain death: a controlled trial. *Arch Neurol.* 1990;47:1066–8.
33. Bernat JL. Brain death occurs only with destruction of the cerebral hemispheres and the brain stem. *Arch Neurol.* 1992;49:569–70.
34. Youngner SJ. Defining death: a superficial and fragile consensus. *Arch Neurol.* 1992;49:570–2.
35. Tintinalli JE, Peacock FW, Wright MA. Emergency department evaluation psychiatric patients. *Ann Emerg Med.* 1994;23:859–62.
36. Huff JS. Dr. C. Miller Fisher's description of acute cerebellar hemorrhage. *J Emerg Med.* 1994;12:521–4.
37. Haines SJ. Decerebrate posturing misinterpreted as seizure activity. *Am J Emerg Med.* 1988;6:173–7.
38. Greenberg DA, Simon RP. Flexor and extensor postures in sedative drug-induced coma. *Neurology.* 1982;32:448–51.
39. Beal MF. Amitriptyline ophthalmoplegia. *Neurology.* 1982;32:1409.
40. Mullally WJ. Carbamazepine-induced ophthalmoplegia. *Arch Neurol.* 1982;39:64.
41. Hamel MB, Goldman L, Teno J, et al. Identification of comatose patients at high risk for death or severe disability. *JAMA.* 1995;273:1842–8.
42. Henneman PL, Mendoza R, Lewis RJ. Prospective evaluation of emergency department clearance. *Ann Emerg Med.* 1994;24:672–7.
43. Herbert M. Assessment for medical clearance. *Ann Emerg Med.* 1995;25:852.
44. Leis AA, Ross MA, Summers AK. Psychogenic seizures: ictal characteristics and diagnostic pitfalls. *Neurology.* 1992;42:92–5.
45. Poeck K. Confusion, psychosis, and neuropsychological symptoms. In: Hacke W, Hanley DF, Einhaupl KM, Bleck TP, Diringer MN, eds. *NeuroCritical Care.* New York, NY: Springer-Verlag; 1994.

9 Headache

DOUGLAS J. GELB, ASHOK HARWANI AND WILLIAM D. FALES

SUMMARY Headache is the presenting complaint of 1–2.5% of all emergency department visits.[1-4] It is the most frequent reason that a patient sees a neurologist,[5] and it is among the top 10 complaints encountered in virtually all medical specialties, including pediatrics.[5] At least 40% of all Americans will have what they consider to be a serious and severe headache at some time during their lives.[6] Epidemiological surveys reveal a high prevalence of headache in both children and adults.[6]

Headache can be the principal symptom of a variety of acute systemic or neurological problems. However, most patients have no generalized disorder underlying the headache, and most headaches managed in the emergency department do not represent serious medial conditions.[1-4]

Patients who visit the emergency department for headache tend to exhibit either the "first-or-worst syndrome," or the "last-straw syndrome."[7,8] Individuals in the first category present to the emergency department because they are alarmed by a headache that is different from or more intense than those experienced in the past. Patients in the second category may have experienced headaches for many years but may not have a personal physician and delay seeking medical evaluation until frustration or exhaustion brings them to the emergency department.

Prehospital Considerations

Prehospital care providers are called infrequently to care for a patient with headache. In an out-of-hospital setting, the focus of evaluation is on vital signs and the level of consciousness. Pain of any type, including headache, commonly results in blood pressure elevation. An attempt to lower an elevated blood pressure in an out-of-hospital setting is generally not recommended. Encephalopathy or focal neurological signs can indicate a hypertensive emergency, but can also be a direct result of primary brain pathology, with hypertension occurring secondarily due to the Cushing's reflex.[9-11] In the latter situation, blood pressure is not reduced acutely, because it can result in extension of the region of brain injury. In general, unless the diastolic blood pressure exceeds 140 mm Hg, blood pressure reduction is deferred until arrival in the emergency department.

Headache by itself is not a life-threatening emergency that needs to be treated in the field. When headache is secondary to underlying conditions such as hypovolemic shock or head injury, the underlying conditions are treated. Prehospital care providers aid greatly in the evaluation of a patient with headache by assessing the patient's environment (e.g., checking for carbon monoxide poisoning), collecting suspected agents and drugs, and obtaining a history from witnesses. Prehospital analgesia for headache is generally not indicated.

Relevant Neuroanatomy and Pathology

Headache differs from most neurological problems in that anatomical localization is often unnecessary and not helpful clinically. Headache can be provoked by a variety of pathological processes, both focal and diffuse. The pain-sensitive structures of the head and scalp include: the skin; its blood supply and appendages; muscles of the head and neck; great venous sinuses and their tributaries; portions of the dura mater at the base of the brain and the dural arteries; intracerebral arteries; cervical nerves; and the trigeminal (V), abducens (VI), and facial (VII) nerves.[12]

In contrast, the skull, choroidal plexus, brain parenchyma, ependymal lining of the ventricles, and major portion of the dura and pia mater are pain-insensitive.[12] Headache is not a sensitive indicator of serious intracranial pathology.

The pain-sensitive structures are affected by several pain-producing mechanisms, including tension, traction, distension, dilation, and inflammation. Tension results from constriction of neck and scalp muscles due to causes such as cervical arthritis, irritating lesions, or emotional distress. Traction can result from an intracranial mass and may be felt at the base of the head. Vascular distension or dilation can manifest as the throbbing pain characteristic of migraine and cluster headache. Inflammation is associated with meningitis, arteritis, or sinusitis. Inflammation is commonly infectious in origin, but can be caused by irritants such as blood.

Many lines of evidence suggest that migraine pain results from abnormal firing of nociceptive neurons in the trigeminal pathway, resulting in vasodilatation and plasma protein extravasation, a process termed *neurogenic inflammation*.[13,14] This involves a complex cascade of events in which serotonin appears to play an important role. The process can be initiated by a variety of internal and external triggers, including noxious stimulation of blood vessels or meninges; therefore, it is likely that the headaches that occur with subarachnoid hemorrhage (SAH), meningitis, and other neurological or systemic diseases are pathophysiologically analogous to migraine. It has been suggested by some experts that the pathophysiology of migraine is the same as that of tension headache.

Emergency Department Evaluation

Headaches are associated with a wide variety of systemic and neurological diseases (Table 9.1). Some headaches represent emergencies, but most headaches are "benign" or "primary," meaning they occur in isolation without association to a more

TABLE 9.1. Differential Diagnosis of Headache

I. Primary headaches
  A. Migraine
  B. Tension
  C. Cluster
  D. Chronic paroxysmal hemicrania
  E. Cranial neuralgias
  F. Exertional headache
II. Secondary headaches
  A. CNS mass lesions
    1. Tumor (primary or metastatic)
    2. Hemorrhage (subdural, epidural, or intraparenchymal)
    3. Abscess
  B. Ischemic stroke
  C. Abnormal CSF dynamics
    1. Obstructive hydrocephalus
    2. Benign intracranial hypertension (pseudotumor cerebri)
    3. Cerebral venous or sinus thrombosis
    4. Spontaneous or post-LP intracranial hypotension
  D. Meningeal irritation
    1. Meningitis (bacterial, viral, fungal, or chemical)
    2. SAH (aneurysm, AVM, trauma, idiopathic)
    3. Carcinomatous or lymphomatous meningitis
  E. Diffuse CNS inflammation
    1. Encephalitis
    2. Vasculitis (temporal arteritis, other systemic or CNS vasculitis)
  F. Head trauma
  G. Nonneurologic intracranial disease
    1. Ophthalmologic (glaucoma, orbital tumors or infections)
    2. ENT (sinusitis, other infections or tumors)
    3. TMJ disease
    4. Dental disease
    5. Arterial dissection (carotid or vertebral)
    6. Cervical spine disease
  H. Systemic disease
    1. Hypertension
    2. Toxic (including prescription drugs)
    3. Metabolic (including hypoxia, anemia, hypoglycemia, hypothyroidism)
    4. Systemic infection or other inflammatory disease
  I. Depression

generalized underlying disease process. Primary headaches are diagnosed and managed on the basis of patient history and physical examination, whereas additional tests are required to diagnose and treat secondary headaches. Because most patients with "primary" headaches have a normal physical and neurological examination, the most important diagnostic tool is a careful and detailed history.[15] The most useful information for determining whether a patient's headache is primary or secondary is whether the patient has experienced similar headaches in the past (Fig. 9.1). This is an issue of pain quality, not pain quantity. The character of the headache is more important than the severity. Traditionally, emergency medicine has taught that a patient who complains of the "worst

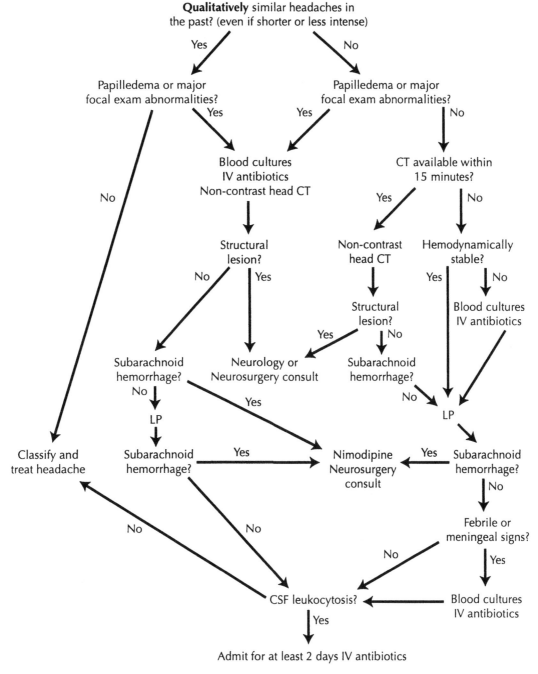

FIGURE 9.1. Diagnostic and therapeutic approach to the patient with headache.

headache ever" needs urgent evaluation for SAH. This dictum must be tempered with common sense. Patients who are sufficiently distressed by their headaches to come to the emergency department want to convey adequately the severity of their pain to the emergency department staff. Patients may honestly report that they have never had a headache like this before; however, further questioning can reveal that the only unusual property of the current headache is its duration, severity, or failure to respond to measures that are usually effective in alleviating symptoms.

Specific details that can help in comparing the current headache to previous headaches include the onset, duration, character, severity, and location of pain. Inquiries about associated symptoms, precipitating factors, and prodromes are made. Important categories of symptom properties are described below.

1. Onset, duration, character, and severity: The acute-onset "thunderclap" headache can suggest SAH. Migraine pain can be pulsating or throbbing. The pain of cluster headache is described as deep and boring, as if a hot poker were being driven into the eye. Tension headache is dull, nagging, persistent, and often described as though a band were wrapped around the head. A change in headache pattern, the presence of unilateral headache that never changes sides ("side-locked headache"), or the occurrence of neurological symptoms during headache (rather than preceding it) suggest a need for neuroimaging.

2. Age of onset: Headache that starts in childhood, adolescence, or the second or third decade of life is frequently migraine. Headache that begins later in life can have an organic etiology such as giant cell arteritis, cerebrovascular disease, or tumor. Tension headache can begin at any age.

3. Location: Approximately 65% of migraine headaches are unilateral.[6] Strictly unilateral orbital pain of brief duration can suggest cluster headache. Tension headache can be bilateral or circumferential. A headache always in the same location can suggest a mass lesion.

4. Course: Headaches that become progressively worse suggest an organic cause. The longer the headache has existed in its present form, the more likely it is to be benign.[16]

5. Prodromes and auras: Significant prodromes such as mood changes or changes in appetite can occur one or two days before a migraine headache. Auras such as scintillating scotomas or paraesthesias precede and define "classic" migraine.

6. Associated signs and symptoms: Relevant accompanying symptoms include fever, nausea, vomiting, photophobia, phonophobia, visual disturbance, numbness, weakness, language difficulty, confusion, dizziness, nasal congestion, rhinorrhea, or ocular injection. Unilateral nasal congestion and eye tearing are associated with cluster headache. Nausea, vomiting, photophobia, and phonophobia are commonly associated with migraine. Teeth grinding and neck tenderness may be seen with tension headache.

7. Precipitating factors: Migraine can be triggered by alcohol, bright lights, fatigue, sleep deprivation or excess, hypoglycemia, stress, and food additives. Migraine can also be provoked by menstruation and relieved by pregnancy. Both exercise and orgasm can trigger migraine, and both can cause an aneurysm to rupture. Frantic pacing, walking, and rocking during the attack strongly suggest cluster headache.

8. Medical and medication history: Alcoholism, trauma, bleeding disorders, and use of anticoagulants are all associated with an increased risk of subdural hematoma (SDH). Medical conditions such as hypertension, hypercapnia, hypoxia, hypothyroidism, metastatic malignancies, anemia, hypoglycemia, and steroid deficiency can all result in headache. A number of medications can elicit headache as a side effect. Common offenders include nitrates, indomethacin, calcium channel blockers, digoxin, and estrogen. Recreational drugs such as nicotine, alcohol, marijuana, and amphetamines can also induce headache. A history of dental procedures, neck manipulations, or other intervention is relevant. Older patients are asked explicitly about recent jaw claudication or symptoms of polymyalgia rheumatica, which may accompany temporal arteritis.

9. Toxic exposures: Patients with prolonged exposure to automobile exhaust, fire, and faulty heat-

ing equipment may complain of headache as an early symptom of carbon monoxide poisoning.

Physical Examination

The scope of a general physical and neurological examination of a patient with headache in the emergency department depends largely on historical findings. For patients whose symptoms are simply an exacerbation of chronic symptoms, a screening examination is sufficient. This includes a review of vital signs, funduscopic examination, pupillary light reflex, eye movements, gait (looking for asymmetry or balance difficulty), limb strength, and deep tendon reflexes. Consistent abnormalities on the screening examination require further evaluation.

The physical examination is directed toward identifying a potential systemic illness. Fever without meningismus can indicate a systemic illness contributing to the headache. Headache due to hypertension generally does not occur until the diastolic pressure is approximately 130–140 mm Hg.[6] Diastolic elevation near 140 mm Hg is associated with changes in mental status or other neurological findings, and represents an emergency situation. Tachycardia and tachypnea occur with headache due to hypoxia, anemia, or carbon monoxide poisoning. More frequently, however, tachypnea reflects pain.

Physical assessment includes palpation and percussion of the sinuses, teeth, temporomandibular joint (TMJ), and pericranial and paracervical muscles. Nuchal rigidity suggests meningeal irritation, either infectious or hemorrhagic in origin. In older patients, the superficial temporal arteries are palpated. An erythematous, papulovesicular rash of the scalp, face, or neck that does not cross the midline is likely to be herpes zoster. Not uncommonly, pain and tenderness precede the rash by several days. Intraocular pressure is measured in order to rule out acute angle closure glaucoma.

Funduscopic assessment can reveal papilledema, which may be the only finding of elevated intracranial pressure (ICP). Subhyaloid and retinal hemorrhages are uncommon, but when present they are virtually diagnostic of acute SAH.[17] Spontaneous venous pulsations on funduscopy, when present, indicate normal ICP.[17]

The relevant aspects of history and physical examinations can be summarized by asking two questions. Does the patient have a long history of similar symptoms? Are there new focal findings on the neurological examination? The specific characteristics of the symptoms are important primarily for determining whether the symptoms are new or chronic, because any given set of symptoms can be produced by a variety of underlying conditions.

Based on the answers to the above questions, patients with headaches are classified into three groups. The first group consists of patients with a long history of similar headaches and no new focal abnormalities on neurological examination. This group includes young patients with classic symptoms of migraine headache, including visual phenomena. Patients in this group have primary headaches, and can be treated without any diagnostic testing.

The second group consists of patients with new symptoms that are likely to be a result of a recognized nonneurological disease (such as glaucoma, hypertensive crisis, or hepatitis). These patients are evaluated and treated for the suspected underlying disease.

The third group includes patients who have new symptoms with no obvious cause, and patients with chronic symptoms but new focal abnormalities on examination. These patients require evaluation for SAH and meningitis (and, in older patients, temporal arteritis).

Diagnostic Testing

Findings of the history and physical examination dictate appropriate diagnostic testing. An erythrocyte sedimentation rate (ESR) is indicated in patients over 50 years of age with a headache in the region of the temporal artery. Most patients with temporal arteritis have an elevated ESR, although a normal value does not exclude it. A complete blood count (CBC) is indicated in patients with fever, meningismus, or suspected anemia. A carboxyhemoglobin level is indicated in patients who have been confined in closed spaces and exposed to smoke or a faulty heater, or when several people from the same home complain of headache. Arterial blood gases (ABGs) are indicated when symptoms, signs, or situations are suggestive of hypoxia or acidosis. Liver function studies and renal indices are obtained when a systemic illness is suspected.

SAH and meningitis are evaluated concurrently because they cannot be reliably distinguished on the basis of the history and physical examination. Fever occurs more frequently and is typically higher in patients with meningitis than in those with SAH.[18–20] Normal body temperature makes meningitis unlikely but not impossible, particularly in an older or an immunocompromised patient.[21–24] Meningeal signs may or may not be present in patients with either SAH or meningitis.[23–26] Focal neurological signs are more common with SAH, but can also occur with meningitis.[21–23] Patients with either condition can have a nonfocal examination.[22,23,26,27]

The diagnosis of meningitis is based on cerebrospinal fluid (CSF) examination. This is also a reliable diagnostic test for SAH. However, SAH can often be detected on a noncontrast computerized tomography (CT) scan and therefore lumbar puncture (LP) is not necessary when SAH is demonstrated. An LP is necessary when a CT scan does not show evidence of SAH, because up to 10% of patients can have normal CT scans in the first five days after SAH, although some studies report higher percentages of missed SAH on CT scanning.[20,26–31] In a study involving a consecutive sample of 350 patients with headache who had CT scanning of the brain, 7 patients (2%) had abnormal scans. All 7 patients had an abnormal physical or neurological examination, or unusual clinical symptoms. The likelihood of a positive CT scan increased over fivefold when only patients with abnormal physical or neurological findings or unusual symptoms received CT scanning, with no apparent increase in the number of missed cases.[32]

The traditionally accepted premise of obtaining a CT scan prior to performing an LP is based on the possibility of brain herniation in the small group of patients with an undiagnosed intracranial mass or raised ICP. Unless the examination provides strong evidence of a mass lesion – specifically, a consistent asymmetry in sensory, motor, or reflex findings, papilledema, alteration of mental status, or cranial nerve lesions – an LP can be performed prior to CT scanning.

A CT scan is considered in the presence of:

1. Worst headache ever, not in quantity, but rather in the quality of the headache
2. Depressed sensorium or cognition
3. Focal neurological deficits
4. Onset with exertion
5. Meningismus
6. Deterioration during observation[33,34]

Emergency CT scanning is also considered in those older than 50 years of age with new onset of headache, sudden onset of headache, or an insidious onset of headache with progressive worsening over weeks or months, or onset with coughing, straining, or sexual activity.

A conservative approach that excludes diagnostic testing (CT scanning and CSF examination) is acceptable in the following situations:

1. None of the above findings
2. Normal vital signs, including temperature
3. Improvement during observation[34]

Magnetic resonance imaging (MRI) has greater sensitivity for vascular disease, tumor, and posttraumatic changes, and is the best method for evaluating chronic headache. MRI has excellent resolution in the posterior fossa, a region that is poorly visualized by CT, and MRI more accurately demonstrates gliosis and demyelination.

Differential Diagnosis and Management

Published classifications of headache include those of the Ad Hoc Committee on Classification of Headache[35] and the International Headache Society.[36] However, a simpler classification has been formulated (Table 9.2).[37] A distinction between emergent, urgent, and nonurgent causes of headache is made (Table 9.3).[15]

Subarachnoid Hemorrhage

SAH is among the frequently missed serious causes of headache. SAH affects nearly 30,000 persons annually in the United States and has an overall mortality rate of approximately 50%. Of surviving patients, only half eventually have a good outcome, and less than one-third return to their premorbid neurological state.[38] Trauma, or rupture of an intracranial aneurysm or arteriovenous malformation are the three most frequent causes of SAH.

TABLE 9.2. Classification of Headache

Tension Type	Vascular	Traction & Inflammatory
Anxiety	Migraine With aura Without aura	Mass lesions (e.g., tumor edema, hematoma, cerebral hemorrhage)
Depressive equivalents and conversion reactions	Complicated Hemiplegic Ophthalmoplegic Basilar artery	Diseases of eye, ear, nose, throat, and teeth Arteritis, phlebitis, and cranial neuralgias Occlusive vascular disease
Cervical osteoarthritis	Cluster Toxic vascular	Atypical facial pain
Chronic myositis	Hypertensive	Temporomandibular joint disease

Source: Adapted from Diamond and Dalessio.[37]

Clinical Presentations. The classic presentation of SAH is sudden onset of a severe ("thunderclap") headache, frequently described by the patient as "the worst headache I have ever had." This is followed by neck stiffness, confusion, and neurological signs. Atypical presentations of SAH include syncope, confusion, coma, or a migrainelike headache. Warning symptoms precede major SAH in 40–60% of cases. These occur within 6–21 days of a major SAH, due to aneurysmal expansion causing cranial nerve palsies (especially cranial nerve III), localized head pain, and visual field defects, or sentinel bleeds characterized by generalized headache with or without nausea, vomiting, photophobia, or meningismus. The probability of eventual morbidity and mortality is much higher in patients who have experienced an unrecognized warning "leak," and who subsequently have aneurysmal rupture, than in patients who are in good condition after the initial SAH.[39]

Emergency CT scanning is the initial procedure of choice for diagnosis of SAH. Normal CT scans are common two or more days after initial hemorrhage, and in patients without neurological deficit. A yellow supernatant liquid (xanthochromia), obtained by centrifuging a bloody CSF sample, can help differentiate SAH from a traumatic LP (no xanthochromia) (see Chapter 4, "Lumbar Puncture").

Various electrocardiogram (EKG) changes (peaked or symmetrically inverted T waves or U waves, prolongation of QRS complexes, prolonged QT interval, and dysrhythmias) can occur in association with SAH and can confound interpretation of clinical data.

Patients with SAH require supportive care and an aggressive evaluation for the source of the hemorrhage so that measures can be taken to prevent rebleeding.[26,27,30,31,40] While awaiting hospitalization, patients are kept at quiet bed rest. Sedation may be necessary but is kept to a minimum to avoid complicating the neurological assessment. Nimodipine (60 mg orally every 4 hours) is beneficial in preventing brain injury and improving outcome after SAH.[41] Use of prophylactic anticonvulsant medication may be of benefit, but its routine use in the emergency department is not recommended. An optimal timing of angiography and surgery is not established.

Migraine Headaches

Migraine headaches are characterized by unilateral throbbing pain associated with nausea, vomiting, photophobia, phonophobia, and sometimes vi-

TABLE 9.3. Common Causes of Headache Presenting in the Emergency Department

I. Emergent causes
   A. Intracranial hemorrhage – subarachnoid hemorrhage, subdural, epidural, or intracerebral hematoma
   B. Meningitis or encephalitis
   C. Severe hypertension with encephalopathy
   D. Disorder of oxygenation or respiration: hypoxia, hypercarbia, carbon monoxide poisoning
II. Urgent causes
   A. Vascular – migraine, cluster, cerebrovascular accident, arteriovenous malformation, altitude sickness, giant cell arteritis
   B. Mass – brain tumor, abscess, arteriovenous malformation
   C. Potential head trauma or chronic subdural hematoma
   D. Secondary to systemic disorder, hypoglycemia, fever, hypothyroid, anemia
   E. Miscellaneous – glaucoma, benign intracranial hypertension
III. Less urgent causes
   A. Muscle contraction (tension)
   B. Secondary to diet or medications
   C. Fatigue, postexertion, postcoital
   D. Post trauma
   E. Post lumbar puncture
   F. Sinusitis without complications
   G. Myofascial pain syndrome

Source: Brillman JD. Headache. In: Hamilton GC, Trott AT, Sanders AB, Strange GR, eds. *Emergency Medicine: An Approach to Clinical Problem-Solving.* Philadelphia, Pa: WB Saunders Co; 1991:830–46.

sual phenomena or other focal neurological symptoms. The temporal artery may appear dilated and pulsating. During the postheadache phase, the skull can remain tender and the patient can feel exhausted.

The severity of a migraine attacks can range from moderate to severe to incapacitating. The acute attack typically lasts 4–24 hours.[42] Prolonged attacks (lasting 72 hours or longer) are called *status migrainosus.*

Migraine headaches are diagnosed in approximately 22% of patients who complain of headache.[43] About 75% of migraine headaches occur without auras (common migraine) while 20% occur

with an aura (classic migraine). The most common auras are visual, including scotomas (blind spots), fortification spectra, and photopsia (flashing lights). Other auras can include paresthesias, visual and auditory hallucinations, vertigo, syncope, and hyperosmia. These symptoms usually disappear prior to the headache phase. A painless migraine is referred to as *migraine sine cephalgia* or *migraine equivalent.* Less than 5% of migraine headaches are considered complicated migraines, which include ophthalmoplegic, hemiplegic, and basilar artery varieties.

Ophthalmoplegic migraine is usually seen in young adults and is relatively rare. The third cranial nerve is most frequently involved, followed by the sixth and fourth cranial nerves. A dilated, outwardly deviated eye with ptosis is the common presentation. The pain is moderate in intensity and ipsilateral. Ophthalmoplegic migraine can mimic symptoms of a dissecting carotid aneurysm. Hemiplegic migraine is uncommon. It is characterized by unilateral motor and sensory symptoms ranging from mild hemiparesis to hemiplegia. The symptoms can last longer than the headache. This is a diagnosis of exclusion. Basilar artery migraine can have a prodrome consisting of vertigo, tinnitus, dysarthria, ataxia, unsteadiness, syncope, stupor, bilateral visual blurring, and bilateral paresthesias. It occurs primarily in young women. Because of the presenting symptoms, patients are often misdiagnosed as illicit drug or alcohol users.

Treatment. The two categories of medications, abortive and prophylactic, are used to treat migraine headaches (Table 9.4). Abortive medications have greater relevance to emergency medicine because these agents eliminate or alleviate headaches that have already begun. Prophylactic medications are taken on a regular basis to prevent or reduce the frequency of recurrent headaches. The use of prophylactic medications is appropriately managed in an outpatient setting, but a prophylactic medication can be started in the emergency department in a patient with a long history of migraine headaches.

Most patients seeking emergency care for migraine have not responded to first- or second-line home treatment: a dark, quiet room; nonsteroidal anti-inflammatory drugs with or without caffeine; oral ergotamines; oral opiates; and oral or rectal

TABLE 9.4. Medications for Treatment of Headaches

I. Abortive agents
A. Oral, sublingual or rectal

Medication	Dose
Aspirin	325–1950 mg
Acetaminophen	325–1300 mg
Naproxen	500–1000 mg
Ibuprofen	400–800 mg
Indomethacin	25–50 mg
Ketorolac	10 mg
Ergotamine tartrate/caffeine	1–3 mg ergotamine
Isometheptene/acetaminophen/ dichloralphenazone	325–975 mg acetaminophen
Sumatriptan	25–100 mg
Aspirin/butalbital/caffeine	325–650 mg aspirin
Acetaminophen/butalbital/caffeine	325–650 mg acetaminophen
Dexamethasone	4–8 mg
Ergotamine tartrate (sublingual)	2 mg
Ergotamine tartrate/caffeine (suppository)	0.5–2 mg ergotamine

B. Parenteral

Medication	Dose
Dihydroergotamine	0.5–1 mg IV (premedicate with 10 mg metoclopramide or prochlorphenazine)
Chlorpromazine	12.5–37.5 mg IV (slowly) or 25–50 mg IM
Prochlorphenazine	10 mg IV
Metoclopramide	10 mg IV
Sumatriptan (subcutaneous)	6 mg SQ
Ketorolac	30–60 mg IM
Dexamethasone	12–20 mg IV or IM may follow with prednisone taper: 60 mg × 1 d; 40 mg × 1 d; 20 mg × 1 d
Hydrocortisone	100–250 mg IV over 10 minutes may follow with prednisone taper: 60 mg on the first day; 40 mg on the second day; 20 mg on third day
Butorphanol	2 mg IM or intranasally
Oxygen	100% by mask at 8–10 l/min for 30 minutes

II. Selected prophylactic agents

Medication	Dose
Naproxen	250 mg bid–tid
Propanolol	20 mg tid–80 mg qid
Amitriptyline	25 mg qhs–150 mg qhs

phenothiazines. Frequently, parenteral medications are indicated, because severe nausea and vomiting make oral administration impossible or because pain has not responded to medications that the patient usually finds effective. The three agents most frequently used are sumatriptan, dihydroergotamine (DHE), and chlorpromazine.[7,33,44–48]

Sumatriptan, a specific 5-hydroxytryptamine (5-HT) receptor agonist, alleviates pain by constricting distended, edematous arteries and by decreasing release of vasoactive peptides, which, in turn, minimizes sterile inflammation within involved cerebral blood vessels. Sumatriptan is effective when administered subcutaneously, orally, or intranasally during an attack of migraine. In three trials, one of which involved self-administration of the drug, a subcutaneous dose of 6 mg resulted in improvement in 70–77% of patients within 1 hour of treatment, and in 81–86% of patients within 2 hours of treatment.[49–51] Nausea and vomiting were relieved in most patients within 1–2 hours of treatment, and the need for other analgesic medications was greatly reduced in patients treated with sumatriptan compared with those receiving placebo (12–20% versus 44–61%, respectively). A second subcutaneous injection of sumatriptan 1 hour after the first did not improve the outcome. Headache recurred in 38–46% of patients within 24 hours, probably related to the short half-life of the drug. A second dose can be tried in case of recurrence. The maximum dose consists of two 6 mg injections within 24 hours, with each administration separated by at least 1 hour.

Sumatriptan is initially given under medical supervision to those at risk for unrecognized coronary artery disease (CAD), such as postmenopausal women, men over 40 years of age, and patients with risk factors for CAD. The drug is contraindicated in patients with a history of myocardial infarction, symptomatic ischemic heart disease, Prinzmetal's angina, or hypertension. Pharmacy costs are about $30 per injection,[43] which makes this agent among the more expensive options to treat migraine. Oral and intranasal sumatriptan are alternative formulations available for use.[43]

As emergency treatment for migraine has deemphasized use of narcotic analgesic medications, there has been renewed interest in dihydroergotamine (DHE), another serotonin receptor agonist. It has fewer side effects than related ergotamine preparations (e.g., cafergot), although nausea, vomiting, diarrhea, and ischemic symptoms can be problematic. Up to 90% of attacks stop when the drug is given intravenously, but up to 26% of patients require additional doses because of recurrent headache.[52–54] In trials, DHE was given in combination with a phenothiazine, which is also beneficial when given alone. DHE is considered superior to both meperidine plus hydroxyzine and to butorphanol in controlled trials.

DHE can be administered by the intravenous, intramuscular, or subcutaneous route.[43] As with other ergotamines, it is contraindicated in patients with CAD, peripheral vascular disease, or uncontrolled hypertension. Dependency and rebound phenomena do not occur with DHE.

In addition to their role as antiemetics when administered with other antimigraine medications, metoclopramide, chlorpromazine, and prochlorperazine are themselves effective in reducing or eliminating migraine pain in most patients.[44,45,47] One study reported headache relief in 67% of patients given a 10-mg dose of metoclopramide intravenously, a nonphenothiazine central dopamine antagonist.[55] In other trials, chlorpromazine given in three intravenous injections of 0.1 mg per kilogram of body weight 15 minutes apart was more effective than meperidine in combination with dimenhydrinate.[56] Prochlorperazine, given in an intravenous dose of 10 mg, was found to be superior to placebo in another trial.[57] All three drugs offer an alternative to narcotics, DHE, and sumatriptan. Infrequent side effects include dystonia, tardive dyskinesia, drowsiness, nausea, vomiting, dizziness, and hypotension. The mechanism by which these dopamine-antagonists relieve headache remains to be determined. Adrenergic blockade, anti-5-HT receptor activity, antiemetic action, and modulation of pain systems have been hypothesized.

A simple analgesic or nonsteroidal anti-inflammatory drug is appropriate for mild to moderate attacks, with ergotamine or sumatriptan for moderate to severe attacks. Attacks that are severe, prolonged, and unresponsive to self-administered medication are treated in the emergency department. Treatment begins with sumatriptan given subcutaneously or DHE given intravenously or intramuscularly. When these measures fail, metoclopramide, prochlorperazine, or chlorpromazine can be used. Frequent acute attacks and intractable pain occasionally require hospitalization. In these cases, DHE given intravenously for 3–4 days along with intravenous fluids can be effective.[58]

Corticosteroids can also be effective, although the evidence is mainly anecdotal.[7,33,44,46] Parenteral corticosteroids administered in the emergency department, followed by a brief course of oral prednisone (60 mg on the first day, 40 mg on the second day, and 20 mg on the third day), may be particularly effective in "breaking" the headache in patients with a recent history of continuous headache for two weeks or longer.[44]

Use of narcotic analgesics to treat migraine headaches in the emergency department is generally avoided. A patient with chronic, recurrent headaches is at risk of developing chemical dependency. When used, the dose of narcotic is sufficient to control pain. A typical combination of meperidine and hydroxyzine is widely used.

Tension Headache

Tension headaches are typically described as a bilateral sensation of pressure or tightness, often occipital, nuchal, or involving the entire head. Many patients have features of migraine and tension headache. On examination, there can be scalp tenderness or palpable spasm of involved muscles. Treatment consists of mild analgesics such as acetaminophen, aspirin, or nonsteroidal anti-inflammatory drugs (NSAIDs), and occasionally sedatives and/or muscle relaxants. Narcotics are generally avoided. Many of the medications that are effective in treating migraine are also effective in treating tension headache. There is continued debate whether there is a difference in the pathophysiology of migraine and tension headache.

Cluster Headache

Distinct from patients with migraine, 90% of patients with cluster headaches are males, without any familial predisposition. Cluster headaches are diagnosed primarily on the basis of their distinctive temporal features.[13,59,60] Patients experience clusters of daily headaches for four to eight weeks, separated by headache-free intervals lasting months to years. Within these clusters, headaches can occur from once a day up to several times a day, and are common at night. One of the headaches usually occurs

at the same time each day. The headaches typically have an explosive onset and last from 30–120 minutes, with an average duration of 45 minutes. Headaches are unilateral and occur almost always on the same side of the head. Cluster headaches are unlike migraines, in which the affected side may vary from one headache to the next. Ipsilateral tearing and redness of the eye, rhinorrhea, nasal congestion, and occasionally an ipsilateral Horner's syndrome can be associated with cluster headaches. Infrequently migraine headaches can have these characteristics. Therefore, cluster headaches are not diagnosed unless the typical temporal features are present.[13,59,61] Vasodilators, particularly alcohol, can precipitate attacks, and sublingual nitroglycerine administered during the cluster period is a reliable provocative test.

Medications used to treat migraine headaches are also effective for treating cluster headaches. Sumatriptan and inhalation of 100% oxygen are the two most reliable treatment options for cluster headaches. Ergot agents tend to be ineffective.[13,47,59–61] Instillation of 5–10% cocaine solution or 4% lidocaine solution into the ipsilateral nostril (anesthetizing the sphenopalatine ganglion) may be effective.

Given the brief duration of cluster headaches, they often resolve by the time the patient undergoes evaluation in the emergency department. Consequently, there is often no need to abort the acute headache. Instead the goal is to abort the cluster, that is, to prevent the recurrence of headaches on subsequent days. Prophylactic agents used for migraine headaches can be tried, but methysergide and verapamil are used most often.[13,59–61] A standard alternative approach is to prescribe prednisone, 40–80 mg a day for a week followed by a rapid taper over several weeks.[13,59–61] Intranasal application of capsaicin ipsilateral to the headache has been advocated for prophylaxis but requires further trials.[47,60,61] Other prophylactic medication such as lithium has been advocated for use between clusters.

Chronic Paroxysmal Hemicrania

Chronic paroxysmal hemicrania is a rare condition characterized by headaches that resemble cluster headaches except for a very different temporal profile. These attacks last an average of 13 minutes (range, 3–46 minutes) and recur frequently throughout the day (4–38 attacks a day, average 14). The headaches usually occur daily throughout the year, with no tendency to cluster. The headaches are usually treated with indomethacin.[13,59,60] Other medications used for migraine headache can be tried.

Trigeminal Neuralgia (Tic Doloreaux)

Headaches can at times be located in the face. The diagnosis is based on the characteristics of the pain and the accompanying symptoms. Trigeminal neuralgia is a distinctive facial pain syndrome characterized by sudden, severe jabbing pains, usually in the distribution of the second and third branches of the fifth cranial nerve. The pain is described as excruciating, often like an electric shock. Each episode of pain lasts only seconds to minutes, but multiple episodes can occur, producing pain for hours. Trigger points are usually around the lips, ala nasae, nasolabial fold, or upper eyelid, and attacks are precipitated when these points are stimulated by pressure, facial movements, or emotional excitement. The simple act of shaving, teeth brushing, face washing, eating, or drinking can cause an attack.

Trigeminal neuralgia, usually a benign condition, primarily affects individuals over 50 years of age. It can be associated with structural or inflammatory lesions of the fifth cranial nerve, so a dental evaluation and MRI of the brainstem are indicated, especially in younger patients. Parenteral analgesics are commonly required for pain control in the emergency department. First-line treatment consists of the use of carbamazepine, starting at a dose of 100 mg two or three times per day, and gradually increasing as necessary.[62] Baclofen or clonazepam can be added when carbamazepine monotherapy fails.[62] Use of phenytoin, amitriptyline, valproate, and clonazepam is also advocated.[62] When medical therapy fails, selective sectioning or decompression of the Gasserion ganglion through a posterior fossa craniotomy may be necessary.

Other Causes of Facial Pain

Glossopharyngeal neuralgia is similar to trigeminal neuralgia but occurs much less frequently.[13,63] The pain typically begins in the oropharynx and extends upward and backward toward the ear. It is treated with the same medications used for trigeminal neuralgia.

TMJ disease, also known as Kostin's syndrome, is considered when headaches are provoked or exacerbated by chewing. Associated features include localized facial pain in front and back of the ear, muscle tenderness, joint crepitus and limited jaw motion, facial tenderness, and easy dislocation of the TMJ. Treatment is directed toward relieving the muscle spasm and inflammation. In addition to the medications used for migraine/tension headaches or trigeminal neuralgia, these patients may require modification of diet, jaw prostheses, or even oral surgery.[13]

Acute sinusitis frequently presents with localized headache or facial pain overlying and surrounding the involved sinus or sinuses. Fever and chills are frequently present. Many patients report upper respiratory tract symptoms and posture-related changes in discomfort. Commonly, a history of pain or pressure on awakening is reported. These symptoms resolve as the day progresses, presumably as a result of posture-related drainage. Physical examination usually reveals localized facial tenderness with percussion or palpation over the involved sinus or sinuses. Purulent material can be observed surrounding the nasal turbinates. Although sinus radiographs sometimes demonstrate opacification, an air-fluid level, or mucosal thickening, they are frequently normal in patients with acute sinusitis.

Headache from Central Nervous System Infection

Headache, fever, and a stiff neck suggest the presence of meningitis or encephalitis. An emergency LP is indicated for diagnostic purposes. When historical or physical findings suggest increased ICP or a mass lesion, diagnostic LP is preceded by CT scan of the brain. When clinically indicated, antibiotic therapy is initiated prior to diagnostic studies.

The presentation of a brain abscess is similar to that of an expanding intracranial mass. In addition to headache, occurrence of fever, nausea, vomiting, and seizure is common. An emergency CT scan of the brain precedes LP when brain abscess is suspected. Treatment usually consists of surgical drainage, administration of appropriate antibiotics, and supportive care.

Temporal Arteritis

Also called giant cell arteritis, temporal arteritis is an inflammatory disease predominantly of the extracranial portions of the cerebrovascular circulation. It occurs very rarely in individuals under 50 years of age, and typically presents with malaise, weight loss, low-grade fever, and headache. Since it is commonly found in association with polymyalgia rheumatica, patients can also complain of proximal joint or muscle pains.

The most important laboratory finding is a markedly elevated ESR, usually greater than 60, and frequently as high as 100. Temporal artery biopsy is diagnostic when it reveals granulomatous arteritis. Temporal arteritis is rarely fatal, but a severe complication is permanent visual loss, which can be bilateral, due to optic nerve ischemia from inflammation of the ciliary arteries. Therapy is instituted immediately in patients with suspicious historical or physical findings associated with an elevated ESR. Prednisone, in dosages of 60–100 mg per day, is recommended for initial treatment to prevent visual loss. NSAIDs are administered for pain relief. Long-term (i.e., six months) corticosteroid therapy is usually indicated. For this reason, it is important that the patient is referred for temporal artery biopsy within three to five days. However, the initiation of prednisone is not delayed for biopsy.

Headache Associated with Mass Lesions

Epidural Hematoma. A typical history is that of head injury and a brief period of unconsciousness, followed by a return to normal mental status. Subsequent expansion of the hematoma over a period of minutes to hours pushes the dura inward. This causes a severe, diffuse, constant headache, pupillary dilation, hemiplegia, and eventually obtundation and brain herniation when not treated surgically. Epidural hematoma carries a 25–50% mortality rate, largely because of delays in diagnosis. Immediate neurosurgical consultation is required.

Subdural Hematoma. SDH is characterized by depression of mental status disproportionate to focal findings, with a headache of variable quality. Chronic SDH is frequently seen in the elderly after a forgotten minor head injury. Atraumatic SDHs have been reported but are rare. Symptoms are vague, and include general weakness and frequent falls. Patients with acute SDH are often too obtunded to complain of headache. CT scanning generally confirms the diagnosis.

Brain Tumors. Almost two-thirds of patients with a brain tumor complain of headache. Brain tumors above the tentorium typically produce pain referred to the frontal region or vertex, while infratentorial lesions cause pain in the occipital region. A new or unfamiliar headache associated with nausea and vomiting, headache (pain) upon awakening, and pain that is exacerbated with the Valsalva maneuver can indicate an intracranial mass.[64] Vomiting that precedes headache by weeks is suggestive of posterior fossa tumors. The initial examination is frequently without focal findings. Diagnosis is made by CT scanning without and with contrast.

Postconcussive Headache

Postconcussive headache follows trauma by hours to days. Associated symptoms include vertigo, nausea, vomiting, difficulty in concentration, and mood alterations. Duration of symptoms is variable and correlates poorly with the severity of head injury. Physical examination and CT scanning are normal. These headaches are usually self-limiting, but NSAIDs may be beneficial.

Post–Dural-Puncture Headache

The typical post–dural-puncture ("spinal") headache is described as severe, dull, nonthrobbing pain. It is usually fronto-occipital in location, is aggravated by standing, and improves by lying supine. It occurs within 48–72 hours after LP, and can be associated with nausea, vomiting, dizziness, tinnitus, or visual changes. The persistent leakage of CSF from the dura, and subsequent traction upon intracranial pain-sensitive structures is considered to be the etiology of spinal headaches.

Female gender and an age between 20 and 40 years are independent risk factors for spinal headache.[65,66] The incidence of spinal headache is directly proportional to the diameter of the needle used. A 36% incidence of headache using a 22-gauge needle versus a 12% incidence using a 26-gauge needle was observed in one study.[67] The incidence of headache also depends on bevel alignment and the design of the needle tip.

Although supine position and bed rest do not prevent such headaches, they decrease the severity of symptoms once the headache has occurred. Correcting hypovolemia and administering analgesics are the primary treatments of mild spinal headache.

Methylxanthines, such as caffeine, theophylline, or their derivatives, are effective in diminishing the symptoms in 75–85% of patients.[65] When conservative measures fail, an epidural patch can tamponade the dural leak and is 90–100% effective.[66]

Benign Intracranial Hypertension

Pseudotumor cerebri or idiopathic intracranial hypertension (see Chapter 27, "Idiopathic Intracranial Hypertension") is a condition in which CSF pressure is elevated without the presence of an intracranial mass lesion or obstruction to CSF pathways. Usually idiopathic, the condition has been described as a side effect of vitamin A, tetracycline, or steroid use. The cause is uncertain but likely due to defective CSF absorption by the arachnoid villi. Typically, patients are young, obese women and present with generalized headache and papilledema. The neurological examination is usually normal, with the exception of papilledema, although unilateral or bilateral sixth nerve palsies can be present. The CT scan is normal or shows small ventricles. CSF pressure is elevated. Repeated LPs with evacuation of measured quantities of CSF in order to reduce CSF pressure may be utilized but has unproven long term benefits. A diuretic such as acetazolamide is also used. In selected patients, a CSF shunt system may be required to prevent blindness.

Toxic Metabolic Headaches

Toxic metabolic headaches are nonrecurrent, nonmigrainous, throbbing headaches. Fever is an extremely common cause of headache. However, the possibility of meningeal infection is considered. Foods containing tyramine, monosodium glutamate, or sodium nitrate can precipitate throbbing headache of a migrainous or nonmigrainous nature. Toxic metabolic headaches are common with withdrawal of caffeine-containing beverages such as coffee, tea, and cola. Both ingestion and withdrawal from alcohol can result in headaches. The latter cause is more frequent and results from breakdown of ethanol to acetaldehyde, a potent vasodilator. Commonly used medications, such as oral contraceptives, indomethacin, and nitroglycerine, can result in headache. Hypoglycemia may cause throbbing headache as an early symptom. Hypoxia, anoxia, and hypercapnia can dilate cerebral vessels with resultant headache.

Carbon monoxide poisoning can cause a diffuse, pulsatile headache accompanied by nausea, vomiting, dizziness, and blurred vision. The headache worsens in severity as serum carbon monoxide concentration rises, until obtundation occurs. High-altitude headache, probably related to cerebral edema, can occur in nonacclimatized mountain climbers at 10,000–12,000 feet above sea level.

Headache secondary to postictal vascular distension can occur after a generalized seizure. When the headache character is different from prior postictal headaches, further investigation is warranted. Severe anemia can result in headache, caused by relative lack of oxygen and pronounced vasodilation.

Definitive treatment of most toxic metabolic headaches is removal of the underlying cause, with analgesic supplementation, as needed.

Miscellaneous Causes of Headache

Acute narrow-angle glaucoma presents with severe headache, associated with nausea, vomiting, blurred vision, and colored haloes around light. Physical examination reveals ciliary injection, an edematous cornea and a semidilated, vertically oval, sluggishly reactive pupil. Shiotz or applanation tonometry reveals elevated pressure.

Postcoital headache is a male-dominated (M:F = 4:1) syndrome. This headache is very abrupt in onset, occurs periorgasmically, and subsides in a few minutes after coitus is interrupted. These headaches are usually benign events, but SAH can present in a similar manner, and prudent clinical judgment prevails in the management of these episodes.

Pediatric Headaches

Headache is a common presenting symptom in children. In a study of 8993 schoolchildren, headache prevalence increased from 39% at 6 years of age to over 70% by age 15. Migraine prevalence, equal in boys and girls, is approximately 4%.[68] The history includes information on pregnancy, labor, delivery, growth and development, academic performance, behavior, and any previous neurological problems.[69] A headache accompanied by fever, lethargy, meningeal signs, or other neurological abnormalities is investigated appropriately. Muscle contraction is the most common cause of chronic headache in the pediatric population. Migraine in children usually resolves within a few hours and is typically relieved by vomiting. Migraine variants without headache are more common in children than in adults.[68] Some children experience cyclical vomiting, and many have a history of motion sickness. In very young children (2–6 years), alarming episodes of paroxysmal vertigo can occur. Organic causes of vertigo are excluded before the symptom is attributed to migraine.

Sinusitis is suspected in children with respiratory symptoms and an acute or chronic headache. Systemic illnesses such as upper respiratory infections also cause headaches. Resolution of the headache parallels improvement in the systemic illness.

PEARLS AND PITFALLS

- Focus on the "unprecedented" headaches, not the "worst" headaches.
- Headache can represent a minor or catastrophic illness.
- SAH and bacterial meningitis cannot be distinguished on clinical grounds.
- LP can be performed safely in most cases without obtaining a CT scan of the brain. Patients with severe headache associated with papilledema, focal neurological deficits, or alteration of mental status require neuroimaging prior to LP.
- The most reliable way to distinguish SAH from a traumatic spinal tap is to examine the CSF for xanthochromia.
- Temporal arteritis is considered in a patient over 50 years of age with severe headache of recent onset.
- Most migraine headaches can be aborted with parenteral sumatriptan, dihydroergotamine, or dopamine receptor antagonists (chlorpromazine, prochlorperazine, and metoclopramide).
- Hypertension is evaluated and managed cautiously in patients with headache. Headache can be a manifestation of a hypertensive emergency; however, hypertension can also result from primary brain pathology, in which case aggressive treatment can sometimes be harmful.
- When bacterial meningitis is suspected, parenteral antibiotics are not delayed for a CT scan or for any other reason. If a CT scan is required prior to LP (because of papilledema or major fo-

cal abnormalities), a dose of empirical antibiotics is administered. An LP is performed as soon as possible, adding antibiotic inhibitors to the culture medium.

- Normal body temperature does not exclude bacterial meningitis, especially in older patients.
- A normal CT scan of the brain does not exclude the diagnosis of SAH.

REFERENCES

1. Dhopesh V, Anwar R, Herring C. A retrospective assessment of emergency department patients with complaint of headache. *Headache.* 1979;19:37–42.
2. Dickman RL, Masten T. The management of non-traumatic headache in a university hospital emergency room. *Headache.* 1979;19:391–6.
3. Leicht MJ. Non-traumatic headache in the emergency department. *Ann Emerg Med.* 1980;9:404–9.
4. Barton CW. Evaluation and treatment of headache patients in the emergency department: a survey. *Headache.* 1994;34:91–4.
5. Samuels MA. The splitting headache: listen carefully. *Emerg Med.* 1991;23;24:22–36.
6. Henry GL. Headache. In: Rosen P, Barkin RM, Braen CR, et al., eds. *Emergency Medicine – Concepts and Clinical Practice.* 3rd ed. St. Louis, Mo: CV Mosby; 1992:1751–65.
7. Edmeads JF. Emergency management of headache. *Headache.* 1988;28:675–9.
8. Callaham M, Raskin NH. Management of acute headache in the emergency department. ACEP Monograph; 1992.
9. Healton EB, Brust JC, Feinfeld DA, Thomson GE. Hypertensive encephalopathy and the neurologic manifestations of malignant hypertension. *Neurology.* 1982; 32:127–32.
10. Calhoun DA, Oparil S. Treatment of hypertensive crisis. *N Engl J Med.* 1990;323:1177–83.
11. Elliott WJ. Malignant hypertension. In: Hall JB, Schmidt GA, Wood LDH, eds. *Principles of Critical Care.* New York, NY: McGraw-Hill Book Co; 1992:1563–71.
12. Dalessio DJ. *Wolff's Headache and Other Head Pain.* 6th ed. New York, NY: Oxford University Press; 1993.
13. Raskin NH. *Headache.* 2nd ed. New York, NY: Churchill Livingstone; 1988.
14. Moskowitz MA. Neurogenic inflammation in the pathophysiology and treatment of migraine. *Neurology.* 1993;43(suppl 3):S16–S20.
15. Silberstein SD. Evaluation and emergency treatment of headache. *Headache.* 1992;32:396–407.
16. Dalessio DJ. Diagnosing the severe headache. *Neurology.* 1994;44(suppl 3):S6–S12.
17. Little N. Acute head pain. *Emerg Med Clin North Am.* 1987;5:687–98.

18. Sengupta RP, McAllister VL, Gates P. Differential diagnosis. In: Sengupta RD, McAllister VL, eds. *Subarachnoid Haemorrhage.* Berlin, Germany: Springer-Verlag; 1986:79–92.

19. Maurice-Williams RS. *Subarachnoid Haemorrhage: Aneurysms and Vascular Malformations of the Central Nervous System.* Bristol, England: Wright; 1987:83–100.

20. Weir B. Headaches from aneurysms. *Cephalalgia.* 1994;14:79–87.

21. Overturf GD. Pyogenic bacterial infections of the CNS. *Neurol Clin.* 1986;4:69–90.

22. Roos KL, Tunkel AR, Scheld WM. Acute bacterial meningitis in children and adults. In: Scheld WM, Whitley RJ, Durack DT, eds. *Infections of the Central Nervous System.* New York, NY: Raven Press, Ltd; 1991.

23. Durand ML, Calderwood SB, Weber DJ, et al. Acute bacterial meningitis in adults. A review of 493 episodes. *N Engl J Med.* 1993;328:21–8.

24. Ashwal S. Neurologic evaluation of the patient with acute bacterial meningitis. *Neurol Clin.* 1985;13:549–77.

25. Behrman RE, Meyers BR, Mendelson MH, Sacks HS, Hirschman SZ. Central nervous system infections in the elderly. *Arch Intern Med.* 1989;149:1596–9.

26. Kassell NF, Torner JC, Haley EC, Jane JA, Adams HP, Kongable GL. The international cooperative study on the timing of aneurysm surgery, I: overall management results. *J Neurosurg.* 1990;73:18–36.

27. Kistler JP, Gress DR, Crowell RM, Pile-Spellman J, Heros RC. Management of subarachnoid hemorrhage. In: Ropper AH, ed. *Neurological and Neurosurgical Intensive Care.* 3rd ed. New York, NY: Raven Press, Ltd; 1993:291–307.

28. Tourtellotte WW, Metz LN, Bryan ER, DeJong RN. Spontaneous subarachnoid hemorrhage. Factors affecting the rate of clearing of the cerebrospinal fluid. *Neurology.* 1964;14:301–6.

29. Macdonald A, Mendelow AD. Xanthochromia revisited: a re-evaluation of lumbar puncture and CT scanning in the diagnosis of subarachnoid haemorrhage. *J Neurol Neurosurg Psychiatry.* 1988;51:342–4.

30. Weaver JP, Fisher M. Subarachnoid hemorrhage: an update of pathogenesis, diagnosis, and management. *J Neurol Sci.* 1994;125:119–31.

31. Miller J, Diringer M. Management of aneurysmal subarachnoid hemorrhage. *Neurol Clin.* 1995;13:451–78.

32. Mitchell CS, Osborn RE, Grosskreutz SR. Computed tomography in the headache patient: is routine evaluation really necessary? *Headache.* 1993;33:82–6.

33. Rapoport AM, Silberstein SD. Emergency treatment of headache. *Neurology.* 1992;42(suppl 2):S43–S44.

34. Edmeads JF. Challenges in the diagnosis of acute headache. *Headache.* 1990;30(suppl 2):537–40.

35. Ad Hoc Committee on Classification of Headache. Classification of headache. *JAMA.* 1962;179:717–18.

36. Headache Classification Committee of the International Headache Society. Classification and diagnostic criteria for headache disorders, cranial neuralgias and facial pain. *Cephalalgia.* 1988;8(suppl 7):1–96.

37. Diamond S, Dalessio DJ, eds. *The Practicing Physician's Approach to the Headache Patient,* 5th ed. Baltimore, Md: Williams & Wilkins; 1992.

38. Fontanarosa PB. Recognition of subarachnoid hemorrhage. *Ann Emerg Med.* 1989;18:199–205.

39. Duffy GP. The "warning leak" in spontaneous subarachnoid hemorrhage. *Med J Aust.* 1983;1:514–16.

40. Meyer FB, Morita A, Puumala MR, Nichols DA. Medical and surgical management of intracranial aneurysms. *Mayo Clin Proc.* 1995;70:153–72.

41. Pickard JD, Murray GD, Illingworth R, et al. Effect of oral nimodipine on cerebral infarction and outcome after SAH: British aneurysm nimodipine trial. *Br Med J.* 1989;298:636–42.

42. Diamond S. Head pain: diagnosis and management. *Clin Symp.* 1994;46:2–34.

43. Caesar R. Acute headache management: the challenge of deciphering etiologies to guide assessment and treatment. *Emerg Med Reports.* 1995;16:117–27.

44. Spierings ELH. Management of acute headache in the emergency department. *Neurology Chronicle* 1993;3: 1–5.

45. Raskin NH. Acute and prophylactic treatment of migraine: practical approaches and pharmacologic rationale. *Neurology.* 1993;43(suppl 3):S39–S42.

46. Foley JJ. Pharmacologic treatment of acute migraine and related headaches in the emergency department. *J Emerg Nurs.* 1993;19:225–30.

47. Kumar KL. Recent advances in the acute management of migraine and cluster headaches. *J Gen Intern Med.* 1994;9:339–48.

48. Ferrari MD, Haan J. Acute treatment of migraine attacks. *Curr Opin Neurol* 1995;8:237–42.

49. Ferrari MD. The subcutaneous sumatriptan international study group. Treatment of migraine attacks with sumatriptan. *N Engl J Med.* 1991;325:316–21.

50. Sumatriptan Auto-Injector Study Group. Self-treatment of acute migraine with subcutaneous sumatriptan using an auto-injector device. *Eur Neurol.* 1991;31: 323–31.

51. Cady RK, Wendt JK, Kirchner JR, Rothrock JF, Skaggs H Jr, Sargent JD. Treatment of acute migraine with subcutaneous sumatriptan. *JAMA.* 1991;265:2831–5.

52. Callaham M, Raskin N. A controlled study of dihydroergotamine in the treatment of acute migraine headache. *Headache.* 1986;26:168–71.

53. Saadah HA. Abortive headache therapy in the office with intravenous dihydroergotamine in the treatment of acute migraine headache. *Headache.* 1992;32: 143–6.

54. Klapper JA, Stanton J. Current emergency treatment of severe migraine headaches. *Headache.* 1993;33:560–2.

55. Tek DS, McLellan DS, Olshaker JS, Allen CL, Arthur DC. A prospective, double-blind study of metoclopramide hydrochloride for the control of migraine in

the emergency department. *Ann Emerg Med.* 1990; 19:1083–7.

56. Lane PL, McClellan BA, Baggoley CJ. Comparative efficacy of chlorpromazine and meperidine with dimenhydrinate in migraine headache. *Ann Emerg Med.* 1989;18:360–5.

57. Jones S, Sklar D, Dougherty J, White W. Randomized double-blind trial of intravenous prochlorperazine for the treatment of acute headache. *JAMA.* 1989;261: 1174–6.

58. Raskin NH. Repetitive intravenous dihydroergotamine as therapy for intractable migraine. *Neurology.* 1986;36:995.

59. Kudrow L. Diagnosis and treatment of cluster headache. *Med Clin North Am.* 1991;75:579–94.

60. Stovner LJ, Sjaastad O. Treatment of cluster headache and its variants. *Curr Opin Neurol.* 1995;8:243–7.

61. Mathew NT. Cluster headache. *Neurology.* 1992;42 (suppl 2):22–31.

62. Green MW, Selman JE. Review article: *The Medical Management of Trigeminal Neuralgia. Headache.* 1991; 31:588–92.

63. Dalessio DJ. Diagnosis and treatment of cranial neuralgias. *Med Clin North Am.* 1991;75:605–15.

64. Hoffman GL. Headache. In: Tintinalli JE, Krome RL, Ruiz E, eds. *Emergency Medicine – A Comprehensive Study Guide.* 3rd ed. New York, NY: McGraw-Hill Book Co; 1992:789–92.

65. Leibold RA, Yealy DM, Cappola M, Cantees KK. Post-dural-puncture headache: characteristics, management, and prevention. *Ann Emerg Med.* 1993;22: 1863–70.

66. Morewood GH. A rational approach to the cause, prevention and treatment of postdural puncture headache. *Can Med Assoc J.* 1993;149:1087–93.

67. Tourtellotte WW, Henderson WG, Tucker RP, et al. A randomized, double-blind clinical trial comparing the 22 versus 26 gauge needle in the production of the post-lumbar puncture syndrome in normal individuals. *Headache.* 1972;12:73–8.

68. Bille B. Migraine in school children. *Acta Pediatr.* 1962;51(suppl 136):3–151.

69. Silberstein SD. Twenty questions about headaches in children and adolescents. *Headache.* 1990;30:716–24.

70. Brillman JD. Headache. In: Hamilton GC, Trott AT, Sanders AB, Strange GR, eds. *Emergency Medicine: An Approach to Clinical Problem-Solving.* Philadelphia, Pa: WB Saunders Co; 1991:830–46.

10 Weakness

GEORGE A. SMALL AND LYNN BROWN

SUMMARY Few complaints in emergency medicine are as ill-defined and difficult to evaluate as weakness. The chief complaint of weakness requires a focused history and physical examination to localize the cause and to generate a rational differential diagnosis. Determination of the distribution of symptoms, directed questioning regarding associated symptoms, and the presence of upper or lower motor neuron signs usually results in an expeditious differential diagnosis. Weakness due to brain or spinal cord lesions requires acute intervention. Neuromuscular junction and myopathic causes of weakness tend to present insidiously, and impending respiratory failure is not always apparent on examination. A low forced vital capacity, excessive drooling, and increased respiratory rate with normal arterial blood gases are indications for admission and close observation, and possible ventilatory support.

Introduction

Weakness is defined as a condition involving muscles that cannot exert a normal force.[1] This is in contrast to *fatigue,* a vague complaint that is best defined as a diminution in strength with repetitive actions. Most patients respond affirmatively to questions about whether they are weak, because they may interpret pain, cramping, fatigue, depression, and psychiatric issues as weakness. It is important that there is a correct understanding by the patient and the emergency physician when the terms *weakness* and *fatigue* are used. The inability to perform a specific normal activity suggests weakness, and can be readily distinguished from loss of stamina or endurance (Fig. 10.1). General questions about difficulties in combing one's hair, climbing stairs, reaching with hands over head to arrange shelves, squatting, standing, or carrying heavy objects can elicit evidence of proximal upper or lower extremity weakness. Questions regarding tripping over objects or curbs while walking, difficulty buttoning one's clothes, or writing or performing other fine motor tasks with the hands can provide evidence of distal upper or lower extremity weakness. Complaints of choking, double vision, drooping eyelids, or slurred speech can provide objective evidence of impaired function of the brainstem, cranial nerves, or cranial muscles resulting in weakness. Thus a well-taken patient history can yield a focused differential diagnosis that can avoid unneeded and expensive laboratory testing.

Emergency Department Evaluation

Medical History

Onset. Acute onset of weakness refers to a progression of symptoms within minutes or hours, and is more frequently associated with vascular, metabolic, or toxic etiologies. Rapid onset of weakness refers to a beginning and progression of weakness within the first 24 hours, and is usually indicative of metabolic or toxic disorders, stroke, acute polyneuropathies, and the periodic paralyses. Subacute weakness is that which progresses over the course of less than a week and commonly occurs with disorders involving the peripheral nerve or the neu-

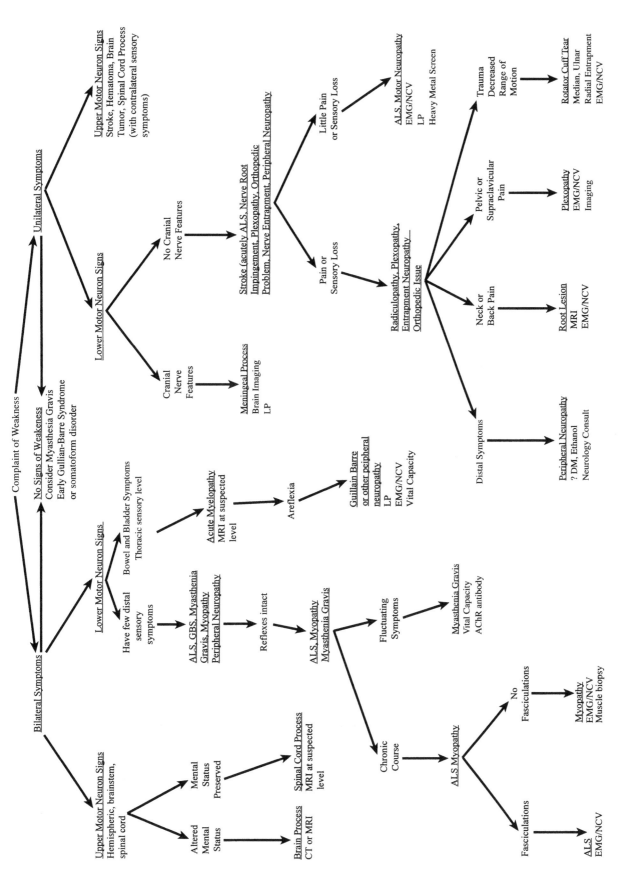

FIGURE 10.1. Diagnostic approach to weakness.

romuscular junction. Slowly progressive weakness evolves over the course of weeks and months, sometimes even a year or more, and is more likely to be associated with chronic myopathy and polyneuropathy. When the weakness is unilateral, spinal cord or brain dysfunction from slow-growing neoplasms is suspected.

Acute-onset symptoms resulting in generalized weakness are frequently due to metabolic or toxic disorders of muscle or the neuromuscular junction. Sudden alterations in critical electrolytes resulting in hypokalemia, hypocalcemia, hypermagnesemia, or hypophosphatemia can cause weakness with a proximal muscle predominance, or quadriplegia and respiratory compromise. Toxins, either synthetic or elaborated by organisms such as *Clostridium botulinum,* can alter neural transmission to the point of moderate to severe quadriparesis with respiratory compromise. Stroke is the main vascular cause of acute onset of weakness.

Rapid-onset weakness can occur in those disorders associated with acute-onset weakness and acute inflammatory myopathies (especially viral or parasitic), and acute polyneuropathies such as Guillain-Barré syndrome or acute porphyric neuropathy. In addition, muscle weakness caused by defective neuromuscular transmission, as in myasthenia gravis and tick paralysis, can occur over a 24-hour period.

Subacute weakness includes disorders of neuromuscular transmission, Guillain-Barré syndrome, and acute porphyric neuropathy. The toxin elaborated by the diphtheria bacterium can produce subacute weakness; however, this problem is virtually unknown in developed nations where immunization programs are routine.

Slowly progressive proximal weakness occurs in polymyositis, dermatomyositis, and steroid-resistant inflammatory myopathy – the latter called inclusion body myositis, a disorder that occurs primarily in the elderly, resulting in proximal upper and lower extremity weakness, favoring weakness of the finger flexors. These disorders are insidious, and frequently only an approximation of onset time can be obtained from the patient. These patients typically present after stressful events such as surgery or infection. The initial manifestation of these disorders can be unexpected respiratory failure. Muscular dystrophies, primary disorders of motor nerves such as spinal muscular atrophies, and am-

yotrophic lateral sclerosis are considered when symptoms have been present for months, years, or lifelong. Insidious peripheral neuropathies that usually have a distribution of distal, greater-than-proximal weakness are typically due to diabetes and alcoholism.

Slowly progressive distal weakness is usually secondary to peripheral nerve or anterior horn cell disorders, especially diabetic and alcoholic polyneuropathy and amyotrophic lateral sclerosis. The commonly encountered distal myopathy is myotonic dystrophy (the muscular dystrophy most common in adults).

Slowly progressive cranial musculature weakness demonstrated by difficulty in speaking, coughing, or swallowing is more typical of amyotrophic lateral sclerosis and myasthenia gravis. Patients with other myopathies – such as dominantly inherited oculopharyngeal muscular dystrophy, myotonic dystrophy, polymyositis, and dermatomyositis – present to the emergency department less commonly.

Location. Location of symptoms is divided into three categories: proximal, distal, and cranial. Each of these locations is further subdivided into symmetrical and asymmetrical categories. Proximal weakness is typical of inherited diseases of motor neurons, the rare spinal muscular atrophies. Inherited myopathies in this category are rarely encountered in the emergency department. Patients generally report proximal muscle weakness as trouble combing their hair, arising from a chair, toilet, or bathtub, or climbing stairs. All these motions require force from the hip girdle or periscapular musculature and can be referred to as proximal. Patients can perform the Gower's maneuver when arising from the floor – utilizing one or more supports as they "walk" themselves up their own bodies by placing their hands on their knees and thighs and finally onto a nearby object in order to stand. Scapular winging is noted as shoulder girdle weakness progresses due to a disease process of nerve or muscle. Inspection may reveal a trapezius hump formed by high-riding scapulae, downsloping clavicles, and loss of muscle mass in the neck.

Distal weakness is found when patients complain of difficulty with manipulating small objects, typing, buttoning clothes, or dragging a foot or tripping over a curb or a high-pile rug. Patients with distal weakness who present to the emergency department because of a broken bone or a contusion may later be diagnosed with a primary nerve or muscle problem; occasionally, this problem is incorrectly attributed to old age or clumsiness. Frequent falls or stumbles can be associated with a marchlike gait due to foot drop from nerve or muscle weakness. Distal weakness without sensory loss is frequently found in patients with amyotrophic lateral sclerosis. Distal weakness accompanied by sensory loss is characteristic of peripheral neuropathy or a mononeuropathy such as a peroneal neuropathy at the fibular head. Unilateral upper or lower extremity proximal or distal weakness can be associated with a brain or spinal cord process such as stroke or neoplasm.

Cranial weakness affecting the extraocular, facial, and oropharyngeal muscles, frequently occurring as ptosis, ophthalmoparesis, and diplopia can suggest two disorders of the neuromuscular junction: myasthenia gravis and botulism. Dysphagia occurs with these disorders and amyotrophic lateral sclerosis. Patients with brainstem or meningeal processes such as stroke, neoplasia, or carcinomatous meningitis can present with isolated cranial musculature weakness.

Duration. Symptom duration is important but can be difficult to establish accurately in the emergency department. Frequent relapses and remissions suggests myasthenia gravis, periodic paralysis, or multiple sclerosis.

Radiation. Radiation of stabbing, "electric-like" pain is likely to be associated with nerve trauma or entrapment that can also result in weakness. This weakness is usually evident to the examining physician. However, pain is usually not associated with the weakness of most neuromuscular disorders. Muscle cramps are a hallmark of amyotrophic lateral sclerosis and can be misrepresented as numbness or pain by the patient. Symptoms such as cramping, or "charley horse," can alert the emergency physician to disorders of the motor neuron or metabolic myopathies.

Intensity. The degree of weakness is documented for the benefit of other examiners and to provide evidence of improvement or worsening in the patient's condition. A correct diagnosis may be made only several days or weeks after an initial emergency department evaluation. Objective evidence of fluctuating strength suggests disorders of the neuromuscular junction, somatoform disorders, or malingering.

The Medical Research Council (MRC) of Great Britain 0–5 scale is the most frequently used documentation format for grading weakness. It requires the examiner to have sufficient experience to understand strength differences among patients related to age, sex, and debilitation. Utilization also requires a highly motivated subject. Although the scale is a crude form of measurement, it provides a baseline of the patient's weakness. Each muscle group is evaluated separately and is given a numerical designation: 5 indicates normal; 4 indicates the ability to oppose gravity plus resistance; 3 indicates the ability to move fully against gravity but not against resistance; 2 indicates the ability to move with gravity eliminated; 1 indicates trace movement; and 0 indicates no movement.

Associated Symptoms. Symptoms that can be associated with weakness include pain and cramping, stiffness, muscle twitching, atrophy, and hypertrophy. The collagen-vascular diseases and inflammatory myopathies are likely to produce myalgia, which is best defined as spontaneous muscle pain or tenderness, and muscle pain to touch. However, the absence of these symptoms does not exclude the diagnosis of an inflammatory myopathy. Polymyalgia rheumatica is considered in older patients complaining of pain, achiness, and stiffness. This disease does not cause true weakness, however. A high sedimentation rate, normal neurological examination, and rapid clinical response to low-dose steroids usually confirm the diagnosis. Muscle cramps are prolonged involuntary contractions of muscle fibers and can be defined by their characteristic electrical discharges on electromyography. Although usually benign, they occur with hypothyroidism, overuse, hypocalcemia, hypomagnesemia, metabolic or respiratory alkalosis, amyotrophic lateral sclerosis, and certain metabolic myopathies. Sensory symptoms suggest peripheral nerve disorders but can be associated with disorders of the brain and spinal cord. Intermittent muscle pain associated with exercise can be associated with disorders of substrate metabolism such as glycogen storage diseases or disorders of fatty acid metabolism. Dark urine that tests positive for blood with no red blood cells observed by microscopy is assessed for myoglobulin. Myoglobinuria can result from the muscle breakdown associated with some metabolic disorders, and occasionally in polymyositis and dermatomyositis.

Relieving Factors. Patients typically describe weakness improving with rest. However, it is important to determine whether this represents normal physiological fatigue or improved strength, which occurs in myasthenia gravis after muscle rest. Double vision or ptosis that is inapparent or minimal on awakening and appears or worsens throughout the day is myasthenia gravis, until proven otherwise.

Precipitating Factors. The patient's medical history is important in generating an accurate differential diagnosis of weakness in the emergency department. A history of risk factors for stroke, including smoking, hypertension, hypercholesterolemia, diabetes, and congestive heart failure, provides important information. Diuretic use with or without poor nutrition can result in electrolyte disturbances resulting in weakness. A psychiatric history, especially of somatoform disorders, can lead to an important distinction between organic and nonorganic causes of weakness. A history of rheumatoid arthritis, lupus, cancer, hypo- or hyperthyroidism, adrenal insufficiency, Cushing's syndrome, or parathyroid disorders can help to formulate a reasonable differential diagnosis. Knowledge of the patient's human immunodeficiency virus (HIV) status is important in evaluating weakness, because Guillain-Barré syndrome, chronic inflammatory demyelinating polyneuropathy (CIDP), myelopathy, and myopathy occur with higher frequency in these patients.

Family medical history is critical in determining whether the patient has a hereditary cause of weakness, including autosomal dominantly inherited myotonic muscular dystrophy and autosomal dominantly inherited peripheral neuropathies formerly known as the Charcot-Marie-Tooth diseases. X-linked inheritance of muscle weakness can suggest Duchenne's muscular dystrophy or its less severe variant, the Becker form of muscular dystrophy, which is compatible with longer life. Metabolic disorders of muscle, including glycogen and lipid storage diseases, are frequently autosomal recessive dis-

orders. A family history of endocrine disorders is relevant. Multiple sclerosis and amyotrophic lateral sclerosis are inherited rarely.

Knowledge of current medication use can help exclude toxic peripheral nerve, neuromuscular junction, or muscle disorders, and disorders of the muscle membrane and spinal cord. Nitrous oxide abuse with or without associated vitamin B_{12} deficiency can cause an acute myelopathy. Cocaine and amphetamine ingestion can result in cerebral hemorrhage and stroke, with resulting weakness. Amiodarone, cisplatinum, Dapsone, disulfiram, isoniazid, metronidazole, pyridoxine, and vincristine can cause polyneuropathy with varying sensory and motor findings. Diuretic use can be associated with acute areflexic or hyporeflexic quadriplegia, as previously described. Cholesterol-lowering agents with 3-hydroxy-3-methylglutaryl (HMG) CoA-reductase activity cause a reversible myopathy associated with myotonic discharges recorded by electromyography. D-penicillamine can cause an acquired autoimmune neuromuscular junction disorder indistinguishable from myasthenia gravis.

Insect envenomations can result in an acute neuromuscular junction disorder with areflexia, as in tick paralysis, mimicking Guillain-Barré syndrome. Botulism results in a descending paralysis of cranial, then somatic and respiratory musculature with pupillary dilatation. When multiple cases of this clinical syndrome occur concomitantly, a search for a common source of the ingested botulinum toxin follows. A history of overseas travel in areas with known toxins from sea life result in an accurate diagnosis of paralysis resulting from these poisons.

Social History

The topic of drug abuse and alcohol abuse is reviewed. Alcohol abuse results in a high frequency of peripheral neuropathy and myopathy. Pentazocine use can cause myopathy.

Physical Examination

In the emergency department, the most serious presentation of weakness is usually that of acute respiratory failure of unknown cause. The three most common primary neurological causes of acute respiratory failure are previously unrecognized amyotrophic lateral sclerosis, myasthenia gravis, and Guillain-Barré syndrome. Each of these diseases is discussed below. Respiratory failure due to a neuromuscular cause is a form of restrictive pulmonary disease. This is distinct from respiratory failure due to chronic obstructive pulmonary disease (COPD). In COPD, due to a primary airway problem, the P_{CO_2} rises, heralding respiratory failure. In neuromuscular diaphragmatic and intercostal muscle weakness, ventilation–perfusion mismatch usually occurs over a period of days or weeks. Respiratory failure is not reflected in arterial blood gases until extremely late in the course of respiratory muscle failure. The precipitous rise in P_{CO_2} occurs with much greater rapidity and is not a reliable indicator of when to provide ventilatory support. A rapidly rising respiratory rate or a forced vital capacity of less than 1.0/l in a 60-kg patient (<15 cc/kg) indicates the likely need of endotracheal intubation.

Specific Conditions

The following causes of weakness commonly encountered in the emergency department are described to facilitate the localization of lesions in the neuraxis to the cerebral hemispheres, brainstem, spinal cord, nerve roots, peripheral nerves, neuromuscular junction, or muscles (see Chapter 18, "Neuromuscular Disorders"). Decisions regarding admission and monitoring are based on the cause and severity of the weakness.

Cerebral Hemispheric Lesions. Patients with primary intracranial hemorrhage, ischemic stroke, or expanding neoplasms commonly present to the emergency department with unilateral weakness of the face, arm, and leg. Abrupt onset signifies cerebral vascular disease of either ischemic or hemorrhagic cause. These unilateral symptoms can be accompanied by sensory impairment. Although hyporeflexia usually occurs acutely, within several hours spasticity, hyperreflexia, and extensor plantar responses (Babinski sign) can be present contralateral to the lesion. Patients with glioblastoma multiforme and other neoplasms, including metastases and slow-growing astrocytomas, typically present with focal seizures, headache, and an altered mental status worsening over days to weeks. Headache is usually present with neoplasia, but not with thrombotic or embolic ischemic cerebral vascular disease. Headache, nausea, and vomiting are typical indicators of

primary intracranial hemorrhage. In HIV-positive patients, slowly progressive unilateral weakness with hyperreflexia requires a computerized tomography (CT) scan of the brain with contrast to assess for toxoplasmic encephalitis or primary central nervous system (CNS) lymphoma. In the non-HIV positive population, contrast imaging can be used when primary CNS neoplasia or brain abscess is suspected.

Brainstem. Patients with slowly evolving mass lesions in the brainstem or primary cerebellar hemorrhages usually do not present with unilateral or bilateral weakness, but with clumsiness, vertigo, and double vision. When accompanied by weakness, these symptoms are commonly associated with profound alterations in mental status due to the proximity of the ascending reticular activating system to the corticospinal tracts subserving voluntary muscle movement. An appropriate history, CT scanning, or magnetic resonance imaging (MRI) is usually sufficient to distinguish cerebral vascular disease from primary CNS hemorrhage, or neoplasia.

Spinal Cord. The hallmark of myelopathy resulting in weakness includes bilateral symptoms with hyperreflexia, a Babinski sign, and urinary urgency. Sensory symptoms accompany the weakness of cervical or thoracic myelopathy. Back pain is a typical accompaniment at the level of the spinal cord lesion, whether it is from an extradural lesion, an intradural extramedullary lesion, or an intramedullary lesion. The most frequent cause of weakness of spinal cord origin is extradural lesions, especially a severe central or eccentric cervical intervertebral disc herniation. Thoracic disc herniations are rare. Secondary causes include severe spinal trauma with spinal cord contusion or secondary disc herniation, gunshot and stab wounds, and metastases from breast, lung, or prostate cancer. Intradural extramedullary lesions typically occur in the thoracic spinal cord in middle-aged women due to compression from meningiomas, schwannomas, or metastases. Primary intramedullary tumors include ependymomas, astrocytomas, and metastases. Patients with slow-growing neoplasms or structural problems present with back pain, urinary urgency, and bilateral leg weakness or quadriparesis with upper motor neuron signs. Initial spine radiographs can be helpful in suggesting a primary cause such as metastasis or osteomyelitis. However, MRI is the neuroimaging modality of choice for establishing lesion at the appropriate level of the spinal column. MRI is available to many emergency departments as the initial imaging study to diagnosis these pathologies. Gadolinium-enhanced MRIs are performed for specific diagnosis.

Transverse myelitis can be considered a primary intramedullary inflammatory process that can result in severe disability. The typical patient is a young woman who has experienced a viral syndrome in the preceding month followed by back pain and typical signs of myelopathy. The term *transverse* is a misnomer, as the inflammatory process is clearly three-dimensional and can be patchy in nature. MRI reveals spinal cord hyperintensity and patchy enhancement in areas of blood–brain barrier breakdown. After MRI is performed, a lumbar puncture (LP) is required to demonstrate a CSF cellular response with high protein, high immunoglobulin content, and oligoclonal band synthesis. In one study, 15% of such patients developed clinically definite multiple sclerosis. Transverse myelitis requires admission to the hospital and high-dose intravenous corticosteroids for 7–10 days followed by a prednisone taper to minimize the sequelae of inflammation.

Anterior Horn Cell Disorders. These devastating causes of weakness *without* sensory disturbances are commonly separated into hereditary and acquired forms. Hereditary forms are rare and are not discussed here. Acquired disorders of the anterior horn cell[3] include postinfectious motor neuron degenerations such as polio, which has been virtually eradicated. An enterovirus, the polio virus typically causes a gastroenteritis followed rarely by a primary degeneration of spinal cord motor neurons (anterior horn cells) resulting in asymmetrical muscle wasting, fasciculations, and weakness. In North America, susceptible individuals include occasional infants exposed to the oral Sabin polio vaccine and to nonimmunized caregivers of recently immunized infants. There is no known treatment for acute poliomyelitis. Supportive care is provided after most of the nerve degeneration has occurred. Radiation to the spinal column has been reported to cause primary anterior horn cell dysfunction with hyporeflexia, wasting, and fasciculations months to years after irradiation. Knowledge of radiation doses causing such weakness has allowed radiation oncologists to minimize the likelihood of radiation-induced motor neuron disease.

The most frequently encountered anterior horn cell disorder in the emergency department is amyotrophic lateral sclerosis (Lou Gehrig's disease). Patients with undiagnosed amyotrophic lateral sclerosis can present to the emergency department with a diagnosis of "failure to thrive" or with severe respiratory failure. Families commonly bring elderly patients with weak, wasted muscles to the emergency department when those individuals can no longer walk or swallow. These patients are examined completely undressed in order to observe areas of fasciculations, which represent spontaneous contractions of abnormal motor units. Patients typically deny that their muscles are twitching unless it is pointed out to them by the physician. Common areas to observe fasciculations include the dorsal small hand muscles, triceps, periscapular muscles, biceps, quadriceps, and gastrocnemius muscles. Hyperreflexia in weak, wasted muscles with normal vibration, proprioception, and light touch sensation, and upper motor neuron signs including a hyperactive jaw jerk and a Babinski sign, confirm the diagnosis of amyotrophic lateral sclerosis. Electromyography and nerve conduction studies are eventually performed to confirm the clinical impression. Weight loss is usually due to a primary loss in muscle mass due to the lack of trophic influences from fewer surviving motor nerves, or severe dysphagia resulting in poor caloric intake. Amyotrophic lateral sclerosis usually begins with a foot drop or severe unilateral hand weakness. It progresses regionally so that when one arm is affected, the next limb most likely affected is the other arm. Similarly, when the problem begins in one lower extremity, the other lower extremity typically becomes affected. In addition, the disease can begin in the cranial musculature, characterized by regurgitation, dysphagia, and a change in voice. The patient commonly carries a tissue much of the time to blot away saliva that can no longer be swallowed.

In summary, diffuse weakness, fasciculating muscles, and hyperactive reflexes in weak, wasted limbs without sensory disturbances strongly suggests the possibility of amyotrophic lateral sclerosis.

Nerve Root Disorders. Acute inflammatory demyelinating polyneuropathy, also known as Guillain-Barré syndrome, is the most common primary lesion of nerve roots to present to the emergency department. Two to four weeks after experiencing a flulike upper respiratory or gastrointestinal syndrome, patients describe diffuse aching, and occasionally back pain. A rapid progression of weakness, usually proximal, extends to the distal muscles in the upper and lower extremities. Sensory loss is minor and usually of the large fiber type. Proprioceptive senses are lost. The patient finds it difficult to stand or walk, and occasionally complains of electriclike sensations in the limbs (paresthesias). Bilateral facial weakness occurs in more than 50% of individuals. Swallowing can become a problem. Shortness of breath generally heralds respiratory failure. The primary problem is a restrictive lung deficit resulting in ventilation–perfusion mismatch, decreasing the patient's vital capacity imperceptibly until a high respiratory rate ensues. The only criteria necessary for the clinical diagnosis of Guillain-Barré syndrome are weakness of a fairly symmetrical distribution, and hyporeflexia or areflexia. Patients present to the emergency department with acute respiratory failure or with an inability to stand or walk. A bedside vital capacity is obtained immediately and cardiac monitoring is instituted because the disease causes severe dysautonomia with orthostatic hypotension and life-threatening arrhythmias. CSF commonly reveals an elevated protein without a cellular response in the first week. These patients are admitted to the intensive care unit, where frequent neurological examinations are performed and ventilatory assistance is immediately available. Patients with a vital capacity of less than 25 cc/kg or those who cannot stand require plasmapheresis.

Motor Neuropathy. Isolated pathology of motor nerves distal to the immediate nerve exit zone of the spinal column is rare and is usually due to heavy metal intoxication, particularly lead. Patients with this disorder typically do not present to the emergency department. A known exposure to lead, as in solder or paint fumes, is usually elicited. The disease typically causes bilateral wrist drop prior to distal leg weakness. A high index of suspicion to exposure to lead and measurement of urinary lead excretion are required for diagnosis.

Sensory Motor Peripheral Neuropathies. These disorders affect sensory and motor nerves in the periphery, manifesting as weakness in the feet prior to the arms, and as sensory symptoms of paresthesias, total sensory loss, or burning sensations. The most common sensory motor peripheral neuropathies encountered in the emergency department include subacute to chronic diabetic peripheral neuropathy and alcoholic peripheral neuropathy.

Primarily a problem in the outpatient setting, diabetic peripheral neuropathy can mimic an acute lumbar radiculopathy with the sudden onset of back pain radiating down the posterior thigh and calf into the sole of the foot. In addition, acute unilateral femoral neuropathy is frequent among the elderly. Sudden excruciating thigh pain that follows knee extensor weakness and thigh atrophy is common in poorly controlled diabetics. The pathophysiology of acute diabetic femoral neuropathy and radiculopathy is likely the result of nerve infarction from atherosclerosis of the vasa nervorum.[4] Although this condition is very painful, the patient can generally be reassured of improvement. In the case of femoral neuropathy, gradual return of strength occurs over several weeks to months. Prudent use of nonsteroidal anti-inflammatory agents, physical therapy, temporary use of a cane, and reassurance about the return of function aids clinical improvement.

Patients with distal symmetrical peripheral neuropathy due to diabetes or alcoholism generally present to the emergency department only after falls caused by tripping from poor foot dorsiflexion. Ankle dorsiflexion weakness and poor vibratory and toe position sense are uniform signs of these disorders. Nutritional support with B-complex vitamins and abstinence from alcohol improves alcoholic polyneuropathy. Strict normoglycemia can retard all forms of diabetic peripheral nerve disease.

When diabetes and alcohol use are not an issue, toxic neuropathy from chemotherapy, paraproteinemia, heavy metal exposure, and collagen vascular diseases are considered. After gait stability is assessed, the evaluation of potential causes of peripheral neuropathy is performed by the patient's primary care physician or neurologist. Electrophysiological testing separates axonal from demyelinating processes.[2]

Neuromuscular Junction Disorders. Myasthenia gravis and botulism are two of the most difficult-to-recognize and potentially life-threatening causes of weakness. Because both diseases can produce rapidly progressive pharyngeal and diaphragmatic dysfunction, a high index of suspicion is necessary for a quick and efficient assessment of a patient's imminent risk of respiratory failure with these conditions.

The *Clostridium botulinum* bacillus produces a toxin present in poorly canned legumes or other root vegetables, where the anaerobic organism can thrive. A portion of the toxin enters the human presynaptic neuromuscular nerve terminal, irreversibly preventing quanta of acetylcholine (ACh) from being released to bind to postsynaptic ACh receptors, thereby preventing muscle contraction. Severe weakness results from a large quantity of ingested toxin and irreversible "short circuiting" of neuromuscular transmission, which requires resprouting of neuronal axons to form new neuromuscular junctions, a process that can take over four months.

Alternatively, myasthenia gravis does not prevent ACh release. ACh receptor antibodies form a complex with ACh receptors postsynaptically and prevent muscle contraction by decreasing muscle membrane potentials, which are inadequate to initiate action potentials. Botulism is considered a prototype presynaptic neuromuscular junction disorder; myasthenia gravis is considered a prototypical postsynaptic neuromuscular junction disorder.

Botulism becomes apparent when ptosis and double or blurry vision due to a lack of pupillary constriction brings the patient to medical attention. Stridor, dysphagia, quadriparesis, and diaphragmatic respiratory failure ensue. Myasthenia gravis can occur with an equally rapid onset over a period of hours; however, it does not affect pupillary size. A history of fluctuating double vision or lid drooping over the previous months likely occurs with myasthenia gravis, whereas botulism presents within hours of ingestion of the toxin. A history of multiple individuals displaying the same symptoms (having shared a meal, typically at a picnic of home-canned goods) makes the diagnosis of botulism very likely.

Respiratory failure is the most severe result of these disorders. Although antitoxin can be administered for botulism, patients typically require respiratory assistance for months before nerve sprouting can create new neuromuscular junctions and return strength to respiratory and limb muscles. Once respiratory failure has occurred from upper respiratory failure or diaphragmatic weakness in myasthenia gravis, plasmapheresis or intravenous immunoglobulin can return function over a period of days or weeks.

It is important to remember that because cranial nerve weakness can herald sudden respiratory failure with myasthenia gravis or botulism, a detailed history and subsequent therapeutic intervention and monitoring are crucial.

Myopathies. Rarely acute, the most common myopathic disorders to present to the emergency department include polymyositis, dermatomyositis, steroid myopathy, and alcoholic myopathy.

Patients with any of these disorders present with the prototype distribution of proximal muscle weakness.[5] Patients complain of a chronic course of difficulty climbing stairs, arising from a seated position, getting off a toilet, or getting out of a bathtub. In addition, they have problems combing their hair and reaching for objects on shelves. They generally do not trip over curbs or high-piled rugs or have difficulty buttoning clothes until late in the disease process. No sensory loss occurs, but cramping can be a sensory symptom. Swallowing can become a problem with polymyositis or dermatomyositis. Double vision, ptosis, or facial weakness is unlikely to occur. The patient can present to the emergency department with repeated falls, bruises, or broken bones. The presence of reflexes and the demonstration of proximal muscle weakness in a fairly symmetrical distribution about the shoulders and hip girdle without sensory loss generally allows for an accurate diagnosis in the emergency department. An elevated creatine phosphokinase (CPK) or aldolase level helps confirm the diagnosis. However, in patients with chronic myopathy, these levels can be normal. Ultimately, an electromyogram or muscle biopsy is necessary for definitive diagnosis of these disorders. When the patient's gait is stable, and the diagnosis is corroborated by a consistent clinical presentation and an abnormal CPK level, referral to a neurologist is necessary to help distinguish these disorders from others. A history of corticosteroid use or obvious Cushingoid features can help in diagnosing exogenous toxic steroid myopathy or endogenous Cushing's syndrome. A history of chronic alcoholism helps to specify a cause of the disorder. Corticosteroid therapy generally does not confound a diagnosis of polymyositis or dermatomyositis prior to muscle biopsy. Dermatomyositis is a humorally mediated B-cell antibody disorder, correctly described as an autoimmune vasculopathy that affects the skin, causing an erythematous rash over the extensor surfaces of the fingers, diffuse erythema over the chest, and a purplish hue to the periorbital area. Polymyositis is a T-cell-mediated disorder that causes the same distribution of weakness as dermatomyositis, without the rash. The alcoholic patient with proximal muscle weakness generally appears cachectic and has a normal CPK level. Abstinence from alcohol and nutritional support are the best treatments.

Severe electrolyte disturbances including hypophosphatemia and hypokalemia can cause an acute quadriparesis with areflexia. Muscle biopsy reveals myopathic features. This is a reversible syndrome and occurs in patients with laxative abuse or diuretic use.

The only distal myopathy of any considerable prevalence is myotonic muscular dystrophy. Typical patients are young adults or teenagers who present with problems buttoning clothes or tripping. They can show excessive frontal balding for age, in a male pattern whether male or female. Mild ptosis and thinning of the sternocleidomastoid muscles are apparent, and percussion myotonia can be elicited over the thenar muscles. Hand grip is commonly prolonged, which can be tested by shaking the patient's hand. Personality disorders and mental retardation occur commonly, although not uniformly. Patients with this disease rarely present to the emergency department. A family history of at least one parent with a similar problem is usually obtained.

PEARLS AND PITFALLS

■ Weakness implies an inability to perform usual activities due to loss of muscle, nerve, or upper motor neuron function, not a loss of stamina or endurance.

■ One of the most common presentations of weakness is gait instability with frequent falls.

■ Sialorrhea is a serious sign of possible dysphagia from botulism, myasthenia gravis, or one of the myositides.

■ A patient presenting with paresthesias, nonspecific sensory symptoms, or aches and pains approximately one month after a viral syndrome may have Guillain-Barré syndrome.

■ Limb muscle strength is tested by separate muscle groups to determine whether there is a proximal or distal distribution to weakness, thus narrowing the differential diagnosis.

■ Hyperactive reflexes in weak, wasted limbs suggest combined nerve root and spinal cord injury from arthritis or amyotrophic lateral sclerosis, until proven otherwise.

■ Hip girdle weakness may be the only sign on examination in a weak patient who has myopathy or Guillain-Barré syndrome.

■ Bedside spirometry frequently elicits low forced vital capacities due to a poor seal of the patient's lips on the device.

■ Shoulder separations and partial rotator cuff tears can mimic unilateral proximal upper extremity weakness. MRI revealing the tear or nerve conduction velocity studies verifying normal nerve and muscle function can prevent the misdiagnosis of an orthopedic condition as a neurological condition.

REFERENCES

1. Lewis P, Rowland MD, eds. *Merritt's Textbook of Neurology.* 9th ed. Baltimore, Md: Williams & Wilkins; 1995.
2. Sethi RK, Thompson LL. *The Electromyographer's Handbook.* 2nd ed. Boston, Mass: Little, Brown and Co; 1989.
3. Swanson PD, ed. *Signs and Symptoms in Neurology.* Philadelphia, Pa: JB Lippincott Co; 1984.
4. Dyck P, Thomas PK, eds. *Peripheral Neuropathy.* 3rd ed. Philadelphia, Pa: WB Saunders Co; 1993.
5. Engel AG, Franzini-Armstrong C, eds. *Myology.* 2nd ed. New York, NY: McGraw-Hill Book Co; 1994.

11 Dizziness

KEVIN M. KELLY AND STEVEN A. TELIAN

SUMMARY The emergency department evaluation of dizziness or vertigo is based on a careful history and physical examination. In general, simple clinical information can determine whether dizziness or vertigo is due to a disorder of the peripheral vestibular system, the central nervous system, or nonvestibular systems. Supportive evidence of the clinical diagnosis can be obtained in the emergency department from laboratory studies indicated from the clinical data. The rational management of dizziness or vertigo in the emergency department is directed at identifying and correcting the underlying abnormality whenever possible, ruling out serious underlying causes for the presenting symptoms, providing symptomatic therapy, treating any associated trauma, and promoting vestibular compensation when indicated. Disposition of the patient is determined by the cause and severity of symptoms, response to treatment, and indications for additional evaluation and therapy.

Introduction

The evaluation of patients with the complaint of "dizziness" is a frequent occurrence in the emergency department. The word *dizziness* is a nonspecific term used by patients and health care professionals to describe a disturbed sense of well-being, usually perceived as an altered orientation in space. It is often difficult for the patient to describe accurately the quality of the sensation, which can suggest different entities such as an emotional disorder, presyncope, disequilibrium, or vertigo.[1] *Vertigo* is defined as an illusion of movement of oneself or one's surroundings. It is usually experienced as a sensation of rotation or, less frequently, as undulation, linear displacement (pulsion), or tilt.[2] Although vertigo usually suggests a vestibular disorder that can involve the inner ear or brain, this symptom itself cannot reliably localize the disorder.[3] Dizziness or vertigo can result from numerous disorders of the human balance system, which is extremely complex. Abnormalities can occur peripherally, where visual, proprioceptive, and vestibular information is obtained, or centrally, where this information is integrated.[2] Despite the inherent complexities, the emergency department evaluation of dizziness or vertigo can be simplified by a systematic approach in history taking, physical examination, and laboratory testing. A useful diagnostic method is to determine whether the patient's symptoms are due to a disorder of the vestibular system or nonvestibular systems.[3] At times it can be difficult to distinguish a primary vestibular disorder from a nonvestibular disorder that affects the vestibular system secondarily. Nevertheless, differentiating vestibular from nonvestibular disorders provides a conceptual framework to localize the abnormality anatomically, to determine its cause, and to judge the potential seriousness of the disorder.

* This chapter has been adapted from *Principles and Practice of Emergency Medicine*, 4th ed., G. Schwartz, ed. (Baltimore: Williams & Wilkins, in press), with permission.

132

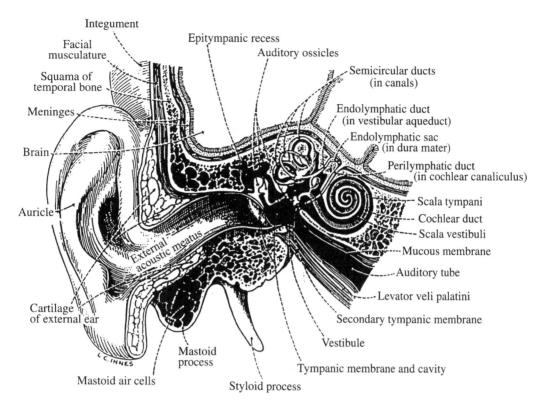

FIGURE 11.1. Vertical section of the ear illustrating the vestibular sensory organs. (Reprinted with permission from Anson BJ and Donaldson JA: *Surgical anatomy of the temporal bone.* Philadelphia: WB Saunders Co, Philadelphia, 1981.)

Anatomy

Dizziness or vertigo is frequently caused by a disorder of the vestibular system. The vestibular system is organized into peripheral and central components. A brief description of the basic anatomy of the peripheral and central vestibular systems is given below.

Peripheral Vestibular System

The peripheral vestibular system is composed of bilateral sensory organs, their afferent fibers, and brainstem efferent fibers that innervate the sensory organs. Figure 11.1 shows the location of the vestibular sensory organs within the inner ear. They are located in the *bony labyrinth*, which is a series of hollow channels connecting into a round chamber, called the *vestibule*, within the petrous portion of the temporal bone. The sensory organs within the bony labyrinth are three *semicircular canals*, the *utricle*, and the *saccule*, together constituting the *membranous labyrinth*. The semicircular canals are ring-shaped tubes aligned at right angles to each other, one in the horizontal plane (horizontal) and the other two in the vertical plane orthogonal to each other (superior and posterior). Each of the semicircular canals is able to interpret angular acceleration of the head relative to the plane of that canal by changes within the *crista ampullaris,* a neuroepithelial receptor organ in the ampullated end of the canal that is adjacent to the vestibule. *Hair cells* within the cristae sense displacement of fluid within the canals during head acceleration and transduce the stimulus into a generator potential. The utricle and saccule, commonly referred to as "otolithic organs," are saclike structures that communicate with each other and with the fluids of the cochlea. The utricle and saccule sense linear inertial forces (gravity) as well as linear head accelerations. They contain the *maculae*, receptor organs that consist of a gelatinous material containing calcium carbonate crystals (*otoliths*) overlying a membrane containing sensory hair cells. The hair cells sense displacement of the otolithic membrane

133

during linear acceleration of the head and transduce the stimulus to a generator potential similar to that of the hair cells within the cristae.

The fluid within the membranous labyrinth that bathes the vestibular sensory organs is called *endolymph*. The membranous labyrinth is surrounded by a continuous space within the bony labyrinth containing a chemically distinct second fluid type called *perilymph*. The perilymph and the endolymph fluid compartments are continuous with those inside the cochlea, the auditory sensory organ. The perilymph is derived from blood vessels located within the perilymphatic space, with possible contributions from a filtrate of cerebrospinal fluid (CSF), reaching the perilymphatic space from the posterior fossa through a small bony channel known as the cochlear aqueduct (see Fig. 11.1). Perilymph chemically resembles extracellular fluid, having low potassium and high sodium concentrations. The endolymph is believed to be produced in specialized cells of the cochlea and vestibular labyrinth. The endolymph resembles intracellular fluid, having high potassium and low sodium. The vestibular sensory organs communicate with each other by anatomical connections that allow for the passage of endolymph. The semicircular canals are connected by five openings to the utricle, which is also connected to the *endolymphatic duct*. After leaving the utricle, the endolymphatic duct proceeds posteriorly to become the *endolymphatic sac*, a specialized portion of the posterior fossa dura adjacent to the temporal bone where resorption of endolymph takes place. The saccule is connected by the saccular duct to the endolymphatic duct and thus communicates indirectly with the utricle. The saccule is also connected to the cochlea by the ductus reuniens.

The hair cells of the vestibular sensory organs are innervated by afferent bipolar cells of the *vestibular ganglion* (Scarpa's ganglion), located in the *internal auditory canal* of the petrous portion of the temporal bone. The central processes of these cells form the *superior and inferior vestibular nerves,* which occupy the posterior half of the internal auditory canal. Afferent fibers from the cochlea form the auditory nerve that occupies the anteroinferior part of the internal auditory canal. The vestibular nerves and the auditory nerve emerge from the internal auditory canal and combine to constitute the *eighth cranial nerve.* As these nerves exit the internal auditory canal, there is a rotation of the nerve bundle so that the vestibular fibers constitute the upper half of the eighth nerve in the cerebellopontine angle. The facial nerve accompanies the eighth nerve, running anterior to it within the cerebellopontine angle and into the anterior superior quadrant of the internal auditory canal. Afferent vestibular axons enter the brainstem and synapse mostly in the vestibular nuclei, with a small component of fibers synapsing within the cerebellum directly. Efferent fibers from neurons located bilaterally near the lateral vestibular nucleus travel through the vestibular nerve to make synaptic contact with vestibular hair cells or their afferent nerve endings. These efferent fibers provide tonic inhibition of the receptors and the afferent nerve endings and thereby modulate and gate their activity.

The blood supply of the vestibular sensory organs and the nerves within the internal auditory canal originates from the *anterior inferior cerebellar artery* (*AICA*), which arises from the basilar artery. As the AICA enters the temporal bone, it forms branches that perfuse the vestibular ganglion cells and their fibers. The AICA gives rise to the *labyrinthine artery,* which divides into two main branches after entering the inner ear: the *anterior vestibular* artery and the *common cochlear artery.* The anterior vestibular artery supplies the utricle, the ampullae of the superior and horizontal semicircular canals, and a small part of the saccule. The common cochlear artery gives rise to the *posterior vestibular artery,* which supplies the ampulla of the posterior semicircular canal and the inferior aspect of the saccule.

Central Vestibular System

The central vestibular system includes the vestibular nuclei and their central nervous system (CNS) connections. The major connections of the vestibular nuclei of clinical importance are those to the cerebellum, ocular motor nuclei, spinal cord, and reticular formation. Connections among these structures are commonly referred to as "vestibular pathways." There are four *vestibular nuclei* (superior, medial, lateral, and inferior) situated in the dorsolateral part of the pons and medulla. The medial, lateral, and inferior vestibular nuclei constitute the major central termination of afferent fibers innervating the utricle and saccule. The superior, medial, and lateral vestibular nuclei receive afferent fibers innervating the semicircular canals. In addition, some of these fibers terminate in the flocculonodular lobe, or *vestibulocerebellum,* and the vermian cortex of the cerebellum. Efferent fibers of the vermis project ipsilaterally to the vestibular nuclei and to the cerebellar fastigial nucleus, which sends fibers to the contralateral vestibular nuclei. Thus each side of the cerebellum influences the vestibular nuclei bilaterally. The vestibular—cerebellar interactions are important in the maintenance of equilibrium and locomotion.

Axons from neurons in the vestibular nuclei travel through the *median longitudinal fasciculus* (*MLF*), a large fiber bundle pathway lying along the floor of the fourth ventricle, to make direct synaptic connections with the ocular motor nuclei (third, fourth, and sixth cranial nerve nuclei). The vestibular nuclei, MLF, and ocular motor nuclei are part of the neuronal circuitry that underlies the *vestibuloocular reflex* (*VOR*). The VOR is primarily a response to brief, rapid head movements, automatically producing compensatory eye movements in the opposite direction, thereby maintaining stable retinal images.[4] There are other anatomical pathways that interconnect the vestibular nuclei with the *paramedian pontine reticular formation* (*PPRF*), a cellular region located lateral to the sixth cranial nerve nucleus. The PPRF receives input from the contralateral frontal gaze center and drives the ipsilateral sixth cranial nerve nucleus to produce rapid eye abduction ipsilaterally. The sixth cranial nerve nucleus sends axons through the MLF to drive concomitantly the contralateral third cranial nerve nucleus, thereby producing rapid conjugate horizontal eye movements.

The vestibular nuclei send projections to the spinal cord by the *lateral and medial vestibulospinal tracts.* The lateral vestibulospinal tract originates primarily from the lateral vestibular nucleus; its main action is to produce contraction of extensor (antigravity) muscles and relaxation of flexor muscles of the limbs. The medial vestibulospinal tract arises mainly from the medial vestibular nucleus and provides direct inhibition of motor neurons of the neck and axial muscles. The vestibulospinal tracts are important in vestibular reflex reactions and in the maintenance of posture.

The vestibular nuclei send fibers to the pontomedullary region of the reticular formation, which constitutes the central core of the brainstem extending from the caudal medulla to the rostral midbrain. The reticular formation contains distinct nuclei as well as others that are not clearly defined. Axons of neurons within the medial, magnocellular area of the reticular formation form the *reticulospinal tracts,* which travel the length of the spinal cord and terminate on spinal motor neurons and interneurons. The reticulospinal tracts are important in regulating motor activity and the flow of afferent signals in the spinal cord.

The blood supply of the central vestibular system originates primarily from the posterior circulation. The vestibular nuclei and the vestibulocerebellum are supplied by the *vertebral arteries,* which ascend along the ventrolateral aspects of the medulla and unite at the pontomedullary junction to form the *basilar artery.* The basilar artery runs along the ventral aspect of the pons and ends at the caudal midbrain. A *posterior inferior cerebellar artery* (*PICA*) arises from each vertebral artery approximately 1 cm inferior to the basilar artery and supplies the lateral surface of the medulla and part of the surface of the cerebellar hemisphere ipsilaterally.

History and Physical Examination

History

A carefully obtained history is critical in the evaluation of a patient's complaint of dizziness or vertigo. This is important diagnostically because vertigo usually results from vestibular system disorders, whereas nonvertiginous dizziness usually results from nonvestibular system disorders. Symptom description can also differentiate peripheral from central vestibular system disorders. Special attention is paid to the quality and time course of symptoms, associated symptoms, predisposing factors, precipitating factors, and exacerbating or mitigating factors.[2,3] Table 11.1 lists general properties of dizziness in vestibular and nonvestibular system dysfunction. Table 11.2 lists properties of vertigo

TABLE 11.1. Properties of Dizziness Due to Vestibular and Nonvestibular System Dysfunction

Property	Vestibular	Nonvestibular
Description	Spinning, whirling, rotating, off-balance	Lightheaded, faint, dazed, floating
Time course	Episodic or constant	Episodic or constant
Associated symptoms	Nausea, vomiting, pallor, diaphoresis, hearing loss, tinnitus	Paresthesias, palpitations headache, syncope
Predisposing factors	Congenital inner ear anomaly, ototoxins, ear surgery	Syncope due to cardiovascular disease, psychiatric illness
Precipitating factors	Head or body position changes, ear infection or trauma	Body position changes, stress, fear, anxiety, hyperventilation

and associated symptoms due to peripheral and central vestibular system dysfunction.

Symptom Quality. The patient should accurately describe the symptoms experienced in his or her own words so that the examiner has a firm impression of the symptom quality. This information can distinguish different types of dizziness from vertigo. If the patient's description of symptoms is not clear, the patient can be asked if the symptoms resemble nervousness, confusion, weakness, lightheadedness, faintness, imbalance, or a sensation of spinning or whirling. The patient should specify whether one symptom gave rise to another. Symptom intensity is graded as mild, moderate, or severe.

Symptom Time Course. Symptom onset is described as sudden or insidious. Symptom duration is estimated as lasting seconds, minutes, hours, days, or longer. Symptoms are described as episodic or constant. The time course of symptom intensity includes the time to peak intensity, peak intensity duration, and the time of decreasing intensity.

Associated Symptoms. Numerous symptoms can be associated with dizziness or vertigo. Autonomic symptoms of nausea, vomiting, pallor, and diaphoresis often occur with vestibular disorders due to the numerous connections between brainstem

vestibular and autonomic centers. The symptoms are generally more severe when the vestibular abnormality is peripheral than when it is central. These symptoms also can occur in other forms of dizziness where lightheadedness, shortness of breath, or palpitations may be prominent.

Symptoms associated with dizziness or vertigo can be due to the anatomical location of the abnormality and can occur in different combinations. Hearing loss, tinnitus, pressure, pain, hyperacusis (hypersensitivity to loud sounds), and diplacusis (distortion of pitch perception in one ear) are associated with inner ear lesions; hearing loss, tinnitus, and facial weakness with internal auditory canal lesions; hearing loss, tinnitus, facial weakness and/or numbness, and extremity incoordination with cerebellopontine angle lesions; diplopia, dysarthria, dysphagia, hiccups, perioral numbness, and extremity weakness and numbness with brainstem lesions; imbalance and incoordination with cerebellar lesions.

Other symptoms experienced with dizziness or vertigo can involve vestibular or nonvestibular systems depending on anatomical or physiological involvement. Headache can be associated with systemic illness or an intracranial process such as hemorrhage, mass lesion, or infection. Alteration or loss of consciousness can be associated with presyncope, syncope, hyperventilation, seizures, or

TABLE 11.2. Properties of Vertigo and Associated Symptoms Due to Peripheral and Central Vestibular System Dysfunction

Symptom	Vestibular System Dysfunction	
	Peripheral	Central
Vertigo		
Onset	Sudden	Insidious
Quality	Spinning, rotation	Disequilibrium
Intensity	Severe	Mild to moderate
Occurrence	Episodic	Constant
Duration	Seconds, minutes, hours, or days	Weeks or longer
Exacerbation by head movement	Moderate to severe	Mild
Nausea and vomiting	Severe	Mild
Imbalance	Mild	Moderate
Ear pressure or pain	Occasional	None
Hearing loss	Frequent	Rare
Tinnitus	Frequent	Rare
Neurologic symptoms	Rare	Frequent

vertebrobasilar insufficiency. Falling can be associated with labyrinthine disorders, vertebrobasilar insufficiency, syncope, seizures, or posterior fossa mass lesions.

Predisposing Factors. The patient's medical, surgical, and psychiatric history, family history, recent general health, medications, and substance abuse history are reviewed carefully. The medical and psychiatric history can reveal that symptoms are recurrent and attributable to a particular disease state that has been identified previously. Surgery may have been performed to treat a specific disorder associated with dizziness or vertigo. In other patients, symptoms can develop following surgery. In any case, the medical, psychiatric, and surgical history is not overlooked, because it can provide important information for diagnosis and management. The patient's family history is reviewed because several vestibular disorders have a genetic predisposition. These include migraine, Meniere's disease, and otosclerosis. The patient's recent general health is reviewed for any abnormality such as infection, mood disturbance, or trauma. Symptoms are detailed, and

the clinician ascertains whether the underlying cause was determined and whether any treatment was prescribed. Medication use is frequently associated with dizziness or vertigo and is reviewed carefully. Particular attention is paid to any new prescriptions, and to the use of antihypertensives, hypoglycemics, diuretics, or known ototoxins. Possible drug interactions or drug synergism is questioned. The patient is asked directly if any controlled substances or street drugs have been used and, if so, whether previous use was associated with similar symptoms.

Precipitating Factors. A detailed account of the circumstances at the onset of symptoms is elicited from the patient. General considerations include whether the patient was at rest, engaged in normal activity, exercising, straining, or sleeping at the time of onset. The patient is asked to identify any event that seemed to precipitate symptoms. It is determined whether symptoms occurred with preceding anxiety, fear, or excitement; before or after eating; with coughing, sneezing, straining at stool, or after urinating, or with overexertion or overheating.

Movements of the head and/or body are frequently associated with the onset of dizziness or vertigo. These movements include turning over in bed, sitting up from a lying position, standing up from a sitting position, looking up by extending the neck, bending over, and straightening up.

Exacerbating or Mitigating Factors. Head and body positions or movements as described above can exacerbate or mitigate dizziness or vertigo. Worsening dizziness or vertigo with movement is a general characteristic of peripheral and central vestibular system disorders. Worsening symptoms with standing are often due to a nonvestibular disorder, and can precede syncope. Symptoms may improve in vestibular disorders with either visual fixation or closing the eyes. Dizziness associated with peripheral neuropathy, posterior column disease, or cerebellar disease is generally less severe with eyes open. Vertigo worsened by loud noise (Tullio phenomenon), change in pressure in the ear canal, or Valsalva maneuvers suggests a disorder of inner ear fluid mechanics, such as Meniere's disease, otosyphilis, or perilymph fistula. Nonvertiginous dizziness worsened by Valsalva maneuvers can precede syncopal states, as described above. Exercise-induced worsening of symptoms can occur with perilymph fistula, other peripheral or central vestibular disorders, or nonvestibular disorders such as cardiopulmonary disease. Exacerbations of demyelinating disease can occur with exercise and can affect vestibular or nonvestibular CNS pathways.

General Physical Examination

A general physical examination is performed to assess the condition of the patient and to find physical signs that may be related to the underlying cause of dizziness or vertigo. General inspection of the patient can reveal apparent weakness or anxiety, tremulousness, relative immobility, instability, or vomiting. Vital signs can give evidence of infection, hypotension or hypertension, arrhythmias, or respiratory and/or metabolic disturbances. In particular, the patient is assessed for orthostatic hypotension and hyperventilation. The skin can reveal decreased turgor with dehydration, edema with fluid retention, pallor with anemia, a rash with infection, cyanosis with hypoxemia, or diaphoresis and pallor with autonomic nervous system changes. Abrasions, ecchy-

moses, or lacerations suggest trauma. The sinuses can be tender to percussion or the oropharynx erythematous, findings associated with local infection. The neck can reveal jugular venous distension or carotid bruits with cardiovascular disease, or a decreased range of motion with severe osteoarthritis.

Special attention is paid to the otoscopic examination of the external auditory canal and the tympanic membrane. The external auditory canal is inspected for cerumen, erythema, bloody or purulent otorrhea, CSF leak, or foreign body. The tympanic membrane can show amber or erythematous discoloration with middle ear disease, myringosclerosis from previous otitis media, evidence of prior trauma, retraction pockets, or cholesteatoma. Pneumatic otoscopy can be performed by attaching a rubber bulb to an obturator or speculum of an otoscope, applying positive and negative pressure, and assessing the mobility of the tympanic membrane. Diminished mobility can occur with perforations, middle ear fluid, and thickening of the tympanic membrane. Vertigo or nystagmus in response to pressure changes in the ear canal during pneumatic otoscopy increases the suspicion of a disorder of inner ear fluid mechanics, as listed above.

Auscultation of the lungs can reveal decreased breath sounds with exacerbations of chronic obstructive pulmonary disease, asthma, or infection, rales can be heard with pulmonary edema and congestive heart failure. Auscultation of the heart can reveal arrhythmias or murmurs of acquired heart disease underlying inadequate cerebral perfusion and hypoxia or embolism. The abdomen can be tender with infection or gastrointestinal hemorrhage resulting in hypotension; a rectal examination can give evidence of blood in the stool. Abnormalities of the musculoskeletal system can suggest hereditary degenerative disorders.

Neurological Examination

Following completion of a general physical examination, a focused neurological examination is performed to assess mental status, the functioning of cranial nerves, motor and sensory systems, and deep tendon reflexes. Particular attention is directed to the neuro-otologic examination of patients with a suspected vestibular disorder. Repeat examinations may be necessary for patients with severe vertigo or vomiting.

Mental Status. The mental status of the patient is determined as alert, confused, lethargic, stuporous, or comatose. Typically, patients presenting to the emergency department with the complaint of dizziness or vertigo are alert. Some may have an abnormal mental status at the time of presentation, which can deteriorate depending on the nature of the disorder (e.g., CNS infection or mass lesion, toxic or metabolic encephalopathies). Evidence of an abnormal affect or a thought disorder is investigated. Anxiety, agitation, panic attacks, or depression can result in complaints of dizziness. However, it is important to recognize that vestibular disorders can cause indistinguishable symptoms.

Cranial Nerves. The cranial nerve examination is focused and thorough. Each optic nerve disk is examined by ophthalmoscopy. Bilateral optic disk edema, or papilledema, is due to increased intracranial pressure. Following ophthalmoscopy, an evaluation of the patient's visual function begins by testing corrected visual acuity in each eye. Decreased acuity can be seen with optic nerve, optic chiasm, or optic tract lesions. Visual field testing by confrontation can localize abnormalities along the visual pathway (e.g., homonymous hemianopia and macular sparing occur with an occipital lobe lesion). Abnormalities of pupillary size can suggest focal impairments (e.g., a miotic pupil in Horner's syndrome can occur in lesions affecting the vestibular nuclei that are in close proximity to sympathetic pathways) or generalized effects (e.g., bilateral miosis or mydriasis due to drug effect). An abnormality of pupillary reaction (e.g., afferent pupillary defect) can be related to multiple sclerosis or a compressive lesion such as pituitary tumor.

Ocular alignment and the range of ocular movements are assessed carefully. A *skew deviation,* or vertical misalignment of the eyes, and head tilt can be seen in patients with the complaint of vertical diplopia. This can be due to a fourth cranial nerve palsy or an otolith disorder involving peripheral or central vestibular pathways.[5] *Smooth pursuit* movements are tested with the patient visually following a slowly moving finger. Abnormalities of pursuit can indicate central disorders (e.g., impaired downward tracking in cerebellar degeneration or craniocervical junction anomalies). Saccadic breakdown of pursuit movements becomes extremely common with ad-

vancing age. *Saccades* are rapid eye movements associated with changes in ocular fixation or eye position within the orbit. Dysmetria, or undershooting or overshooting of saccadic eye movements, is pathological if it persists with repeated testing (e.g., hypermetria with a midline cerebellar lesion).

The evaluation of *nystagmus* is extremely important in the evaluation of a patient with a possible vestibular system disorder. Nystagmus is an involuntary rhythmic pattern of eye movements consisting of slow and fast components occurring in opposite directions. It is caused by physiological activation of the VOR, or by pathology in the peripheral or central vestibular system, and generally cannot be compensated by orbital eye movements.[2] When the nystagmus is not particularly intense, it may be suppressed by gaze fixation. By convention, the direction of the fast component designates the direction of nystagmus. *Physiological nystagmus* occurs in healthy individuals and can be induced by head rotation, caloric irrigations, and rapidly moving (optokinetic) stimuli in the visual field. Two to three beats of "end point nystagmus" is a normal finding when the eye position is moved eccentrically in the orbit to the extremes of ocular range of motion. *Pathological nystagmus* suggests an underlying abnormality and can be characterized as one of several types: *spontaneous* (eyes in primary position), *gaze-evoked* (induced by changes in gaze position), *positional* (not present in seated position but present in some other head positions), and *rapid positioning* (appears only with sudden changes in body position).[2] Although quantitative aspects of nystagmus cannot be evaluated with bedside testing, the clinical evaluation is important to determine whether pathological nystagmus occurs and under what conditions.

In testing for pathological nystagmus, the eyes are examined in primary position and during horizontal and vertical gaze. Spontaneous nystagmus can be visualized with the patient fixating his or her vision at a distant object. Spontaneous nystagmus that is inhibited with visual fixation can be demonstrated by ophthalmoscopic visualization of the fundus of one eye while the patient covers the other eye. Nystagmus is seen as slow, unidirectional, drifting retinal movement with brief, jerking movements in the opposite direction. Another method of assessing spontaneous nystagmus involves the use of *Frenzel glasses,* which consist of 20-diopter mag-

TABLE 11.3. Properties of Nystagmus Due to Peripheral and Central Vestibular System Dysfunction

Nystagmus	Vestibular System Dysfunction	
	Peripheral	Central
Spontaneous		
Quality	Horizontal or combined torsional	Vertical, horizontal, torsional
Fixation	Inhibits, unless severe	Little effect
Direction	Unidirectional	May change direction
Gaze-evoked		
Type	None, although gaze in direction of fast phase intensifies nystagmus	Symmetrical, asymmetrical, dysconjugate, rebound (disappears or reverses)
Rapid positioning		
Quality	Torsional, never vertical	Horizontal or vertical
Latency	2–20 seconds	None
Duration	<30 seconds	>30 seconds
Direction	To downward ear	Up or variable, reversing
Fatigability	Usual	Unusual
Head position	One position	More than one position
Associated symptoms	Vertigo, nausea, vomiting	May have none

nifying lenses and an internal light source so that the examiner can easily visualize the patient's eyes. When used in a darkened room, Frenzel glasses prevent visual fixation, allowing for improved visualization of nystagmus. Gaze-evoked nystagmus can be assessed by having the patient change eye position by fixating on a target 30 degrees to the left, right, up, and down, and holding the eye position for 20 seconds.[2] Positional nystagmus can be identified by placing the patient into right ear down and left ear down positions to see if nystagmus appears. Rapid positioning nystagmus can be induced by the Hallpike or Nylen-Barany maneuver (see Chapter 6, "Electronystagmography").[3] These are relatively synonymous eponyms for a series of maneuvers that produce rapid changes in head position relative to gravity. Classically, the patient is taken rapidly from sitting erect to a supine position, with the head extended and hanging over the edge of the table by 45 degrees in the center position. This position is maintained for 30 seconds, after which the patient is rapidly brought back to sitting erect. The maneuver is repeated with an additional 45-degree rotation of the head to the left and repeated again with head rotation to the right. The patient is observed for nystagmus in the head-hanging and sitting positions. In clinical use, it is best to ask the patient which of these positions is most likely to produce vertigo and perform that maneuver first. If nystagmus is observed, the movement is repeated to determine whether the response is fatigable, that is, less intense on the repeat trial. Table 11.3 lists properties of spontaneous, gaze-evoked, and rapid positioning nystagmus due to peripheral and central vestibular system dysfunction.

Bedside assessment of VORs can be done by the *doll's eyes* (oculocephalic) and *cold caloric* tests. These tests are most useful in the assessment of a comatose patient. The doll's eyes maneuver consists of rapidly moving the patient's head back and forth in the horizontal or vertical plane but is not performed when there is possible cervical spine injury. Conjugate compensatory eye movements indicate normal functioning of the vestibulo-ocular pathways. Dysconjugate eye movements suggest abnormalities of the MLF, ocular motor neurons, or the extraocular eye muscles. An absent oculocephalic reflex suggests a toxic or metabolic disorder, or a large lesion of the brainstem tegmentum. Cold caloric testing is performed by infusing ice water against the tympanic membrane of each ear alternately. The external auditory canal must be free of cerumen. The patient's head is tilted 30 degrees up from the supine position to bring the horizontal semicircular canal into an orientation that is parallel to the gravitational vector. The test is not performed when there is evidence of a ruptured tympanic membrane. In a comatose patient, 50 ml of ice water is used and an abnormal reflex can localize a lesion to the brainstem (slow phase of nystagmus is defective) or to the cerebral hemispheres (intact slow phase bilaterally, absent fast phase bilaterally). In an alert patient, a crude test of relative vestibular responsiveness can be performed. The examiner infuses 1–2 ml of ice water into the patient's ear canal. The normal result is a burst of nystagmus within 30 seconds to 1 minute after infusion, with the fast phase beating away from the ear that was stimulated. The duration of nystagmus (usually 1–3 minutes) is recorded for each ear and compared. A difference of more than 20% suggests vestibular paresis on the side of the decreased response. However, information obtained in this manner rarely affects acute management decisions. Ice water in the ear is uncomfortable, and the evoked vertigo can be very unpleasant for the patient, especially when dizzy. Generally, the caloric exam is deferred until a more standardized, objective electronystagmogram (ENG) examination can be performed.

The corneal reflex tests the functional integrity of the trigeminal and facial nerves. An abnormal reflex can be associated with afferent or efferent pathways, and can suggest brainstem pathology such as a cranial nerve schwannoma. A unilateral facial paralysis is due to an ipsilateral abnormality in the temporal bone, facial nerve, or brainstem. Seventh cranial nerve schwannomas are rare, but can produce vestibular dysfunction when the internal auditory canal (IAC) is involved.

Eighth cranial nerve function subserving hearing is evaluated by testing auditory threshold by presenting a minimal stimulus to each ear, such as the rubbing of fingers, a whispered word, or a watch tick. Tests using a tuning fork vibrating at 256 or 512 Hz can differentiate conductive from sensorineural hearing loss. In the Weber test, the vibrating tuning fork is applied to the middle of the forehead and the sound is normally heard in both ears. In conductive hearing loss, the sound is localized to the affected ear, and to the normal ear in sensorineural hearing loss. In the Rinne test, the vibrating fork is applied to the mastoid area until the sound extinguishes, and then held at the external auditory meatus. Air conduction is greater than bone conduction normally. In conductive hearing loss of the external or middle ear, bone conduction is greater than air conduction. In sensorineural hearing loss, the reverse is true, although air and bone conduction can be quantitatively reduced. Eighth cranial nerve schwannomas of the IAC or cerebellopontine angle rarely produce a facial paralysis prior to treatment.

Palatal elevation and the gag reflex test the integrity of the glossopharyngeal and vagus nerves. The gag reflex is tested carefully to minimize the possibility of vomiting. Absent reflexes suggest impairment of the medulla. Tongue deviation with protrusion can be due to impairment of a cerebral hemisphere or a hypoglossal nerve lesion. Tongue deviation to the right suggests impaired function of the left cerebral hemisphere or the right hypoglossal nerve.

Motor System. Motor function is assessed initially by inspection of the patient. Tremor can be due to basal ganglial disease, cerebellar disease, or anxiety. Carpopedal spasm is seen with hyperventilation. Atrophy, fasciculations, and decreased strength occur with lower motor neuron impairments. Increased resistance to passive manipulation of the joints and weakness suggest contralateral upper motor neuron impairment. Decreased resistance to passive manipulation is seen in cerebellar disease. Abnormal cerebellar tests in an appendage generally suggest ipsilateral cerebellar hemisphere impairment, although unilateral dysmetria can be a sign of an acute ipsilateral disturbance of peripheral vestibular function. Abnormalities of station and gait not related to weakness can localize impairments to the midline cerebellum or to the vestibular system.

Sensory System. Sensory function impairments such as paresthesias or numbness can result in abnormal responses to testing by light touch or pinprick. Paresthesia or numbness that is generalized or occurs in the distal extremities bilaterally and around the mouth suggests hyperventilation. A "stocking glove" distribution pattern suggests a peripheral neuropathy. When unilateral, these abnormalities can suggest an ipsilateral mononeuropathy, radiculopathy or plexopathy, or contralateral cerebral hemisphere impairments. Impaired proprioception and vibration sense can suggest posterior column disease. Impaired proprioception can be tested with the *Romberg test,* which assesses the patient's ability to maintain balance with the feet together and the eyes closed. Significant swaying or inability to maintain the posture is a positive test sign. Repeated falling to one side can be seen with a severe acute unilateral labyrinthine disorder, although most patients with isolated unilateral vestibular disorders can perform the Romberg test without difficulty.

Deep Tendon Reflexes. Deep tendon reflex testing can reveal decreased reflexes (e.g., Achilles tendon reflex) in peripheral neuropathy. Increased reflexes can be seen in contralateral upper motor neuron impairment. Pendular reflexes can be seen in cerebellar disease.

Provocative Tests

Provocative tests are procedures or maneuvers that attempt to reproduce a patient's symptoms and thereby suggest mechanisms responsible for them. These tests can be especially useful for patients with unclear histories and/or normal clinical examinations.

Hyperventilation. Hyperventilation is frequently the cause of presyncopal dizziness. When hyperventilation is suspected from the patient's history, the patient is asked to hyperventilate for 1–3 minutes. Breathing should be rapid and deep, and encouragement is offered to promote a good effort by the patient. Following hyperventilation, the patient is asked to describe the way he or she feels, and to judge whether any unusual sensations resemble the previously experienced dizziness.

Carotid Sinus Massage. The carotid sinus is sensitive to stretch, and massage of a hypersensitive carotid sinus can cause bradycardia or decreased arterial pressure resulting in dizziness or syncope. The carotid sinus is located at the bulb of the carotid bifurcation. It is localized by palpating the carotid bulb below the angle of the mandible anterior to the sternocleidomastoid muscle. The patient is seated, and each carotid sinus is massaged alternately for 15 seconds without significant compression of the carotid artery. Blood pressure and pulse are recorded, and the patient is asked if he or she has experienced any symptoms. A modest drop in blood pressure and pulse without associated symptoms is normal. Carotid sinus massage is contraindicated in patients with known cardiovascular disease.

Valsalva Maneuver. The Valsalva maneuver is performed by having the patient forcibly exhale against a closed glottis, causing decreased cardiac output and cerebral hypoxia. The Valsalva maneuver can result in dizziness or syncope, vertigo can worsen with a perilymph fistula or a craniocervical junction anomaly (e.g., Arnold-Chiari malformation).

Fistula Test. A perilymph fistula can result from otological trauma, barotrauma (e.g., SCUBA diving incidents), or stapedectomy surgery. Fistulas produce disordered fluid mechanics within the inner ear, and can lead to vertigo or disequilibrium, with or without hearing loss. In cases where a perilymph fistula is suspected, pneumatic otoscopy is performed as described above by applying positive and negative pressures to the tympanic membrane. The applied pressure can stimulate one of the semicircular canal cristae, resulting in a transient burst of nystagmus and vertigo. The nystagmus can occur toward or away from the involved ear. A false-positive fistula test can be seen in Meniere's disease or otosyphilis.

Head Shaking. Patients with compensated vestibular disorders can develop nystagmus after quickly shaking the head for 10 cycles in the horizontal plane. Unilateral peripheral lesions are in the direction of the slow phase of the nystagmus.[2]

Fukuda Stepping Test. When a patient is able to perform the eyes-closed Romberg test, the Fukuda stepping test can identify and help to lateralize an acute or chronically uncompensated peripheral vestibular lesion. In this test, the patient extends the arms, closes the eyes, and marches in place. The examiner stands close by to ensure safety and to assist the patient's stability when necessary. Any rotation beyond 90 degrees within 50 steps suggests a paretic lesion on the side to which the patient turned or, less typically, an irritative lesion on the opposite side. The test sensitivity improves when head shaking is performed between eye closure and the initiation of marching in place. It is important to perform the testing in a relatively quiet room so that the patient cannot use auditory cues for orientation.

Differential Diagnosis

The differential diagnosis of dizziness or vertigo can be approached by determining whether the disorder is due to an abnormality of the vestibular system or of nonvestibular systems. Table 11.4 lists categories and common examples of nonvestibular system disorders. Table 11.5 lists vestibular system disorders and some nonvestibular disorders that can affect the vestibular system secondarily by virtue of anatomical or physiological involvement. Disorders common to Tables 11.4 and 11.5 suggest that a disorder may variably affect vestibular and nonvestibular systems. Vestibular system disorders[6] of particular importance to emergency department management are described.

Benign Positional Vertigo

Benign paroxysmal positional vertigo (BPPV) (also known as benign positional vertigo) is a condition characterized by brief periods of vertigo induced by position changes of the head. Onset is usually in middle age;[2] it is the most common cause of vertigo assessed in clinical practice.[2,3] Vertigo is often precipitated by rolling over in bed, getting in or out of bed, bending over, or extending the neck. It typically lasts for only a few seconds, always less than 1 minute.[7] The patient may recognize a critical head position that reproduces the vertigo. Following the first attack or a flurry of episodes, lightheadedness and nausea may persist for hours to days.

The pathophysiology of BPPV is not fully known, although an abnormality of the posterior semicircular canal is strongly supported by clinical and experimental evidence. It is likely that dislodgement of cal-

TABLE 11.4. Differential Diagnosis of Dizziness or Vertigo: Nonvestibular System Disorders

Systemic disorders
  Cardiovascular presyncope
    Hypovolemia
    Postural hypotension
    Vasovagal
    Carotid sinus
    Postmicturition
    Posttussive
    Vasodilators
    Autonomic nervous system dysfunction
    Addison's disease
    Brady/tachyarrhythmias
    Heart block
    Congestive heart failure
    Valvular heart disease
  Medications
  Hyperventilation
  Chronic obstructive pulmonary disease
  Infection
  Hypoglycemia
  Hyperglycemia
  Anemia
  Alcohol
  Street drugs
Ophthalmological disorders
  Glaucoma
  Lens implant
  Refractive errors
  New prescription lenses
  Acute ocular muscle paralysis
Neurological disorders
  Headache
    Sinus
    Muscle contraction
    Migraine
  Concussion
  Complex partial seizures
  Dementia
  Peripheral neuropathy
  Paraneoplastic cerebellar dysfunction
Psychiatric disorders
  Anxiety
  Panic attack
  Depression
  Psychogenic seizure
  Conversion reaction
  Malingering

TABLE 11.5. Differential Diagnosis of Dizziness or Vertigo: Vestibular System Disorders

Peripheral causes
  Middle ear
    Infection
      Viral
      Bacterial
    Otosclerosis
    Cholesteatoma
    Tumors
      Glomus tympanicum or jugulare
      Squamous cell carcinoma
  Inner ear
    Benign positional vertigo
    Vestibular neuronitis
    Meniere's disease
    Labyrinthitis
      Infection
      Autoimmune disorder
    Vascular disorders
      Vertebrobasilar insufficiency
        Labyrinthine
          Anterior inferior cerebellar
          artery
      Hemorrhage
        Labyrinthine
        Bleeding diathesis
    Systemic disorders
      Diabetes
      Uremia
    Trauma
      Perilymph fistula
    Ototoxins
      Alcohol
      Salicylates
      Antiepileptics
      Aminoglycosides
      Loop diuretics
      Cinchona alkaloids
        Quinidine
        Quinine
      Heavy metals
        Cisplatin

Cranial nerve
  Infection
  Collagen vascular disease
  Tumor
    Schwannoma
    Neurofibroma
    Meningioma
    Metastasis
Central causes
  Cerebrovascular disorders
    Vertebrobasilar insufficiency
      Posterior fossa
        Basilar artery
        Posterior inferior cerebellar artery
    Hemorrhage
      Cerebellar
    Basilar migraine
    Vascular loop
  Mass lesions
    Tumor
      Brainstem
        Glioma
      Cerebellum
        Medulloblastoma
    Abscess
  Metabolic disorders
    Alcoholic cerebellar degeneration
  Infection
    Meningitis
    Encephalitis
  Developmental disorders
    Malformations of the inner ear
    Craniocervical junction
      Arnold-Chiari malformation
  Hereditary disorders
    Friedreich's ataxia
    Refsum's disease
    Olivopontocerebellar atrophy
  Complex partial seizures
  Demyelinating disease
  Trauma

cium carbonate crystals from the otolithic membrane in the utricle results in gravity-sensitive particles settling onto the cupula (*cupulolithiasis*) or floating freely in the membranous portion (*canalolithiasis*) of the posterior semicircular canal. BPPV can be the sequela of head injury or degeneration due to aging. Secondary forms of BPPV can follow viral labyrinthitis, vestibular neuronitis, vascular disease of the inner ear, or any cause of peripheral vertigo.

Diagnosis is based on history and supported by a positive rapid positioning test (Hallpike maneuver). The patient with classic BPPV demonstrates torsional rotatory nystagmus, with a fast horizontal component that beats toward the ear that is placed downward. The nystagmus has the following additional features to support the diagnosis of BPPV: (1) it is latent, beginning 2–5 seconds after assuming the provocative position; (2) it is transient, disappearing within 20–30 seconds; (3) it has a crescendo and decrescendo in intensity; and (4) it fatigues with repeat trials, usually with complete resolution by the fourth repetition of the Hallpike maneuver. The dependent ear is generally the one that causes the symptoms, although bilateral disease can occur. Although the nystagmus of BPPV can be recorded with ENG, the pattern can be difficult to interpret due to the torsional nature of the nystagmus. Therefore, the diagnosis is best made by direct visual inspection of the eyes by the clinician. Frenzel glasses are unnecessary because the nystagmus intensity is usually great enough to prevent suppression by visual fixation. Most patients with BPPV note resolution of symptoms without treatment. Although vestibular suppressants can provide temporary relief of associated nausea and lightheadedness, they usually do not prevent the motion-provoked spells of vertigo. Therefore, proper management includes discouraging the long-term use of such medications. Conventional vestibular rehabilitation training exercises are effective in treating this condition. A unique therapeutic procedure that can provide immediate relief of BPPV, the particle repositioning maneuver, has been developed (Figure 11.2).[8,9] The procedure involves slowly bringing the patient's head through a series of movements designed to permit the removal of the offending particulate material from the posterior semicircular canal. The rare patient who does not respond to conservative therapy is a candidate for surgical therapy. Selective sectioning of the ampullary nerve of the posterior semicircular canal is effective but technically demanding. A simpler procedure that interrupts endolymphatic flow within the posterior semicircular canal is safe for hearing and very effective in resolving vertigo due to BPPV.[10]

Vestibular Neuronitis

Vestibular neuronitis (also known as acute vestibulopathy, acute vestibular neuritis, vestibular neurolabyrinthitis[2]) is a condition typically characterized by sudden, severe vertigo associated with nausea and vomiting in the absence of auditory symptoms. Symptoms usually peak within 24 hours, and patients can remain relatively immobile because symptoms often worsen with head movement. There can be truncal unsteadiness, imbalance, and difficulty focusing vision. Symptoms subside in several days and resolve within several weeks to 3 months. Recovery from any acute peripheral lesion depends on the process of vestibular compensation within the CNS. During the compensation process, patients can have a sense of disequilibrium that is aggravated by rapid head movements. In general, vestibular neuronitis is a benign condition characterized by one episode of symptoms. However, 20–30% of patients have at least one recurrent attack of vertigo.[11] There are several other more serious conditions that can mimic vestibular neuronitis.[12]

Vestibular neuronitis is likely the result of a systemic viral illness or an isolated viral infection that affects the vestibular labyrinth and/or the vestibular ganglia. Small vessel disease in the elderly has also been implicated. In most patients, the cause is not determined. Vestibular neuronitis is a diagnosis of exclusion, based on a compatible history, signs of an acute unilateral vestibular loss (vertigo and spontaneous nystagmus, usually with the fast phase away from the abnormal ear), and the absence of any central findings on the neurological examination, imaging studies, or the ENG. Often, the ENG will show a caloric weakness on the affected side. Management includes the short-term use of antihistamines or anticholinergics, an antiemetic, and/or a benzodiazepine for tranquilization as needed. Corticosteroids appear to reduce the intensity and duration of acute symptoms when administered early in the disease.[13] The patient is encouraged to avoid prolonged immobility. Vestibular training exercises are

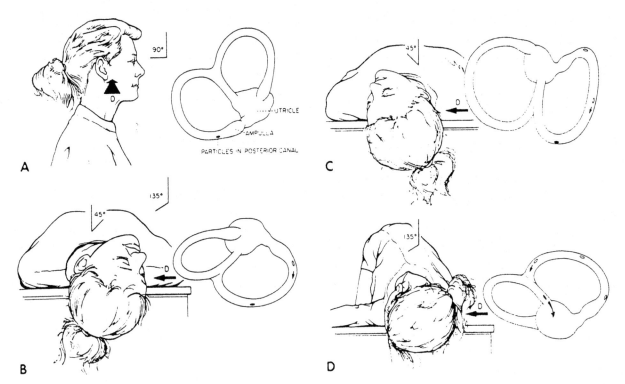

FIGURE 11.2. Particle repositioning maneuver for the right ear (A–D). The left side of each drawing shows the position of the patient. The arrow (D) represents the direction of view of the labyrinth depicted on the right side showing the relative position of the labyrinth and the movement of particles (dark oval, new position; open oval, previous position) in the posterior semicircular canal. (A) Patient sitting lengthwise on table. (B) Patient in Hallpike position placing the undermost (affected) ear in the earth-vertical axis. Nystagmus is exhibited in this position, possibly associated with vertigo. This position is maintained until the nystagmus is resolved. (C) Head is rotated to the left with the head turned 45 degrees downward. (D) Head and body are rotated until facing downward 135 degrees from the supine position and maintained for 1–2 minutes before the patient sits up. During B–D, particles gravitate in the posterior semicircular canal through the common crus and into the utricle. (Reprinted with permission from Parnes LS, Price-Jones RG: Particle repositioning maneuver for benign paroxysmal vertigo. *Ann Otol Rhinol Laryngol* 1993;102:325–331.)

undertaken and vestibular suppressant medication is discontinued as soon as the severe initial symptoms have improved.

Labyrinthitis

Labyrinthitis is a condition characterized by inflammation or infection of the labyrinthine system. The symptoms of acute labyrinthitis are identical to those of vestibular neuronitis, except that hearing loss accompanies the vertigo. The degree of auditory and/or vestibular symptoms depends on the extent and severity of inner ear involvement. Labyrinthitis can be caused by numerous agents including viruses, bacteria, spirochetes, and fungi, and possible involvement of systemic allergic or autoimmune diseases. There is a broad range of clinical expression for most specific etiologies.

Viral labyrinthitis (viral neurolabyrinthitis[2]) can occur with a systemic viral illness such as mumps, measles, influenza, or infectious mononucleosis. Commonly, it is due to an isolated infection of the labyrinth and/or the eighth cranial nerve, with the infectious agent unidentified. It can present with severe hearing loss that progresses over hours ("sudden deafness"), accompanied by tinnitus and ear fullness, acute vertigo, or some combination of auditory and vestibular symptoms. Hearing returns to normal in many patients after a variable period of time, usually within one month. Diagnosis is based on history, physical examination, and laboratory evidence of peripheral auditory and/or vestibular dysfunction. Audiometry documents a sensorineural hearing loss. If the vestibular system is involved, caloric responses can be decreased or absent on the involved side. Management consists of vestibular suppressants, antiemetics, and vestibular training exercises as indicated. Corticosteroid use for an anti-inflammatory effect is not of clear benefit in the treatment of this disorder, but it is generally provided empirically if the patient seeks medical care in the first few days of the illness.

Toxic labyrinthitis is a nonspecific disturbance of labyrinthine function that results from the products of inflammation entering the confines of the bony labyrinth. This occurs in response to acute or chronic otitis media, and is not associated with frank suppuration in the labyrinth. Inner ear function frequently returns to normal following treatment of the underlying infection and symptomatic management of the labyrinthine symptoms.

Bacterial labyrinthitis is a more serious infection, with actual suppuration of the labyrinth itself. This condition usually presents with a fulminant course of severe vertigo, nausea, vomiting, and profound hearing loss. There can be associated fever, headache, or pain. Unilateral cases of bacterial labyrinthitis typically originate from infection in the pneumatized spaces of the temporal bone (acute or chronic otitis media, mastoiditis); bilateral cases can result from bacterial meningitis. Diagnosis is commonly based on clinical information. Treatment consists of aggressive parenteral antibiotic therapy with agents that provide adequate penetration of the blood–brain barrier. Surgery can be required for treatment of middle ear or mastoid infection, and to drain the resulting abscess within the labyrinth in the critically ill patient with unilateral suppurative labyrinthitis.

Syphilitic labyrinthitis occurs as a late manifestation of either congenital or acquired syphilis. It begins with deteriorating inner ear function and, when untreated, progresses slowly to profound bilateral loss of auditory and vestibular function. This course is punctuated with episodic fluctuating and progressive sensorineural hearing loss and vertigo. The peak incidence of congenital syphilitic laby-

rinthitis is in the fourth or fifth decade of life. The acquired form peaks in the fifth or sixth decade.[2] Pathological changes consist of an inflammatory infiltration of the labyrinth and osteitis of the otic capsule (osseous boundary of the labyrinth). This condition can occur despite prior treatment of syphilis, and may not be accompanied by neurosyphilis. Diagnosis is based on a history of unexplained vertigo, a course of fluctuating hearing loss, which is often bilateral, and a positive fluorescent treponemal antibody (FTA) test. Penicillin is the treatment of choice. Corticosteroid therapy may provide additional benefit, albeit often temporary, in some cases.

Meniere's Disease

Meniere's disease (endolymphatic hydrops) is characterized by fluctuating hearing loss, tinnitus, and episodic vertigo. Onset of the syndrome is usually in the third or fourth decade of life. The patient typically becomes symptomatic in one ear, with the development of a sensation of fullness or pressure, hearing loss, and tinnitus. Episodes of spontaneous, intense vertigo that peak within minutes and subside over several hours usually follow these symptoms, but can precede them. Nausea, vomiting, diaphoresis, and pallor usually occur. Following an acute attack of vertigo, the patient can feel unsteady for several days. The syndrome follows a remittent course, with relapses having variable severity and periodicity. Tinnitus can resolve or decrease between episodes. When persistent, the tinnitus typically increases in intensity immediately prior to or during a recurrent attack. Hearing loss is reversible in the early stages of the disease, but a gradually worsening residual hearing loss occurs with repeated attacks. Approximately one-third of patients experience symptoms in both ears.[14] The paroxysmal episodes cease spontaneously late in the course of the disease.

The characteristic histopathological finding in Meniere's disease is a distension of the entire endolymphatic system.[2] The increased volume of endolymph likely results from retention of sodium in the endolymphatic compartment and possibly impaired resorption of endolymph due to dysfunction of the endolymphatic duct and sac. The mechanism responsible for the fluctuating course of severe symptoms is not known completely, but may be due to episodic ruptures of the delicate membranes separating endolymph and perilymph, such as Reissner's membrane, located between the scala media and the scala vestibuli in the cochlea. This would result in an admixture of the two fluid compartments and a potassium intoxication of the neural processes that lead to the afferent fibers of the eighth nerve until the fluid balance is restored. Several diseases can result in Meniere's disease, including temporal bone trauma, otological surgery such as stapedectomy, and viral, toxic, bacterial, or syphilitic labyrinthitis. However, the cause is idiopathic in most cases.

Diagnosis is based on a characteristic history and documentation of fluctuating hearing by audiometry. ENG can show a peripheral spontaneous nystagmus acutely and vestibular paresis on caloric testing in chronic cases.[2] Acute management is largely empirical and involves the use of vestibular suppressants and antiemetics. A low-salt diet and diuretic use is recommended for maintenance therapy.[6] Surgical options in refractory cases include endolymphatic shunts and ablative procedures, with the latter providing more reliable results. Surgical ablative procedures include labyrinthectomy and vestibular nerve transection. Chemical labyrinthectomy is sometimes performed with local or systemic application of aminoglycosides.

Perilymph Fistulas

Perilymph fistulas are defects of the otic capsule or its oval or round windows. These defects allow leakage of perilymph from the inner ear into the middle ear space. Perilymph fistulas can occur secondary to congenital defects of the inner ear; following stapedectomy surgery for otosclerosis; following pressure changes in the middle ear associated with nose blowing, sneezing, or barotrauma as in SCUBA diving; or with sudden increases in CSF pressure associated with lifting, coughing, or straining.[2]

Perilymph fistulas are commonly experienced as an audible "pop" in the ear followed by hearing loss and vertigo. Diagnosis is made from the history and supported by a positive fistula test or Valsalva maneuver. Audiometry can show either normal hearing or a sensorineural hearing loss. A small conductive component to the hearing loss is seen rarely. ENG can show spontaneous and/or positional nystagmus. Unilateral caloric hypoexcitability can re-

sult, but calorics are generally normal. Management is conservative except in cases of penetrating otologic trauma, because most perilymph fistulas heal spontaneously. Bed rest, sedation, head elevation, and the avoidance of straining are recommended. Surgical exploration and repair can be indicated with persistent auditory and vestibular symptoms.

Cerebellopontine Angle Tumors

Tumors of the cerebellopontine angle (CPA) typically begin in the internal auditory canal and slowly grow into the CPA, compressing the seventh and eighth cranial nerves. The most common CPA tumor is the vestibular schwannoma (acoustic neuroma), which usually arises from schwann cells of the vestibular nerve but can also arise from the facial, acoustic, or trigeminal nerves. Vestibular schwannomas account for over 90% of tumors of the CPA. Unilateral hearing loss and tinnitus are the most frequently experienced symptoms. Vertigo occurs in less than 20% of patients, and is rarely severe. Diagnosis is based on history and can be supported by clinical information indicating impairment of other adjacent cranial nerves. Magnetic resonance imaging (MRI) is sensitive in identification of tumors smaller than 1 cm.[15] Auditory brainstem response testing is a sensitive screening test for eighth cranial nerve involvement, and is usually abnormal in vestibular schwannomas.[16] With few exceptions, such as small tumors in the elderly, treatment is surgical removal.

Vascular Disease

The vertebrobasilar circulation supplies blood to the labyrinth, eighth cranial nerve, and brainstem. Hypoperfusion of the vertebrobasilar system, or *vertebrobasilar insufficiency* (*VBI*), can lead to widespread or focal ischemia and/or stroke of the vestibular system. VBI is a common cause of vertigo that has an abrupt onset, lasts for minutes, and can occur with nausea and vomiting. Other associated symptoms include diplopia, visual field defects, and headache. The common cause of VBI is atherosclerosis of the subclavian, vertebral, and basilar arteries. Occasionally, VBI can be precipitated by postural hypotension or by decreased cardiac output. VBI due to compression of the vertebral arteries by bony cervical spine spurs is a rare occurrence.[2]

There are several clinical syndromes of abnormalities of the vertebral and basilar arteries and their branches. Certain syndromes are of particular importance in the emergency department evaluation of vertigo. Occlusion of the AICA can result in labyrinthine ischemia or infarction. There is usually a sudden profound loss of auditory and vestibular function. Ipsilateral facial numbness and weakness, ipsilateral Horner's syndrome, ipsilateral cerebellar signs, paresis of lateral gaze, and nystagmus can occur. Occlusion of the PICA, known as the lateral medullary or Wallenberg's syndrome, results in infarction of the lateral medulla. There is usually a sudden onset of vertigo, nystagmus, diplopia, dysphagia, nausea, and vomiting. Ipsilateral abnormalities include Horner's syndrome, palatal paralysis, loss of pain and temperature sensation of the face, facial and lateral rectus weakness, and cerebellar signs. There is contralateral loss of pain and temperature sensation of the body.

Acute management of vertigo due to vascular disease is usually directed at correcting the underlying disorder, whenever possible. General medical stabilization includes oxygenation, control of blood pressure, and fluid balance regulation.

Laboratory Studies

Ordering of laboratory studies in the emergency department for a patient with dizziness or vertigo is guided by information obtained from the history and physical examination. Routine hematological and chemical tests to be considered include a complete blood count with white blood cell differential counts, serum electrolytes, glucose, blood urea nitrogen, and creatinine. Other studies include FTA, cardiac enzymes, carboxyhemoglobin, and ethanol levels. Urine can be obtained for routine and microscopic tests and for a toxicology screen. Arterial blood gases, pulse oximetry, chest radiograph, or electrocardiogram may be required.

Imaging Studies

Imaging studies of the skull and brain may be indicated in the evaluation of a patient with dizziness or vertigo. The two most important imaging techniques used for this purpose are computerized tomography (CT) and MRI. CT scanning is available in most hospitals and can be important diagnostically during evaluation of the patient in the emergency department. MRI is available in some hospitals but its use

during evaluation in the emergency department is limited. When indicated, MRI is obtained following the patient's hospital admission or during an outpatient evaluation. MRI is frequently superior to CT because of its greater sensitivity in demonstrating pathology of brain parenchyma and its lack of bone artifacts. In the evaluation of vertigo, lesions affecting the labyrinthine or peripheral organ are best studied with thin-section high-resolution CT. Retrolabyrinthine or "central" lesions are best studied with MRI. Pathological disorders affecting the labyrinth include cholesteatomas, temporal bone tumors, and fractures. Retrolabyrinthine lesions of the CPA include vestibular schwannomas, meningiomas, epidermoids, cholesterol cysts of the petrous apex, glomus tumors, and ectatic vertebral or basilar arteries.[15] Retrolabyrinthine disorders of the brain that involve vestibular pathways include benign and malignant brain tumors, demyelinating disease (e.g., multiple sclerosis), vascular malformations, ischemic disease of the cerebral gray–white matter junction, and craniocervical abnormalities.[17]

Other diagnostic studies can be performed in the evaluation of the patient with vertigo either in the hospital or on an outpatient basis. Frequently utilized tests are MRA (magnetic resonance angiography) audiometry, brainstem auditory evoked potentials (see Chapter 7), and ENG (see Chapter 6).

Management

The emergency department management of a patient with dizziness or vertigo is guided by the presumptive diagnosis and is directed at correcting the underlying cause whenever possible, providing symptomatic therapy, and promoting vestibular compensation when indicated. Because there are numerous vestibular and nonvestibular system disorders that can cause dizziness, it may not be possible to make a definitive diagnosis during an evaluation in the emergency department. For those disorders that can be diagnosed, some are correctable and others receive symptomatic therapy.

Initial Stabilization

A patient who presents to the emergency department acutely ill with vertigo accompanied by severe nausea and vomiting requires immediate stabilization. These symptoms can cause the patient to be extremely frightened and can compromise the emergency physician's ability to obtain an adequate history and physical examination. The patient is given calm verbal reassurance and is allowed to assume a body position that minimizes symptoms. All unnecessary external stimuli (e.g., excessive light, noise) are removed from the examination room. When tolerated by a vomiting patient, a semiprone position can provide some airway protection against aspiration of gastric contents. Oxygen can be administered by nasal cannulae, and a peripheral intravenous line is established. Oropharyngeal suctioning can be performed when necessary. Any trauma associated with the patient's presentation is treated as a high priority.

Pharmacological Treatment

Pharmacological treatment of vertigo and associated symptoms can be divided into two categories: symptomatic and pathophysiological. Symptomatic treatment in the emergency department generally includes the use of vestibular suppressant and antiemetic medications. The selection and duration of use of specific agents within these medication groups is not standardized. The optimal therapeutic strategy is to reduce severe symptoms while minimizing undesirable side effects and impairment of compensatory vestibular mechanisms. Psychotherapeutic medications can be used to treat underlying anxiety or depression associated with some forms of dizziness. Table 11.6 lists several of these medications, their dosing regimens, and the routes of administration.

Vestibular Suppressants. The main categories of vestibular suppressants are antihistamines, anticholinergics, benzodiazepines, and monoaminergics. These medications are commonly used to suppress vertigo associated with peripheral vestibular disorders. In experimental studies, these medications alter and usually suppress the level of tonic activity in vestibular neurons.[6] Antihistamines suppress vestibular end organs and inhibit central cholinergic pathways. The macular end organs (utricle and saccule) are typically more suppressed than the semicircular canals. Therefore, antihistamines are often more effective in treating motion sickness than acute, severe vertigo. The side effects of antihistamines include dry mouth, drowsiness,

TABLE 11.6. Symptomatic Treatment of Vestibular Disorders: Medications, Dosing, and Routes of Administration

Vestibular suppressants
  Antihistamines
    Meclizine (Antivert) 12.5–25 mg PO q4–6h
    Dimenhydrinate (Dramamine) 50 mg PO, IM q4–6h
    Promethazine (Phenergan) 25–50 mg PO, PR, IM q4–6h
    Cyclizine (Marezine) 50 mg PO, IM q4–6h
    Diphenhydramine (Benadryl) 25–50 mg PO, IM, IV q4–6h
    Astemizole (Hismanal) 10 mg PO qd
  Anticholinergics
    Scopolamine (Transderm Scop) 1 disc delivers 0.5 mg q3d
  Benzodiazepines
    Diazepam (Valium) 5–10 mg PO, IM, IV q4–6h
  Monoaminergics
    Ephedrine 25 mg PO, IM q4–6h
Antiemetics
  Phenothiazines
    Prochlorperazine (Compazine) 5–10 mg PO, IM q6h or 25 mg PR q12h
    Thiethylperazine (Torecan) 10 mg PO, PR, IM q8–24h
    Promethazine (Phenergan) 12.5–25 mg PO, PR, IM, IV q4–6h
  Butyrophenones
    Droperidol (Inapsine) 2.5–5 mg IM, IV
  Benzamides
    Trimethobenzamide (Tigan) 250 mg PO q6–8h or 200 mg PR, IM q6–8h
Psychotherapeutic agents
  Benzodiazepines
    Alprazolam (Xanax) 0.25–0.50 mg PO q8h
    Chlordiazepoxide (Librium) 25–50 mg PO q6–8h
    Diazepam (Valium) 2–10 mg PO q6–12h
    Lorazepam (Ativan) 2–3 mg PO q8–12h
  Tricyclic antidepressants
    Amitriptyline (Elavil) 50–100 mg PO qd
    Imipramine (Tofranil) 50–150 mg PO qd
    Nortriptyline (Pamelor) 25 mg PO q6–8h

Notes: Recommended pharmacological regimen for the vertiginous patient to provide acute and short-term vestibular suppression, control of nausea and vomiting, and sedation:
Diazepam 2–10 mg PO, IM, IV q4–6h
Promethazine 12.5–25 mg PO, PR, IM, IV q4–6h
Dosing and route of administration are determined by body weight, severity of symptoms, and response to therapy. Therapy is intended to provide prompt control, continued relief, and convenience at the lowest effective dose to allow for vestibular compensation.

blurred vision, and urine retention, but are generally well tolerated by patients. Anticholinergics inhibit activation of central cholinergic pathways and are similar to the antihistamines with regard to effectiveness in treating motion sickness and side effects. Benzodiazepines suppress central and peripheral vestibular pathways, provide tranquilization, and are often beneficial when antihistamines and anticholinergics are ineffective. Benzodiazepines can cause confusion, drowsiness, and ataxia and are used judiciously because of abuse potential. Monoaminergics suppress activity within vestibular neurons and can cause hypertension, nervousness, palpitations, and insomnia.

The use of vestibular suppressants is guarded because of their ability to retard CNS compensatory mechanisms needed to restore vestibular balance. Abnormal vestibular inputs must be recognized by the CNS in order for it to initiate adaptive changes. Recognition of a vestibular deficit by the CNS results from the integration of visual, proprioceptive, and vestibular sensory feedback information produced when the patient attempts to use his or her vestibular reflexes. Research in animals and humans suggests that compensation can be affected directly by the experience of the animal or patient immediately after loss of function. Therefore, suppression of vestibular symptoms by medications or immobilization can limit the potential of the CNS to establish, modify, and maintain the compensatory mechanisms necessary for full recovery.[18] Categories of vestibular suppressant medication that influence vestibular compensation in animal studies include anticholinergics (they delay compensation and can produce overcompensation in compensated animals), benzodiazepines (they retard compensation when used chronically, but can accelerate compensation when used acutely to enhance early mobilization), and adrenergics (they produce decompensation). In addition, alcohol can retard compensation or produce decompensation, and caffeine and amphetamines can accelerate compensation.[6]

Antiemetics. The main categories of antiemetic medications are the phenothiazines, butyrophenones, and benzamides. These medications are effective in treating nausea and vomiting by antagonism of dopamine receptors in the chemoreceptor trigger zone of the vomiting center in the lateral reticular formation of the medulla. Phenothiazines can also suppress vestibular nuclei and central vestibular pathways, likely due to their antihistaminic or anticholinergic activity. Side effects include sedation, hypotension, and extrapyramidal symptoms.

Psychotherapeutic Agents. Psychotherapeutic medications include benzodiazepines and tricyclic antidepressants. Benzodiazepines can be used acutely in the emergency department to treat moderately severe anxiety syndromes that cause dizziness. However, continued outpatient use of these medications is under the supervision of the patient's physician because of abuse potential. Tricyclic antidepressant medication can be instituted in the emergency department in consultation with the patient's family physician or psychiatrist to treat major depression that causes dizziness. The side effects of these medications are orthostatic hypotension and anticholinergic symptoms.

Pathophysiological treatment of vertigo is performed under the direction of an otolaryngologist, otologist, or neurologist. Such treatment can involve the use of diuretics, vasodilators, corticosteroids, or antibiotics, depending on the final diagnosis. Diuretics are used to decrease intralabyrinthine fluid pressure in the treatment of Meniere's disease. Commonly used diuretics include hydrochlorothiazide, hydrochlorothiazide-triamterine combinations (Dyazide), and acetazolamide (Diamox). Vasodilators have been used to treat vertigo, as a means to increase perfusion to the labyrinth and brainstem. Efficacy of these agents is not proven, and they are rarely beneficial. Corticosteroids can be used to decrease inflammation and edema in the labyrinth and internal auditory canal. They are frequently used in the treatment of labyrinthitis, vestibular neuronitis, autoimmune ear disease, and Bell's palsy. Generally, 1 mg of prednisone per kilogram of body weight is taken daily for 7–10 days, followed by rapid tapering of the dose. Antibiotics are used to treat bacterial and syphilitic labyrinthitis, and for vestibular ablation in bilateral Meniere's syndrome. Streptomycin is the aminoglycoside of choice for systemic chemical vestibular ablation, although this is rarely performed. Gentamicin is used for intratympanic administration to accomplish unilateral vestibular ablation in refractory cases of Meniere's disease.

Surgical treatment is indicated for some patients with vertigo who do not respond adequately to conservative management. The best surgical candidates are those who have unstable labyrinthine disease that leads to fluctuating or progressively deteriorating inner ear function. Those who experience incomplete recovery from a vestibular disorder due to poor central compensation are poor surgical candidates. It is proper to refer patients with refractory symptoms for a comprehensive evaluation by an otolaryngologist with expertise in disorders and surgery of the vestibular system. Patients rarely require emergency surgery for a vestibular disorder. One example would be the patient with penetrating trauma to the middle ear, resulting in vertigo. Another would be the critically ill patient with suppurative labyrinthitis.

Emergency Treatment of the SCUBA Diver with Vertigo

Transient vertigo during SCUBA diving that resolves with equalization of pressure in the middle ear cleft is known as alternobaric vertigo and requires no treatment except to avoid diving when eustachian tube function may be impaired. Distinguishing between inner ear barotrauma, perilymphatic fistula, and inner ear decompression sickness can be complex, and is best done by an otolaryngologist in consultation with a diving medicine expert.[19]

Vestibular Rehabilitation

Vestibular rehabilitation is an exercise-based physical therapy program designed to facilitate CNS compensatory mechanisms in patients with vestibular pathology.[20,21] Rehabilitative therapy can be beneficial for patients with acute or chronic symptoms of vestibular dysfunction. Patient assessment and the development of a training program are usually done by a properly trained physical or occupational therapist, who designs a customized program tailored to the needs of the individual patient. Generic programs can be helpful, especially for stereotyped conditions such as classic BPPV. The use of a generic program can avoid the trouble and expense of complex vestibular testing and customized rehabilitation therapy. Principles of vestibular training exercises include the following: (1) training tasks exceed the capability of the patient, and task diffi-culty increases progressively with improvement; (2) stimuli elicit symptoms similar to those experienced during normal activities; (3) active head movements that provoke vertigo are practiced without producing overwhelming symptoms; (4) training tasks stress the vestibular apparatus; and (5) when a fixed vestibular deficit is present, the tasks promote improved motor behavior based on proper utilization of available visual and proprioceptive information.[22]

Following an acute vestibular disorder, therapy can be initiated as soon as the patient recovers sufficiently to engage in training exercises. Prolonged bed rest and inactivity are avoided because they often result in poor vestibular compensation. Therapy is directed at improving (1) postural control in sitting, standing, and walking; (2) eye–head coordination for gaze stabilization; (3) head motion tolerance; and (4) physical conditioning.[23] A team approach to rehabilitation that includes the patient's family physician, neurologist, or otologist is most likely to facilitate patient progress and to maintain improvements that allow for an active and productive life.

PEARLS AND PITFALLS

- Carefully obtained clinical information can determine whether dizziness is caused by a disorder of the peripheral or central vestibular system or nonvestibular systems.
- Vertigo usually suggests a vestibular system disorder but cannot reliably localize it.
- The neuro-otologic examination is important in assessing a patient with dizziness or vertigo.
- The Hallpike maneuver can diagnose benign paroxysmal positional vertigo; the particle repositioning maneuver can treat it.
- Symptomatic treatment of severe vertigo in the emergency department usually includes vestibular suppressant and antiemetic medications.
- Unexplained dizziness or vertigo may require referral of the patient to an otolaryngologist or neurologist.
- Vestibular rehabilitation is exercise-based physical therapy designed to facilitate CNS compensa-

tory mechanisms in patients with vestibular pathology; prolonged bed rest, inactivity, or use of vestibular suppressant medication can result in poor vestibular compensation and a less-than-desired clinical outcome.

REFERENCES

1. Weiss HD. Dizziness. In: Samuels MA, ed. *Manual of Neurology: Diagnosis and Therapy.* Boston, Mass: Little, Brown and Co; 1991.

2. Baloh RW, Honrubia V. *Clinical Neurophysiology of the Vestibular System.* 2nd ed. Contemporary Neurology Series. Philadelphia, Pa: FA Davis Co; 1990.

3. Smith DB. Dizziness: a clinical perspective. In: Kaufman AI, Smith DB, eds. *Neurologic Clinics: Diagnostic Neurotology.* Philadelphia, Pa: WB Saunders Co; 1990;8.

4. Adams RD, Victor M. *Principles of Neurology.* New York, NY: McGraw-Hill Book Co; 1989.

5. Leigh RJ, Zee DS. *The Neurology of Eye Movements.* Philadelphia. Pa: FA Davis Co; 1983.

6. Zee DS. The management of patients with vestibular disorders. In: Barber HO, Sharp JA, eds. *Vestibular Disorders.* Chicago, Ill: Yearbook Medical Publishers; 1988.

7. Baloh RW, Honrubia V, Jacobson K. Benign positional vertigo. Clinical and oculographic features in 240 cases. *Neurology.* 1987;37:371.

8. Epley JM. The canalith repositioning procedure for treatment of benign paroxysmal positional vertigo. *Otolaryngol Head Neck Surg.* 1992; 107:399–404.

9. Parnes LS, Price-Jones RG. Particle repositioning maneuver for treatment of benign paroxysmal positional vertigo. *Ann Otol Rhinol Laryngol.* 1993; 102:325–31.

10. Parnes LS, McClure JA. Posterior semicircular canal occlusion in the normal hearing ear. *Otolaryngol Head Neck Surg.* 1991;104:52–7.

11. Coats AC. Vestibular neuronitis. *Acta Otolaryngol.* 1969; 251 (suppl):1.

12. Disher MJ, Telian SA, Kermink JL. Evaluation of acute vertigo: unusual lesions imitating vestibular neuritis. *Am J Otol.* 1991;12:227–31.

13. Ariyasu L, Byl FM, Sprague MS, Adour KK. The beneficial effect of methylprednisolone in acute vestibular vertigo. *Arch Otolaryngol Head Neck Surg.* 1990;116: 700–3.

14. Wladislavosky-Waserman P, Facer GW, Mokri B, Kurland LT. Meniere's disease: a 30-year epidemiologic and clinical study in Rochester, MN, 151–1980. *Laryngoscope.* 1984;94:1098.

15. Seibert CE, Dreisbach JN. Neuroradiology of vestibular pathways. In: Kaufman AI, Smith DB, eds. *Neurologic Clinics: Diagnostic Neurotology.* Philadelphia, Pa: WB Saunders Co; 1990;8.

16. Telian SA, Kileny PR, Kemink JL, Niparko JK, Graham MD. Normal auditory brainstem response in acoustic neuroma. *Laryngoscope.* 1989;99:10–14.

17. Dobben GD, Valvassori GE. Imaging studies in patients with central vestibular disorders. In: Kaufman AI, Smith DB, eds. *Neurologic Clinics: Diagnostic Neurotology.* Philadelphia, Pa: WB Saunders Co; 1990;8.

18. Peppard SB. Effect of drug therapy on compensation from vestibular injury. *Laryngoscope.* 1986;96:878–98.

19. Arthur DC, Margulies RA. A short course in diving medicine. *Ann Emerg Med.* 1987;16:689–701.

20. Shumway-Cook A, Horak FB. Rehabilitation strategies for patients with vestibular deficits. *Neurol Clin.* 1990;8:441–57.

21. Shepard NT, Telian SA. Programmatic vestibular rehabilitation. *Otolaryngol Head Neck Surg.* 1995;112: 173–82.

22. Zee DS. Treatment of vertigo. In: Johnson RT, ed. *Current Therapy in Neurologic Disease.* Philadelphia, Pa: BC Decker Inc; 1985.

23. Shumway-Cook A, Horak FB. Rehabilitation strategies for patients with vestibular deficits. In: Kaufman AI, Smith DB, eds. *Neurologic Clinics: Diagnostic Neurotology.* Philadelphia, Pa: WB Saunders Co; 1990;8.

24. Anson BJ, Donaldson JA. *Surgical anatomy of the temporal bone.* Philadelphia, Pa: WB Saunders Co; 1981.

12 Seizures

KEVIN M. KELLY, JAMES P. VALERIANO,
AND JERALD A. SOLOT

SUMMARY The emergency department evaluation of seizures is based primarily on history taking and physical examination. In many cases, the history is incomplete and examination of the patient is difficult. However, carefully obtained clinical information can result in a focused differential diagnosis and a correct identification of the cause of the seizure. Confirmation of the clinical diagnosis is often achieved by examination of blood counts, serum chemistries, serum antiepileptic drug (AED) levels, a toxicology screen, and cerebrospinal fluid, imaging studies of the skull and brain, and an electroencephalogram. The rational treatment of seizures in the emergency department consists of stopping the seizures with AEDs, identifying and correcting the underlying abnormality, treating resultant trauma, and providing appropriate therapy to prevent seizure recurrence. Disposition of the patient begins by presenting and discussing relevant information with the patient's primary care physician or neurologist, and by arranging hospitalization or outpatient follow-up care. The patient, when competent, is informed of the cause of the seizures, the determined need for AEDs and their potential side effects, and any restrictions to activities of daily living, including the state's law regarding driving privileges. This information is documented carefully in the medical record. (Credit information for this chapter can be found on p. 172.)

Introduction

A patient who has had a seizure is frequently evaluated and treated in the emergency department. The seizure can be due to epilepsy or to nonepileptic causes. There are an estimated 2.5 million people with epilepsy in the United States, and current data indicate that the prevalence of active epilepsy ranges from 4–10 in 1000.[1,2] These data, combined with the large number of patients who have seizures from nonepileptic causes, indicate that seizure occurrence is relatively frequent and results from diverse causes. Although many patients who have a seizure do not need emergency department care, some present to the emergency department critically ill and require immediate, definitive management. Advances in the understanding of the causes

and types of seizures in the use of new antiepileptic drugs (AEDs) have enhanced the emergency physician's ability to diagnose the cause of a patient's seizures accurately and to treat both the underlying abnormality and the seizures in a rational and systematic fashion.

Epileptic Seizures

There are various types of seizures, epilepsies, and epileptic syndromes. The classification and terminology of epileptic seizures that is used currently was established by the Commission on Classification and Terminology of the International League Against Epilepsy in 1970 and revised in 1981. The International Classification of Epileptic Seizures

TABLE 12.1. International Classification of Epileptic Seizures

I. Partial (focal, local) seizures
    A. Simple partial seizures
        1. With motor signs
        2. With somatosensory or special sensory symptoms
        3. With autonomic symptoms or signs
        4. With psychic symptoms
    B. Complex partial seizures
        1. Simple partial onset followed by impairment of consciousness
        2. With impairment of consciousness at onset
    C. Partial seizures evolving to secondarily generalized seizures
        1. Simple partial seizures evolving to generalized seizures
        2. Complex partial seizures evolving to generalized seizures
        3. Simple partial seizures evolving to complex partial seizures evolving to generalized seizures
II. Generalized seizures (convulsive or nonconvulsive)
    A. Absence seizures
        1. Typical absences
        2. Atypical absences
    B. Myoclonic seizures
    C. Clonic seizures
    D. Tonic seizures
    E. Tonic-clonic seizures
    F. Atonic seizures (astatic seizures)
III. Unclassified epileptic seizures

(Table 12.1) is based on clinical and electrophysiological properties of the ictal event that categorize it as one of two fundamental groups of seizure: *partial* or *generalized.* A partial seizure has clinical or EEG evidence indicating a focal onset in one cerebral hemisphere. A generalized seizure has no evidence of focal onset and therefore appears to begin simultaneously from both cerebral hemispheres. The International Classification of Epilepsies and Epileptic Syndromes (ICE) distinguishes epilepsies with partial seizures from epilepsies with generalized seizures.[3] Additionally, the ICE distinguishes epilepsies of unknown cause, or idiopathic (primary), from those of known etiology, or *symptomatic* (secondary), and those that are *cryptogenic,* that is, the cause is not known but the epilepsy is presumed to be symptomatic. Idiopathic epilepsies and syndromes are considered to have a possible hereditary predisposition, whereas symptomatic epilepsies and syndromes are considered a consequence of a known or suspected disorder of the central nervous system (CNS). Many of the different types of idiopathic and symptomatic epilepsies are listed in Table 12.2, the differential diagnosis of seizures. A basic understanding of the types of partial and generalized seizures listed in Table 12.1 is important for the evaluation and treatment of seizures in the emergency department.

Partial Seizures

Partial seizures are divided into *simple* (without impairment of consciousness) and *complex* (with impairment of consciousness). Simple partial seizures are classified by the type of symptom experienced by the patient. These include motor, sensory, autonomic, and psychic events. The EEG shows a restricted area of electrical discharge over the contralateral cerebral cortex corresponding to the body area involved. A simple partial seizure with motor signs is a focal motor seizure that can occur in any body area (e.g., clonic activity of digits). If the abnormal electrical discharge causing the seizure spreads to contiguous cortical areas, a sequential involvement of body parts occurs in a "march" (e.g.,

TABLE 12.2. Idiopathic and Symptomatic Epileptic Disorders and Causes of Provoked Seizures

Idiopathic epileptic disorders
  Benign neonatal familial convulsions
  Benign myoclonic epilepsy in infancy
  Childhood and juvenile absence epilepsy
  Juvenile myoclonic epilepsy
  Epilepsy with grand mal seizures on
  awakening
Symptomatic epileptic disorders
  Genetic disorders
  Metabolic disorders
    Amino acid and protein
      Phenylketonuria
      Porphyria
    Lipid
      Gangliosidoses
        Tay-Sachs disease
        Gaucher's disease
      Ceroid lipofuscinoses
    Vitamin
      Pyridoxine deficiency
  Myelin disorders
    Krabbe's disease
    Adrenoleukodystrophy
  Phakomatoses
    Tuberous sclerosis
    Neurofibromatosis
    Sturge-Weber syndrome
  Progressive myoclonic epilepsies
    Lafora body disease
    Unverricht-Lundborg syndrome
  Acquired disorders
    Brain anoxia
      Perinatal
      All ages
      Stroke
    Brain trauma
      Perinatal
        Subdural hematoma
        Subarachnoid hemorrhage
        Intraventricular hemorrhage
      All ages
        Contusions
        Lacerations
        Hematomas
    Brain tumors

CNS infections
  Prenatal and perinatal
    Toxoplasmosis
    Rubella
    Herpes
    Syphilis
    Cytomegalovirus
    Meningitis
  Older
    Meningitis
    Encephalitis
    Abscess
    Syphilis
    HIV
Degenerative disorders
  Alzheimer's disease
  Multiple sclerosis
Malformations
  Arteriovenous malformation
Causes of provoked seizures
  Metabolic disorders
    Uremia
    Hepatic insufficiency
    Hypoglycemia
  Electrolyte disorders
  Acid–base disorders
  Connective tissue and inflammatory disorders
    Systemic lupus erythematosis
    Rheumatic fever
    Vasculitis
  Endocrine disorders
    Infections
    Meningitis
  Vascular
    Ischemic stroke
    Subarachnoid hemorrhage
    Intracerebral hemorrhage
  Toxic disorders
    Substances of abuse
    Medications
    Environmental toxins
  Head trauma
    Contusion
    Hematoma
  Pregnancy

Source: Adapted from Engel J Jr. *Seizures and Epilepsy.* Philadelphia, Pa: FA Davis Co; 1989.

clonic activity of digits spreading to the wrist and then to the elbow). This type of seizure is known as a *Jacksonian seizure.* Other types of focal motor seizures include head turning or speech arrest. When focal motor seizures are continuous, the condition is known as *epilepsia partialis continua,* a form of *status epilepticus* (SE), which is a condition characterized by a seizure that lasts longer than 30 minutes or when a patient has two or more consecutive seizures without regaining consciousness. A simple partial seizure with somatosensory symptoms is a focal sensory seizure, usually consisting of paresthesias (tingling, pins-and-needles sensations) or numbness. These symptoms may also undergo a progression, or march, as in focal motor seizures. A simple partial seizure with special sensory symptoms includes elaborate visual or auditory experiences, olfactory sensations (e.g., unpleasant odor), or gustatory sensations (e.g., metallic taste). A simple partial seizure with autonomic symptoms can include pallor, flushing, diaphoresis, piloerection, and pupil dilatation. A simple partial seizure with psychic symptoms is a disturbance of higher cerebral function usually occurring with impairment of consciousness (i.e., complex partial seizures). The psychic symptoms include distorted memories such as *déja vu* (the sensation that the present situation has already been experienced) and *jamais vu* (a familiar visual experience is not recognized). Other symptoms include dreamy states, intense fear or terror, illusions, and structured hallucinations.

The word *aura* has been used traditionally to describe the sensory, autonomic, or psychic symptoms perceived by the patient before the onset of impaired consciousness and/or a motor seizure. Actually, an aura is itself a simple partial seizure that may or may not progress to another seizure type. Prodromal symptoms of prolonged mood changes, uneasiness, or premonitions are usually not auras. *Postictal paralysis* (Todd's paralysis) can occur following a simple partial seizure. Focal motor seizures are followed occasionally by paralysis or weakness of the muscles involved in the seizure. The paralysis usually resolves within 48 hours, although it may persist for much longer periods. Less commonly, focal sensory seizures that have associated paresthesias may be followed by postictal numbness in the same body distribution. The numbness is the sensory equivalent of a postictal

paralysis. The cause of these postictal phenomena is thought to be transient, reversible biochemical alterations in the neurons involved in the seizure activity. Postictal phenomena that persist for weeks or months have been associated with complex partial SE,[4] and the long reversal time of the postictal deficits may be caused by structural or functional reorganization of those neurons involved in the prolonged seizure activity.

A simple partial seizure may progress to a complex partial seizure, which also can occur spontaneously. A complex partial seizure includes impairment of consciousness, which refers to the patient's abnormal awareness and responsiveness to environmental stimuli. The initial features of the seizure include an arrest reaction or motionless stare usually followed by *automatisms,* which are relatively coordinated motor activities occurring during the period of impaired consciousness. The automatism may be a continuation of motor activity that was present at the time of seizure onset (e.g., continuing to drive a car) or an apparently purposeful activity such as scratching, lip smacking, or fumbling with clothing. The seizure is usually brief, lasting from seconds to minutes, and there is a period of postictal confusion. The EEG shows unilateral or bilateral discharges in temporal or frontotemporal regions either focally or diffusely. *Complex partial SE* is a series of complex partial seizures without intervening return to full responsiveness.[5] Because some complex partial seizures do not originate in the temporal lobe, the commonly used terms *temporal lobe seizure* and *psychomotor seizure* are not truly synonymous with complex partial seizure and should be avoided. A partial seizure, simple or complex, can evolve into a generalized tonic-clonic seizure and is then referred to as a "partial seizure secondarily generalized." The EEG shows focal discharges in one cerebral hemisphere evolving into generalized, bilaterally synchronous discharges.

Generalized Seizures

Generalized seizures are divided into convulsive (major motor) or nonconvulsive (brief loss of consciousness or minor motor) types. Generalized convulsive seizures include *tonic, clonic,* and *tonic-clonic* types. Generalized tonic seizures typically occur in childhood and typically include impaired consciousness, muscle contraction of the face and trunk, flexion of the upper extremities, flexion or extension of the lower extremities, and postictal confusion. Generalized clonic seizures usually begin in childhood and include impaired consciousness, bilateral limb jerking, and postictal confusion. Generalized tonic-clonic seizures, commonly referred to as *grand mal* seizures, are characterized by a sudden loss of consciousness and tonic and clonic phases. The tonic phase lasts 10–20 seconds and begins with brief flexion, eyelid opening, upward movement of the eyes, and elevation and external rotation of the arms. More prolonged extension follows involving the back and neck, a cry may occur, the arms extend, and the legs extend and rotate externally. At this point, the patient becomes apneic. The clonic phase lasts about 30 seconds and begins by brief, repetitive relaxations of the tonic rigidity, creating pronounced flexor spasms of the face, trunk, and limbs. This clonic jerking gradually decreases in rate until it ceases. Following this, there is muscular flaccidity, respirations resume, and there may be incontinence. Consciousness returns gradually and the patient awakens in a confused state. Fatigue and headache are common. The EEG during the tonic phase shows a generalized rhythm of 10 Hz or more, decreasing in frequency and increasing in amplitude to include generalized polyspike or polyspike-and-wave discharges. In the clonic phase, this rhythm is associated with muscle contraction and is interrupted repetitively by slowing or EEG silence associated with the periods of muscle relaxation. The EEG pattern of polyspike or polyspike-and-wave discharges alternating with slowing is displayed as rhythmic muscular jerking in the patient. After the clonic phase, the EEG shows diffuse slowing corresponding to the postictal period.

Generalized nonconvulsive seizures include *absence, myoclonic, tonic,* and *atonic* types. Generalized absence seizures, commonly referred to as *petit mal* seizures, typically are 5–10-second episodes of loss of consciousness characterized by staring and unresponsiveness. Clonic movements, changes in postural tone, automatisms, and autonomic phenomena commonly accompany absence seizures. The patient quickly resumes normal consciousness, has no postical confusion, and is generally unaware of the episode. The EEG typically shows generalized, bilaterally synchronized 3-Hz spike-and-wave discharges. Continuous absence seizures are known as *absence SE.* Generalized myoclonic seizures are bilaterally synchronous jerks that can be single or repeated in trains. The muscles involved may be few and restricted to a body part (e.g., the face) or extensive, involving all limbs. Most myoclonic seizures occur with no impairment of consciousness. The EEG shows generalized, bilaterally synchronous polyspike-and-wave or spike-wave discharges that may not be time-locked with the muscle jerks. Generalized tonic seizures that are brief are considered nonconvulsive, in contrast to the longer generalized tonic seizures, which are classified as convulsive. Generalized atonic seizures, commonly referred to as *drop attacks,* consist of a sudden loss of tone in postural muscles, often resulting in a fall. There is brief, mild impairment of consciousness and little postictal confusion. The EEG shows polyspike-and-wave discharges or suppression of electrical activity.

Pathophysiology

An epileptic seizure is the clinical manifestation of abnormal paroxysmal activity of groups of neurons in the cerebral cortex. The electrical discharges of these neurons are excessive and/or synchronous and can propagate to other cortical or subcortical areas by specific anatomical pathways. The clinical features of an epileptic seizure often reflect the functional properties of the cortical areas involved in seizure activity. The neuronal mechanisms involved in human seizure activity are understood incompletely. Much has been learned from studies of animal hippocampal and neocortical tissue. Seizure activity can be induced in these tissues by electrical stimulation or application of convulsant drugs. These techniques can cause partial seizures when applied to focal areas of one brain hemisphere and generalized seizures when applied to both hemispheres or to diffuse areas. Information from these and other types of experiments has provided a basic understanding of the neuronal mechanisms that initiate, propagate, and terminate seizure activity.

Studies of Epileptic Seizures in Humans

In partial seizures, it is likely that ictal discharges from an *epileptogenic zone* are contained by synaptic inhibition, local spread occurs by nonsynaptic events caused by rapid neuronal firing, and propagation to intrahemispheric and interhemispheric areas occurs by preferential anatomical routes.[6] Although not proven, an independent epileptogenic *mirror focus* may develop in a homotopic site in the contralateral hemisphere as a result of frequent epileptiform discharges carried across connecting fiber tracts. Secondarily generalized seizures have propagation patterns that are not uniform among patients, presumably because of diffuse or multifocal regions capable of generating epileptiform discharges. Although there has been no direct demonstration in humans, convulsive generalized seizures are thought to involve the brainstem in the tonic phase, and the forebrain in the clonic phase. Absence seizures may result from cortical inhibition by synchronized diencephalic input.[7]

Prehospital Care

Most seizures that occur in an out-of-hospital setting do not result in the patient going to the emergency department for evaluation. This is because most seizures occur in patients with epilepsy who recognize that their seizures are usually self-limited and do not require immediate evaluation. However, some seizures are severe or life-threatening and require immediate evaluation and management. Management of airway, breathing, and circulation is addressed first. Management of SE by emergency medical services personnel essentially follows the same guidelines as in the emergency department. When emergency medical services personnel are called for a patient who has had a seizure, information obtained in the field is frequently important for establishing a diagnosis and a treatment plan. The patient is usually transported to the emergency department for evaluation, and the emergency physician is updated as needed. Conditions that can require transport to the hospital include seizures that last for several minutes without evidence of abatement, failure to regain consciousness after a seizure, serial seizures, seizures resulting in significant injury, new or severe seizures in pregnancy, medical conditions such as diabetes, or seizures occurring at the extremes of age.

Emergency Department

History. Patients assessed in the emergency department can be postictal, or experiencing a recurrent seizure. It is the responsibility of the emergency physician to evaluate the seizure by obtaining pertinent information regarding the patient's medical, surgical, neurological, and psychiatric history. This information is obtained from all available sources including patient, family, friends, witnesses to the seizure, emergency medical services personnel, the patient's physician, and hospital records. A history of a seizure disorder is especially important and ideally provides information regarding the patient's age at seizure onset, the cause and type of the seizure(s), the frequency of seizures, the last known seizure occurrence, and the use of AEDs.

When little information is available about the patient, descriptions of the seizure and the circumstances of its occurrence are extremely important in determining the cerebral localization of the epileptogenic lesion, the seizure type, and its likely cause. Obtaining accurate details of the seizure occurrence is often difficult or impossible to achieve. The seizure may not have been witnessed, and the patient may be unable to provide information. Whenever possible, detailed descriptions of the seizure should be elicited by careful inquiry of the patient and any witness to the seizure. Important information includes the occurrence of a prodrome or aura, the features of the clinical seizure (e.g., autonomic changes, alteration of consciousness, arrested body movements, automatisms, the temporal sequence of tonic and/or clonic movements affecting one or both sides of the body, tongue biting, incontinence), and postictal symptoms. When AEDs are used, recent drug or dosage changes and the patient's compliance with medication taking should be determined. Associated factors that may be important include chronic disease states, intercurrent illness, stress, sleep deprivation, menses, pregnancy, the use of other medications, alcohol or drug ingestion, or withdrawal.

General Physical Examination. A careful general physical examination is performed to assess the condition of the patient and to find physical signs that may be related to the underlying cause of the seizure, AED therapy, or resultant trauma, old or new. Vital signs can give evidence of infection, hypotension or hypertension, arrhythmias, and respiratory or metabolic disturbances. The skin may reveal decreased turgor with dehydration, a rash with infection or connective tissue disorders, cyanosis with hypoxemia, hirsutism with chronic phenytoin therapy, contusions, lacerations, scarring from seizure-related injury, characteristic abnormalities of the phakomatoses, or congenital ectodermal disorders. These include axillary freckling, café-au-lait spots, and neurofibromas associated with neurofibromatosis; facial sebaceous adenoma, ash leaf spots, and shagreen patches associated with tuberous sclerosis; and port wine stain of the face associated with Sturge-Weber syndrome. The head may reveal microcephaly, macrocephaly, or facial asymmetry, suggesting abnormal cerebral development or injury. A tense fontanelle can be seen in infection or hydrocephalus. Auscultation of the head for bruits may suggest an arteriovenous malformation (AVM). There may be evidence of trauma or previous neurological surgery such as craniectomy for tumor or AVM removal or aneurysm clipping, or placement of a ventriculoperitoneal shunt for hydrocephalus. The sinuses may be tender to tap and the tympanic membranes or oropharynx may be red – findings associated with infection. The mouth may reveal gingival hypertrophy with chronic phenytoin therapy, lacerations or scarring of the tongue and buccal mucosa, or a smell of alcohol. The neck may be stiff, and positive Brudzinski's or Kernig's sign suggests meningeal irritation from infection or subarachnoid hemorrhage. The limbs may be asymmetrical, suggesting lateralized cerebral injury. Auscultation of the heart may reveal arrhythmia or murmurs of acquired heart disease underlying inadequate cerebral perfusion and hypoxia or embolism. Auscultation of the lungs may reveal decreased ventilation in several disease states including exacerbations of chronic obstructive pulmonary disease and asthma resulting in cerebral hypoxia, infection resulting in cerebral abscess, and tumor resulting in cerebral metastasis. The abdomen may be rigid with infection or hemorrhage, resulting in hypotension or shock. Hepatomegaly may be associated with liver insufficiency and an encephalopathic state. There may be urinary or fecal incontinence.

Neurological Examination. Following completion of a general physical examination, a focused neurological examination assesses mental status, functioning of the cranial nerves, motor and sensory systems, and deep tendon reflexes.

Abnormal findings may be from ictal or postictal states of complex partial or generalized seizures, the patient's interictal condition, toxic or metabolic encephalopathies, or intracranial injury. Prolonged bizarre behavior with alteration of consciousness may represent complex partial SE and not delirium or a psychotic event.[6] Prolonged lethargy and decreased mental status may represent absence SE rather than a postictal state.[5] Reversible memory impairment occurs frequently with complex partial and generalized convulsive seizures.[6] Isolated findings such as aphasia suggest focal brain abnormalities.

Cranial nerve examination is focused and thorough. The optic nerve may show papilledema, suggesting increased intracranial pressure. Abnormalities of pupil size may suggest focal impairments (e.g., a nonreactive dilated pupil in transtentorial herniation) or generalized effects (e.g., bilateral miosis or mydriasis from drug effect). An afferent pupillary defect may be related to multiple sclerosis or a compressive lesion such as pituitary tumor. Tonic deviation of the eyes may represent an ictal event and can localize the abnormality (e.g., a right hemisphere seizure tonically drives the eyes to the left). Nystagmus may be due to AED intoxication. Abnormal visual field testing can localize abnormalities along the visual pathway (e.g., a superior quadrantic visual field defect is related to a posterior temporal lobe lesion). The corneal reflex tests the patency of the trigeminal and facial nerves, and an abnormal reflex may be associated with brainstem pathology such as cranial nerve schwannomas. A central facial paresis is caused by a contralateral cerebral hemisphere abnormality and may represent a postictal paralysis. The vestibular system can be tested by the oculocephalic (doll's eyes) reflex and, when abnormal, the oculovestibular (caloric) reflexes. The oculocephalic reflex should not be performed when there is a possible cervical spine injury. An abnormal oculocephalic reflex is seen with barbiturate overdose (absent reflex with preserved pupillary function) and with lesions of the brainstem tegmentum (asymmetrical or no reflex). The oculovestibular reflex should not be performed in patients with a ruptured tympanic membrane. An abnormal oculovestibular reflex can localize a lesion to the brainstem (slow phase of nystagmus is defective) or to the cerebral hemispheres (intact slow phase bilaterally, absent fast phase bilaterally). A normal reflex is seen in hysterical coma. The gag reflex tests patency of the glossopharyngeal and vagus nerves. It should be tested carefully to minimize the possibility of vomiting. An absent reflex may suggest impairment of the medulla. Tongue deviation with protrusion can be caused by impairment of a cerebral hemisphere or the hypoglossal nerve. Tongue deviation to the right suggests impaired function of the left cerebral hemisphere or the right hypoglossal nerve.

Motor function should be assessed initially by inspection of the patient. An abducted lower extremity suggests focal weakness that may be related to stroke in the contralateral cerebral hemisphere or to postictal paralysis. Tremors may be related to alcohol withdrawal states, and fasciculations can occur in severe dehydration. Myoclonus may be caused by toxic, metabolic, or infectious disturbances. Tonic rigidity or clonic movements occur with ongoing seizure activity.

Decorticate or decerebrate rigidity elicited by a noxious stimulus indicates coma. Brain injury associated with decorticate posturing is generally more rostral with less severe supratentorial impairment than with decerebrate rigidity, which is correlated with deeper or more severe but still primarily supratentorial dysfunction. Abnormalities of station and gait not related to weakness can localize impairments to the cerebellum or the vestibular system.

Sensory function impairments such as paresthesias or numbness may result in abnormal responses to testing by light touch or pinprick. When focal, these abnormalities suggest ipsilateral mononeuropathy, plexopathy, radiculopathy, or contralateral brain impairment, including ongoing simple partial seizure activity or a postictal equivalent.

Muscle stretch reflexes may be decreased in postictal paralysis or increased because of contralateral upper motoneuron impairment, which also underlies a plantar extensor response. A decreased rate of reflex relaxation (a "hung-up" reflex) suggests hypothyroidism.

Differential Diagnosis

Epileptic Seizures

The emergency department evaluation of a seizure is directed toward determining whether the seizure is due to epilepsy or nonepileptic causes. When a seizure has the characteristics of a partial or generalized seizure, represents a chronic condition, and has no identifiable cause or a cause that cannot be cured by specific treatment, the seizure is caused by epilepsy.[6] This distinguishes *provoked seizures,* due to a transient reversible insult (e.g., minor head trauma), from *recurrent provoked seizures,* which can be cured by definitive therapy of an underlying disease state (e.g., resection of a brain tumor).[6] The causes of epileptic seizures are diverse and numerous. Table 12.2 lists categories and representative types of idiopathic and symptomatic epileptic disorders and causes of provoked seizures.

Nonepileptic Paroxysmal Events

Paroxysmal events from nonepileptic causes are frequently confused with epileptic seizures, and their accurate identification is important for appropriate management. Nonepileptic paroxysmal events that cannot be distinguished from epileptic seizures on clinical features alone are studied by appropriate tests, including EEG. Nonepileptic paroxysmal events have been classified as being inducible by systemic, neurological, or psychiatric disorders.[6] Examples of these disorders, which occur commonly in the emergency department, are listed in Table 12.3 and described below.

Systemic Disorders. Systemic disturbances include syncope, breath holding, hyperventilation, and toxic and metabolic disturbances.[6] Syncope is a relatively frequent event and is related to a sudden decrease in cerebral blood flow. Decreased cerebral perfusion can be caused by numerous factors, which have been categorized as follows: (1) decrease in cardiac output (e.g., hypovolemia, decreased venous tone), (2) reflex syncope, caused by an inappropriate decrease in systemic vascular resistance and/or heart rate (e.g., vasovagal, carotid sinus, postmicturition syncope), (3) sudden decrease in systemic vascular resistance (e.g., vasodilator drugs, autonomic nervous system dysfunction), (4) arrhythmias (e.g., bradyarrhythmias, tachyarrhythmias, heart block).[8] After a syncopal episode, the patient usually falls to the ground, can display tonic and clonic movements lasting only a few seconds, and has a prompt return to consciousness. These brief tonic and clonic movements reflect decerebrate rigidity and are commonly called *syncopal*

TABLE 12.3. Nonepileptic Paroxysmal Events

Systemic disorders
  Syncope
    With decreased cardiac output
    Reflex syncope
    With decreased systemic vascular resistance
    With arrhythmias
  Breath holding
  Hyperventilation
  Toxic and metabolic disturbances
    Alcohol and drug withdrawal
    Hepatic and renal failure
Neurologic disorders
  Cerebrovascular disorders
    Transient ischemic attacks
    Stroke
    Migraine
      Classical
      Complicated
      Equivalent
    Transient global amnesia
  Narcolepsy
  Movement disorders
    Paroxysmal dyskinesias
    Hemifacial spasm
  Sensory disorders
    Trigeminal neuralgia
    Positional vertigo
    Acute labyrinthitis
    Meniere's disease
Psychiatric disorders
  Psychogenic seizures
  Intermittent explosive disorders
  Dissociative states
    Fugue states
    Psychogenic amnesia
    Depersonalization disorders

Source: Adapted with permission from Engel J Jr. *Seizures and Epilepsy.* Philadelphia, Pa: FA Davis Co; 1989 and Dohrmann ML and Cheitlin MD. Cardiogenic syncope: seizure versus syncope. *Neurol Clin.* 1986;4:549–62.

seizures or *convulsive syncope.* They can occur with prodromal diaphoresis and vertigo, are frequently associated with stress (such as the death of a relative), and do not require treatment.

Breath holding in infants and children can also result in syncope and is common between 6 and 18 months of age. It is often precipitated by frustration,

fear, or surprise followed by autonomic phenomena and loss of consciousness. Brief syncopal seizures may follow and do not require treatment.

Hyperventilation occurs most frequently in adolescents and adults and is usually precipitated by anxiety or stress. The increased frequency and/or depth of respirations can produce significant symptoms in virtually all organ systems and is frightening to the patient. Typical symptoms include shortness of breath, lightheadedness, and perioral and phalangeal tingling. Carpopedal spasm and loss of consciousness may occur. Seizures are infrequent but can occur in susceptible patients or those with a history of epilepsy. Treatment of hyperventilation consists of rebreathing expired air, calm reassurance of the patient, and sedation when indicated.

Toxic and metabolic disturbances can result in transient neurological dysfunction that may be difficult to distinguish from some features of seizure activity. Toxic disturbances that are frequently seen in the emergency department are caused by alcohol and psychomimetic drugs. Alcoholic blackouts are periods of amnesia that occur during and after periods of heavy ethanol consumption. Delirium tremens (DTs) occurs within 48 hours of cessation of drinking and is characterized by confusion, hallucinations, tremor, and autonomic changes. Psychomimetic drugs can cause altered awareness and responsiveness, hallucinations, and autonomic changes. Aspects of alcoholic blackouts, DTs, and drug intoxication can resemble features of complex partial seizures. Metabolic disturbances such as hepatic and renal failure can create lethargy and confusion, which may be mistaken for ictal or postictal phenomena.[6]

Neurological Disorders. Neurological disturbances include cerebrovascular, sleep, movement, and sensory disorders.[6] Cerebrovascular disorders include transient ischemic attacks (TIAs), stroke, migraine, and transient global amnesia.[6] TIAs are focal, reversible neurological symptoms caused by local brain ischemia and are experienced most frequently by the elderly. Stroke is brain injury caused by a cerebral vascular insult and can be the reason for provoked seizures (e.g., secondary to embolic stroke) and epileptic seizures (e.g., secondary to scar formation in the area of stroke). Classic migraine is a vascular headache preceded by transient visual and other sensory and/or motor prodromes.[8]

Focal neurological symptoms that occur in classic migraine can suggest a partial seizure; however, headache following a partial seizure is not common. Complicated migraine is migraine headache followed by prolonged neurological deficits including mental aberrations. These impairments can be difficult to distinguish from those related to partial seizures or TIAs. Migraine equivalents are focal neurological or visual symptoms that occur without accompanying or subsequent headache. These symptoms usually occur in a patient with a history of migraine headaches. Transient global amnesia is an episode lasting approximately 20 minutes to several hours characterized by a sudden loss of memory and apparent confusion with repetitive questions. These symptoms occur without other neurological symptoms or signs. After the episode, there is permanent amnesia concerning the event.

Narcolepsy is a condition characterized by hypersomnia, cataplexy (sudden drop attacks, with preserved consciousness usually precipitated by emotional factors), sleep paralysis, and hallucinations with sleep onset or awakening. Different combinations of these symptoms occur in patients. Although narcolepsy can usually be distinguished from seizure disorders by clinical features, polysomnography with EEG may be necessary for diagnosis.

Movement disorders that occur as paroxysmal events can resemble epileptic seizures. Paroxysmal dyskinesias include familial and acquired types. Familial types begin in childhood and are characterized by choreoathetotic and/or dystonic posturing that can be either brief (minutes) and precipitated by sudden movement or longer (hours) and often preceded by prodromal abnormal sensations in the affected limbs. Acquired types include the tonic spasms of multiple sclerosis and the choreoathetosis of cerebral palsy, hypoparathyroidism, and thyrotoxicosis.[6] Hemifacial spasm consists of irregular contractions of one side of the face, including blinking, and is related to facial nerve pathology. Although hemifacial spasm may resemble a partial motor seizure clinically, the EEG is normal.

Sensory disorders with paroxysmal features include those that are characterized by pain (e.g., trigeminal neuralgia) and vertigo (e.g., positional vertigo, acute labyrinthitis, and Meniere's disease). Hearing loss and tinnitus in Meniere's disease can be present for long periods of time but not well recognized by the patient prior to an episode of vertigo. The specific symptoms and precipitants of these sensory disorders generally distinguish them as nonepileptic paroxysmal events.

Psychiatric Disorders. Psychogenic disturbances include psychogenic seizure, intermittent explosive disorders, and dissociative states.[6] Intermittent explosive disorders (episodic dyscontrol) are episodic or impulsive violent behaviors resulting in personal assault or destruction of property without significant precipitating psychosocial stress. Generalized impulsivity or aggressiveness is not exhibited between episodes.[9] Typically, they occur in patients with minimal brain dysfunction or a history of traumatic brain injury. The directed aggression of these episodes distinguishes them from stereotyped, aggressive epileptic ictal behavior, which is relatively rare.

Dissociative states include fugue states, psychogenic amnesia, and depersonalization disorders. Fugue states involve sudden, unexpected travel from familiar environments, assumption of a new identity, inability to recall one's previous identity, and amnesia concerning the event following recovery. Disorientation can occur. Psychogenic amnesia is a sudden inability to recall important personal information that is too extensive to be explained by ordinary forgetfulness. Depersonalization disorder involves the perception or experience of one's own reality being temporarily lost or changed.[9] Features of fugue states, psychogenic amnesia, and depersonalization disorder can resemble some of the cognitive features of complex partial SE, particularly memory loss. The specific nature of the abnormality seen in dissociative states generally distinguishes them from epileptic seizures. However, EEG may be required for definitive diagnosis.

Laboratory Studies and Procedures

Laboratory evaluation of a patient who has had a seizure is guided by information obtained from the history and physical examination. Patients with a new-onset seizure are assessed for underlying systemic abnormalities that can cause or predispose to the occurrence of a seizure. Hematological testing is a complete blood count with white blood cell (WBC) differential counts. Chemistries include a capillary blood sugar level upon arrival in the emergency department, followed by serum sodium, potassium, chloride, bicarbonate, calcium, magnesium, and glucose levels. Blood urea nitrogen, creatinine, serum glutamic-oxaloacetic transaminase (SGOT), alkaline phosphatase, total bilirubin, and ethanol levels can be helpful. When indicated, urine is obtained for routine and microscopic tests and for a toxicology screen. An electrocardiogram (EKG) can be helpful with cardiac disease, and a chest radiograph can be obtained when infection is suspected. Patients with known seizure disorders who have had an isolated seizure followed by rapid and complete recovery and a normal neurological examination may not require laboratory studies other than serum AED levels, especially when medication noncompliance is suspected.

Computerized tomography (CT) of the brain is available in most hospitals, and its judicious use is important in seizures associated with neurodegenerative disease, major brain malformations, intracranial hemorrhage, space-occupying lesions, or head trauma. CT scanning with bone windows can be indicated to assess for penetrating wounds or depressed skull fractures, and has largely replaced the need for skull radiographs. Magnetic resonance imaging (MRI) of the brain is available in many hospitals and has greater sensitivity than CT in demonstrating certain types of abnormalities (e.g., temporal lobe abnormalities in patients with partial seizure disorders).[10] The use of MRI is usually not helpful during the evaluation of a patient in the emergency department. The EEG is the single most useful study in assessing the cause of seizures. Although its use is also limited in the emergency department, it should be considered in patients with an unexplained and prolonged impaired level of consciousness.

Lumbar puncture is performed when CNS infection is suspected and there are no signs of increased intracranial pressure. An opening pressure is recorded and CSF is obtained for blood counts, including a WBC differential count, protein, glucose, Gram stain, acid-fast bacilli, cryptococcal antigen, Venereal Disease Research Laboratory test (VDRL), bacterial cultures, and counterimmunoelectrophoresis or agglutination assays for bacterial antigens. Treatment of suspected meningitis or encephalitis is instituted immediately. It is important to note that the CSF may reveal pleocytosis after a single simple or complex partial seizure, a generalized tonic-clonic seizure, or SE. After a single partial or generalized tonic-clonic seizure, concentrations of CSF WBC's have been found to be as high as 12/ml with less than or equal to 2% polymorphonuclear leukocytes.[11] In SE, the concentration of CSF WBCs can be as high as 80 cells/ml and the percentage of polymorphonuclear leukocytes without bands can be as high as 92%. Pleocytosis can also be associated with increased protein concentration. The mechanisms involved in causing pleocytosis are not known but likely include breakdown of the blood–brain barrier or release of chemotactic factors into the CSF. Treatment of suspected CNS infection is not withheld because of the possibility that the observed pleocytosis is simply due to seizure occurrence.

Management

The emergency department management of a patient with a seizure is commonly determined by the cause, type, severity, and frequency of the seizure. At times, treatment of the seizure precedes diagnosis of its cause. When identified, the underlying cause of seizures is treated, and AEDs are used when indicated. AEDs are chosen on the basis of their clinical effectiveness in treating specific epileptic syndromes or seizure types. Commonly prescribed AEDs and their associated clinical indications, dosing requirements, and therapeutic serum concentrations are given in Table 12.4.

Status Epilepticus

SE can be nonconvulsive or convulsive. Nonconvulsive SE includes absence SE, simple partial SE, and complex partial SE. These conditions are encountered relatively infrequently in the emergency department and are not as immediately serious as convulsive (generalized tonic-clonic) SE. The diagnosis of nonconvulsive SE is often difficult to make unless the patient has a history of such episodes. EEG may be necessary to confirm the diagnosis. Absence SE is treated with diazepam, 0.3 mg/kg

TABLE 12.4. Antiepileptic Drugs, Clinical Indications, Dosing Requirements, and Therapeutic Serum Concentrations

Drug	Seizure Types	Daily Dosing	Therapeutic Levels
Phenytoin	Partial, tonic-clonic	3–8 mg/kg	10–20 µg/ml
Carbamazepine	Partial, tonic-clonic	15–25 mg/kg	8–12 µg/ml
Phenobarbital	Tonic-clonic, partial	2–6 mg/kg	15–40 µg/ml
Primidone	Tonic-clonic, partial	10–20 mg/kg	5–15 µg/ml
Valproic acid	Tonic-clonic, myoclonic Absence, partial	15–60 mg/kg	50–100 µg/ml
Ethosuximide	Absence	10–30 mg/kg	40–100 µg/ml
Clonazepam	Myoclonic	0.03–0.3 mg/kg	0.01–0.05 µg/ml
Felbamate	Partial; generalized (Lennox-Gastaut)	~3600 mg/day	Not defined
Gabapentin	Partial	~4800 mg/day	Not defined
Lamotrigine	Partial	~400 mg/day	Not defined
Topiramate	Partial	~400 mg/day	Not defined
Tiagabine	Partial	~40 mg/day	Not defined

given intravenously (<5 mg per minute), followed by an initial dose of ethosuximide or valproic acid, 20 mg/kg per day, in three divided doses. Simple partial SE and complex partial SE can be treated with the same AED regimens as in convulsive SE, but aggressive treatment is usually not necessary or warranted.

Convulsive SE is a medical emergency requiring prompt and focused treatment. Treatment of convulsive SE must be aimed at controlling the seizures while proceeding with the evaluation to establish their cause. Failure to stop the seizures of convulsive SE can cause significant morbidity or mortality, which is directly related to the duration of ongoing seizure activity.[6] Descriptive details of management of convulsive SE are given below and summarized in Table 12.5.

Management of convulsive SE begins by placing the patient in a left lateral decubitus position in the middle of a gurney. The head is supported and protected from injury during convulsions. An adequate airway is established immediately. When the teeth are not clenched, the oropharynx is suctioned and an oral airway inserted. Insertion of other hard objects between the teeth, including a padded tongue blade, is not advised because of potential dislodge-

ment and local trauma. Oxygen can be administered by nasal cannula or face mask. A nasogastric tube can be placed for continuous vomiting. Endotracheal intubation is considered when there is evidence of compromised ventilation despite implementation of these procedures. Endotracheal intubation can be performed by the orotracheal route when the patient's teeth are not clenched and there is little movement or resistance by the patient. When the patient is having generalized tonic-clonic seizures, endotracheal intubation can be performed by the nasotracheal route to provide controlled ventilation and airway protection. When nasotracheal intubation fails, rapid sequence intubation is performed (see Chapter 25, "Neuroanesthesiology"). Briefly, a neuromuscular blocking agent can be given to achieve paralysis and facilitate intubation while pressure is applied over the cricoid cartilage to prevent regurgitation and aspiration of gastric contents. After muscle relaxation, endotracheal intubation can be performed safely and ventilations begun. Paralysis is maintained for a total of three to five minutes. It is important to remember that paralysis can mask ongoing seizure activity in the brain.

While the patient's airway is being secured, blood pressure is measured and EKG monitoring be-

TABLE 12.5. Management of Convulsive Status Epilepticus

Place patient on left side to prevent aspiration.
Establish airway and administer oxygen.
Obtain blood pressure and begin ECG monitoring.
Establish a peripheral IV line with isotonic saline in right arm.
Place a nasogastric tube for persistent vomiting.
Obtain blood for laboratory tests including a capillary blood glucose level.
Consider thiamine, 100 mg IV, followed by glucose, 50 g IV.
Benzodiazepine treatment:
   Administer diazepam, 0.3 mg/kg IV (<5 mg/min), repeating the dose once if necessary (0.5 mg/kg
   PR when there is no IV access), *or*
   Administer lorazepam, 0.1 mg/kg IV (<2 mg/min), *or*
   Consider midazolam, 0.1–0.2 mg/kg IV bolus. Continuous IV infusion, 0.05–4.0 mg/kg per hour, can follow as needed.
Phenytoin/fosphenytoin treatment:
   If seizures continue, administer phenytoin 15–20 mg/kg IV (<50 mg/min), with continuous
   monitoring of blood pressure and ECG, *or*
   Administer fosphenytoin, 15–20 mg PE/kg IV (150 mg PE/min), with continuous monitoring of blood pressure and ECG.
Barbiturate treatment:
   If seizures continue, administer phenobarbital, 20 mg/kg (<100 mg/min), with continuous monitoring of vital signs, *or*
   Induce general anesthesia with pentobarbital, 5–15 mg/kg IV, given slowly to achieve EEG burst suppression,
   followed by 0.5–3.0 mg/kg per hour to maintain burst suppression. The rate of pentobarbital infusion should be
   lowered every 2–4 hours to determine if seizure activity has ended.

gun. When convulsions have stopped, a peripheral intravenous line is established in the right arm with plastic catheters, and is protected against movement and subcutaneous infiltration during clonic motor activity. Blood is drawn for a capillary blood sugar, complete blood count; serum electrolytes including Na^+, Ca^{2+}, and Mg^{2+}; serum glucose, urea nitrogen, and creatinine; serum AEDs or other potentially neuroactive medications; and a toxicology screen. After blood drawing is complete, the intravenous line is kept open with isotonic saline. Thiamine, 100 mg by intravenous push, is given to protect patients with thiamine deficiency against a possible exacerbation of Wernicke's encephalopathy precipitated by administration of glucose. Wernicke's encephalopathy occurs in chronic alcoholics or patients with chronic malnutrition and is relatively common among patients with SE.[12] Glucose, 50 g (50 ml of 50% dextrose in water), by intravenous push, can be given for treatment of potential hypoglycemia. Only rarely does hypoglycemia cause SE. Administration of thiamine and glucose does not pose a risk to patients who are not deficient in them.

Use of Medications in Status Epilepticus

A benzodiazepine is the first class of drug to be administered in treating SE. Benzodiazepines have a rapid onset of clinical action, probably because of increasing GABAergic inhibition of neurons by enhancing the binding of GABA to its receptor and by enhancing GABA receptor currents. The available benzodiazepines for intravenous treatment of SE are diazepam, lorazepam, and midazolam. Diazepam and lorazepam are effective anticonvulsants and similar in their ability to control SE,[13] whereas midazolam may be superior in terminating refractory SE.[14–16] Selection of a particular benzodiazepine is determined by availability, pharmacokinetic differences, and side effects profile.

Diazepam. Diazepam enters the brain within 10 seconds, can stop seizures in 1 minute, and has a half-life of 15 minutes.[17] Diazepam, 0.3 mg/kg (<5 mg per minute), by intravenous push, is given commonly as 10 mg in 2 minutes, repeating the dose once when necessary.[6] When there is no intravenous access, it can be administered rectally, with absorption taking place within minutes. Following the use of diazepam, observable seizure activity may cease. Because the effectiveness of diazepam is brief, it must be followed immediately by a longer-acting AED. Sedation is the most common side effect. Hypotension and respiratory depression can also occur; therefore, the drug must be administered cautiously and vital signs monitored continuously.

Lorazepam. Compared to diazepam, lorazepam has a smaller volume of distribution, a longer duration of action, but a longer onset of action. It enters the brain within 2–3 minutes, can stop seizures in less than 5 minutes, and has a half-life of 12–14 hours, during which it can maintain effective antiepileptic activity.[17] Lorazepam, 0.1 mg/kg (<2 mg per minute), by intravenous push, has become increasingly popular for the initial management of SE.[18] After the use of lorazepam, observable seizure activity may cease. Although lorazepam can effectively control seizures for many hours, a second AED is usually given, as with diazepam, to provide additional antiepileptic activity and begin the transition to maintenance therapy.[18] An advantage of lorazepam use is the time it allows the emergency physician to determine the need and the amount of additional AED therapy. The side effects of lorazepam are essentially the same as those of diazepam.

Midazolam. Midazolam is a water-soluble benzodiazepine with high lipophilicity at physiological pH. It has short-acting anxiolytic, sedative-hypnotic, muscle relaxant and anticonvulsant properties. Clinically, midazolam is approximately three to four times more potent per milligram than diazepam. It has been shown to be effective in terminating SE in patients who failed treatment with diazepam, lorazepam, phenytoin, and phenobarbital.[14–16] Midazolam, 0.1–0.2 mg/kg, by intravenous push, can be followed by a continuous intravenous infusion of 0.05–0.40 mg/kg per hour, which can be continued for hours to days as needed. Although midazolam can be administered intramuscularly when intravenous access is difficult to obtain, the intravenous route is preferred for more rapid absorption and clinical effect.[14] Continuous cardiovascular monitoring is necessary. Mild to moderate hypotension can

be associated with use of midazolam, and can be treated with fluid or pressors as needed.

Phenytoin. Phenytoin, a hydantoin, is an effective AED, probably because of its ability to reduce neuronal sustained high-frequency repetitive firing of action potentials. Phenytoin can be given after the use of diazepam or lorazepam. Phenytoin enters the brain within 1 minute, can stop seizures in 15–30 minutes, and has a half-life of 24 hours.[17] Phenytoin, 15–20 mg/kg (<50 mg per minute), by intravenous push, is given with continuous monitoring of ECG and blood pressure because it can cause cardiac arrhythmia and hypotension, respectively. Cardiac arrhythmias and hypotension occur largely due to the effects on the atrioventricular conduction system by propylene glycol, the diluent for phenytoin. Therefore, the use of phenytoin is relatively contraindicated in patients with known cardiac conduction abnormalities. Cardiac arrhythmias and hypotension can often be corrected by decreasing the rate of phenytoin infusion. Phenytoin can usually be given safely to patients who have been on maintenance phenytoin therapy before a serum phenytoin level is available. Significant toxicity does not occur unless the patient's serum phenytoin level is more than 20 μg/ml.

Phenytoin can also be the first AED given, without use of a benzodiazepine. In general, phenytoin has little effect on the patient's level of consciousness. Using it alone can be advantageous in situations requiring continuous neurological assessment of the patient's mental status, for example, in patients with severe head trauma or intracerebral hemorrhage.[6] The disadvantage of using it in this manner is the time required to stop seizures (15–30 minutes). When seizure activity has not stopped after the use of a benzodiazepine and/or phenytoin, the patient usually requires intubation. Phenobarbital is routinely given as the third-line agent.

Fosphenytoin. Fosphenytoin is a phosphorylated pro-drug of phenytoin. It is cleaved by tissue phosphatases into phenytoin.[19] The antiepileptic mechanism of action of fosphenytoin is that of phenytoin, over which it has some important clinical advantages. Fosphenytoin is water soluble and, therefore, does not need to be diluted with propylene glycol. As described previously, it is felt that the propylene glycol diluent is primarily responsible for the cardiac arrhythmias and hypotension that potentially attend intravenous infusion of phenytoin. Because propylene glycol is not used with fosphenytoin, rates of infusion of the drug can be approximately three times faster than that of phenytoin. Because 3 mg of fosphenytoin are converted by the body into 2 mg of phenytoin (3:2 ratio), 150 mg of fosphenytoin can be given in 1 minute (expressed as 150 mg of phenytoin equivalents (PE) when ordering fosphenytoin).[20] Fosphenytoin is converted to phenytoin in vivo, taking approximately 10–15 minutes. Therefore, infusing 1500 mg of fosphenytoin at a rate of 150 mg PE takes 10 minutes, whereas a phenytoin load of 1500 mg given intravenously at 50 mg per minute takes 30 minutes. The full in vivo conversion of fosphenytoin to phenytoin adds 10–15 minutes to the infusion time, resulting in a marginal savings in time. However, phenytoin is frequently given more slowly than 50 mg per minute, thus increasing the time saved by using fosphenytoin. Regardless, the safety factor is increased substantially with use of fosphenytoin.

Water solubility makes fosphenytoin suitable for intramuscular administration, resulting in rapid absorption and therapeutic loading levels in 30–45 minutes.[21] Phenytoin cannot be given intramuscularly due to poor absorption and the tendency to form sterile abscesses. Because fosphenytoin is supplied at a concentration of 75 mg/ml (50 PE/ml), one drawback of intramuscular loading is that 20 ml of solution is used to deliver 1 g of PE, requiring at least two injections. However, 10-ml injections can be given safely. Maintenance daily dosing of fosphenytoin, in the range of 300 mg of phenytoin, requires only a 6-ml injection.

In summary, fosphenytoin has distinct clinical advantages compared with phenytoin in that intravenous loading doses can be administered more quickly and with a substantially greater margin of safety. Cardiac monitoring should still be used with intravenous loading of fosphenytoin. Fosphenytoin given intramuscularly can be used either for loading doses or for maintenance therapy. However, intramuscular loading should not be used to treat convulsive SE due to the increased time required to obtain therapeutic phenytoin levels compared with intravenous administration.

Phenobarbital. Phenobarbital, a barbiturate, is another effective AED due to its enhancement of GABA receptor currents. Phenobarbital can be given when phenytoin or fosphenytoin has not been effective after 30 minutes. Phenobarbital enters the brain in 20 minutes, can stop seizures in 20 minutes, and has a half-life of 50–100 hours.[17] Phenobarbital, 20 mg/kg (<100 mg per minute), by intravenous push, can be given until seizures stop by administering half of the dose over 10 minutes and repeating it as needed. Severe respiratory depression and hypotension can occur with high doses of phenobarbital, requiring continuous monitoring of vital signs. When seizures have not stopped after the use of phenobarbital, pentobarbital coma is used.

Pentobarbital. When seizures have not been controlled with diazepam or lorazepam, phenytoin or fosphenytoin, or phenobarbital, induction of coma by pentobarbital is usually undertaken next. This step involves an anesthesiologist and EEG monitoring to assess the desired aim of burst suppression or EEG silence. Pentobarbital's anesthetic effect may be mediated by several mechanisms that decrease neuronal activity, including enhancement of GABAergic inhibition, inhibition of neuronal sustained repetitive firing, and inhibition of high-threshold calcium currents. Pentobarbital also lowers cerebral oxygen consumption and brain lactate content. Pentobarbital's peak antiepileptic effect is achieved in 15 minutes and has a half-life of 15–60 hours. Pentobarbital, 5–15 mg/kg, given intravenously, is given slowly to achieve EEG burst suppression and is followed by 0.5–3.0 mg/kg per hour to maintain burst suppression. The patient can be kept in an EEG burst suppression pattern for days, when necessary, and the rate of pentobarbital infusion lowered every 2–4 hours to determine when seizure activity has ended. The major side effect of pentobarbital is hypotension, which can be reversed with saline infusion or pressors.

Propofol. Propofol is a relatively new anesthetic compound. Its mechanism of action appears to be an enhancing allosteric modulation of the $GABA_A$ receptor at a site distinct from the binding sites for benzodiazepines or barbiturates. Propofol has not been used extensively to treat SE, but it can be effective in terminating SE when benzodiazepines or barbiturates have failed. Dosing regimens have varied, but a standard regimen consists of a loading dose of 1–3 mg/kg followed by a maintenance infusion of 50–125 μg/kg per minute. As with other anesthetics used in treating SE, the dose is titrated using EEG monitoring to ensure suppression of all ictal activity and maintenance of a burst suppression pattern. Propofol has the advantage of a very short half-life, and patients can recover more quickly from prolonged intravenous infusions than with benzodiazepines or barbiturates.

Gestational Epilepsy

Some women experience seizures only during pregnancy. This condition is known as gestational epilepsy, and may be due to changes in hormonal, metabolic, or systemic factors during pregnancy. Serum levels of AEDs frequently decrease during pregnancy and may be the result of one or several factors including decreased drug compliance, increased volume of distribution, decreased absorption, decreased protein binding, and increased elimination. Noncompliance and increased elimination of AEDs are the most important reasons for decreased serum levels of AEDs and increased seizure frequency. When protein binding is reduced, free serum AED levels are often more reliable than the total serum level. For patients who present to the emergency department after experiencing a first seizure, the need for and selection of an AED should be determined after discussion with the patient's obstetrician and/or family physician. In general, complex partial seizures and generalized tonic-clonic seizures are commonly treated with carbamazepine or phenobarbital. SE is treated as described previously.

Preeclampsia is a condition characterized by the development of hypertension with proteinuria and/or edema after the 20th week of gestation or within 48 hours after delivery. Preeclampsia may evolve into eclampsia, a serious disorder of pregnancy occurring almost exclusively in the second half of gestation. Eclampsia essentially reflects the neurological consequences of hypertensive encephalopathy[6] and is characterized by hypertension, seizures, coma, proteinuria or persistent edema, or both.[12] Treatment of eclampsia has not been standardized; however, control of seizures may be achieved by treatment of hypertension, and definitive therapy requires termination of the pregnancy. Hypertension is defined as more than 140/90 mm Hg or increases of 30 mm Hg systolic or 15 mm Hg diastolic above midtrimester readings. Blood pressure should be reduced to 140 to 150 mm Hg systolic and 90–100 mm Hg diastolic by hydralazine, 5–10 mg, by intravenous push every 20 minutes or a continuous intravenous infusion or by nitroprusside, 3 mg/kg, by a continuous intravenous infusion.[12] When nitroprusside is used, thiocyanate levels must be obtained. Many feel that nitroprusside use is relatively contraindicated because of the potential accumulation of toxic concentrations of cyanide in utero. Propranolol, 1–5 mg, by intravenous push, may be required to block reflex tachycardia. When seizures continue despite adequate treatment of hypertension, then electrolytes, especially sodium, and metabolic parameters should be assessed. When seizures continue after normalization of metabolic abnormalities, phenytoin, 15–18 mg/kg (50 mg per minute), by intravenous push, should be started. When phenytoin is not effective, diazepam, 5–10 mg, by intravenous infusion over 5 minutes, should be given and lumbar puncture and CT of the brain performed.[12]

The practice of treating seizures in the preeclamptic or eclamptic patient with magnesium sulfate ($MgSO_4$) remains controversial. There is little evidence that $MgSO_4$ affects central epileptogenic mechanisms.[22] It has effects at the neuromuscular junction, including diminished presynaptic release of acetylcholine (ACh) and decreased postsynaptic sensitivity to ACh. This can cause neuromuscular blockade, which could mask continued epileptic activity.[6] The treatment of choice for seizures in the eclamptic patient is appropriate AED therapy, which poses little to no risk to the fetus in late pregnancy.[6] Treatment of seizures with $MgSO_4$ routinely, however, is a bolus of 4–6 g given intravenously followed by an infusion of 1–2 g per hour given with hydralazine therapy. Therapeutic serum levels of $MgSO_4$ are 6–8 mEq/l. Increased serum levels of $MgSO_4$ are associated with loss of reflexes (more than 8 mEq/l) and respiratory arrest (usually more than 1 mEq/l). *Careful and continuous monitoring is essential when magnesium sulfate is used.* Adverse reactions can occur at lower than "therapeutic" serum levels. Deaths have occurred from inadequate monitoring.

Alcohol Withdrawal Seizures

Alcohol withdrawal seizures are generalized tonic-clonic convulsions that usually occur within 48 hours after cessation of ethanol ingestion, with a peak incidence between 13 and 24 hours. The seizures are usually brief, occur as a single episode or in bursts of two or more, and can evolve into SE.[23] These seizures typically occur in chronic alcoholics or after episodes of binge drinking. Other causes of generalized seizures that may occur during alcohol withdrawal include head trauma, subdural hematoma, meningitis, and metabolic derangements,[12] and should be evaluated as indicated. Partial seizures that occur during the withdrawal period suggest focal brain injury – old or new – and require evaluation.

The standard treatment of alcohol withdrawal seizures is based on the principle of providing a medication with cross-tolerance to alcohol. Because these seizures are usually brief and limited in number, a benzodiazepine such as chlordiazepoxide (Librium), 50–100 mg given intravenously, or diazepam, 5–10 mg given intravenously, can be administered to treat an ongoing seizure. These medications can be repeated at regular intervals (chlordiazepoxide every 1–2 hours orally or intravenously, diazepam every 15–20 minutes orally or intravenously) as indicated to suppress other withdrawal symptoms and continued for several days on a tapering schedule. Patients are assessed carefully for hypotension and respiratory depression. Patients who have a history of epileptic seizures should have serum levels obtained for their prescribed AEDs and supplemented as needed to achieve therapeutic serum concentrations. Patients with seizures refractory to benzodiazepine treatment or those with a history of epileptic seizures not currently treated can be given a loading dose of phenytoin, 15–18 mg/kg given intravenously (50 mg per minute with ECG monitoring) or orally (2–3 split doses over 6 hours), respectively. Alcohol withdrawal seizures that evolve into SE should be treated as described previously.

Disposition of Patients Following a Seizure

The disposition of a patient who has experienced a seizure is largely based on the cause and the severity of the seizure. New-onset seizures may or may not require treatment with an AED. A decision to treat with an AED is best made after discussing the patient's case with his or her primary care physician or a neurologist. Usually, patients can be discharged safely when the seizure is brief, nonfocal, and uncomplicated, the neurological examination is normal, and the diagnostic evaluation is unremarkable. Patients are usually admitted to the hospital for further evaluation and management when there has been SE, trauma-induced seizures, identification of a space-occupying CNS lesion or infection, anoxia, or a serious toxic or metabolic derangement. Typically, patients admitted to the hospital are started and maintained on an AED during their hospitalization.

Medicolegal Issues

A patient who has experienced a seizure must be informed of the cause of the seizure, the determined need for AEDs and their potential side effects, reasonable restrictions on activities of daily living, and the state's law regarding restriction of driving privileges. This information is documented clearly in the medical record for potential medicolegal issues.

For patients with seizures, there are no uniform restrictions on activities of daily living that might be of potential harm to them or others. The range of activities must be determined for each patient based on the type of seizures experienced, the associated functional impairment, and the degree of seizure control achieved with AEDs. In general, patients with seizures are encouraged to lead full and active lives. They are advised to develop regular routines for sleeping, eating, working, and medication taking, and to avoid excessive exertion, sleep deprivation, excessive use of alcohol and caffeine, and undue stress. Excessive use of alcohol can increase the risk of seizure recurrence during a withdrawal period. Excessive use of caffeine can make seizures more difficult to control. Common sense and good judgment should dictate avoidance of certain activities that may pose substantial risk to the patient or others. These include driving, swimming, bathing, and working at heights or with heavy machinery or power tools. Patients with seizures may be able to swim but should never swim alone. High-risk sports such as sky diving, hang gliding, or rock climbing should probably be avoided.

The laws for restriction of driving privileges after a seizure with impairment of consciousness vary among different states. It is important that the emergency physician know the laws of the state so that the patient can be informed accurately. Generally, patients who experience a seizure are not permitted to drive for 6–12 months. Most neurologists consider a patient capable of driving without serious risk posed to the patient or others when the patient is seizure-free for 1 year and compliant with the prescribed AEDs. In patients with seizures who have no history of seizures associated with impairment in consciousness or significant motor dysfunction (e.g., simple partial seizures), driving may be considered safe when the patient can drive without difficulty during a seizure. Patients experiencing only nocturnal seizures may not need to have their licenses suspended. When seizures have been well controlled on an AED regimen and drug withdrawal is undertaken, it is reasonable to recommend against driving during the withdrawal period or for 6 months, whichever is longer.

Some states require that the physician responsible for treating the seizures report that information to the agency responsible for issuing drivers' licenses. Most states hold the patient responsible for providing information about his or her condition to the appropriate authority when applying for a driver's license. Specific information regarding drivers' license restrictions can be obtained from each state's department of motor vehicles.

Documentation on the emergency department medical record of the patient who has had a seizure includes common side effects of AEDs, informing the patient of the state laws regarding driving restrictions, and potential risks. When an AED is not initiated in the emergency department, or is delayed, the reasons are documented. For example, when the seizure has been a single, isolated event, treatment with an AED may not be initiated. This decision is made with the patient's physician, and appropriate follow-up determined.

PEARLS AND PITFALLS

- Patients evaluated in the emergency department following a seizure may be postictal, normal, or experiencing a recurrent seizure.
- Patients who appear confused or postictal may be experiencing absence or complex partial SE.
- Convulsive SE is a medical emergency associated with high morbidity and mortality.
- Although used infrequently in the emergency department, an EEG can diagnosis ongoing seizure activity in a patient with a prolonged period of impaired consciousness.
- Syncope can be difficult to distinguish from seizure.
- The diagnosis of psychogenic seizures is made cautiously after a thorough neurological examination and focused diagnostic evaluation are normal; many patients with psychogenic seizures have epilepsy.
- Alcoholics can have epilepsy; patients with epilepsy can drink alcohol.
- It is important that the emergency physician knows the state's law regarding restriction of driving privileges for patients who have experienced a seizure.

REFERENCES

1. Hauser WA, Hesdorffer DC. Epilepsy: frequency, causes and consequences. New York: NY: Demos Publications; 1990.
2. Sander JWAS, Shorvon SD. The epidemiology of the epilepsies. *J Neurol Neurosurg Psychiatry.* 1996;61: 433–43.
3. Commission on Classification and Terminology of the International League Against Epilepsy: Proposal for revised classification of epilepsies and epileptic syndromes. *Epilepsia.* 1989;30:389–99.
4. Engel J Jr, Ludwig BI, Fetell M. Prolonged partial complex status epilepticus: EEG and behavioral observations. *Neurology.* 1978;28:863–9.
5. Porter R. *Epilepsy: 100 Elementary Principles.* London, England: WB Saunders Co; 1989.
6. Engel J Jr. *Seizures and Epilepsy.* Philadelphia, Pa: FA Davis Co; 1989.
7. Gale K, Browning RA. Anatomical and neurochemical substrates of seizures. In: Dichter MA, ed. *Mechanisms of Epileptogenesis: The Transition to Seizure.* New York; NY: Plenum Press; 1988;111–52.

8. Dohrmann ML, Cheitlin MD. Cardiogenic syncope: seizure versus syncope. *Neurol Clin.* 1986;4:549–62.

9. American Psychiatric Association. *Diagnostic and Statistical Manual of Mental Disorders.* 4th ed. (DSM-IV). Washington, DC: American Psychiatric Association; 1994.

10. Kuzniecky R, de la Sayette V, Ethier R., et al. Magnetic resonance imaging in temporal lobe epilepsy: pathologic correlations. *Ann Neurol.* 1987;22:341–7.

11. Devinsky O, Nadi SN, Theodore WH, Porter RJ. Cerebrospinal fluid pleocytosis following simple, complex partial, and generalized tonic-clonic seizures. *Ann Neurol.* 1988;23:402–3.

12. Fernandez RJ, Samuels MA. Epilepsy. In: Samuels MA, ed. *Neurology: Diagnosis and Therapy.* 4th ed. Boston: Little, Brown and Co; 1991;82–118.

13. Treiman DM. Pharmacokinetics and clinical use of benzodiazepines in the management of status epilepticus. *Epilepsia.* 1989;30(suppl 2):S4–S10.

14. Kumar A, Bleck TP. Intravenous midazolam for the treatment of refractory status epilepticus. *Crit Care Med.* 1992;20:483–8.

15. Rivera R, Segnini M, Baltodano A, Perez, V. Midazolam in the treatment of status epilepticus in children. *Crit Care Med.* 1993;21:991–4.

16. Parent JM, Lowenstein DH. Treatment of refractory generalized status epilepticus with continuous infusion of midazolam. *Neurology.* 1994;44:1837–40.

17. Treiman DM. General principles of treatment: responsive and intractable status epilepticus in adults. *Adv Neurol.* 1983;32:377–84.

18. Treiman DM. The role of benzodiazepines in the management of status epilepticus. *Neurology.* 1990;40 (suppl 2):34–42.

19. Browne TR, Kugler AR, Elder MA. Pharmacology and pharmacokinetics of fosphenytoin. *Neurology.* 1996; 46(suppl 1):S1–S7.

20. Allen FH Jr, Runge JW, Legarda S, et al. Safety, tolerance, and pharmacokinetics of intravenous fosphenytoin (Cerebyx) in status epilepticus. *Epilepsia.* 1995; 36(suppl 4):90.

21. Uthman BM, Wilder BJ, Ramsay RE. Intramuscular use of fosphenytoin: an overview. *Neurology.* 1996;46 (suppl 1):S24–S28.

22. Sibai BM, Spinnato JA, Watson DL, et al. Effect of magnesium sulfate on electroencephalographic findings in preeclampsia-eclampsia. *Obstet Gynecol.* 1984;64: 261–6.

23. Adams RD, Victor M, Ropper AH. *Principles of Neurology.* 6th ed. New York, NY: McGraw-Hill Book Co; 1997.

*This chapter has been adapted from *Principles and Practice of Emergency Medicine,* 4th ed., G. Schwartz, ed. (Baltimore: Williams & Wilkins, in press), with permission.

13 Gait Disturbance

JON BRILLMAN AND KATHLEEN COWLING

SUMMARY Human locomotion is a complex neural activity achieved after the first year of life. It can be compromised or lost due to aging, illness, or injury. The coordination of sensory input with integral central processing and motor output is the essential structure of gait. In this chapter, problems related to gait are outlined as they pertain to emergency medicine.

Introduction

Abnormalities of gait have diverse causes and can be difficult to diagnose because of the complexity of coordinating sensory, motor, visual, vestibular, and cerebellar inputs into the gait cycle. A person's station and gait is unique and reflects gender, age, body habitus, mood, and culture, enough so that an acquaintance can be recognized at a distance based solely on his or her gait. At the biomechanical level, gait can be subdivided into kinematics, kinetics, and kinesiology. Kinematics is how the limb segments move with respect to each other. Kinetics refers to the joint forces involved in the motion.[1] Kinesiology is the study of muscle functions of the limb in motion. These distinctions are important for researchers, but a more practical designation is more useful to clinicians.

The gait cycle is a combination of phases designated as *stance* and *swing*. The stance phase is that part of the cycle that begins with heel strike and continues to "toe off." Swing involves the motion from "toe off" to just before heel strike. A full gait cycle starts with a heel strike and ends just before the next heel strike of the same foot, referred to as *stride* (see Fig. 13.1). The dynamics are such that "toe off," the point during the stride separating the stance phase from the swing phase, occurs at 60% of the gait cycle. "Toe-off" provides the force necessary for forward propulsion during the swing phase. The body is actually falling forward until stopped by the contralateral limb's heel strike. Knee flexion and ankle dorsiflexion provide toe clearance that is necessary for the limb in swing to be successful and smooth. Concurrently, the stance limb requires stability of hip extensors to resist passive flexion forces as the center of gravity is moved forward. Integrating these forces into a smooth and rapid cadence requires stability of single limb support, rapid swing, and necessary range of motion at each of the involved joints. Fixing a single joint such as with ankle fusion significantly alters the entire stride. Some authors describe walking as a rhythmic series of controlled falls that are halted by each step.[2-4] Using this concept, it is easy to understand that disrupted gait frequently results in falling.[5]

Walking is defined as gait that permits double stance, with both feet on the ground for up to 25% of the cycle. As gait velocity increases, this percentage decreases until there is no point in the cycle when both feet are touching the ground at the same time, designated as running. Normal gait is learned by humans at about 1 year of age. Normal gait is generated by an erect head, stable trunk, and feet that clear the ground, and does not require conscious forethought. Abnormal gait results from changes in the mechanisms that provide upright position, balance, and forward stepping movements.

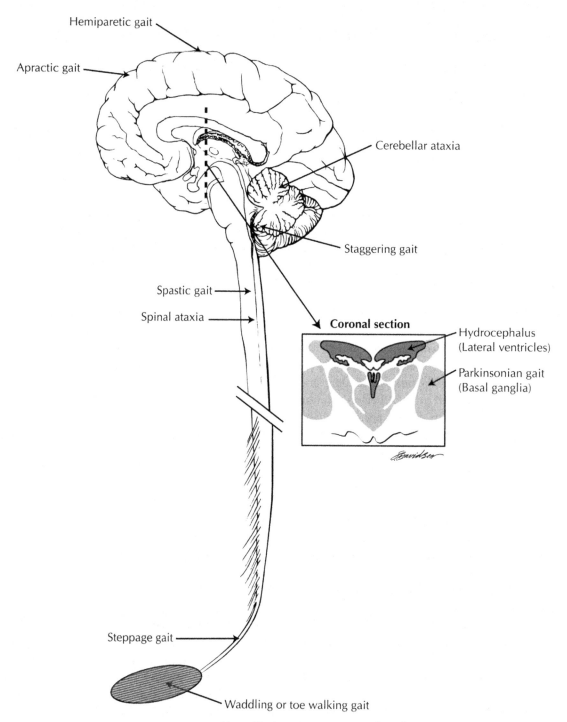

Hemiparetic gait

Apractic gait

Cerebellar ataxia

Staggering gait

Spastic gait

Spinal ataxia

Coronal section

Hydrocephalus
(Lateral ventricles)

Parkinsonian gait
(Basal ganglia)

Steppage gait

Waddling or toe walking gait

FIGURE 13.1. Sites of lesions in various gait disorders.

Emergency Department Evaluation

The patient arriving at the emergency department typically does not present complaining of gait disturbance. Weakness, headache, or manifestations from falls secondary to a gait abnormality are the common chief complaints.[6] A detailed history of a problem with gait is crucial for determining its cause. The differences between acute, subacute, and chronic gait disturbances are especially significant when distinguishing vascular disease from degenerative disease as the cause.

Physical examination of gait often begins by observing the patient approach the examination area. After performing the rest of the screening neurological examination to determine if weakness, abnormal position sense, visual impairment, or labyrinthine disorder is involved, gait can be assessed. Observation of station and regular walking – including stride height, length, base width, stops, starts, turns, walking on toes and heels, and tandem (heel-to-toe) walking – constitutes the basic examination. Testing of station begins by asking the patient to stand erect with feet close together. The patient is observed with his or her eyes open and closed. Unsteadiness with eyes open suggests cerebellar disease. Steadiness with eyes open and unsteadiness with eyes closed (Romberg sign) indicates disease of the dorsal columns of the spinal cord. Specific cerebellar testing, such as finger-to-nose and heel-to-shin coordination movements, helps determine whether there is appendicular ataxia, a sign of ipsilateral cerebellar hemisphere involvement. In general, assessment of gait in the emergency department can be performed adequately by simple observation of the patient walking and the associated truncal or upper extremity movements.

Differential Diagnosis

Gait disturbances commonly observed in the emergency department are classified according to cause and frequency of occurrence in Table 13.1. The different types of gait disturbance are described below with regard to neuroanatomical localization and specific neurological disorders (Fig. 13.1).

Senescent Gait (Early Gait Apraxia)

This gait is observed commonly in patients of advanced age and is characterized by small, uncertain steps. Generally, the foot is planted flat without springing from the heel to the ball of the foot and there is reduced associated arm movement. Patho-

TABLE 13.1. Classification of Gait Disorder by Etiology*

Etiology	1980–1982**	1990–1993	Total	%
Myelopathy	8	12	20	18.5
Parkinsonism	5	7	12	11.1
Hydrocephalus	2	4	6	5.6
Multiple infarcts	8	8	16	14.8
Cerebellar degeneration	4	4	8	7.4
Sensory deficits	9	11	20	18.5
Toxic/metabolic	3	0	3	2.8
Psychogenic causes	1	3	4	3.7
Other causes	3	2	5	4.6
Unknown causes	7	7	14	13.0

* *n* =108 patients.
** Data from Sodarsky L, Ronthal M. Gait disorders among elderly patients. *Arch Neurol.* 1983;40:740–3. © American Medical Association.

logically, this gait disturbance may be partially due to cerebral atrophy. However, decreased mobility of the joints, tightness of the hamstrings, and decreased proprioceptive input caused by mild peripheral neuropathy may be involved.[7]

Advanced Senescent Gait (Late Gait Apraxia)

Typically, patients with advanced senescent gait are demented. These patients may have Alzheimer's disease, severe cerebral atrophy of other causes and associated communicating hydrocephalus, or subcortical arteriosclerotic encephalopathy (Binswanger's disease). Their steps are extremely small and tenuous, and frequently the feet seem to be stuck to the floor. Balance is impaired, patients may be tipped over backward or forward. When asked to get out of bed to walk, they have a great deal of difficulty assuming an upright posture, and frequently position and reposition their feet, or oscillate in an attempt to maintain balance. Many patients with advanced gait apraxias are unable to walk and are wheelchair-bound.

Parkinson's Disease and Parkinsonian Conditions

The gait of patients with Parkinson's disease and related disorders is fairly stereotyped but can be confused with a senescent gait. Generally, there is flexion of all limbs and the trunk (universal flexion), and a tendency to lean forward and accelerate in walking, a disturbance of gait referred to as *festination*. There is usually a loss of associated arm swing that is unilateral initially but becomes bilateral. Patients and their families report the patient's tendency to shuffle, but not always in early disease. Generally, the patient has severe postural instability and can be easily tipped over. In advanced stages of the disease, there is a tendency for the patient to get stuck in doorways and not be able to place the lower limbs through an aperture. The turn is slow and automaton-like with very small, hesitant steps. Once an about-face is accomplished, the patient may have difficulty getting started again. Patients with other Parkinson's disease–like (parkinsonian) syndromes, such as progressive supranuclear palsy, commonly have axial dystonia, with a tendency of the body to arch slightly backward. They can have an "astonished" facial appearance, rather than a hy-

pomimic appearance, which is characteristic of patients with Parkinson's disease. Other extrapyramidal disorders such as Shy-Drager syndrome, olivopontocerebellar degeneration, and cortico-basal ganglionic degeneration are parkinsonian but can have features of gait apraxia. At times, it is extremely difficult to distinguish these various disorders.[8] Neurological consultation is obtained, because idiopathic Parkinson's disease can be treated medically.

Hemiparetic Gait

The most frequent cause of hemiparetic gait is cerebral infarction. Patients with hemiparesis have arm flexion in the upper extremity, adduction of the arm held closely to the body, flexion of the fingers, and hyperextension of the foot with an equinovarus deformity. The leg is commonly stiff and spastic. In order to avoid tripping, the patient swings the leg out in a so-called circumducting fashion. This type of gait is most commonly observed in patients with a spastic hemiparesis.

Spastic Gait

Patients with spastic gait generally have problems involving the spinal cord. In elderly individuals, this can be due to cervical spondylotic myelopathy or tumors of the spine, either primary or metastatic. Demyelinating disorders, particularly with involvement of the cervical spinal cord, are a common cause of spastic gait in younger individuals. Under these circumstances, the patient is frequently "wooden-legged" or stiff, with minimal or no flexion of the knees while walking. When combined with cerebellar impairment as in multiple sclerosis, or involving the ascending cerebellar pathways of the spinal cord, titubation (oscillation of the head and body) or wide-based gait can be present. These are commonly referred to as *spastic-ataxic gaits*. Severe spastic paraparesis is observed in patients with congenital abnormalities such as cerebral palsy and may have associated severe adductor spasm and "scissoring" of gait. Typically, this can be identified by the sound of the thighs or clothing rubbing together during walking.

Ataxic Gait

Ataxia refers to disordered balance and is not associated with a specific neuroanatomical localization. Patients with cerebellar injury due to infarction, hemorrhage, metastasis, tumor, or demyelination have ipsilateral appendicular ataxia when the cerebellar hemisphere is involved, or ataxic gait when the cerebellar vermis is involved.[9] Ataxic gait is usually broad-based and often associated with titubation. Swaying is present when the patient's eyes are open, and is worse when the eyes are closed. Mild forms of cerebellar ataxia, particularly in midline (vermian) cerebellar disorders, can be detected by tandem gait testing, in which the patient walks a straight line touching heel-to-toe. When cerebellar hemisphere involvement is present, there is dystaxia and dysmetria, commonly demonstrated by finger-to-nose testing or heel-to-shin testing. Ataxia can be seen with dorsal column dysfunction, such as in vitamin B_{12} deficiency (Romberg sign), or with a severe large fiber peripheral neuropathy involving the lower extremities.

Patients with ataxia due to impaired joint position sense (sensory ataxia), from either posterior column disease or peripheral nerve disorders involving the lower extremities, may have a prominent Romberg sign. Patients with sensory ataxia are particularly impaired if visual input is diminished, and typically they fling their legs abruptly forward and outward to variable lengths and heights. This gait is referred to as "haughty gait" and was described for tabes dorsalis; however, now it is more often observed in patients with spinocerebellar degenerations, multiple sclerosis, and spondylotic cervical myelopathy.

Staggering Gait

Staggering gait is observed commonly in the emergency department. It is characteristic of alcoholic intoxication and can be seen in sedative drug intoxication. The term *drunken* is applied to this type of gait, but it is different from a cerebellar ataxic gait. The gait is wide-based, or narrow-based with pitching and reeling to one side or the other, a loss of balance, and a need to grasp and hold onto objects.[10] Intoxicated patients can reel backward, sideward, or forward, with a tendency to propel in the direction in which they get started. The accompanying features of intoxication, including the smell of alcohol, slurred speech, and disordered behavior, are characteristic of patients with staggering gait.

Steppage Gait

Steppage gait is observed in patients who have a foot drop due to a peripheral neurological disorder. It is usually unilateral and is due to an injury of the common peroneal nerve at the level of the fibular head in the lateral portion of the knee. Injury to this nerve can be due to direct trauma, for example, compression by a knee-high cast or stretching of the nerve associated with a lithotomy position during childbirth or hemorrhoidectomy. It is observed commonly in cachectic, bedridden patients. Other causes include diabetic mononeuritis multiplex or are idiopathic. The steps are normal, but the advancing foot cannot be dorsiflexed and has to be elevated by excessive flexion of the hip and knee so the foot can clear the ground, curbsides, or steps. When applied to the ground, foot slaps make an audible noise. Occasionally, foot drop results from an L5 radiculopathy due to a herniated L4–5 disc, and is usually associated with sciatic nerve distribution pain.[11] Bilateral foot drop suggests a more severe disease process such as Charcot-Marie-Tooth disease, amyotrophic lateral sclerosis, and polio.

Waddling Gait

Waddling gait is characteristic of patients who have hip girdle weakness. It is seen in hip dislocations usually in adults, and is characteristic of polymyositis or muscular dystrophy. Patients with a waddling gait shift their weight from side to side in an exaggerated fashion. When a leg is planted down, the opposite hip rises. The trunk tends to incline to the side of the patient's step. Alteration in trunk movements results in the waddling feature.

Hysterical Gait

Hysterical gait cannot be explained satisfactorily by a specific neuroanatomical localization or disease process. As is the case with other hysterical disorders, associated features of emotional disturbance are elicited in a nonthreatening manner by the examiner. Gait may be bizarre, pitching and starting to one side or the other, wavering suddenly from left to right, or with twirling motions with the arms outstretched and flopping about (astasia-abasia).[12] Frequently, patients suddenly topple or fall into a position where they may take a step and push the other leg. In hysterical hemiparesis, there is absence of circumducting gait, hyperactive deep tendon reflexes, and a Babinski sign. A diagnosis of hysterical gait is not made when there is objective evidence of nervous system dysfunction.

Antalgic Gait

Antalgic gait results from a shortened stance phase of a painful limb. Osteoarthritis is a common cause.[13] Sometimes called *coxalgic gait,* it commonly refers to hip disease and the compensatory gait of decreased stride length and stance phase that minimizes discomfort in the hip joint.

Gait Disturbance in Children

Pediatric considerations of gait disturbance range from a limp secondary to an orthopedic problem to cerebellar ataxia. Acute focal weakness is usually a sign of serious disease. Sickle cell anemia, leukemia, and congenital heart disease can present with leg weakness resulting from ischemia. Lower extremity weakness can be due to traumatic brain or spinal cord injury, infection such as local abscess in the brain or spinal cord, botulism, or Guillain-Barré syndrome.[14,15] Tick paralysis, which results from a tick bite that releases a neurotoxin, typically develops within a week after the bite and can cause ascending paralysis and cerebellar symptoms. Removal of the tick and supportive care are the only treatments required.

The most common cause of cerebellar ataxia in the pediatric population is a postinfectious process, most frequently seen following varicella infection.[16] Most children developing a postinfectious cerebellar ataxia have nystagmus, headache, nausea, vomiting, and occasional nuchal rigidity. These symptoms can occur one week before and up to three weeks after the development of the rash. Other common infections that cause ataxia are due to polio, coxsackievirus, Epstein-Barr virus, measles, mumps, rubella, mycoplasma, and echoviruses.[17] Cerebrospinal fluid can be normal or show a lymphocytic pleocytosis and elevated protein level. Greater than 90% of patients recover completely from this form of ataxia. Another form of ataxia in the pediatric population is secondary to immunizations. Typically, this is a temporary gait disturbance observed after administration of the measles, mumps, and rubella vaccine. Another cause of ataxia in the pediatric population is that of drug intoxication. The most frequently involved agents are anticonvulsants, sedatives, and exposure to heavy metals, for example, lead and organic solvents. Sniffing of paint, glue, and gasoline is a significant cause of sickness and death in young people. The effects of inhaling these chemicals include delirium, seizures, ataxia, irreversible encephalopathy, and death.[18]

Toe walking is observed almost exclusively in children. It occurs commonly in Duchenne's muscular dystrophy due to replacement of the gastrocnemius muscle by collagen and fat. Spasticity of the lower extremities can manifest itself initially with toe walking. Palpation of the muscular tone allows the examiner to distinguish between upper and lower motoneuron lesions associated with gait disturbances. Some children walk on their toes as an affectation and have no neurological disorder. They outgrow this and walk normally in one to two years.

Management and Disposition

Patients presenting with a gait disturbance are assessed for treatable causes such as hypoglycemia, drug toxicity, or infection when indicated. Most patients with acute-onset ataxia are admitted to facilitate further evaluation. Patients presenting with simple accidental drug overdoses or a postictal state can be observed in the emergency department and, when improved, discharged with appropriate supervision. Acute or subacute gait disturbances require urgent evaluation, which may include CT scanning or MRI of the brain and spine, and neurological consultation.

PEARLS AND PITFALLS

- Patients with acute or subacute gait disturbance of unknown cause are hospitalized for further investigation.
- Acute paraparesis or ataxia associated with ascending sensory alterations represents an inflammatory or compressive lesion of the spinal cord, such as a plaque of multiple sclerosis or tumor, respectively.

■ Similar symptoms in the setting of decreased or absent deep tendon reflexes suggest Guillain-Barré syndrome.

■ Chronic gait disorders usually can be evaluated in a nonurgent fashion.

■ When a gait abnormality is likely to lead to a fall with subsequent injury, a gait assist device with instruction on its use or supervision is indicated.

REFERENCES

1. Cochran GVB. *A Primer of Orthopedic Biomechanics.* New York, NY: Churchill Livingstone; 1981.
2. Grimm RJ. Disorderly walks. *Neurol Clin.* 1984;2:615–31.
3. Isaacs B. Gait and balance. In: Pathy MSJ, ed. *Principles and Practice of Geriatric Medicine.* New York, NY: Wiley; 1985;695–7.
4. Nutt JG, Marsden CD, Thompson PD. Human walking and higher-level gait disorders, particularly in the elderly. *Neurology.* 1993;43:268–79.
5. Sudarsky L. Gait failure. *Emerg Med Clin North Am.* 1987;5:677–85.
6. Dejong RN, Haerer AF. Case taking and the neurologic examination. In: Joynt RJ, ed. *Clinical Neurology.* Philadelphia, Pa: JB Lippincott Co; 1994;47–9.
7. Murray MP, Kory RC, Clarkson BH. Walking patterns in healthy old men. *J Gerontol.* 1969;24:169–78.
8. Cardoso F, Jankovic J. Movement disorders. *Neurol Clin.* 1993;11:625–33.
9. Connolly AM, Dodson WE, Prensky AL, Rust RS. Course and outcome of acute cerebellar ataxia. *Ann Neurol.* 1994;35:673–9.
10. Schiller F. Staggering gait in medical history. *Ann Neurol.* 1995;37:127–35.
11. Wagner JH. *Neurologic Disorders of Ambulatory Patients: Diagnosis and Management.* Philadelphia, Pa: Lea & Febiger; 1989.
12. Quane T, Chambers CV. Conversion disorder presenting as gait disturbance in an adolescent. *Arch Fam Med.* 1995;4:805–7.
13. Olsson E. Gait analysis in hip and knee surgery. *Scand J Rehabil Med.* 1986;15(suppl):1–55.
14. Dodge PR, Pomeroy SL. Transverse myelitis or myelopathy. In: Feigin RD and Cherry JD, eds. *Pediatric Infectious Diseases.* Philadelphia, Pa: WB Saunders, 1987.
15. Fagin DH. Weakness. In: Reisdorff EJ and Roberts HR, eds. *Pediatric Emergency Medicine.* Philadelphia, Pa: WB Saunders; 1993.
16. Bhende MS. Ataxia. In: Reisdorff EJ and Roberts HR, eds. *Pediatric Emergency Medicine.* Philadelphia, Pa: WB Saunders; 1993.
17. Cherry JD. Enteroviruses. In: *Pediatric Infectious Diseases.* Philadelphia, Pa: WB Saunders, 1987.
18. Goodheart RS, Dunne JW. Petrol sniffer's encephalopathy. *Med J Aust.* 1994;160:178–81.
19. Sudarsky L, Ronthal M. Gait disorders among elderly patients. *Arch Neurol.* 1983;40:740–3.

THREE SPECIFIC NEUROLOGICAL CONDITIONS

14 Central Nervous System Infections in Adults

PAUL BLACKBURN, OLIVER W. HAYES, AND GREG FERMANN

SUMMARY Central nervous system (CNS) infections are serious but relatively infrequent. The presentation varies from nonspecific constitutional symptoms to an array of neurological findings. The potential for rapid clinical deterioration and permanent neurological sequelae requires prompt consideration of the diagnosis, and urgent and sometimes empirical treatment of suspected CNS infections. CNS infections can be due to a variety of causes with either an acute or insidious onset. This chapter reviews the epidemiology, clinical presentation, approaches to diagnosis, and emergency department therapy of CNS infections in adults.

Introduction

Central nervous system (CNS) infections have a variety of forms, ranging from acute and rapidly fatal bacterial meningitis to slowly progressive infectious processes from mycobacterial, fungal, or viral agents. Viral and bacterial meningitis are the most frequent CNS infections encountered in the emergency department (see Table 14.1). Differentiating *encephalitis* from *meningitis* on a clinical basis is not always possible in the emergency department. Patients who present with encephalitis commonly have altered mentation; those with headache, fever, and meningismus generally have meningitis.

The cumulative risk for the most common CNS infections in patients 80 years of age and younger is 2.3% for men and 1.5% for women.[1] Clinical outcome depends on expeditious and appropriate therapy because mortality from bacterial disease occurs most commonly in the first 48 hours of the therapy.

The CNS infections discussed are a collection of processes that can have various clinical presentations to the emergency department. A careful history documents the course and the pace of the illness, exposures to infectious agents, and factors that increase susceptibility to CNS infections. The physical examination is directed toward the identification of systemic infection and localization of neurological dysfunction. Clinical assessment is supplemented by cerebrospinal fluid (CSF) analysis and neuroimaging studies. Empirical antibiotic therapy and supportive care are initiated promptly while awaiting definitive diagnosis and treatment.

Anatomical Considerations in Central Nervous System Infections

The pathogenesis and clinical course of CNS infections is affected by the anatomy of the brain and the spinal cord. The CNS is relatively well protected from infection by the scalp, skull, and meninges that shield the brain from extracranial sources of infection. The blood–brain barrier helps prevent hematogenous spread to the brain. Most infectious agents reach the CNS by hematogenous spread from extracranial sources or by retrograde propagation of infected thrombi within emissary veins. Because of the rigid confines of the skull and the spinal column, physiological responses to infections such as inflammation, hemorrhage, hydrocephalus, and

Sid M. Shah and Kevin M. Kelly, eds., *Emergency Neurology: Principles and Practice.* Copyright © 1999 Cambridge University Press. All rights reserved.

TABLE 14.1. Central Nervous System Infections in Adults

1. Meningitis
   a. Aseptic
   b. Bacterial
   c. Chronic or recurrent
   d. Fungal
   e. Rickettsial
   f. Tuberculous
2. Abscess, empyema, and effusion
   a. Intraparenchymal
   b. Extraparenchymal
3. Encephalitis
   a. Viral encephalitis
4. Other conditions
   a. HIV-related CNS infections
   b. Lyme disease
   c. Neurosyphilis
      (1) Syphilis of the brain
      (2) Syphilis of the spinal cord
   d. Sarcoidosis
   e. Tetanus
   f. Cerebral brucellosis
   g. Protozoan infections
   h. Psittacosis and lymphogranuloma venereum

edema can produce brain herniation due to increased intracranial pressure (ICP), or spinal cord compression.

Prehospital Management

The primary considerations in the prehospital care of patients with suspected CNS infections are airway management and hemodynamic support. When mental status is altered, finger-stick glucose determination is obtained. Pulse oximetry is a helpful adjuvant. Seizures occur in 30% of adults with meningitis and are treated in the field with anticonvulsant agents such as benzodiazepines.

Emergency Department Evaluation and Management

Bacterial Meningitis

Acute bacterial meningitis is a significant cause of morbidity and mortality. Of the 25,000 individu-als who contract bacterial meningitis in the United States annually, nearly 30% are adults.[2] Approximately 70–85% of cases are caused by *Hemophilus influenzae, Neisseria meningitidis,* or *Streptococcus pneumonia.*[2,3] The organisms most frequently associated with community-acquired adult meningitis are *S. pneumoniae, N. meningitidis,* and *Listeria monocytogenes.*[4] Although the overall incidence of CNS infections has declined in the United States, the incidence in the geriatric population has increased, including infections caused by gram-negative bacilli and *Listeria.*[2,3] Anaerobic organisms cause infection in less than 1% of patients. Infection with multiple organisms occurs in 1% of patients, and is usually secondary to paranasal sinus and ear infections, skull fractures, neurosurgery, and immunosuppression.[3]

Patients at increased risk of meningitis include those with human immunodeficiency virus (HIV) infection, malignancy, alcoholism, sickle cell disease, organ transplantation, neurosurgical procedures, head trauma, splenectomy, and high-dose steroid therapy, and those on hemodialysis.[2] Anatomical factors such as the presence of a CSF leak or fistula, presence of a CNS shunt, accompanying contiguous focus of infection such as sinusitis, otitis media, brain abscess, or recent neurological procedure can jeopardize host defenses and increase the risk of bacterial meningitis.[5] Despite advances in treatment, the morbidity and mortality of bacterial meningitis remain high. Clinical outcome depends on the age, general state of health, severity of the acute illness, and presence of systemic complications.[2]

Pathophysiological Considerations. Nasopharyngeal colonization appears to be crucial in the initiation of bacterial meningitis. Organisms attach to nasopharyngeal epithelial cells and are transported to the bloodstream within phagocytic vacuoles. Upon gaining access to the bloodstream, host defense mechanisms are ineffective, resulting in a virulent, high-grade bacteremia. The exact site of CNS invasion is unknown, but the choroid plexus has been implicated due to its vascularity.[6] Having gained access to the CNS, the bacterial infection quickly results in the high organism densities in CSF that are characteristic of bacterial meningitis. Once established in the CSF, a "secondary bacteremia" of the

CSF can occur, and the host can be continuously reseeded until overwhelmed with infection.[6]

Clinical Presentation. Typical presentation of meningitis includes fever, headache, nuchal rigidity, and altered mental status. However, 15% of patients do not have these typical findings.[2,3] Fewer than 25% of elderly patients complain of a headache, and meningismus is present in approximately a third of the elderly with meningitis.[1] Symptoms such as nausea, vomiting, sweating, myalgias, weakness, and photophobia can be present. Approximately 25% of patients with meningitis present with symptoms less than 24 hours in duration; approximately 50% have a subacute progression over 1–7 days.[2]

A variety of cutaneous signs occur in patients with meningitis. Approximately 33% of patients with meningitis present with dermatological findings. Diffuse maculopapular eruptions that progress to petechiae and purpura occur especially with *N. meningitidis* infection.

Focal neurological findings complicate meningitis in at least 5% of cases.[2] These findings are prevalent when the disease progresses rapidly. Signs of acutely increased ICP can be present (see Chapter 26, "Increased Intracranial Pressure"). The ophthalmological examination can reveal sluggishly reactive or dilated pupils or even ophthalmoplegia (particularly sixth nerve palsy). However, most patients with early meningitis do not have papilledema.[2] When present, it suggests the possibility of brain abscess, subdural empyema, tertiary syphilis, or venous sinus thrombosis. Cranial nerve III and VI palsies are caused by basal exudation and inflammation, and sixth nerve palsies can indicate dangerously elevated ICP.[3] The level of consciousness correlates best with the likely clinical outcome and is closely monitored. The possibility of mortality increases dramatically as consciousness decreases, and approaches 55% for adults in coma.[3] Up to 30% of adult patients with meningitis have seizures. Those with focal seizures are more likely to have a poor prognosis.[5]

Diagnosis. The confirmation of the diagnosis of acute bacterial meningitis is made by the examination of CSF. In the absence of a contraindication (local infection at the puncture site or suspected in-

creased ICP), lumbar puncture (LP) is performed when meningitis is suspected (see Chapter 4, "Lumbar Puncture"). Bleeding diatheses or coagulation defects are corrected prior to LP. ICP, which normally ranges from 80–200 mm of CSF, is elevated in 85% of patients with bacterial meningitis.

The CSF in bacterial meningitis is characterized by a polymorphonuclear pleocytosis, depressed glucose level, and elevated protein level.[7] CSF protein is normally less than 50 mg/dl but is elevated in most patients with meningitis, with values between 200 mg/dl and 500 mg/dl.[2,7] The degree of protein elevation in CSF depends on the severity of the inflammatory response, the organism, age of the patient, and the integrity of the immune system. CSF glucose concentration is normally in the range of 45–65 mg/dl, with a ratio of CSF to serum glucose of approximately 0.6.[2,3,7] A ratio of less than 0.4 is found in approximately 75% of patients with bacterial meningitis.[2,3]

CSF white blood cell (WBC) counts in adults are normally less than 5 cells/ml.[6] With bacterial meningitis, the WBC count can vary greatly but is usually between 1000 and 10,000 cells/ml.[7] In bacterial meningitis, over 90% of CSF samples have a polymorphonuclear pleocytosis.[2] A lymphocytic pleocytosis is present in up to 14% of cases of meningitis and is frequently due to infection with *Listeria monocytogenes*. Normal cell counts can occur at the onset of meningitis, and in those with severe immunocompromise.[4] Table 14.2 lists typical CSF findings in patients with meningitis.

Oral or systemic antibiotics received prior to LP can make diagnostic interpretation of CSF results difficult. Patients treated with oral antibiotics have a reduced number of neutrophils in the CSF, a decrease in the CSF protein concentration, and a decreased yield on Gram stain and culture results. Intravenous antibiotics received two to three days prior to LP diminish the possibility of organism isolation by Gram stain or culture.[2] The interpretation of CSF cell count is also confounded by a traumatic LP when CSF is contaminated with blood. CSF white blood cell (WBC) count is expected to be proportional to the peripheral blood WBCs when all the cells are from introduced blood and there is no true CSF pleocytosis. It has been demonstrated that CSF pleocytosis tends to be significantly lower than expected from this calculation and the danger of missing true CSF pleocytosis is significant.

TABLE 14.2. Characteristic Findings in Cerebrospinal Fluid with Meningitis

	Normal	Bacterial	Viral	Fungal/TB	Abscess
Glucose (mg/dl)	45–65	<40	45–65	30–45	45–65
Protein (mg/dl	<50	>150	>50	>100	>50
Leukocytes (WBC/ml)	0–5	>1000	100–1000	100–500	10–1000
Type	Mononuclear	PMN	Mononuclear	Mononuclear	Indeterminate
CSF:blood glucose ratio	0.6	<0.4	0.6	<0.4	0.6

Note: CSF: cerebrospinal fluid; PMNs: polymorphonuclear neutrophils.

Organisms are detected on Gram stain of the CSF in 60–90% of untreated patients, and in 40–60% of patients treated with antibiotics.[2,7] The diagnostic accuracy of the CSF Gram stain varies with the number of organisms present, the organism type, and the skill of the person conducting the analysis. With fewer than 10^3 bacteria colony forming units, the CSF Gram stains are positive in 25% of cases. This test is positive in 50% of cases of gram-negative meningitis and in less than 50% of cases caused by *Listeria monocytogenes* or anaerobes. CSF cultures are positive in 70–85%, however, they are positive in less than 50% of patients receiving prior antibiotics.[5]

Antigen detection testing by counterimmuno-electrophoresis, coagglutination, or latex agglutination is more sensitive and specific than Gram stain and is recommended. However, the sensitivity of antigen detection tests is usually less than that of culture and can vary from institution to institution. The decision to withhold antibiotic therapy based on negative antigenic testing is not recommended.[4]

Computerized tomography (CT) or magnetic resonance imaging (MRI) of the brain is obtained prior to LP in those patients with altered mental status, focal or lateralizing findings, or seizures. Although the majority of imaging studies are normal for patients with meningitis, clinically important findings on CT scanning can occur when the neurological examination is abnormal, seizures are focal or persistent, or the fever has persisted for longer than seven days.[2] When LP is delayed in order to obtain neuroimaging studies, antibiotics are administered promptly after blood cultures have been obtained.

Treatment. Early antibiotic therapy improves survival rate and reduces adverse neurological sequelae (Table 14.3). Some experts recommend that antibiotic treatment be initiated within 30 minutes of presentation to the emergency department; others have questioned this recommendation.[6] It seems prudent to administer antibiotics to a patient with suspected meningitis as soon as possible, preferably within 30–60 minutes of arrival in the emergency department.

The emergency department management of a patient with suspected bacterial meningitis is similar to that of any other critically ill patient. The initial focus is on achieving hemodynamic stability. Next, obtaining appropriate studies, and providing empirical or definitive antimicrobial therapy is completed in tandem as dictated by the clinical condition of the patient.

The initial choice of antibiotic therapy in meningitis is directed at the common causal agents, including *S. pneumoniae, H. influenzae, N. meningidis,* and *L. monocytogenes.* In patients with immunosuppression, recent neurosurgery, or CSF leak, therapy is directed at *Staphylococcus aureus* and gram-negative bacilli. The eventual antibiotic choice depends on the Gram stain results, antigen testing, culture results, and knowledge of local nosocomial drug resistance patterns. The ideal antibiotic achieves CSF minimal bactericidal concentrations 10–20 times higher than in vitro and is lipid-soluble, although in practice this is rarely a problem due to the blood–brain barrier disruption from meningeal inflammation.[3] Because there has been little change in the age-related prevalence

TABLE 14.3. Initial Antibiotic Therapy for Acute Bacterial Meningitis in Adults

S. pneumoniae	Cefotaxime, ampicillin, penicillin G (plus vancomycin with/without rifampin)
N. meningitidis	Penicillin G, ampicillin, cefotaxime, chloramphenicol
H. influenzae	Cefotaxime, ceftriaxone, ampicillin
S. aureus (methicillin-sensitive)	Nafcillin, oxacillin
S. aureus (methicillin-resistant)	Vancomycin plus rifampin
L. monocytogenes	Ampicillin
Streptococci (group A, B, etc.)	Penicillin G, ampicillin
Gram-negative bacilli	Ceftriaxone, cefotaxime, trimethoprim-sulfamethoxazole
P. auruginosa	Ceftazidime
Anaerobes	Cefotaxime plus metronidazole plus rifampin

Adapted from: Ashwal S. Neurologic Evaluation of the Patient with Acute Bacterial Meningitis. *Neurologic Clinics.* 1995;13(3):549–577.

of bacterial pathogens, third-generation cephalosporins are now considered the initial therapy of choice, often accompanied by ampicillin.[2]

For meningococcal meningitis, penicillin remains the drug of choice.[2,3] For patients with meningococcal meningitis confirmed by culture or Gram stain, treatment is initiated with ampicillin (200 mg/kg per day) or penicillin G (200 mg/kg per day), given by intravenous injection. *Staphylococcus aureus* is suspected in those with ventriculoperitoneal shunts. Nafcillin or oxacillin is usually effective, although in cases of methicillin resistance, vancomycin plus rifampin or metronidazole is indicated. In most cases, it is necessary to remove the shunt in order to eradicate the infection completely.[2,3]

For *S. pneumoniae* meningitis, cefotaxime, ceftriaxone, and penicillin are the drugs of choice. Reports of relative resistance to penicillin have led to the use of cefotaxime as the preferred initial choice of antibiotic therapy. Strains of pneumococci resistant to third-generation cephalosporins have been reported, requiring therapy with cefotaxime or ceftriaxone plus vancomycin.[8,9]

The emergence of beta-lactamase production in *H. influenzae* type B and chloramphenicol-resistant strains of *H. influenzae* (1%) has led to the use of cefotaxime or ceftriaxone as the initial agents of choice. Similarly, ceftriaxone has proven effective against gram-negative meningitis in adults. Because ceftriaxone and other third-generation cephalo-

sporins are ineffective against *Listeria monocytogenes,* ampicillin or penicillin combined with an aminoglycoside, or trimethoprim-sulfamethoxazole (for those with penicillin allergy), is required.[1]

The effectiveness of corticosteroids as adjunctive therapy is not proven; however, experimental studies and anecdotal evidence suggest that the use of corticosteroids may be beneficial.

Chemoprophylaxis for Contacts. Chemoprophylaxis is indicated in susceptible persons in order to prevent the transmission or development of acute bacterial disease. Currently such therapy is recommended for household contacts of patients with meningococcal or Hemophilus meningitis. Individuals experiencing casual contact need not receive prophylaxis unless they have had prolonged close contact with a patient with meningitis before that patient began therapy. Antimicrobial agents for chemoprophylaxis include rifampin (10 mg/kg – up to 600 mg – every 12 hours for 4 days), ceftriaxone (250 mg given intramuscularly in adults, 125 mg in children), ciprofloxacin (one dose of 500 mg or 750 mg), or ofloxacin (one dose of 400 mg).

Brain Abscess

Brain abscess is a suppurative infection involving brain parenchyma. Intracranial suppuration is diagnostically and therapeutically a challenging condition, despite the advances in imaging modalities, organism isolation techniques, neurosurgical advances, and newer antibiotics. Brain abscesses frequently present as confounding emergencies. As with other CNS infections, delay in diagnosis and treatment adversely affects the outcome.[3]

Pathophysiological Considerations. Bacteria can reach the brain by three pathways: (1) seeding from the bloodstream or hematogenous spread, (2) direct extension from an adjacent infectious focus, and (3) implantation during trauma or neurosurgery. In up to 20% of patients with brain abscesses, the source of infection cannot be identified.[3]

Brain abscesses arise as a result of direct spread from a contiguous site of infection in 20–60% of patients.[10] Subacute and chronic otitis media and mastoiditis are the most important predisposing factors. Temporal lobe or cerebellar abscesses are often of otogenic origin. Chronic sinusitis can lead to abscess formation in the frontal lobes and the deeper parts of the temporal lobes. Facial trauma, missile injuries of the head, and craniotomy can be complicated by abscess formation, which may not manifest until years later.

Hematogenous spread is the second most important route of abscess formation. These abscesses are usually multiple and generally in the distribution of the middle cerebral artery. Patients with pulmonary arteriovenous fistula, infective endocarditis, and dental infection are at risk. Patients with cyanotic congenital heart disease are 10 times more prone to develop brain abscess than those without a cyanotic heart disease.[11]

Clinical Presentation. The onset of symptoms and signs is frequently subacute, with nonspecific findings that result in a delay of diagnosis. The size and location of the abscess, the general health of the patient, duration of the illness, and prior treatment can all lead to a variety of clinical presentations. Headache is the most common symptom and is often located on the same side as the abscess. Fever is present in approximately 50% of patients with brain abscesses. Focal neurological signs develop days to weeks after the headache. Specific neurological deficits depend on the site of abscess (Table 14.4). The triad of fever, headache, and focal neurological findings is present in less than 50% of patients.[2,3] Neck stiffness can mimic meningitis. Sei-

TABLE 14.4. Anatomic Location of Brain Abscess and Related Neurological Findings

Location	Signs
Temporal Lobe	Wernike aphasia, homonymous superior quadranopsia, contralateral facial weakness
Frontal Lobe	Mental status change, seizures, positive grasp, suck and snuff reflexes, contralateral hemiparesis (large abscess)
Parietal Lobe	Impaired position sense, two point discrimination and stereognosis focal sensory and motor seizures, homonymous hemianopsia, impaired opticokinetic nystagmus
Cerebellum	Ataxia, nystagmus, ipsilateral arm and leg incoordination with intention tremor
Brain Stem	Facial weakness, dysphagia, multiple cranial nerve palsies, contralateral hemiparesis

Adapted from Hoeprich PD, Jordan MC, Ronald AR (eds). *Infectious Diseases: A Treatise of Infectious Processes.* 5th ed. Philadelphia: Lippincott, 1994.

zures, focal or generalized, can occur. Symptoms such as mental status change and third and sixth cranial nerve deficits can be associated with ICP elevation. Brain abscess is strongly suspected in a patient with known cyanotic heart disease and unexplained headache. As with meningitis, the outcome depends on the patient's level of consciousness at time of presentation.[3]

Diagnosis. A high clinical index of suspicion is a critical factor in the assessment of a patient with suspected brain abscess. A comprehensive history and physical examination is directed toward identifying occult sources of infectious foci. Baseline serological studies and "pancultures" are obtained. These studies are rarely helpful in establishing a diagnosis in the emergency department, but they serve as a baseline for monitoring the disease pro-

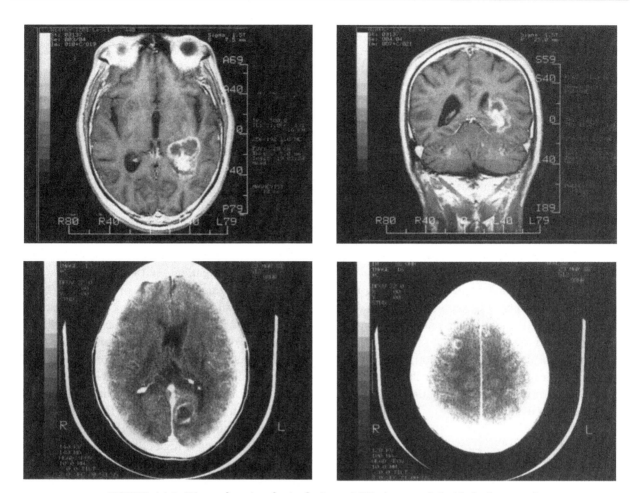

FIGURE 14.1. Ring-enhancing brain lesions. MRI shows a left-sided abscess of *Streptococcus* in axial (A) and coronal sections (B). CT scan shows bilateral *Cryptococcoueas* in axial sections (C, D).

cess. LP is contraindicated because of the possibility of brain herniation.

The diagnostic studies of choice are CT or MRI of the brain, with contrast enhancement. The sinuses and mastoid air cells are inspected for evidence of infection on the imaging studies. CT bone windows can help identify skull fractures and cranial defects. During the earlier stages of abscess formation, CT scanning can be normal. MRI provides more diagnostic information than CT in demonstrating early disease.[12–14] Contrast enhancement of the lesion demonstrates the classic "ring" appearance of the mature encapsulated abscess (see Figure 14.1A–D). Lesions less than 0.5 mm in diameter appear homogeneous rather than ring-enhancing.[13] It is not possible for CT or MRI to provide a specific diagnosis of these lesions, because such diverse conditions as tumors, granulomas, necrotizing encephalitis, infarction, and lymphoma

have similar appearance on the imaging studies. HIV-infected patients with ring-enhancing lesions are presumed to have toxoplasmosis, which is the most frequent cause of focal brain lesions in this population.

Treatment. The goals of therapy are to sterilize the abscess site(s) and to reduce the mass effect. Because surgical drainage of a brain abscess is usually necessary, prompt neurological consultation is obtained. Surgery is indicated for relief of elevated ICP due to space occupation, and biopsy for diagnostic confirmation.[17] The threshold for surgical aspiration is substantially lower in the immunocompromised patient.

Although there are no controlled trials of various antimicrobial therapies for the treatment of brain abscesses, the use of broad-spectrum antibiotics is recommended.[15,16] The antibiotic choice is directed by the presumptive diagnosis of brain abscess and consideration of the ability of the antibiotic to penetrate CSF, the capsule wall, and its activity within the purulent material. The eventual choice of antibiotic therapy depends on the culture and sensitivity reports of the tissue. Current recommendations for empirical treatment while awaiting culture results are a combination of intravenous penicillin G in high dosages (320,000–480,000 units, or 200–300 mg/kg per day) and metronidazole (20–30 mg/kg per day). When staphylococci are suspected (following craniotomy or penetrating trauma), a penicillinase-resistant penicillin or vancomycin (50–60 mg/kg per day) is used.[3] Most experts recommend a 6–12-week course of antibiotics.

Dexamethasone in a loading dose of 10 mg may help reduce the edema surrounding the lesion. The risk of immunosuppression is far outweighed by the benefit obtained by edema reduction. In patients with acute neurological deterioration, measures to decrease ICP are taken (see Chapter 26, "Increased Intracranial Pressure"). Prophylactic anticonvulsants are recommended.[3]

HIV-Related Central Nervous System Infections

Although the CNS infections most commonly associated with HIV infection are toxoplasmosis and cytomegalovirus (CMV), the patient with HIV infection is susceptible to many other infections of the CNS including aseptic meningitis, neurosyphilis, and *M. tuberculosis*.

Toxoplasma gondii is a ubiquitous intracellular protozoan whose definitive hosts are members of the Felidae family (including the domestic cat). Humans and other mammals are incidental hosts. In the United States, the incidence of seropositivity varies between 3% and 30%.[17] *T. gondii* seropositivity in HIV-infected patients is similar to that of the general population in a particular geographical location.[18] In patients with acquired immunodeficiency syndrome (AIDS), the impaired production of lymphokines and gamma interferon, and the lack of specific antibody response and opsonization of *T. gondii* are responsible for reactivation of infection. These changes are seen typically with advanced immunosuppression, and with median CD4 counts of 48 cells/ml. The primary routes of transmission are oral and congenital. Humans become infected typically by the ingestion of undercooked pork or other meat containing tissue cysts.

Clinical Presentation. Patients with toxoplasma encephalitis present with both focal and general complaints. This includes headache (49%), fever greater than 38°C (40%) and abulia, or generalized behavioral slowing (37%). Frequent focal presentations are hemiparesis or hemiplegia (49%), generalized seizures (24%), and cranial nerve palsies (17%).

Diagnosis. Neuroradiology is the primary diagnostic modality for suspected CNS toxoplasmosis. Although 98% of patients with CNS toxoplasmosis have focal abnormalities on CT or MRI of the brain, the characteristics of toxoplasma lesions do not have pathognomonic features and can be similar to those that occur in several other conditions. However, toxoplasmosis is the most frequent cause of focal brain lesions in HIV-infected patients. The initial study of choice is contrast-enhanced brain CT, which frequently shows multiple hypodense, ring-enhancing lesions in the cerebral hemispheres. MRI is of benefit in cases of high clinical suspicion and a negative CT scan.

CSF analysis reveals a mild mononuclear pleocytosis. A slight increase in CSF protein with a small but inconsistent decrease in the glucose can occur. Frequently, the diagnosis can be made only by biopsy, especially in those who demonstrate negative serology, have atypical CT scans, or do not respond to therapy.

Treatment. Confirming the diagnosis of CNS infection with toxoplasmosis can be difficult; therefore, prompt empirical management is initiated. Treatment consists of pyrimethamine (200 mg on day 1, then 50–75 mg per day) and sulfadiazine (4–6 g per day) or clindamycin (2.4–3.6 g per day for 6 weeks). Common side effects of therapy include leukopenia, thrombocytopenia, and anemia. Adverse drug reactions are common and were reported in 62% of patients receiving therapy in one study.[19] Because most patients with HIV infection receive antiretroviral therapy, the nature of adverse drug reactions to the combination of antiretroviral therapy and an antitoxoplasma regimen is not well known.

Cytomegalovirus (CMV) belongs to the herpes family of viruses, which includes herpes simplex I and II, and varicella zoster. These viruses can cause CNS infection in the patient with AIDS. CMV typically infects both immunocompetent and immunocompromised hosts. In immunologically healthy individuals, the disease is often self-limited and asymptomatic, and can be detected only by using CMV antibody assays. Immunosuppressed patients commonly display end organ damage. In the HIV-infected patient, this is represented by multiorgan involvement such as the gastrointestinal system (esophagitis, gastritis and colitis), the eye (chorioretinitis), and the neurological system (meningoencephalitis, ventriculitis, and ascending polyradiculopathy).[20]

Diagnosis. Similar to other CNS infections in the patient with HIV, CMV encephalitis can present as a chronic, indolent process with psychomotor slowing, chronic cephalgia, or progressive ataxia, or as an acute process with encephalopathy, generalized or focal seizures, or hallucinations. Because nonspecific clinical manifestations of CNS pathology are common in most HIV-related infections, the diagnosis is often made on tests of CSF and blood. Radiological studies are often negative or reveal only diffuse white matter changes common to many HIV-related neurological diagnoses. The definitive diagnosis of CMV encephalitis often is made only with surgical specimens obtained at autopsy.

Treatment. The decision to initiate treatment for CMV encephalitis is based on high clinical suspicion while awaiting results of microbiological tests and immunoassays. The current regimen used in CMV encephalitis includes ganciclovir (5 mg/kg every 12 hours, given intravenously). The addition of foscarnet, an inhibitor of DNA polymerase, has proven effective, especially against ganciclovir-resistant strains. Foscarnet is administered intravenously in doses of 60 mg/kg every 8 hours.[28]

Aseptic Meningitis

The term *aseptic meningitis* has been used to describe conditions of acute meningeal irritation that prove to be benign and self-limiting. Aseptic meningitis is currently used in a broader and less precise manner to describe any meningitis for which a cause is not apparent after the initial CSF evalua-tion, especially if it shows a predominately lymphocytic pleocytosis. Other terms used are viral, serous, chemical, sterile, and nonbacterial meningitis.

Aseptic meningitis is a misnomer because up to 70–80% of the cases are caused by viruses.[22] However, the numerous nonviral causes of aseptic meningitis – including tuberculosis, syphilis, Lyme disease, HIV infection, and the fungal meningitis syndromes – are considered when "sterile" CSF is encountered. Certain medications can create an identical clinical picture. The most common offending agents are nonsteroidal anti-inflammatory agents (especially ibuprofen, sulindac, tolmetin, and naproxen), antibiotics (trimethoprim-sulfamethoxazole, metronidazole, ciprofloxacin, penicillin, and isoniazid), and intravenous immunoglobulin therapy.[22–27] Additional causes are intrathecal injections of air, radiological dyes, isotopes, antibiotics, chemotherapeutic agents, steroids, neurosurgical procedures (particularly those involving the posterior fossa), connective tissue diseases, and certain CNS tumors, which can present with acute or recurrent episodes of aseptic meningitis.

Clinical Presentation. The illness typically evolves over hours, with nonspecific symptoms such as fever, malaise, headache, and myalgias. The headache can have various characteristics and is generally described as being different from the "usual headache."[27] Other findings include neck stiffness, photophobia, and irritability. Most patients with viral meningitis remain easily arousable and coherent. However, "encephalitis" is suspected in patients with an altered level of consciousness, seizures, or focal neurological findings. The prognosis for most patients with aseptic meningitis is good, and resolution can be expected within days to two weeks.

Diagnosis. The differential diagnosis of aseptic meningitis includes bacterial and other forms of septic meningitis, subarachnoid hemorrhage, and brain abscess. History includes inquiry of any recent illness, preexisting medical conditions, immunosuppressive disorders, sexual history, HIV risk factors, medications, immunizations, travel, exposure to insect vectors, and animal exposure.[22]

Confirmation of the diagnosis is assisted by the examination of CSF. The opening pressure is generally normal to slightly elevated, and the fluid appears clear to the naked eye. The CSF WBC count varies from 500–1000 cells/ml, predominantly lymphocytes or monocytes. It is not possible to exclude confidently an incipient bacterial meningitis in the presence of predominantly polymorphonuclear CSF pleocytosis and other nondiagnostic CSF parameters. The CSF protein level is normal or minimally elevated, and the CSF glucose level is normal or slightly reduced.[7,22]

In most cases, the offending pathogen is not identified. Accompanying constitutional illness can indicate the etiology. Clinically, the agent usually does not need identification, because the condition is self-limiting and therapy is directed toward the etiology and rarely involves more than symptomatic treatment with analgesics and antiemetics. When medication or "inflammation-induced" aseptic meningitis is suspected, rapid improvement is noted once the offending medication or procedure is withdrawn. Infectious causes (i.e., tuberculous, syphilitic, or Lyme disease) require appropriate antibiotic therapy.

Treatment. The HIV-infected patient who presents with an aseptic meningitis requires special consideration. HIV infection itself can induce aseptic meningitis; however, the immunocompromised state of HIV-infected patients makes them susceptible to numerous CNS infections that mimic the aseptic profile. A serious underlying infection is always considered in the differential diagnosis.

Uncomplicated "viral meningitis" requires symptomatic treatment with the use of analgesics and antiemetics. When identification of the virus is necessary, either viral cultures or identification of IgM antibodies or viral antigens in the CSF can be pursued through appropriate laboratory evaluation.

Tuberculous Meningitis

New cases of tuberculosis (TB) in the United States declined steadily from 1953 (the first year of reporting) to 1985. However, since 1985, the number of new cases have increased. Factors responsible for this trend include the increase in numbers of HIV-infected patients, poor and homeless individuals (among whom tuberculosis rates are 150–300 times higher than the national norm), and immigrants from developing countries.[28] Although the incidence of pulmonary tuberculosis (TB) in the

United States had declined until recently, the number of cases of tubercular CNS infection have remained relatively constant, at about 4000 new cases per year. The rate of extrapulmonary tuberculosis in the United States has risen from 8% to 15% of all cases of TB.

Pathophysiological Considerations. CNS tubercular infection accounts for 15% of extrapulmonary cases, or 0.7% of all clinical cases.[28] CNS tuberculosis can be divided clinically into three categories: (1) meningoencephalitis, (2) intracranial tuberculoma, and (3) spinal tuberculous arachnoiditis. The clinical presentation and the character of illness within each category are highly variable and nonspecific, and overlap with other infections of the CNS, with CNS vascular syndromes, and with CNS space-occupying lesions.[29]

Tuberculous meningitis (*TBM*) is a result of bacteremia that occurs with either primary or reactivated tubercular disease. A small number of mycobacteria are seeded throughout the substance of the brain and meninges, producing isolated miliary tubercles. When a tubercle proliferates, the result is a caseous focus. When the lesion is adjacent to ependyma, it can rupture into the subarachnoid space, leading to meningitis. The probability of a caseous focus rupturing into the CSF is associated with the rate of growth of the lesion. Chronic bacteremia associated with progressive miliary TB greatly increases the probability of developing a juxtaependymal focus.[29]

The pathophysiology associated with TBM is predictable and accounts for the variety of clinical presentations. However, the diagnosis of TBM can be difficult. Clinical presentation consistent with features of tuberculosis and its associated laboratory findings is accompanied by a high index of suspicion for TBM. Delay in both diagnosis and treatment is the most critical factor that leads to poor outcomes. Factors that predispose to TBM are young or advanced age, immunosuppressive drugs, lymphoma, alcoholism, and HIV infection. A family history of tuberculosis is important, as is recent exposure to others with active TB.[29]

Clinical Presentation. The onset of the disease is insidious, with a vague prodrome of constitutional symptoms such as malaise, low-grade fever, and intermittent headache that can be accompanied by personality changes. Within two to three weeks, the clinical picture of meningitis evolves. Protracted headache, meningismus, vomiting, and confusion can be accompanied by cranial nerve palsies and upper motor neuron signs. As the disease evolves, confusion can progress to stupor or coma, and neurological deficits such as seizures and hemiparesis can occur. Atypical presentations include dementia that is slowly progressive over months to years, or a rapidly progressive meningitis that appears indistinguishable from acute bacterial meningitis.

Diagnosis. The key to the diagnosis of TBM is the precise examination and culture of CSF. The opening pressure of LP can be elevated. CSF in TBM is clear or has a ground glass appearance with a delicate weblike clot at the surface. The typical CSF findings are elevated protein level (100–500 mg/dl), diminished glucose level (<45 mg/dl), and a mononuclear pleocytosis with a total WBC count of 100–500 cells/ml. Twenty percent of patients with TBM have a CSF WBC count of 500–1500 cells/ml. The "classic" CSF finding in TBM is pleocytosis with lymphocytic predominance. However, in the early stage of disease the CSF can be acellular or show a predominance of polymorphonucleocytes (PMNs). Such findings can lead to incorrect diagnoses of aseptic meningitis or bacterial meningitis, or a mistaken "therapeutic success" in a patient on antibiotic therapy. A reverse situation can occur with institution of therapy, creating a "therapeutic paradox." The initial mononuclear pleocytosis can shift to a PMN predominance, which is considered pathognomonic of TBM. The CSF examination of HIV-infected patients with TBM does not differ from that of non-HIV-infected patients.[31]

The diagnosis of TBM depends on demonstration of mycobacteria in the CSF by smear or culture. The sensitivity of the acid-fast bacilli (AFB) smear is directly related to the careful collection and preparation of the sample. Guidelines for the proper preparation and examination of CSF specimens for mycobacteria are as follows.[39]

1. Because AFB are most readily demonstrated in a smear of the clot or sediment, the highest yield will be in the last drops of CSF removed by LP. A total of 10–15 ml of CSF is collected.

2. When a clot does not form, 2 ml of 95% alcohol is added to the sample so that the alcohol mixes with only the upper portion of the CSF. This gives a heavy protein precipitate, which on centrifugation carries bacilli to the bottom of the tube.

3. 0.02 ml of centrifuged deposit of CSF is applied to a glass slide in an area not exceeding 1 cm in diameter, and is stained by the standard Kenyon or Ziehl-Neelsen method.

4. 200× and 500× fields of magnification of the smear are examined, preferably by more than one observer.

CT scanning of the brain can demonstrate basilar arachnoiditis, cerebral edema, infarction, ring-enhancing lesions, or hydrocephalus. Hydrocephalus appears to be the most common CT finding in the HIV-infected patient with TBM, followed by meningeal enhancement and parenchymal involvement.[32–33]

Evidence of active tuberculous infection elsewhere in the body is variable, estimated at 20–70% of all patients with TBM. The chest radiograph is examined for hilar adenopathy, a miliary pattern, or upper lobe nodular infiltrates. Positive findings on chest radiograph are noted in the majority of pediatric patients and in approximately 50% of adult patients with TBM. A tuberculin skin test is performed in all patients with suspected active TB. The skin test is positive in up to 80% of patients. A negative test is of no assistance in excluding the diagnosis.[30]

Spinal tuberculosis can arise at any level of the spinal cord by either breakdown of a tubercular focus or extension of TB from adjacent "tubercular" spondylitis. The inflammation is usually confined, and leads to partial or complete encasement of the spinal cord in a gelatinous or fibrous exudate. Variable presentations include combinations of spinal cord and nerve root compression, causing pain, hyperesthesia or paresthesia, lower motor neuron paralysis, and bladder or anal sphincter incontinence. Vasculitis of the anterior spinal artery can lead to spinal cord infarction.[30]

Treatment. The guiding principle of TBM therapy is prompt institution of therapy based on strong clinical suspicion. Prognosis is good when therapy is initiated before focal neurological changes or alterations in the level of consciousness occur. In absence of large, reliable clinical trials of the use and efficacy of different antitubercular agents in TBM, isoniazid remains the drug of choice. It is initiated at 10 mg/kg per day in both adults and children until a favorable clinical course is achieved, at which time the dosage is decreased to 5 mg/kg per day. Pyridoxine in a dose of 50 mg per day is administered concomitantly to avoid isoniazid-induced neurological complications. The rate of hepatotoxicity in adults receiving isoniazid is about 1%, and doubles with the administration of rifampin.[29]

Rifampin penetrates CSF poorly, even in patients with inflamed meninges. With inflamed meninges, CSF levels are approximately 20% of serum, exceeding the inhibitory concentration for sensitive strains.[29] The dosage is 600 mg per day in adults. An intravenous formulation of rifampin is now available.[33]

Pyrazinamide is a small molecule that penetrates CSF well under all conditions. The dose is 25–35 mg/kg per day. The incidence of hepatotoxicity is low when duration of therapy is restricted to less than two months, and pyrazinamide does not contribute to the hepatotoxicity associated with isoniazid and rifampin. However, the only significant toxicity associated with the use of pyrazinamide is myalgias with hyperuricemia and, occasionally, gout.[29]

Streptomycin, similar to other aminoglycosides, penetrates CSF poorly. The dose is 1 g administered intramuscularly daily in adults. Its use is restricted to those with either intolerance to other agents, bacillary resistance, or limited drug resources. Streptomycin is not given intrathecally because of the high likelihood of cranial nerve VIII toxicity.[29]

Ethambutol given in a dose of 15–25 mg/kg reaches the CSF in moderate concentration. The effectiveness of other medications and the toxicity of ethambutol mitigate against its routine use.

Clinical experience and limited trials of the use of corticosteroids favor the selective use of corticosteroids in preventing or treating neurological complications of TBM. Patients without any neurological compromise do well uniformly, and steroid therapy is not warranted. The use of corticosteroids is not recommended in patients with uncertain diagnosis, particularly when fungal CNS infection is suspected.[33]

Current recommendations for treatment of CNS TB are a combination of isoniazid, rifampin, and pyrazinamide for two months, followed by isoniazid and rifampin for an additional seven months. A fourth drug is added (streptomycin or ethambutol) when the patient is more likely to harbor a resistant strain of TB. "Breakthrough" TBM can occur while the patient is undergoing therapy. This is usually the result of mycobacterial strains that are resistant to one or more drugs, and appears when a medication is withdrawn to which the organism is sensitive, allowing regrowth of the resistant strain.[30]

Clinical outcome depends on factors such as the age and general health of the patient, duration of disease, clinical stage of the disease at time of institution of therapy, and the degree of arachnoiditis and vasculitis. Infection with HIV does not appear to affect the clinical manifestations or outcome of TBM.[30]

Three clinical stages of a patient with TBM are described for prognostic measures. Stage 1 consists of patients without any alteration of mental status, with or without meningismus, and absence of focal neurological deficits or hydrocephalus. Stage 2 patients are confused or have focal neurological deficits. In stage 3, patients have profound mental status changes, coma, or profound focal neurological deficits such as dense hemiplegia or paraplegia. The risk of minimal neurological sequelae with a mortality of less than 10% occurs in stage 1 or in early stage 2. Mortality exceeds 50% in patients over 50 years of age, and in stuporous or comatose patients. The incidence of residual neurological deficits after recovering from TBM is estimated to be between 10% and 30%.

Fungal Meningitis

Fungal meningitis is a rare event in immunocompetent hosts, whereas immunocompromised patients (particularly those with impaired cellular immunity) are susceptible to fungal infections. *Cryptococcus neoformans,* the most extensively studied fungal pathogen, commonly affects HIV-infected patients and 7–10% of patients with AIDS in developed nations.[34,35] *Coccidioides immitis,* endemic to the southwest United States, Central America, and portions of South America, can cause meningitis, particularly with disseminated HIV infection.[36] Less common fungal infections include the pathogen *Candida albicans* in patients with poor neurosurgical procedures and in those treated for bacterial meningitis, and aspergillosis in organ transplant patients.[37] Among patients who receive organ transplantation, 1–10% acquire aspergillosis; of these, 10–50% develop CNS involvement.[38]

Pathophysiological Considerations. *Cryptococcus neoformans* is inhaled from environmental sources. It is a ubiquitous monomorphic fungus that is a normal saprophyte of human skin and mucous membranes. Its small size (< 2 μm) is compatible with alveolar deposition where the infection can remain localized or disseminate hematogenously. The T helper cell is crucial in regulating the cell-mediated response, and cryptococcal growth becomes unrestricted if T cells are diminished in number. The predilection of *C. neoformans* for the CNS may be because human brain tissue has little or no inflammatory response to cryptococci. CSF provides a growth medium that lacks anticryptococcal factors and an alternative complement pathway found in serum.

Coccidioides immitis is a dimorphic fungus that grows in dry, dusty soil until mechanical disruption by physical means (wind, rain, soil movement) causes it to be inhaled. Its small size (<5 μm) leads to alveolar deposition and transition of *C. immitis* into its parasitic phase. Local tissue response can be granulomatous, suppurative, or both.[36]

Clinical Presentation. The clinical presentation of fungal meningitis is highly variable, in part because the majority of patients harbor significant underlying diseases. These underlying conditions can obscure or detract from the diagnosis of fungal meningitis. The onset is acute or gradual. Nonspecific findings such as fever, weight loss, night sweats, nausea, and vomiting reflect underlying disease or can be secondary to the fungal illness. Headache, although nonspecific, is present in most patients. Pulmonary symptoms can be present due to the respiratory portal of entry of *Cryptococcus* and *Coccidioides*. Neurological manifestations of fungal disease are protean. Alteration of mental status can manifest as confusion, lethargy, or even coma. Seizures can be generalized or focal. Isolated or com-

bined cranial nerve abnormalities or focal motor deficits can also be present.[38,39]

History taking and physical examination are performed after hemodynamic stability is achieved. A comprehensive neurological examination notes any focal findings. Neurological examination focuses on cranial nerve function in particular. The presence or absence of papilledema is noted. Meningismus is not uniformly present with fungal meningitis, but assessing nuchal rigidity is required.[38,39] Auscultation of the lungs for adventitious sounds is often helpful.

Diagnosis. CT or MRI of the brain, with contrast enhancement, is obtained. The imaging study rarely results in a specific diagnosis, because fungal lesions appear similar to many other diverse conditions. The type and distribution of lesions vary depending on the organisms, progression of the disease state, and underlying immunocompetence. Cryptococcus typically extends from the basilar cisterns along the deep perforating vessels and upward into the brain parenchyma. Mucormycosis is seen frequently in diabetics as a direct intracranial extension from the nasal cavity or paranasal sinuses. Mucormycosis and aspergillosis invade blood vessel walls and can lead to cerebral infarction or hemorrhage.[41]

The CSF findings in fungal disease are similar to those TBM. The pleocytosis is predominantly lymphocytic, although in the severely immunocompromised patient the CSF can be acellular. Protein levels are increased and glucose levels diminished. Identification of the organism by Gram stain or silver stain of CSF sediment is usually not successful.[7] Degree of organism recovery from CSF varies with the causative organism. *Cryptococcus neoformans* is recovered in approximately 72% of cases on the first sampling of CSF and in more than 90% when multiple LPs are performed to obtain additional CSF. *Cryptococcus neoformans* can be detected with India ink preparation in about 50% of cases, but several LPs can be necessary before sufficient fluid is obtained to detect organisms. The percentage of positive identification by India ink preparation increases to 75% in patients with AIDS. *Candida albicans* can be detected in most cases. The optimal volume of CSF required for fungal cultures is about

40–50 ml, similar to that required for identification of AFB. Cultures become positive within two to three days, but more likely require several weeks of growth due to low concentration of organisms and their fastidious nature.

Serological tests are of paramount importance in the diagnosis of *Cryptococcus* or *Coccidioides.* Cryptococcal antigen is detected in 90% of cases and is the single most useful diagnostic test for this condition. False negative results can be encountered when the disease is limited to brain parenchyma. The diagnostic yield of serological testing for *Cryptococcus* is up to 95% in patients with AIDS. Complement fixation tests for *Coccidioides* in CSF are positive in up to 95% of patients.[7] CSF eosinophilia can be a nonspecific but frequent finding with *C. immitis* meningitis according to one small study.[40]

Routine hematological and chemistry profiles are obtained for baseline values. All pertinent cultures are obtained. Specialized culture media and larger volumes of fluid are required. Cryptococcus is readily cultured from CSF and blood. It can also be cultured from urine after prostatic massage.[41]

Treatment. Some of the reasons for poor prognosis of patients with CNS fungal infections despite optimal treatment regimens are underlying immunosuppression, disseminated disease, delay in diagnosis and treatment, varying penetration of CSF by medications, and therapeutic agent toxicity. Eradication of the opportunistic infection is generally not feasible. The mean survival time of patients with untreated CNS coccidioidomycosis is 6 months, with nearly 100% mortality at 2 years.[45] Patients treated with amphotericin B have a mean survival time of 21 months.[39] Organ transplant recipient patients with CNS aspergillosis have a poor response to antifungal therapy and, therefore, a poor prognosis despite appropriate treatment.[38] In addition, adjustment of immunosuppressive therapy can lead to organ rejection and the need for retransplantation. When disease eradication is achieved, recurrence is less likely than in the patient with AIDS.

Cryptococcal meningitis has a poor prognosis despite optimum antifungal therapy. Use of amphotericin B or fluconazole leads to "negative" CSF cultures at 10 weeks in 35–40% of patients. The addition of oral flucystosine (150 mg/kg per day) to oral fluconazole (400 mg per day) results in negative CSF cultures at 10 weeks in almost 75% of patients.[42]

The traditional treatment for most fungal meningitides has been administration of amphotericin B. Although usually administered intravenously, amphotericin B has been given by alternate routes, such as intrathecally and intraventricularly, because its penetration of the CSF is relatively poor.[43] The disadvantages of amphotericin B are its dose-limiting nephrotoxicity and its limited success rate.[44,45] The use of flucytosine as a sole agent or with other antifungal agents has had variable results. The penetration of CSF by flucytosine is better than that of amphotericin B, and the combination of flucytosine and amphotericin B can have a synergistic effect.[42,45] Fluconazole penetrates the CSF and has proven efficacious in treating cryptococcal meningitis.[47,48] Adverse drug reactions are not uncommon in the HIV-infected patient, thus possibly restricting therapy.[48]

Neurosyphilis

Syphilis is a chronic multisystem disease caused by the spirochete *Treponema pallidum.* Neurological syndromes caused by this agent have been well described since the sixteenth century. Myriad clinical syndromes caused by *T. pallidum* have been described in medical literature. The presentation, diagnosis, and treatment of neurosyphilis, with particular reference to the HIV-infected patient, are emphasized here.

Clinical Presentation. Clinical neurosyphilis typically is divided into four syndromes: meningeal, meningovascular, parenchymatous, and gummatous syphilis. These rarely exist as pure entities, and all of them can manifest some degree of meningeal irritation.

Acute meningeal syphilis presents with nonspecific findings such as headache, confusion, nausea, vomiting, and nuchal rigidity. Cranial nerve involvement, particularly nerves VII and VIII, can occur. Sensorineural deafness occurs in up to 20% of patients, but normal hearing usually returns following therapy. CSF abnormalities such as pleocytosis, elevated protein (>45 mg/dl), and mild diminution of CSF glucose levels (glucose <50 mg/dl) are frequent.

Meningovascular syphilis is a result of focal arteritis leading to thrombosis and infarction. Peak occurrence is four to seven years after the primary infection. Neurological deficits include hemiparesis, hemiplegia, aphasia, and seizures, and can occur due to vessel occlusion (stroke). The middle cerebral artery is most involved commonly, followed by the basilar artery. CSF in meningovascular neurosyphilis is uniformly abnormal.

Parenchymatous neurosyphilis of tabes dorsalis and general paresis are rare in the postantibiotic era. Paretic neurosyphilis and tabes dorsalis, referred to as taboparesis, peaks 10–20 years after untreated infection. Paresis presents with subtle loss of cognitive function and behavioral changes that are commonly mistaken for a psychiatric disturbance. The disease can progress to include pupillary changes, hypotonia, dementia, seizures, and, finally, general paresis. Early clinical features of tabes dorsalis include "lightning pains," paresthesias, diminished deep tendon reflexes, progressive ataxia, pupillary abnormalities, optic atrophy, and urinary incontinence. Sensory loss caused by posterior column destruction leads to Charcot's joints and trophic ulcerations. Pupillary abnormalities are common. The classical Argyll Robertson pupil, a small, irregular pupil that accommodates but fails to react to light, occurs in up to 48% of patients.

Gummatous neurosyphilis is the least common syndrome. Gummas, a manifestation of late-stage syphilis, are masses of necrotic tissue surrounded by dense connective tissue with marked vascularity. The clinical presentation is that of an intracranial mass lesion.

Diagnosis. Although direct analysis of dark field microscopy is useful in the diagnosis of primary syphilis, it cannot be utilized with neurosyphilis because of the small number of organisms in the CSF. Serological testing is the standard for confirming the diagnosis of neurosyphilis and when following response to therapy. However, no single laboratory assay is sufficiently sensitive and specific to serve as a definitive test for CNS syphilis. More specific laboratory tests such as the CSF Venereal Disease Research Laboratory test (VDRL) or the fluorescent treponemal antibody–antibody absorption (FTA-ABS) test, combined with nonspecific parameters (CSF pleocytosis, greater than 9 WBCs per high power field, elevated CSF protein, and de-

pressed glucose levels) in the context of history and physical examination, are required to diagnose neurosyphilis accurately.[49]

Depending on the duration of the untreated infection, 30–70% of patients with neurosyphilis have abnormal CSF protein levels, glucose levels, and WBC count. CSF VDRL is reported to have a sensitivity of 30–70%. The wide range of values is a result of the different (variable) timings of LP and differing diagnostic criteria. Unless CSF is contaminated with seropositive blood during the LP, a reactive CSF VDRL indicates past or present neurosyphilis.[50,51]

Concomitant HIV infection modifies the clinical spectrum of neurosyphilis and the response to treatment. Syphilitic meningitis and ophthalmic syphilis is common in HIV-infected patients. Anecdotal evidence suggests that immune response abnormalities in HIV-infected patients may alter the sensitivity of serological tests for syphilis. Additionally, CSF parameters in the HIV-seropositive patient are difficult to interpret due to the CSF pleocytosis and elevated protein levels observed in HIV infection independent of treponemal infection.

Treatment. The treatment of neurosyphilis for both immunocompetent and immunocompromised patients is penicillin G, 12–24 million units per day for 10 days intravenously, given as 2–4 million units every 4 hours. Alternative drug regimens include ceftriaxone. Consensus concerning optimal therapy in the HIV-seropositive patient is not established.

Lyme Disease

Lyme disease is a bacterial infection whose etiological agent is *Borrelia burgdorferi,* a tick-borne spirochete. Lyme disease shares many neurological features with other spirochetal infections such as syphilis, leptospirosis, and relapsing fever. Major target organs of Lyme disease are the skin, heart, eye, joints, and nervous system. This discussion is limited to CNS manifestations of Lyme disease.

Neurological involvement occurs in 10–40% of symptomatic patients with Lyme disease. This involvement is observed during all stages of infection and affects both the central and peripheral nervous systems.

Clinical Presentation. Lyme disease is characterized by three clinical stages. The first stage is characterized by erythema chronicum migrans (ECM), an erythematous eruption at the location of the bite. The second stage occurs when the disease disseminates, producing arthritis and cardiac manifestations. The third stage, and last infectious stage, is characterized by ocular and joint findings. The neurological syndromes associated with Lyme disease can occur during any of the three stages but is generally categorized into those seen early in the infection cycle and those that complicate the late stage of the disease. The three syndromes that characterize early infection are meningoencephalomyelitis, cranial nerve palsies, and radiculoneuritis. The three syndromes that occur during late-stage infection are encephalopathy, polyradiculoneuropathy, and meningoencephalomyelitis.[52]

Early in the disease course, B. burgdorferi seeds the meninges, which produces aseptic meningitis. Fluctuating headache is the most common feature. Neck stiffness and fevers are typically mild. An examination of CSF reveals mononuclear pleocytosis of less than 200 cells/ml. CSF protein is usually less than 100 mg/dl, and CSF glucose levels are rarely depressed. Lyme antibodies are found in 73–92% of patients. In some patients, the disease can progress to produce cognitive changes, and mood and sleep disturbances suggestive of encephalitis. Cranial nerve involvement with meningitis is highly suggestive of Lyme disease. The facial nerve (cranial nerve VII) is involved in 11% of clinical infections, and 33% of these have bilateral facial nerve involvement. The prognosis of Lyme-related Bell's palsy is similar to the idiopathic form. The optic nerve (cranial nerve II) is the second most frequently involved, producing optic neuritis or disc edema. All cranial nerves reportedly have been involved with Lyme disease. Radiculoneuritis or nerve root inflammation, referred to as Bannworth's syndrome, typically causes lancinating extremity pain in a dermatomal distribution.

Syndromes of late-stage infection include encephalopathy, polyneuropathy, and meningoencephalomyelitis. Encephalopathy is characterized by malaise with memory and concentration impairment. Polyneuropathy manifests as distal limb paresthesias and asymmetrical radicular pain. Median nerve involvement at the carpal tunnel has been reported in 25% of late-stage infections.[53] In-

volvement of brain or spinal cord parenchyma is an uncommon late-stage infectious syndrome. Continued or recurrent meningeal involvement is also uncommon.

A number of syndromes have been described anecdotally, but are poorly characterized in the various stages of Lyme disease infection. Experimental studies suggest that B. burgdorferi can seed the CNS without objective CSF findings in patients symptomatic with headache and cranial nerve palsy.[53] A clinical presentation similar to pseudotumor cerebri syndrome can develop in children and adolescents. Stroke syndromes, transient ischemic attacks, vasculitis, and psychiatric syndromes have been attributed to B. burgdorferi. Posttreatment syndromes, which include persistent headache, cognitive difficulties, fatigue, myalgias, and arthralgias, are well described following adequate treatment regimens. Factors that predispose to persistent symptoms include delayed treatment, marked constitutional symptoms with initial infection, and a Jarisch-Herxheimer reaction to antibiotics. This subset of patients does not appear to respond to additional antibiotics.[54]

Diagnosis. The number of organisms in Lyme disease is scant and often tissue-bound; therefore, serological testing is the mainstay of diagnosis. The most useful laboratory evaluation is documentation of antibody response in serum and CSF. Other CSF findings are a mild mononuclear pleocytosis in patients with meningitis. Normal values of CSF occur with peripheral nervous system involvement and encephalopathy. Polymerase chain reaction (PCR) studies on CSF and serum will likely be performed in the future. Neuroimaging is abnormal in 25% of patients with neuroborreliosis, but no unique pattern is noted.

Treatment. The preferred treatment for most neurological syndromes associated with Lyme disease, particularly with abnormal CSF, is ceftriaxone, 2 g administered intravenously every day for a minimum of 2 weeks. Alternative intravenous regimens include ampicillin, cefotaxime, chloramphenicol, doxycycline, and penicillin G. A Jarisch-Herxheimer reaction, which occurs in 10–20% of patients within the first 24–48 hours of treatment, generally responds to antipyretics and anti-inflammatory agents. Antibiotics are not discontinued during a Jarisch-

Herxheimer reaction. Steroids are not administered. Antibiotics do not appear to alter the course of Bell's palsy. Late-stage infection syndromes commonly require protracted therapy.

Patients who have mild peripheral syndromes with negative CSF are treated with oral antibiotics for 30 days. Preferred agents include amoxicillin, 500–1000 mg three times per day (50 mg/kg per day), and doxycycline, 100 mg three times per day or 200 mg two times per day. The chronic sequelae of Lyme disease (headache, fatigue, myalgias, cognitive deficits) are treated symptomatically.

Disposition. It is unlikely that patients presenting acutely with CNS infections can be confidently discharged from the emergency department. The course of infection is unpredictable, and many of the complications occur early in the course of the disease. A period of inpatient observation is prudent, to deliver therapy and to determine the clinical course of the process.

PEARLS AND PITFALLS

- A common pitfall in the emergency department is not to consider CNS infection in the differential diagnosis of many nonspecific and apparently nonurgent clinical conditions. The evolution of CNS infection can be very rapid.
- Although routine diagnostic LP is an invasive procedure, it carries very little risk to the patient. Performing an LP in patients clinically suspected of having CNS infection is appropriate in the emergency setting.
- A careful history is of paramount importance in diagnosing many of the CNS infections; they are associated with specific socioeconomic or environmental etiological factors or with significant underlying patient illness or immunosuppression.
- A comprehensive physical examination can help localize mass lesions or reveal papilledema, nuchal rigidity, and coinfection. For many patients with CNS infections, the examination results are deceptively benign.
- CT scanning and MRI imaging can be very sensitive but nonspecific for CNS infections.

- CSF studies are required in the evaluation of a patient with suspected CNS infection but can be difficult to interpret. In the severely immunocompromised patient, CSF can appear acellular or inappropriately consistent with an aseptic meningitis. A nonspecific lymphocytic pleocytosis can be observed with a variety of conditions, including partially treated bacterial meningitis. Misinterpretations of CSF results can lead to delays in or incorrect diagnosis and treatment.
- Neuroimaging precedes LP in patients with altered mental status, a focal neurological examination, or frequent seizures. Bleeding diatheses and coagulopathies are corrected prior to the diagnostic LP.

REFERENCES

1. Centers for Disease Control. Bacterial meningitis & meningococcemia. United States, 1978. *MMWR.* 1979; 28:277.
2. Ashwal S. Neurologic evaluation of the patient with acute bacterial meningitis. *Neurol Clin.* 1995;13:549–77.
3. Anderson M. Management of cerebral infection. *J Neurol Neurosurg Psychiatry.* 1993;56:1243–58.
4. Segreti J, Harris AA, Levin S. Acute bacterial meningitis. In: Klawans HL, ed. *Textbook Clinical of Neuropharmacology.* New York, NY: Raven Press, Ltd; 1981.
5. Segreti J, Harris AA. Acute bacterial meningitis. *Infect Dis Clin North Am.* 1996;10:797–809.
6. Tunkel AR, Wispelwey B, Scheld WM. Pathogenesis and pathophysiology of meningitis. *Infect Dis Clin North Am.* 1990;4:555–75.
7. Greelee JE. Approach to diagnosis of meningitis: cerebrospinal fluid evaluation. *Infect Dis Clin North Am.* 1990;4:583–95.
8. Drug-resistant Streptococcus pneumoniae – Kentucky and Tennessee, 1993. *MMWR.* 1994;43:23–31.
9. The choice of antibacterial drugs. *Med Lett Drugs Ther.* 1994;36:53–60.
10. Louvois J, Gortvai P, Hurley R. Bacteriology of abscesses of the central nervous system: a multicentre prospective study. *Br Med J.* 1977:981–4.
11. Fishbein CA, Rosenthal A, Fischer EG, et al. Risk factors for brain abscess in patients with congenital heart disease. *Am J Cardiol.* 1974;34:97–102.
12. Davidson HD, Steiner RE. Magnetic resonance imaging in infections of the central nervous system. *AJNR.* 1985;6:499–504.
13. Hasso AN. Current status of enhanced magnetic resonance imaging in neuroradiology. *Invest Radiol.* 1993; 28(suppl 1):S3–S20.

14. Schroth G, Kretzschmar K, Gawehn J, Voigt K. Advantage of magnetic resonance imaging in the diagnosis of cerebral infections. *Neuroradiology.* 1987;29:120–6.

15. Rousseaux M, Lesoin F, Destee A, Jomin M, Petit H. Developments in the treatment and prognosis of multiple brain abscesses. *Neurosurgery.* 1985;16:304–8.

16. Boom WH, Tauzon CV. Successful treatment of multiple brain abscesses with antibiotics alone. *Rev Infect Dis.* 1985;7:189–99.

17. Feldman HA. Epidemiology of toxoplasma infections. *Epidemiol Rev.* 1982;4:204–13.

18. Grant IH, Gold JWM, Rosenblum M, et al. 1990. Toxoplasma gondii serology in HIV infected patients: the development of central nervous system toxoplasmosis in AIDS. *AIDS.* 1990;4:519–21.

19. Porter SB, Sande MA. Toxoplasmosis of the central nervous system in the acquired immunodeficiency syndrome. *N Engl J Med.* 1992;327:1643–8.

20. Behar R, Wiley C, McCutchan JA. Cytomegalovirus polyradiculopathy in acquired immune deficiency syndrome. *Neurology.* 1987;37:557–61.

21. Peters M, Timm U, Schurmann D, et al. Combined and alternating gangcyclovir and foscarnet in acute and maintenance therapy of human immunodeficiency virus-related cytomegalovirus encephalitis refractory to gangyclovir alone. *Clin Invest Med.* 1992;70:456–8.

22. Connolly KJ, Hammer SM. The acute aseptic meningitis syndrome. *Infect Dis Clin North Am.* 1990;4:599–619.

23. Corson AP, Chretien JH. Metronidazole-associated aspetic meningitis. *Clin Infect Dis.* 1994;19:974.

24. Marinac JS. Drug and chemical-induced aseptic meningitis: a review of the literature. *Ann Pharmacother.* 1992;26:813–22.

25. Scribner CL, Kapti RM, Phillips ET, Rickles NM. Aseptic Meningitis and intravenous immunoglobulin therapy. *Ann Intern Med.* 1994;121:305–6.

26. Sekul EA, Cupler EJ, Daladas MC. Aseptic meningitis associated with high-dose intravenous immunoglobulin therapy: frequency and risk factors. *Ann Intern Med.* 1994;121:259–62.

27. Lamonte M, Silberstein SD, Marcelis JF. Headache associated with aseptic meningitis. *Headache.* 1995;35:520–6.

28. Gracey DR. Tuberculosis in the world today. *Mayo Clin Proc.* 1988;63:1251–7.

29. Leonard JM, Des Perez R. Tuberculous meningitis. *Infect Dis Clin North Am.* 1990;4:769–87.

30. Berenguer J, Moreno S, Laguna F, et al. Tuberculous meningitis in patients infected with the human immunodeficiency virus. *N Engl J Med.* 1992;1326:668–72.

31. Castro C, Barros N, Campos Z, et al. CT scans of cranial tuberculosis. *Radiol Clin North Am.* 1995;33:753–69.

32. Villoria MF, de la Torre J, Fortea F, et al. Intracranial tuberculosis in AIDS: CT and MRI findings. *Neuroradiology.* 1992;34:11–14.

33. Alzeer AH, FitzGerald JM. Corticosteroids and tuberculosis: risks and adjunct therapy. *Tuber Lung Dis.* 1993;74:6–11.

34. Chuck SL, Sande MA. Infections with cryptococcus neoforms in the acquired immunodeficiency syndrome. *N Engl J Med.* 1989;321:794–9.

35. Dismukes WE. Cryptococcal meningitis in patients with AIDS. *J Infect Dis.* 1988;157:624–8.

36. Mischel PS, Vinters HV. Coccidioidomycosis of the central nervous system: neuropathological and vasculopathic manifestations and clinical correlates. *Clin Infect Dis.* 1995;2:400–5.

37. Nguyen NM, Yu VL. Meningitis caused by candidal species: an emerging problem in neurosurgical patients. *Clin Infect Dis.* 1995;21:323–7.

38. Torre-Cisneros J, Lopez OL, Kusne S, et al. CNS aspergillosis in organ transplantation: a clinicopathologic study. *J Neurol Neurosurg Psychiatry.* 1993;56:188–93.

39. Vincent T, Galgiani JN, Huppert M, Salkin D. The natural history of coccidioidal meningitis: VA-armed forced cooperative studies, 1955–1958. *Clin Infect Dis.* 1993;16:247–54.

40. Ragland AS, Arsura E, Ismail Y, Johnson R. Eosinophilic pleocytosis in coccidioidal meningitis: frequency and significance. *Am J Med.* 1993;95:254–7.

41. Larsen RA, Bozzette S, McCutchan JA. Persistent cryptococcus neoformans infection of the prostate after successful treatment of meningitis. *Ann Intern Med.* 1989;111:125–8.

42. Larsen RA, Bozzette SA, Jones BE, Haghigh D. Fluconazole combined with flucytosine for treatment of cryptococcal meningitis in patients with AIDS. *Clin Infect Dis.* 1994;19:714–5.

43. Cherry JD, Lloyd CA, Quilty JF, et al. Amphotericin B therapy in children: a review of the literature and a case report. *J Pediatr.* 1969;75:1063–9.

44. Kovacs JA, Kovacs AA, Polis M, et al. Cryptococcosis in the acquired immunodeficiency syndrome. *Ann Intern Med.* 1985;103:533–8.

45. Medoff G, Comfort M, Kobayashi GS. Synergistic action of amphotericin B and 5-fluorocytosine against yeast-like organisms. *Proc Soc Exp Bio Med.* 1971;138:571–4.

46. Arndt CA, Walsh TJ, McCully CL, et al. Fluconazole penetration into cerebrospinal fluid: implications for treating fungal infections of the central nervous system. *J Infect Dis.* 1988;157:178–80.

47. Saag MS, Powderly WG, Cloud GA, et al. Comparison of amphotericin B with fluconazole in the treatment of acute AIDS-associated cryptococcal meningitis. *N Engl J Med.* 1992;326:88–9.

48. Zuger A, Louie E, Holzman RS, Simberkoff MS, Rahal JJ. Cryptococcal disease in patients with the acquired immunodeficiency syndrome. Diagnostic features and

outcome of treatment. *Ann Intern Med.* 1986;104:
234–40.

49. Schenk DN, Hood EW. Neurosyphilis. *Infect Dis Clin North Am.* 1994;8:769–95.

50. Simon RP. Neurosyphilis. *Arch Neurol.* 1985;42:
606–13.

51. Davis LE, Schmitt JW. Clinical significance of cerebrospinal fluid tests for neurosyphilis. *Ann Neurol.* 1989;25:50–5.

52. Halperin JJ, Volkman DJ, Luft BJ, et al. CTS in Lyme borreliosis. *Muscle Nerve.* 1989;12:397.

53. Coyle PK, Deng Z, Schutzer SE, et al. Detection of borrelia burgdorferi antigens in cerebrospinal fluid. *Neurology.* 1993;43:1093.

54. Duttwyler RJ, Volkman DJ, Conaty SM, et al. Amoxicillin plus probenecid versus doxycycline for treatment of erythema migrans borreliosis. *Lancet.* 1990;
336:1404.

15 Viral Encephalitis

EARL J. REISDORFF

SUMMARY Viral encephalitis is considered in any patient in whom a diagnostic evaluation for central nervous system infection is performed. Herpes simplex virus type 1 (HSV-1) encephalitis is treated with acyclovir, which is administered empirically when HSV-1 encephalitis is suspected. Encephalitis that is arthropod-borne (e.g., California and St. Louis encephalitis) tends to be seasonal, and there is no effective antiviral therapy. Human immunodeficiency virus causes a primary encephalitis and may eventually become the most common cause of viral encephalitis in the United States and possibly worldwide.

Introduction

Viral encephalitis is an infectious and inflammatory process involving the brain, and is associated with an altered state of consciousness, impaired cognitive abilities, and cerebrospinal fluid (CSF) pleocytosis. *Encephalitis* is differentiated from *meningitis* primarily on a clinical basis. Patients who have encephalitis are encephalopathic; that is, they have altered cognition. Patients with meningeal inflammation have meningitis. Patients with characteristics of both have *meningoencephalitis*. *Postinfectious encephalitis* is regarded as an autoimmune disorder that typically becomes clinically apparent after the acute phase of illness.

In the United States, 1000–2000 cases of viral encephalitis are reported each year to the Centers for Disease Control.[1] The overall mortality of viral encephalitis is 5–10%. With certain forms of encephalitis, the mortality approaches 70–80%.

The central nervous system (CNS) is commonly exposed to a viral pathogen by hematogenous spread. Direct neuronal migration can occur with rabies encephalitis and probably with certain herpes viruses. The invading virus triggers an inflammatory response with degeneration of parenchymal neurons, primarily affecting the gray matter. Gross inspection of the brain typically reveals edema and small hemorrhages. Cellular inclusions are observed on brain biopsy with herpes simplex virus (HSV), cytomegalovirus (CMV), measles, and rabies.

HSV encephalitis has a tendency preferentially to affect the frontal and temporal lobes of the brain. Eastern equine encephalitis (EEE) has a predilection for the hippocampus. Cerebellar involvement with resultant ataxia can occur with herpes varicella zoster (HVZ) virus as part of the initial infection or resulting from a postinfectious phenomenon. Rabies has a proclivity for involving the brainstem and cortical gray matter. Brainstem encephalitis has been reported with CMV and HSV type 1 (HSV-1).[2] Localized cerebritis can occur with other viruses including the mumps virus, Epstein-Barr virus (EBV), poliovirus, coxsackievirus, echovirus, enterovirus, and measles virus.

Etiology

Encephalitis resulting from infection is most frequently caused by viruses (Table 15.1). The viruses mostly commonly involved are ribonucleic acid (RNA) viruses, which include the "arboviruses" such as St. Louis encephalitis (SLE), EEE, western equine

TABLE 15.1. Viral Causes of Encephalitis

Togavirus (arbovirus)
  Eastern equine encephalitis
  Western equine encephalitis
  Venezuelan equine encephalitis
Flavivirus
  St. Louis encephalitis
  Japanese encephalitis
  Powassan
Bunyavirus (arbovirus)
  California (LaCrosse) encephalitis
Arenavirus
  Lymphocytic choriomeningitis
Reovirus
  California tick fever
Rhabdovirus
  Rabies
Herpes virus
  Herpes simplex I and II
  Herpes varicella zoster
  Ebstein-Barr
  Cytomegalovirus
Picornovirus
  Polioviruses 1–3
  Coxsackieviruses A2, 5, 6, 7, 9
  Coxsackieviruses B1–6
  Enteroviruses (70 and 71)
  Echoviruses 2–4, 6, 7, 9, 11, 14, 16, 18, 19, 30
Paramyxovirus
  Measles virus
  Mumps virus
Adenovirus
  Adenovirus
Retrovirus
  Human immunodeficiency virus

encephalitis (WEE), and California encephalitis (CE). Additional RNA viruses that cause encephalitis are retroviruses (human immunodeficiency virus, HIV, encephalitis), paramyxoviruses (measles encephalitis), and rhabdoviruses (rabies). Some RNA viruses that can cause encephalitis, yet typically produce aseptic meningitis, include the coxsackie virus, echovirus, mumps virus, and lymphocytic choriomeningitis virus. The deoxyribonucleic acid (DNA) virus that most frequently causes encephalitis is HSV-1. Other herpes (DNA) viruses can cause encephalitis. About 13% of cases of encephalitis are due to arboviruses, 12% are herpes viruses, 10% are enteroviruses, 10%

are lymphocytic choriomeningitis, and 5% are other viruses.[3] Thus, in about 50% of cases the cause is nonviral or no etiology is discovered. Encephalitis caused by nonviral pathogens includes infection by bacteria (e.g., *Mycobacterium tuberculosis, Mycoplasma pneumoniae*), fungi (e.g., *Coccidioides immitis, Cryptococcus neoformans*), and protozoa (e.g., *Naegleria fowleri, Toxoplasma gondii*).

Herpes Virus Encephalitis

Herpes simplex virus type-2 (HSV-2) (genital herpes) causes perinatal infection. The constellation of encephalitis, hepatitis, and pneumonitis strongly suggests HSV-2 infection as opposed to bacterial sepsis.[4] HSV-1 is the most common cause of encephalitis from the group of herpes viruses. HSV-1 encephalitis has an annual incidence of about 3 cases per 1 million individuals and accounts for 10–20% of all cases of encephalitis.[5,6] With HSV-1, there is no gender predominance or seasonal pattern of outbreak. Although individuals of all ages are susceptible to HSV-1 infection, 31% of cases of herpes simplex encephalitis occur in children, and 50–55% occur in patients older than 50 years of age.[6,7]

HSV-1 encephalitis is a progressive disease, with a succession from lethargy to deep coma. It is commonly characterized by an altered state of consciousness, abnormal behavior, and seizures. HSV-1 encephalitis can produce olfactory or gustatory hallucinations, memory loss, and anosmia.[7] Focal neurological deficits become evident in at least 60% of patients. Temporal lobe involvement (e.g., speech difficulties and olfactory hallucinations) strongly suggests HSV-1 encephalitis. The mortality rate approaches 70% in untreated patients. Determinants of the outcome include the age of the patient, the duration of illness, and the level of consciousness at the start of therapy. Therefore, prompt initiation of antiviral therapy is essential to optimize the chance of a good recovery.

HVZ encephalitis is rare and occurs largely in immunocompromised patients. The HVZ virus causes primary varicella (chickenpox) and herpes zoster (shingles). HVZ encephalitis can occur from 11 days before to 21 days after the onset of the exanthem.[8,9] Cerebellar ataxia is a common associated finding. It occurs about 1 week following the varicella rash and is likely a limited form of postinfectious encephalitis. The mortality rate of HVZ encephalitis is 15–35%, with up to 30% of survivors having long-term sequelae.[10,11]

Epstein-Barr virus (EBV) encephalitis is rare, although 1–5% of patients with infectious mononucleosis have some form of CNS involvement. Similarly, EBV is the cause in 5% of cases of acute viral encephalitis.[12]

CMV encephalitis presents most often in patients who are immunocompromised.

Arbovirus Encephalitis

The term *arbovirus* is no longer an official taxonomic term. It refers to more than 450 RNA viruses that are transmitted by arthropods, primarily mosquitoes, and sometimes ticks. These viruses are *arthropod-bo*rne, hence the prefix *arbo.*

Included as arboviruses are the alphaviruses, the flaviviruses, and the bunyaviruses. Alphaviruses cause EEE, WEE, and Venezuelan equine encephalitis. The flaviviruses are responsible for SLE, Japanese B encephalitis, yellow fever, the tick-borne encephalitis. Bunyaviruses cause CE (LaCrosse strain). Although arboviruses account for about 10–15% of all cases of encephalitis, in an epidemic year they can cause up to 50% of all cases.[13,14]

St. Louis Encephalitis

During epidemic years, SLE is typically the prevalent arbovirus disease in the United States. In nonepidemic years, CE (LaCrosse strain) is the most common type of viral encephalitis. SLE most commonly occurs in regions bordering the Ohio and Mississippi rivers; outbreaks also occur in the San Joaquin Valley of California.[15] During one epidemic year, about 2000 cases were reported.[16] Even during an epidemic, when 11.5% of the general population was infected, only 1 in 268 infected developed clinically detectable encephalitis.[17]

The clinical presentation of SLE ranges from mild aseptic meningitis to a severe, fulminant, and lethal encephalitis.[18] Headache, vomiting, and lethargy are common. The condition usually lasts one to two weeks. Children tend to recover completely, whereas adults may have permanent mental or motor impairment.

Eastern Equine Encephalitis

EEE is a grave illness, with fatality rates exceeding 55%. EEE occurs sporadically along the east coast of the United States, especially near freshwater marshes (e.g., cranberry bogs). EEE is characterized by the abrupt onset of a high fever, headache, and vomiting. This is followed by a decreased level of consciousness. EEE can produce focal neurological signs, mimicking HSV-1. Mortality is highest among younger children and persons who develop coma.[19] Neurological sequelae are common among survivors and include mental impairment, seizures, and disturbed motor function.

Western Equine Encephalitis

WEE occurs sporadically in rural areas of the western two-thirds of the United States. One of the highest attack rates of WEE occurs in infants younger than 1 year of age. The infant with WEE appears "septic" and has a bulging fontanelle. Older children appear "viremic," as if they have a flulike condition. Behavioral changes (including delirium) occur early in the course of the disease, and the patient can become comatose rapidly. Seizures occur in 90% of infants and 40% of children younger than 4 years of age.[20] Symptoms usually last one to two weeks. The overall mortality of 3–10% usually involves infants; adults typically survive. Children (younger than 2 years of age) who survive can develop mental retardation, seizures, and spasticity. Permanent neurological impairment occurs in 37–64% of surviving infants.[21,22]

California Encephalitis

The term *California encephalitis (CE)* is used to describe most cases of bunyavirus disease, including those specifically caused by the California, LaCrosse, Jamestown, and snowshoe hare strains. The virus that causes CE most frequently is the LaCrosse strain. CE is most common in the upper Mississippi valley.

Children 5–9 years of age are most often affected;[23] 90% of cases are seen in children younger than 15 years of age. A flulike syndrome precedes the headache. As the condition worsens, seizures can develop, and coma may ensue.[24] About 20% of patients develop focal neurological deficits. After three to five days, symptoms begin to resolve, with most children recovering without neurological sequelae. However, up to 15% of affected children develop personality changes and recurrent seizures. Death from CE is rare.

Japanese Encephalitis

Japanese encephalitis (JE) is the most common arbovirus encephalitis in the world, occurring most frequently in Asia. The initial symptoms of JE are malaise, fever, and headache, followed by meningismus, confusion, and delirium. There is a high incidence of fever, coma, and seizures.[25] A masklike facies and brainstem dysfunction ensue. Mortality rates are 25%, and long-term neurological sequelae occur in 50–70% patients.[26–28] Childhood vaccination programs have markedly decreased JE rates in Japan and Korea.[29] Recommendations for the vaccination of foreign travelers must balance the exposure risk against the high incidence of allergic responses to the vaccine.[30,31]

HIV Encephalitis

HIV causes immune suppression, which leads to opportunistic CNS infections and CNS lymphoma. HIV can attack the brain directly, causing *HIV encephalitis* (multinucleated giant cell encephalitis) and *HIV leukoencephalopathy* (progressive diffuse leukoencephalopathy). HIV encephalitis is characterized by dementia, weakness, and spasticity. Involuntary movement disorders and seizures can occur.[32]

Early in the course of HIV infection, the CNS is invaded, resulting in an initial inflammatory reaction.[33] With HIV encephalitis, there is diffuse white matter disease with an inflammatory cell infiltrate and marked neuronal destruction.[34] Of AIDS patients at autopsy, 10% demonstrate HIV encephalitis; other forms of viral encephalitis are seen in another 22% of these patients.[35] Among patients with AIDS, brain biopsy has demonstrated viral encephalitis in 11% of patients with an identifiable brain lesion.[36] Treatment with zidovudine (AZT) can help both children and adults with HIV encephalitis.[37,38] HIV encephalitis may eventually become the most common viral CNS infection worldwide.

Other Viral Causes

Enteroviral encephalitis occurs primarily in children, during the summer and early fall months. Although enteroviruses cause 30–50% of all cases of viral (aseptic) meningitis, they account for less than 5% of all cases of encephalitis. Children (other than neonates) usually recover without sequelae. *Measles* (rubeola) can cause encephalitis, but childhood immunizations have greatly reduced the incidence of measles encephalitis. Nonetheless, measles encephalitis has occurred as a consequence of measles immunization; the incidence is estimated to be 1 case per 1 million doses. Symptoms of measles encephalitis begin 1–8 days after the appearance of a rash, but it can be delayed for up to 3 weeks. Typically, the patient appears to be recovering from the primary measles infection when the encephalitis abruptly occurs. Seizures occur in 50% of patients, and neurological morbidity (mental retardation, epilepsy, behavioral changes, paralysis) occurs in 20–50% of patients. Mortality is 10%.[39]

Mumps encephalitis is usually mild, typified by fever, headache, nausea, vomiting, nuchal rigidity, and lethargy.[40–43] The prognosis is typically favorable.

The *rabies virus* causes encephalitis that is almost always fatal. It is characterized by an initial state of headache, fever, and dysesthesia at the inoculation site.[44] The patient becomes progressively agitated with painful muscular spasms. Ultimately, seizures, coma, apnea, and death occur. Rabies is present in the saliva of infected dogs, cats, foxes, skunks, raccoons, bats, and other domestic and wild animals.

Lymphocytic choriomeningitis (*LCM*) *virus* infection is caused by exposure to rodents, and typically resembles influenza. LCM encephalitis is usually mild, although it can be associated with arthritis, orchitis, parotitis, and cerebellar incoordination. Death or neurological sequelae is rare. Encephalitis has also been reported with EBV, CMV, and *parainfluenza virus type 3*.

Emergency Department Evaluation and Differential Diagnosis

Clinical Evaluation

History. Viral encephalitis can present as a headache with mild mental status changes or as a fulminant disease with severe neurological consequences including death. The incubation period varies for different pathogens; for the arboviruses, it is usually 2–15 days.

Viral encephalitis can be preceded by a 1–4 day prodrome of fever, chills, headache, pharyngitis, conjunctivitis, myalgias, and malaise. Once encephalitis is apparent clinically, vomiting, dizziness, and

TABLE 15.2. Clinical Findings in Patients with Biopsy-Proven Herpes Simplex Encephalitis

Historical Findings	
Alterations of consciousness	97%
Fever	90%
Headache	81%
Personality change	71%
Seizures	67%
Vomiting	46%
Hemiparesis	33%
Memory loss	24%
Physical Findings	
Fever	92%
Personality change	85%
Dysphasia	76%
Autonomic dysfunction	60%
Hemiparesis	38%
Seizures	38%
Cranial nerve deficits	32%
Visual field loss	14%
Papilledema	14%

Source: Whitley RJ, Soong SJ, Linneman C Jr, et al. Herpes simplex encephalitis – clinical assessment. *JAMA.* 1982; 247:317.

impaired cognition occur. Ataxia, tremors, mental confusion, speech difficulties, stupor, hyperexcitability, delirium, convulsions, and coma can follow.

Rapid clinical deterioration suggests HSV-1 or EEE infection. Bizarre behavior, memory loss, olfactory or gustatory hallucinations, personality changes, and anosmia are associated with HSV-1 (Table 15.2). With HSV-1, headache occurs in 81% of patients, dysphasia in 76%, seizures in 67%, autonomic dysfunction in 60%, and ataxia in 40%.[7] Focal paralysis, cranial nerve paralysis, and aphasia are also associated with HSV-1.

The history investigates events leading to the patient's behavioral change; recent or recurrent fever or infectious illness; systemic conditions; and the presence of headache, vomiting, meningeal irritation, seizures, irritability, or lethargy. SLE and EEE tend to have higher rates of infection among children. The time of year is considered because some of the encephalitides have a seasonal predilection of

occurrence. Arbovirus encephalitides (SLE, CE, WEE, and EEE) occur most often in the summer months and subside in autumn. Enteroviral encephalitis peaks during the summer and fall months. Varicella encephalitis typically begins in the winter months, peaks in the spring, and is lowest during summer and fall. Mumps and HSV-1 encephalitis occur year-round.

Physical Examination. Fever and mental status changes are hallmarks of encephalitis. The patient can be drowsy or even comatose. Gross motor aberrations can include hemiplegia, ataxia, and involuntary muscle movements. Cranial nerve palsies can occur, especially in patients with HSV-1 encephalitis. Focal neurological disturbances occur in 80% of patients with HSV-1 encephalitis, and in 20% of patients with CE. Lymphocytic choriomeningitis can be accompanied by arthritis, orchitis, or parotitis.

In all cases, the skin is inspected for evidence of trauma, a rash, or needle marks. An abnormal pupil size can suggest drug or toxin exposure. Funduscopy is performed to identify papilledema (increased intracranial pressure) and retinal hemorrhages (trauma, subarachnoid hemorrhage, carbon monoxide toxicity). Fixed deviation of the eyes in a lateral direction suggests focal seizure (irritative lesion) or stroke (destructive lesion). The gag response is assessed to determine protection of the patient's airway. Examination of the neck examination may or may not reveal meningeal signs.

Diagnostic Evaluation

Encephalitis is rarely diagnosed in the emergency department. Definitive diagnosis rests on antibody testing, recovery of viral DNA from the CSF, or brain biopsy with viral culture. Nevertheless, presumptive evidence for encephalitis can be obtained by lumbar puncture (LP), neuroradiological imaging, and common laboratory studies.

Lumbar Puncture. Viral encephalitis is characterized by CSF pleocytosis with a lymphocytic or mononuclear cell predominance. This type of pleocytosis can occur with other conditions (e.g., cryptococcal or mycobacterial infection). Early in the disease process, viral encephalitis can have a neutrophilic predominance, although a neutrophilic pleocytosis usually suggests a bacterial infection. In most patients, CSF protein levels are modestly elevated and the glucose level is normal.

When viral encephalitis is suspected, the CSF is cultured for viruses and bacteria, including mycobacteria. CSF cultures for fungi are obtained when the patient is immunocompromised or when directed by other CSF findings. Antigen assays for cryptococcus and toxoplasmosis are performed. Normal CSF studies suggest a metabolic or toxic encephalopathy, but do not exclude early viral encephalitis. Although CSF studies can assist in directing suspicion toward or away from HSV-1, the considerable overlap in values prohibits distinction between herpetic and nonherpetic viral encephalitis. Polymerase chain reaction (PCR) studies to retrieve HSV DNA can be performed when HSV-1 is suspected. When the treating institution does not have PCR technology, the CSF is sent to an appropriate laboratory.

HSV-1. Abnormal CSF findings are present in 90–95% of patients with HSV-1 encephalitis.[45] A CSF pleocytosis, with a median white blood cell (WBC) count of 130 (cells/ml) is usually evident. Red blood cells in the CSF (up to 500 cells/ml) due to necrotizing frontotemporal lesions is characteristic, and occurs in 75–85% of patients. CSF protein is elevated in 80% of cases with a median protein concentration of 80 mg/dl. The glucose concentration is normal. In adults, HSV-1 is rarely isolated from the CSF; cultures are negative in more than 95% of patients.

Arboviruses. SLE usually has a CSF lymphocytic pleocytosis of 50–500 cells/ml and a protein concentration of 50–100 mg/dl. The glucose concentration is normal. Successful CSF culture of the SLE virus is rare.[46] EEE typically causes an elevated CSF pressure and 200–2000 cells/ml, 50% of which are neutrophils. The peripheral WBC count with EEE can be as high as 66,000 cells/ml.[47] WEE has a mixture of neutrophils and lymphocytes in the CSF; later in the course of the illness, only lymphocytes may be observed. CE shows primarily lymphocytic pleocytosis, commonly 50–200 cells/ml.

Other viruses. The CSF lymphocytic pleocytosis observed with rubeola encephalitis rarely exceeds 100 cells/ml; the protein concentration is commonly 50–200 mg/dl; and the glucose concentration is normal. When HIV infections are associated with a progressive encephalopathy, both the virus and antigen commonly are detected in the CSF.[48]

Viral Detection. Detection of viruses in the CSF is variable. Enteroviruses, mumps, adenoviruses, HVZ virus, and CMV can be detected in the CSF. Viral antigens or antibodies can be detected in the CSF by enzyme-linked immunosorbent assays. SLE virus, coxsackievirus, and echovirus have been cultured from the oropharynx. In addition, HSV immunoglobulin G and immunoglobulin A detection by enzyme-linked immunosorbent assay allows for the diagnosis of HSV encephalitis. This method has limited success until the second week of illness.[49] Monoclonal antibodies can detect HSV-specific glucoproteins, but the sensitivity is poor early in the course of HSV-1 disease.[50]

New assays using PCR technology for the detection of the HSV-1 virus in the CSF appear promising.[51,52] The PCR technique employs the amplification of DNA strands from HSV-1 to allow for ready detection. The primary advantage of this technique is the ability to detect HSV-1 in the CSF early in the course of the illness, as early as 24 hours after the onset of symptoms.[53–55] When compared to other methods of viral detection, PCR is the most specific, rapid, and sensitive.[55] Nonetheless, the mishandling of CSF specimens can potentially cause a false-negative result.[56] In one study, PCR detected 129 of 130 serologically or brain biopsy–confirmed cases of HSV-1 encephalitis.[57]

Laboratory Studies. Laboratory studies that are immediately available in the emergency department are minimally helpful in establishing the diagnosis of viral encephalitis. The greatest benefit of ancillary laboratory studies is in confirming or excluding other causes of acute encephalopathy. Definitive tests such as serial antibody titers, viral blood cultures, or viral CSF cultures are obtained even though results are unavailable to the emergency physician. A complete blood cell (CBC) count is obtained. A leukocytosis can suggest sepsis. Blood cultures can exclude or confirm bacteremia. The CBC can demonstrate lead-induced basophilic stippling. Serum sodium, glucose, and blood urea nitrogen (BUN) studies can exclude metabolic causes for lethargy. A "drug screen," specific drug analyses, and a carboxyhemoglobin level can be useful in

TABLE 15.3. Differential Diagnosis of Viral Encephalitis

Infectious	Lead encephalopathy
Nonviral encephalitis	Substances of abuse
Mycobacterium tuberculosis	Sedative-hypnotic agents
Mycoplasma pneumoniae	Narcotics-opiates
Rickettsia rickettsii	Anticholinergic toxicity
Lyme disease *(Borrelia burgdorferi)*	Alcohols
Leptospirosis	Mushroom poisoning (amatoxins,
Treponema pallidum	monomethylhydrazine)
Coccidioides immitis	Valproate toxicity
Naegleria fowleri	Other causes
Toxoplasma gondii*	Tumors
Cryptococcus neoformans*	Leukemia
Listeria monocytogenes	Lymphoma
Meningitis	Cerebral vascular event
Viral	Hydrocephalus with shunt
Bacterial (including mycoplasma,	malfunction
mycobacterium, rickettsia)	Postictal state
Fungal	Infantile botulism
Protozoa	Reye's syndrome
Brain abscess	Cat scratch disease
Subdural–epidural empyema	SIADH
Sepsis	Hypoglycemia
Trauma	Hyperglycemic hyperosmolar coma
Epidural hematoma	Uremic encephalopathy
Subdural hematoma	Collagen vascular disease
Subarachnoid hemorrhage	Alcohol withdrawal syndrome
Concussion – closed head injury	Hyperammonemia
Toxins	Chronic encephalitis (Rasmussen's
Carbon monoxide	syndrome)

* Seen more frequently in immunodeficient patients.

eliminating toxic etiologies (Table 15.3). Hepatic transaminases and an ammonia level can be useful in the evaluation for Reye's syndrome.

Neuroradiology. Brain imaging excludes mass lesions and findings associated with cerebral trauma (e.g., subdural hematoma). In some cases, neuroimaging can reveal signs of *T. gondii* infection or cerebral edema.

Most cases of viral encephalitis have no pathognomonic CT or MRI findings. Cerebral edema, obstructive hydrocephalus, and multifocal or disseminated lesions support the diagnosis of viral encephalitis. Conversely, HSV-1 encephalitis frequently is associated with CT abnormalities, which typically develop between days 3 and 11 of the illness. The CT scan can show edema, mass effect, or hemorrhage, often with hypodense enhancing lesions in the temporal or frontal lobes (Figs. 15.1 and 15.2).[58–60] However, HSV-1 can demonstrate diffuse or multifocal involvement, lacking temporal lobe localization.[61] MRI is more sensitive and is the study of choice to evaluate suspected viral encephalitis (Fig. 15.3).

Electroencephalography. Electroencephalography (EEG) is typically abnormal, especially for patients with HSV-1. With HSV encephalitis, spike and slow-wave activity or periodic lateralized epileptiform discharges arising from the temporal lobe occurs in most patients (see Chapter 3 "Electroencephalography").[62] EEG is rarely used in the

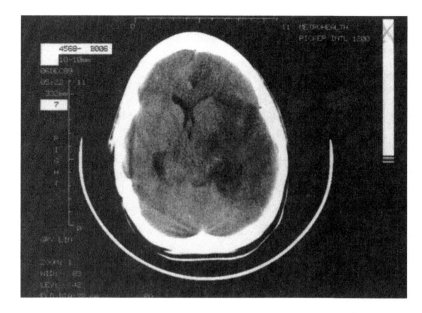

FIGURE 15.1. This noncontrast CT study of a patient with herpes simplex encephalitis demonstrates a large low-density area in the left temporoparietal region with mass effect (courtesy of Judith E. Simon, MD, Department of Radiology, Metro-Health Medical Center, Cleveland, Ohio).

emergency department, and clinical decisions required in the acutely ill patient suspected of having viral encephalitis are not contingent on EEG results.

Brain Biopsy. Brain biopsy is the definitive test for diagnosing HSV encephalitis.[63] Biopsy can confirm HSV encephalitis and establish alternative diagnoses for other conditions in almost 50% of patients. However, these alternative diagnoses may not require any specific treatment.[64] The need for brain biopsy to confirm the diagnosis has diminished with improved immunological and PCR techniques for detecting HSV-1, toxoplasmosis, and

cryptococcus, and improved neuroimaging techniques. The results of brain biopsy, an inpatient procedure, are not available to the emergency physician.

Differential Diagnosis

The differential diagnosis for viral encephalitis is extensive (Table 15.3). Trauma can be excluded by the history, a physical examination showing no external injury, and a normal neuroimaging study. Toxin-induced encephalopathy can be caused by carbon monoxide, sedative-hypnotic agents, narcotic opiates, valproic acid toxicity (with or without

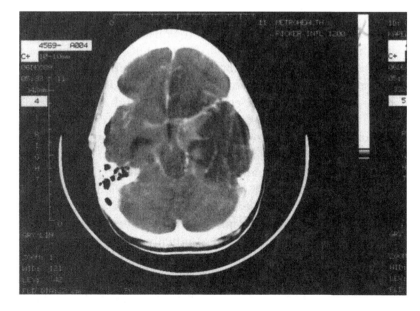

FIGURE 15.2. The contrast-enhanced (CT) study demonstrates peripheral enhancement suggesting meningeal involvement in this patient with herpes simplex encephalitis (courtesy of Judith E. Simon, MD, Department of Radiology, Metro-Health Medical Center, Cleveland, Ohio).

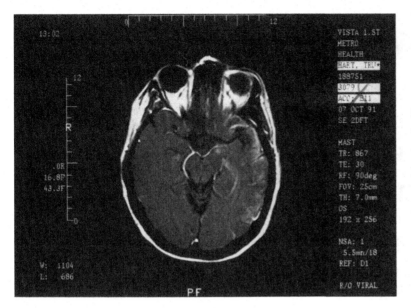

FIGURE 15.3. This MRI study demonstrates increased signal in the left temporoparietal region indicative of herpes simplex encephalitis (courtesy of Judith E. Simon, MD, Department of Radiology, MetroHealth Medical Center, Cleveland, Ohio).

hyperammonemia), isoniazid poisoning, certain mushroom toxins (e.g., ibotenic acid or monomethylhydrazine), and anticholinergic agents. Lead encephalopathy is suspected by detection of lead in the blood, radiographic evidence of lead deposition in bone, a bluish "lead line" in the gums, or basophilic stippling.

A clinical response to naloxone suggests narcotic toxicity. Alcohol intoxication (e.g., ethanol, ethylene glycol, and methanol) is excluded by quantitative assay. Other considerations in the differential diagnosis include endocrine disorders involving glucose metabolism and syndrome of inappropriate antidiuretic hormone. Uremic encephalopathy can be determined by measuring the serum BUN. In children, Reye's syndrome is suggested by elevation of the hepatic transaminases and serum ammonia levels. Other diagnostic considerations include testing for collagen vascular disease, CNS neoplasms, cerebral vascular events, or rare entities such as infantile botulism.

Toxoplasma gondii is a protozoan that causes encephalitis. *T. gondii* encephalitis occurs almost exclusively among immunocompromised patients. Almost one-third of AIDS patients who are seropositive for *T. gondii* ultimately develop toxoplasmic encephalitis.[65] Similarly, patients who develop toxoplasmic encephalitis are almost always chronically infected with *T. gondii*.[66] Fever occurs in 10–47% of AIDS patients with toxoplasmic encephalitis; 44–56% have a headache.[67,68]

Viral encephalitis can be difficult to distinguish from aseptic meningitis. An alteration in cognitive function is characteristic of viral encephalitis, not aseptic meningitis. Fungal encephalitis, bacterial encephalitis, and bacterial meningitis need to be excluded when making a diagnosis of viral encephalitis.

Emergency Department Management and Disposition

Therapeutic Intervention

General Supportive Care. Most emergency department care for patients with viral encephalitis is symptom-specific and supportive. Specific interventions include airway protection, ICP regulation, and seizure control. The obtunded or comatose patient requires intubation. Elevation of the head of the bed and hyperventilation can decrease ICP in patients with cerebral edema. Fluid restriction and mannitol (0.5 g/kg of 20% solution over 20 minutes) is considered. Although use of dexamethasone in meningitis is increasing, its use in viral encephalitis remains controversial. The initial intravenous solution is 0.9% normal saline at one-half the maintenance rate. Seizures are controlled with benzodiazepines (diazepam, 0.2 mg/kg given intravenously, up to 5 mg per dose) initially, followed by phenytoin loading (15–20 mg/kg given intravenously, up to 1 g). Phenytoin loading is no faster than 1 mg/kg per minute, not to exceed 50 mg per minute. Further supportive care addresses thermoregulation, maintaining electrolyte balance, and eventually nutritional maintenance.

Early in the emergency department evaluation, bacterial meningitis must be excluded as a diagnostic possibility. Meningeal irritation and CSF analysis is sometimes helpful in differentiating the two processes (see Chapter 4, "Lumbar Puncture"). Until bacterial meningitis can be excluded, empirical treatment with ceftriaxone (50–100 mg/kg intravenous infusion) and possibly dexamethasone is considered.

Antiviral Therapy. Most viruses causing encephalitis have no specific treatment. HSV-1 encephalitis is the notable exception. Therefore, the emergency physician must determine the likelihood of HSV-1 infection. Acyclovir (10 mg/kg intravenous infusion) administered every 8 hours for 10–14 days is the treatment of choice.[69] Among untreated patients 30–70% die and only 2.5% regain normal neurological function.[70] When treated with acyclovir, patients younger than 3 years of age have a mortality rate of 6%. In addition to reducing mortality, acyclovir significantly improves the outcome of surviving patients.[71] Relapse occurs in up to 27% of children treated for 10 days.[72] Theoretically, higher doses of acyclovir (15 mg/kg per dose) for longer periods of treatment can decrease the relapse rate.

Acyclovir is indicated in the treatment of HVZ encephalitis and has in vitro activity against EBV, CMV, and human herpes virus type 6.[73] The regimen of acyclovir for HVZ encephalitis is the same as that for HSV-1.[74]

The success of acyclovir therapy is contingent upon the patient's condition at the start of therapy. The level of consciousness at the onset of therapy is a critical prognostic factor. Most patients who are diagnosed early can be expected to survive and resume nearly normal neurological function.[75] Complications of acyclovir therapy include rash, gastrointestinal upset, thrombophlebitis, and occasionally a mild azotemia.

Other antiviral agents can improve the course of certain viral CNS infections. Gancyclovir can be given to patients with CMV encephalitis. Similarly, AZT, dideoxycytidine, and dideoxyinosine can help patients who have HIV encephalitis and HIV leukoencephalopathy. However, the efficacy of these agents in patients with HIV encephalitis has not been established.

Disposition. All patients with a presumptive diagnosis of viral encephalitis are admitted to the hospital. Patients who are obtunded require intensive care monitoring. Urgent consultation is required with a critical care specialist, infectious disease specialist, or neurologist. When HSV-1 encephalitis is suspected by the emergency physician, acyclovir therapy is initiated immediately. In the encephalopathic patient, a CSF pleocytosis and elevated CSF protein level without an identifiable pathogen is considered to be caused by HSV.[5]

PEARLS AND PITFALLS

- The absence of red blood cells in the CNS does not exclude the diagnosis of HSV-1 encephalitis.
- The absence of focal neurological findings does not exclude the possibility of HSV-1 encephalitis.
- Acyclovir is administered in the emergency department when HSV encephalitis is suspected.
- Acyclovir has minimal adverse effects, and its efficacy is optimized when administered early in the course of encephalitis.
- A "negative" LP does not exclude a viral CNS infection.
- LP should be repeated when a patient is sent home from the emergency department and returns more than 24–48 hours later with a progression of symptoms.
- Tuberculous meningitis is considered in the differential diagnosis of HSV encephalitis.

REFERENCES

1. Centers for Disease Control. Summary of notifiable diseases, United States, 1990. *MMWR* 1991;39:55.
2. Hall WA. Infectious lesions of the brain stem. *Neurosurg Clin North Am.* 1993;4:543–51.
3. Dyken PR. Viral diseases of the nervous system. In: Swainman KF, ed. *Pediatric Neurology: Principles and Practice.* St. Louis, Mo: CV Mosby; 1989:482.
4. Overall JC. Herpes simplex virus infection of the fetus and newborn. *Pediat Ann.* 1994;23:131–6.
5. Whitley RJ. Viral encephalitis. *N Engl J Med.* 1990; 323:242–50.

6. Koskiniemi M, Vaheri A. Acute encephalitis of viral origin. *Scand J Infect Dis.* 1982;14:181.

7. Whitley RJ, Soong SJ, Linneman C Jr, et al. Herpes simplex encephalitis – clinical assessment. *JAMA.* 1982;247:317.

8. Johnson R, Milbourn PE. Central nervous system manifestations of chickenpox. *Can Med Assoc J.* 1970;102:231.

9. McKendall RR, Klawans J. Nervous system complications of varicella-zoster virus. In: Vinken PJ, Bruyn GW, eds. *Handbook of Clinical Neurology.* Amsterdam: North-Holland Publishing Co. 1978:166–84.

10. Mateos-Mora M, Ratzan KR. Acute viral encephalitis. In: Schlossberg D, ed. *Infections of the Nervous System.* New York, NY: Springer-Verlag, 1990:105–34.

11. Barnes DW, Whitley RJ. CNS disease associated with varicella zoster virus and herpes simplex virus infection: pathogenesis and current therapy. *Neurol Clin.* 1986;4:265–83.

12. Kennard C, Swash M. Acute viral encephalitis. Its diagnosis and outcome. *Brain.* 1981;104:129–48.

13. Rennels MB. Arthropod-borne virus infections of the central nervous system. *Neurol Clin.* 1984;2:241.

14. McGowan JR Jr, Bryan JA, Gregg MB. Surveillance of arboviral encephalitis in the United States, 1955–1971. *Am J Epidemiol.* 1973;97:199.

15. Reisen WK, Meyer RP, Milby MM, et al. Ecological observations on the 1989 outbreak of St. Louis encephalitis virus in the southern San Joaquin Valley of California. *J Med Entomol.* 1992;20:472–82.

16. Centers for Disease Control. St. Louis encephalitis in the United States, 1975. *J Infect Dis.* 1977;135:1014.

17. Marfin AA, Bleed DM, Lofgren JP, et al. Epidemiologic aspects of a St. Louis encephalitis epidemic in Jefferson County, Arkansas, 1991. *Am J Trop Med Hyg.* 1993;49:30–7.

18. Barrett FF, Yow MD, Phillips CA. St. Louis encephalitis in children during the 1964 epidemic. *JAMA.* 1965;193:381.

19. Przelomski MM, O'Rourke E, Grady FT, et al. Eastern equine encephalitis in Massachusetts: a report of 16 cases. *Neurology.* 1988;38:736.

20. Tyler KL. Diagnosis and management of acute viral encephalitis. *Semin Neurol.* 1984;4:480–9.

21. Menzies DW, Grocott HC, Huston AF, et al. Western equine encephalitis. *Epidemiol Bull (Canada).* 1986;12:27.

22. Earnest MP, Goodlishian JA, Claverley JR, et al. Neurologic, intellectual, and psychologic sequelae following Western encephalitis. *Neurology.* 1971;21:969.

23. Johnson KP. The pathogenesis of viral infections of the nervous system. *Neurol Clin North Am.* 1984;2:179.

24. Chun RWM, Thompson WH, Grabow JD, et al. California arbovirus encephalitis in children. *Neurology.* 1968;18:369.

25. Kumar R, Mathur A, Kumar A, et al. Clinical features and prognostic indicators of Japanese encephalitis in children to Kucknow (India). *Indian J Med Res.* 1990;91:321.

26. Burke DS, Leake CJ. Japanese encephalitis. In: Monath TP, ed. *The Arboriviruses: Epidemiology and Ecology, III.* Boca Raton, Fl: CRC Press; 1988:63–92.

27. Vaughn DW, Hoke CH. The epidemiology of Japanese encephalitis: prospects for prevention. *Epidemiol Rev.* 1992;14:197–221.

28. Kumar R, Mathur A, Singh KB, et al. Clinical sequelae of Japanese encephalitis in children. *Indian J Med Res.* 1993;97:9–13.

29. Igarashi A. Epidemiology and control of Japanese encephalitis. *World Health Stat Q.* 1992;45:299–305.

30. Canada Communicable Disease Report National Advisory Committee on Immunization (NACI). Statement on Japanese encephalitis vaccine. 1993;19:160–4.

31. Mulhall BP, Wilde H, Sitprija V. Japanese B encephalitis vaccine. Time for a reappraisal? *Med J Aust.* 1994;160:795–7.

32. Belman AL, Lantos G, Horoupian D, et al. AIDS: calcification of the basal ganglia in infants and children. *Neurology.* 1986;36:1192.

33. Gray F, Hurtel M, Hurtel B. Early central nervous system changes in human immunodeficiency virus (HIV)-infection. *Neuropathol Appl Neurobiol.* 1993;19:3–9.

34. Giangaspero F, Scanabissi E, Baldacci MN, et al. Massive neuronal destruction in human immunodeficiency virus (HIV) encephalitis. A clinico-pathological study of a pediatric case. *Acta Neuropathol (Berlin).* 1989;78:662.

35. Wiester OD, Leib St. L, Brüstle O, et al. Neuropathology and pathogenesis of HIV encephalopathies. *Acta Histochem.* 1992;Suppl-Band XLII:S107–14.

36. Nielsen CJ, Gjerris F, Pedersen H, et al. Brain biopsy in AIDS: diagnostic value and consequence. *Acta Neurochir (Wien).*1994;127:99–102.

37. Pizzo PA, Eddy J, Falloon J, et al. Effect of continuous intravenous infusion of zidovudine (AZT) in children with symptomatic HIV infection. *N Engl J Med.* 1988;319:889–96.

38. Schmidt FA, Bigley JW, McKinnis R, et al. Neuropsychological outcome of Zidovudine (AZT) treatment of patients with AIDS and AIDS-related complex. *N Engl J Med.* 1988;319:1573–8.

39. Peltola H, Heinonen OP. Frequency of true adverse reactions to measles-mumps-rubella vaccine. A double-blind placebo-controlled trial in twins. *Lancet.* 1986;1:939.

40. Azimi PH, Cramblett HS, Haynes RE. Mumps meningocephalitis in children. *JAMA.* 1969;207:509.

41. Johnstone JA, Ross CAC, Dunn M. Meningitis and encephalitis associated with mumps infection: a 10-year survey. *Arch Dis Child.* 1972;47:647.

42. Jubelt B. Enteroviral and mumps virus infections of the nervous system. *Neurol Clin North Am.* 1984;2:187.

43. Mumps Surveillance. Centers for Disease Control. Atlanta, GA. Dept. of Health, Education, and Welfare, Public Health Service, 1978.

44. Binder LS. Rabies. In: Tintinalli JE, Krome RL, Ruiz E, eds. *Emergency Medicine. A Comprehensive Study Guide.* 3rd ed. New York, NY: McGraw-Hill Book Co., 1992:527–9.

45. Koskiniemi M, Vaheri A, Taskinen E. Cerebrospinal fluid alterations in herpes simplex virus encephalitis. *Rev Infect Dis.* 1984;6:608.

46. Work TH. Arbovirus diseases of North America. In: Vinken PJ, Bruyn GW, eds. *Textbook of Pediatric Infectious Diseases.* Philadelphia, Pa: WB Saunders Co; 1981;1065–82.

47. Krugman S, Katz SL, Gershon AA, et al. *Infectious Diseases of Children.* 8th ed. St. Louis, Mo: CV Mosby; 1985:36.

48. Michaels J, Sharer LR, Epstein LG. Human immunodeficiency virus type 1 (HIV-1) infection of the nervous system: a review. *Immunodefic Rev.* 1988;1:71.

49. van Loon AM, van der Logt JTM, Heessen FWA, et al. Diagnosis of herpes simplex virus encephalitis by detection of virus-specific immunoglobulins A and G in serum and cerebrospinal fluid by using an antibody-capture enzyme-linked immunosorbent assay. *J Clin Microbiol.* 1989;27:1983–7.

50. Lakeman FD, Koga J, Whiteley RJ. Detection of antigen to herpes simplex virus in cerebrospinal fluid from patients with herpes simplex encephalitis, with clinicopathlogical correlation. *Radiology.* 1978;129:409.

51. Aslanzadeh J, Osmon DR, Wilhelm MP, et al. A prospective study of the polymerase chain reaction for detection of herpes simplex virus in cerebrospinal fluid submitted to the Clinical Virology Laboratory. *Mol Cell Probes.* 1992;2:367–73.

52. Aslanzadeh J, Skiest DJ. Polymerase chain reaction for detection of herpes simplex virus encephalitis. *J Clin Pathol.* 1994;47:554–5.

53. Aslanzadeh J, Garner JG, Feder HM, Ryan RW. Use of polymerase chain reaction for laboratory diagnosis of herpes simplex virus encephalitis. *Ann Clin Lab Sci.* 1993;23:196–202.

54. Rowley AH, Whiteley RJ, Lakeman FD, Wolinsky SM. Rapid detection of herpes-simplex-virus DNA in cerebral spinal fluid of patients with herpes simplex encephalitis. *Lancet.* 1990;335:440–1.

55. Guffond T, Dewilde A, Lobert PE, et al. Significance and clinical relevance of the detection of herpes simplex virus DNA by the polymerase chain reaction in cerebrospinal fluid from patients with presumed encephalitis. *Clin Infect Dis.* 1994;18:744–9.

56. Uren EC, Johnson PDR. Montanaro J, et al. Herpes simplex virus encephalitis in pediatrics: diagnosis by detection of antibodies and DNA in cerebrospinal fluid. *Pediatr Infect Dis J.* 1993;12:1001–6.

57. DiVincenzo JP. Mild herpes simplex encephalitis diagnosed by polymerase chain reaction: a case report and review. *Pediatr Infect J.* 1994;13:662–4.

58. David JM, Davis KR, Kleinman GM, et al. Computed tomography of herpes simplex encephalitis, with clinicopathological correlation. *Radiology.* 1978;129:409.

59. Greenburg SB, Taber L. Septimus E, et al. Computerized tomography in brain biopsy-proven herpes simplex encephalitis. *Arch Neurol.* 1981;38:58.

60. Taccone A, Gambaro G, Ghiorzi M, et al. Computerized tomography (CT) in children with herpes simplex encephalitis. *Pediatr Radiol.* 1988;19:9.

61. Schlesinger Y, Butler RS, Brunstrom JE, et al. Expanded spectrum of herpes simplex encephalitis in childhood. *J Pediatr.* 1995;126:234–41.

62. Upton A, Gumpert J. Electroencephalography in the diagnosis of herpes-simplex encephalitis. *Lancet.* 1970;1:650–2.

63. Kohl S, James AR. Herpes simplex virus encephalitis during childhood. Importance of brain biopsy diagnosis. *J Pediatr.* 1985;107:212.

64. Fishman MA. Brain biopsy in herpes simplex encephalitis. *Acta Paediatr Jpn.* 1992;34:344–9.

65. Grant IH, Gold JMW, Armstrong D. Risk of CNS toxoplasmosis in patients with AIDS. 26th Interscience Conference on Antimicrobial Agents and Chemotherapy, New Orleans, LA, September 28–October 1, 1986.

66. Luft DJ, Brooks RJ, Conley FK, et al. Toxoplasmic encephalitis in patients with AIDS. *JAMA.* 1984;252:913.

67. Haverkos HW. Assessment of therapy for toxomplasma encephalitis. The TE study group. *Am J Med.* 1987;82:907.

68. Navia BA, Petito CK, Gold JW, et al. Cerebral toxoplasmosis complicating the acquired immune deficiency syndrome: clinical and neuropathological findings in 27 patients. *Ann Neurol.* 1986;19:224.

69. Whitley RJ, Alford CA, Hersch MS, et al. Vidarabine vs. acyclovir therapy in herpes simplex encephalitis. *N Engl J Med.* 1986;314:144.

70. Whitley RJ, Arvin A, Corey L, et al. Vidarabine versus acyclovir therapy of neonatal herpes simplex virus. *Pediatr Res.* 1986;20:323A.

71. Skoldenberg B, Forsgren M, Alestig K, et al. Acyclovir versus vidarabine in herpes simplex encephalitis. Randomized multicentre study in consecutive Swedish patients. *Lancet.* 1984;2:707.

72. Kimura H, Aso K, Kuzushima K, et al. Relapse of herpes simplex encephalitis in children. *Pediatrics.* 1992;89:891–4.

73. Wagstaff AJ, Faulds D, Goa KL. Acyclovir [sic]. A reappraisal of its antiviral activity, pharmacokinetic properties and therapeutic efficacy. *Drug Evaluation.* 1994;47:153–205.

74. Chernoff AE, Snydman DR. Viral infections in the intensive care unit. *New Horizons.* 1993;2:279–301.

75. Tenser RB. Herpes simplex and herpes zoster. Nervous system involvement. *Neurol Clin.* 1984;2:215.

16 Cerebrovascular Disease

MICHAEL R. FRANKEL AND MARC CHIMOWITZ

SUMMARY   Acute stroke is a common neurological emergency. The ability to diagnose stroke accurately and to treat patients appropriately is especially important in the emergency department. With the advent of new acute stroke therapies, rapid recognition and triage of these patients has become more important than ever before.

Introduction

Cerebrovascular disease is the third leading cause of death and the number one cause of adult disability in the United States. Approximately 550,000 individuals experience a stroke each year in the United States, with an estimated cost of greater than $30 billion each year.

Strokes are broadly classified as ischemic or hemorrhagic. Approximately 85% of strokes are ischemic and 15% are hemorrhagic. Ischemic strokes are divided into several categories including cardioembolic, lacunar, and atherosclerotic. Each of these subtypes accounts for about 25% of ischemic stroke, with the remaining 25% being of undetermined causes. Unusual causes constitute about 5% of cases. Hemorrhagic causes include intracerebral hemorrhage or hematoma (ICH) and aneurysmal subarachnoid hemorrhage (SAH), the former occurring about twice as often as the latter. *Hemorrhagic infarction* is a term reserved for cerebral infarcts that become hemorrhagic when perfusion to the ischemic area is restored. The hemorrhage is usually petechial and commonly asymptomatic.

Transient symptoms often precede an ischemic stroke. Patients with a stroke due to atherosclerotic disease have a history of a transient ischemic attack (TIA) 50% of the time, whereas those with lacunar stroke or cardioembolism have a neurological warning only 25% and 5% of the time, respectively. Most TIAs last less than 15 minutes, some can last for hours.[1] Urgent evaluation of patients with TIAs is essential to identify the cause and to institute stroke preventive therapy (e.g., carotid endarterectomy, anticoagulation).

Similarly, recognition of the warning leak (also called *sentinel hemorrhage*) of aneurysmal SAH is extremely important. It is estimated that this occurs 25–50% of the time in the few days or weeks preceding a fulminant hemorrhage.[2] The warning leak causes a sudden severe headache, unlike previous headaches, often without neurological signs. Because symptoms usually resolve spontaneously or with simple analgesic medication, patients may not be evaluated for SAH. Prompt recognition and urgent evaluation are essential. Unlike SAH and ischemic stroke, ICH almost always occurs without warning.

Prehospital Management

The most important aspect of prehospital care of the patient with acute stroke is early recognition of its symptoms and signs, and rapid transport to the emergency department. The phrase "time is brain" was introduced to emphasize the narrow therapeutic window for the treatment of acute stroke and reflects the same urgency required for treating myocardial ischemia, where "time is heart muscle."[3]

Focal cerebral ischemia manifests in a finite number of ways. In general, the symptoms begin abruptly and include any of the following: weakness and/or numbness, usually on one side of the body; difficulty speaking; loss of vision; inability to walk; or severe headache. ICH presents with similar symptoms and signs and is often difficult to distinguish from cerebral infarction clinically. However, certain accompanying signs, such as a depressed level of consciousness early in the course of the stroke, implicate ICH rather than cerebral infarction.

Aneurysmal SAH usually presents with sudden severe headache. Accompanying symptoms and signs of SAH include headache (90%), nausea and vomiting (80%), syncope (33%), neck stiffness (20%), hemiparesis (15%), coma (10%), and confusion (10%).[4]

The prehospital management of these entities is similar. Attention to adequate airway protection, respiration, oxygenation, and circulatory function is essential. Hypoglycemia can cause confusion and rarely hemiparesis, and needs to be corrected immediately when present. Most patients with acute ischemic stroke do not require ventilatory support outside of the hospital. In contrast, patients with ICH or SAH can have a profound change in level of consciousness and require early ventilatory support.

Cardiac arrhythmias can occur in some patients with ischemic stroke, SAH, or ICH, requiring continuous cardiac monitoring. Supplemental oxygen is needed when there is low oxygenation saturation (<95%) or when respiratory function is compromised. There is no evidence that supraphysiological levels of oxygenation provide any therapeutic benefit.

Hypertension is common in the setting of acute ischemic stroke and does not automatically require immediate antihypertensive therapy. When a cerebral artery is blocked acutely, a zone of ischemia is created. In general, this zone will have a gradient of reduced blood flow, with the greatest reduction in the center of the zone and the least reduction in the periphery. The ischemia impairs the brain's ability to autoregulate the flow of blood locally, a phenomenon that normally occurs in order to maintain a constant blood flow to the brain under varying systemic blood pressures (Fig. 16.1). In the ischemic zone, the relationship between blood flow and systemic blood pressure is linear; any reduction in blood pressure will create a corresponding reduction in local blood flow, causing areas with the potential for reversible ischemia to be forced into irreversible ischemia and subsequent tissue infarction. In short, the patient with mild to moderate weak-

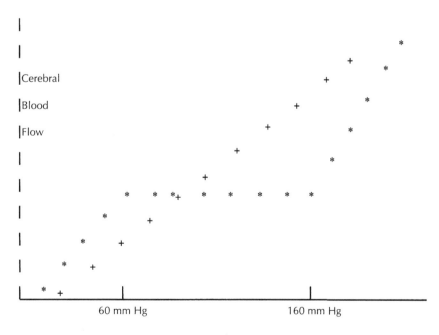

FIGURE 16.1. Graph of cerebral autoregulation.

*: Normal.

+: Disrupted autoregulation after cerebral injury.

215

ness may become paralyzed when blood pressure is lowered. In general, treatment of hypertension in the acute ischemic stroke setting is not recommended unless there is concomitant cardiovascular decompensation related to elevated afterload or suspected acute aortic dissection. When the blood pressure requires treatment, use of labetalol is recommended.

The management of elevated blood pressure in acute ICH is controversial.[5] Most ICHs are related to poorly controlled hypertension with subsequent rupture of a small penetrating artery and the evolving formation of a parenchymal hematoma over minutes to one to two hours. Some patients have continued hematoma growth in the first few hours after the onset of symptoms.[6] This phenomenon may be related to inadequate blood pressure reduction and continued bleeding; however, this has not been established. Blood pressure reduction may not be as deleterious to local cerebral blood flow as it is in acute ischemia, because the underlying mechanism of tissue injury is different. However, blood pressure reduction can produce global blood flow reduction in patients with elevated intracranial pressure (ICP). Therefore, patients suspected of having increased ICP based on a reduced level of consciousness or vomiting do not have their blood pressure lowered in the absence of an ICP monitor. Because ischemic stroke cannot be reliably differentiated from ICH on clinical grounds alone, the prehospital management of elevated blood pressure in suspected ICH is similar to that recommended above for suspected ischemic stroke.

Recommendations regarding the management of blood pressure following SAH are based on the cumulative experience of patients' clinical courses following aneurysmal rupture. The risk of rebleeding after aneurysmal rupture is higher in the first 24 hours than any other 24-hour period after presentation, and the mortality rate is over 50% when rebleeding occurs. It is likely that elevated blood pressure contributes to rerupture and subsequent rebleeding.[7] Therefore, it is important to lower elevated blood pressure to normotensive levels in the patient with suspected SAH. Blood pressure reduction in patients suspected of having elevated ICP is avoided unless the ICP is known.

The prehospital management of seizures in the patient with acute stroke is similar to the management in other patients. The use of lorazepam to treat seizures (2-mg increments given intravenously for adults every three to five minutes until the seizure stops; maximum dose, 0.1 mg/kg) is indicated for patients with generalized convulsions lasting longer than two minutes or for patients with more than one seizure in a short period of time (more than one per hour).

The most important aspect of prehospital management after stabilization in the field is rapid transport. The sooner patients are treated, the greater the potential benefit. Equally important is ensuring that a family member comes with the patient or is available by phone for discussion with the medical staff. Time of stroke onset has become critical for therapeutic decision making in the emergency department and often can be provided only by a family member. A further critical element for many acute stroke teams involved in the rapid treatment of patients has been their early notification by the paramedics in the field or en route. This allows the emergency department to prepare for the patient's arrival and to alert the radiology department to the need for a CT scan of the brain immediately following the patient's arrival.

The placement of an 18-gauge intravenous catheter en route helps to save valuable time after arrival in the emergency department. The key elements of prehospital management of the patient with suspected acute stroke are: stabilize, transport, bring family member or phone number of eyewitness, monitor blood pressure/pulse/cardiac rhythm, obtain chemstrip, notify the emergency department of estimated time of arrival and suspected stroke, and insert large-bore intravenous catheter.

Emergency Department Evaluation and Differential Diagnosis

The initial evaluation quickly defines whether the patient has evidence of acute global or focal cerebral dysfunction (see below, under "Initial Examination"). Brief questioning of the patient and family is essential to determine the onset of symptoms, and other relevant medical history. It is imperative to know the patient's baseline functional status in order to determine accurately whether deficits are acute or chronic.

Patients with acute global cerebral dysfunction have a clouded consciousness, as in delirium tremens or postictal agitation, or a depressed level of consciousness such as that seen with a toxic or metabolic encephalopathy, or sepsis. Most patients with ischemic stroke or ICH have focal findings, which are usually easy to identify. However, some central nervous system (CNS) lesions can give rise to a confusional state without focal findings. Examples of these include acute lesions in the nondominant temporal or parietal lobe (agitated delirium) or thalamus (somnolence/confusion). Additionally, patients with SAH can be confused or somnolent without focal findings.

Patients with ischemic stroke typically present with sudden symptoms; however, symptoms can evolve over several hours or, rarely, a few days. In contrast, a cerebral tumor or abscess usually does not present suddenly; rather, the symptoms evolve over weeks or months. The history is essential in helping to narrow the differential diagnosis. The differential diagnosis of acute focal cerebral dysfunction includes cerebral ischemia, ICH, Todd's paralysis, SAH, contusion, subdural/epidural hematoma, hypoglycemia, cerebral venous thrombosis, encephalitis, tumor, abscess, and psychogenic causes.

Some patients with epilepsy, especially those with underlying structural injury such as a previous stroke, have focal cerebral dysfunction following a seizure. Todd's paralysis refers to a transient focal weakness that occurs after a seizure. A history of these episodes is important to differentiate them from acute stroke.

As mentioned above, patients with ICH present with symptoms and signs similar to focal cerebral ischemia – with some notable exceptions. Patients with ICH have focal signs and are more likely to have a depressed level of consciousness early in their course. When sufficiently awake to converse, they are more likely to complain of headache than are patients with ischemia. Signs of increased ICP often accompany large hemorrhages and include vomiting, headache, and somnolence. Most ICHs are due to accelerated hypertension, frequently characterized by extremely high blood pressure (>200/110). The causes of ICH are: trauma, hypertension, vascular malformation, amyloid angiopathy (>60 years old, lobar), aneurysm, hemorrhagic transformation of infarct, coagulopathy, vasculitis, cerebral venous thrombosis, brain tumor, and abscess.

Spontaneous or nontraumatic SAH is most often (70–80%) due to aneurysmal rupture. Arteriovenous malformations are responsible for 5–10%, and the remainder have no abnormality on angiography. The differential diagnosis of SAH includes malformation (brain or spinal cord), head trauma, ICH with extension into the subarachnoid space, cerebral sinus thrombosis, pituitary apoplexy, coagulopathies, vasculitis, idiopathic perimesencephalic hemorrhage, and drugs (cocaine or amphetamines). Until proven otherwise, SAH is suspected in any patient with an unusually severe headache, especially when the onset is sudden. These headaches are usually described as the worst headache of the patient's life. Typically, they have no associated focal findings and are frequently misdiagnosed as migraines or tension headaches, or as a symptom of a viral illness. When an incorrect diagnosis is made, the patient may present at a later time with rebleeding or vasospasm.

Initial Examination

The purpose of the examination is to determine whether there is evidence of a stroke, what part of the brain is affected, and whether the patient is a candidate for urgent intervention such as thrombolytic therapy. A brief, focused neurological examination that enables accurate localization of the lesion can be performed in less than 10 minutes. The key elements of the examination to be assessed are listed in Table 16.1.

Mental status is tested by initially evaluating level of consciousness. Most patients with focal cerebral ischemia are awake or easily aroused to voice. The exception to this rule is the uncommon, dramatic presentation of basilar artery thrombosis, which can cause unresponsiveness and quadriplegia. In general, patients with focal findings, such as hemiparesis, combined with a depressed level of consciousness are more likely to have ICH or SAH than acute ischemia. Occasionally, this combination of findings is seen following a seizure (Todd's paralysis) or with hypoglycemia. Head trauma can produce hemiparesis and impaired consciousness because of cerebral contusion or subdural or epidural hematoma.

Language function is assessed quickly to determine if aphasia is present. This is done by assessing

TABLE 16.1. Key Elements of the Initial Neurological Examination

---

Mental status
  LOC: awake/alert, disoriented, somnolent but
  arousable to voice or pain
  Aphasic?
  Neglect?
Cranial nerves
  Pupillary asymmetry, abnormal extraocular muscle
  movements, visual field defect, facial weakness?
Motor
  Hemiplegia?
  Hemiparesis?
  Quadriplegia/paresis?
Coordination
  Ataxia?
Sensory
  Mild, moderate, or profound hemibody sensory loss?

---

comprehension, expression, repetition, and naming. Comprehension tests dominant temporal lobe function and is easily assessed by questioning the patient about the recent history of the problem. A specific request such as "Place your right thumb on your left ear" provides the examiner with a very useful and quick assessment of comprehension. Asking the patient to describe why he or she has come to the emergency department tests for the presence of an expressive aphasia. Patients with expressive aphasia have difficulty producing free-flowing speech. This can range from muteness to mild problems such as finding the correct words. These patients are usually quite frustrated with their speech difficulty. Asking the patient to repeat a short phrase tests the integrity of the connections between Wernicke's area, in the temporal and parietal lobes, and Broca's area, in the posterior frontal lobe. Testing for naming ability helps detect mild aphasia when the patient's comprehension and repetition skills seem intact. Asking the patient to name several objects or parts of objects is a good screen for aphasia, because almost all patients with aphasia have impaired naming ability. Neologisms or altering the names of objects (paraphasic errors) are useful clues to the presence of an aphasia. Wernicke's aphasia can occur in isolation and is important to distinguish from an episode of

mania. Similarly, Broca's aphasia needs to be differentiated from hysteria.

Determining the presence of neglect is important. Nondominant parietal lobe dysfunction (right hemisphere in right-handed patients) can produce signs of neglect and is especially profound when both frontal and parietal lobes are involved. These patients can be paralyzed on the left side due to right frontal lobe injury and may be unaware of their deficit. The examiner asks a patient with left hemiplegia, "Is your left arm weak?" The patient with neglect responds, "no." The neglect may be so severe that the patient denies possession of the affected limbs. The examiner holds up the patient's paralyzed left arm and positions it in the normal right visual field and asks, "Whose arm is this?" The patient may respond, "yours" or "I don't know." The patient's lack of concern over his or her weakness can cause the inexperienced examiner to misdiagnose the patient as having conversion disorder. More important, lack of insight into the patient's problem often translates into delayed recognition by family, paramedics, and emergency department staff. This syndrome is usually due to hemispheric ischemia, however, ICH can also produce hemi-neglect.

Brief *cranial nerve examination* includes checking for pupillary symmetry and reactivity. A Horner's syndrome (ptosis, miosis, anhydrosis) suggests an ipsilateral carotid dissection or lateral medullary infarct. Visual fields can be assessed rapidly in cooperative patients by looking for a field defect contralateral to the suspected lesion. The visual field examination is one of the most important parts of the neurological examination in patients with stroke. Visual field deficit implies an occipital or tempoparietal infarct, and essentially excludes small vessel disease as a potential cause of the stroke: Eye movements are assessed by looking for conjugate horizontal gaze preference or skew deviation (vertical malalignment). Patients are asked to follow the examiner's finger in the vertical and horizontal plane. Facial symmetry is assessed by asking patients to smile and to raise their eyebrows. Upper motorneuron, or central facial, weakness produces weakness of the lower face on smiling and relative sparing of the forehead with eyebrow raising. Lower motorneuron or peripheral facial weakness involves the upper and lower face. Dysarthria should be evident while discussing the patient's symptoms. Assessing for symmetry of palatal elevation and tongue protrusion can also be performed quickly.

Examination of *motor function* can be performed in a fast and effective manner. It is not necessary to examine every muscle in the extremities. Asking the patient to hold both arms up with the wrists extended for a count of 10 provides sufficient information. Asymmetrical downward drift of the arm or hand usually implies significant weakness. The patient is asked to raise each leg individually for a count of 5 while the examiner looks for downward drift. Noxious stimuli to an obviously weak limb helps to determine any residual strength and is helpful in patients unable to cooperate. In stuporous or comatose patients, this may induce decorticate or decerebrate posturing.

The physician tests the patient's *coordination* by asking the patient to touch finger-to-nose and heel-to-shin to evaluate for ataxia. Ataxia cannot be detected in patients with severe weakness.

The *sensory examination* is performed by observing for a response to pinprick using an unused safety pin on the patient's face, arm, trunk, and leg on the affected side. Position sense in a finger and toe is assessed when time permits. Depending on the patient's level of cooperation, a sensory examination can be too time-consuming to perform during the brief initial examination, it should not take more than one minute during the initial encounter.

Testing the *deep tendon reflexes* is usually not helpful in the patient with acute stroke and can be skipped during the initial encounter. Acutely, reflexes on the hemiparetic side may be increased, decreased, or unaffected.

The *plantar response* is usually, but not always, extensor (Babinski sign) on the hemiparetic side.

Testing *gait* is necessary in all patients with suspected stroke, unless there is suspicion of postural hypotension (e.g., a patient with dehydration) or the patient has obvious severe weakness. Gait ataxia may be the only sign of cerebellar infarct or hemorrhage.

Ischemia Stroke: Anatomy and Pathophysiology

Anterior Circulation

The internal carotid arteries (ICAs) supply 80% of cerebral blood flow; the remainder comes from the vertebral arteries in the posterior circulation. The common carotid arteries bifurcate into external and internal branches several centimeters below the angle of the jaw. The ICA is most frequently affected by atherosclerosis at its origin. A bruit can be heard in patients with arterial narrowing, but it is neither a sensitive nor specific finding. However, in a patient with an ipsilateral hemispheric ischemic event, a bruit suggests carotid stenosis. Carotid palpation is of little clinical value. Some patients with acute ICA occlusion or dissection have an ipsilateral Horner's syndrome. This is due to injury of the sympathetic fibers that travel with the ICA. Neck pain is a common accompaniment in patients with acute ICA dissection.

Proximal ICA stenosis is the presumed etiology of ischemic stroke in at least 20% of patients, and it causes stroke by at least two mechanisms: (1) local thrombosis with distal hypoperfusion; and (2) artery-to-artery embolization (platelets/fibrin). The latter is probably more frequent, and both mechanisms occur more commonly in patients with higher grades of stenosis. Complete occlusion of the ICA can result in embolization to the middle cerebral artery (MCA). When collateral flow is poor through the circle of Willis, complete ICA occlusion can lead to distal hypoperfusion and ischemic injury. This usually produces a watershed area of infarction that can sometimes be recognized clinically as a distinct syndrome of contralateral proximal arm and leg weakness. Dominant hemispheric watershed infarcts can cause an unusual aphasia (transcortical) with the distinguishing feature of retained ability to repeat phrases.

The ICA does not have extracranial branches. Intracranially, the ICA gives rise to the ophthalmic artery. Amaurosis fugax, also called transient monocular blindness, is due to intra-arterial embolization from the proximal ICA, or hypoperfusion. Emboli can be observed occasionally within the retinal arterioles and are helpful in determining etiology. A dilated funduscopic examination is usually necessary to find these refractile elements. The differential diagnosis of transient monocular blindness includes ophthalmic or central retinal artery embolism, temporal arteritis, migraine, and psychogenic causes. Central retinal artery occlusion usually causes permanent monocular blindness. Funduscopic findings are a pale retina and cherry red macula (see Chapter 20, "Neuro-opthamology").

The distal intracranial ICA divides into the MCA and anterior cerebral artery (ACA). The MCA provides most of the blood supply to the ipsilateral hemisphere including the internal capsule, Broca's area, Wernicke's area, optic radiations through the temporal and parietal lobes, and precentral and postcentral gyri. The distal ICA (beyond the branch to the ophthalmic artery) and the proximal MCA or ACA can develop atherosclerotic stenosis and lead to stroke by the same mechanisms as the proximal ICA (artery-to-artery embolism or hypoperfusion). Intracranial stenosis of these vessels, and intracranial vertebral and basilar arteries, causes ischemic stroke in 5–10% of cases. More frequently, however, these vessels are occluded by a proximal embolic source, usually the heart, aorta, or ICA. With complete occlusion of the ICA or MCA, the resultant neurological deficit is often profound, consisting of contralateral hemiplegia, typically with a gaze preference away from the hemiplegia, global aphasia (dominant hemisphere), neglect (nondominant hemisphere), and homonymous hemianopia. Gaze deviation can occur during or after a seizure, or from brainstem injury.

The first portion of the MCA gives rise to multiple, very small, penetrating arteries that pierce the deep portions of the hemispheres to supply the internal capsule. These penetrating arteries are affected by long-standing hypertension or diabetes, and show deposition of lipid and hyaline material (lipohyalinosis) in the vessel wall.[8] In situ thrombosis is the usual mechanism of occlusion. Pathologically, the infarct is observed as a small, deep hole (*lacunar infarct*). When it involves the internal capsule, the resultant neurological deficit is pure motor hemiparesis or hemiplegia. The deficit is devoid of sensory findings (although patients commonly report some minor subjective sensory symptoms) and affects the contralateral face, arm, and leg to a similar degree. There is no cortical dysfunction; that is, there is no aphasia, neglect, cortical sensory loss (agraphesthesia, astereognosis), or visual field loss. Distal to the origins of the lenticulostriate arteries, the MCA divides into two major divisions: (1) the anterior division supplies the frontal convexity, and pre- and postcentral gyri; and (2) the posterior division supplies the temporal and parietal convexities. Occlusion of the posterior division in the dominant hemisphere causes a fluent aphasia (Wernicke's aphasia) and hemianopia without a motor deficit. Occlusion of the anterior division in the dominant hemisphere causes an expressive aphasia (Broca's aphasia), and contralateral face and arm weakness.

Occlusion of the ACA (usually from an embolus) produces contralateral leg weakness and numbness, and downward drift of the proximal arm with attempts at sustained extension. Occasionally, in the right-handed patient, left ACA occlusion produces left arm apraxia due to involvement of the corpus callosum (anterior disconnection syndrome). The patient is unable to perform learned motor skills on request using the left hand, such as saluting or hammering an imaginary nail, due to a disconnection between the language area of the left hemisphere and the right motor cortex. Information arriving in the language area cannot get to the right motor cortex. There is no apraxia of the right arm because the continuity between the language area and the left motor cortex is intact.

Posterior Circulation

The vertebral arteries arise from the subclavian arteries. Atherosclerosis of the vertebral origin is becoming an increasingly recognized cause of stroke.[9] The vertebral artery can be narrowed at several points along its long extracranial and intracranial course. It receives collateral supply in the neck by several cervical arteries that can reconstitute the vertebral artery distally if it is occluded proximally. Each intracranial vertebral artery gives rise to a posterior inferior cerebellar artery (PICA), which supplies the posterior and inferior portions of the cerebellum and lateral medulla. Cerebellar infarction produces ipsilateral ataxia, dysequilibrium, and vertigo. Cerebellar swelling occurs two to four days after infarction and can lead to life-threatening brainstem compression when the infarct is large. This is important to recognize because surgical evacuation of infarcted cerebellar tissue can prevent death and often allows for a full recovery.

Infarction of the lateral medulla produces a constellation of findings that include: ipsilateral ataxia; diminution or loss of pain and temperature sensation on the ipsilateral face and contralateral arm, trunk, and leg; vertigo; nystagmus; ipsilateral palatal dysfunction and Horner's syndrome; hoarseness; hiccups; and, occasionally, difficulty with airway protection due to the ipsilateral vocal cord and pharyngeal weakness. The key to diagnosing a *lateral medullary infarction* is recognizing hemiataxia and the unique pattern of sensory loss. In most cases, vertebral occlusion at the origin of the PICA causes inferior cerebellar and lateral medullary infarcts, whereas an isolated lateral medullary infarct can be caused by occlusion of a small penetrating branch of PICA. Usually, patients with vertebral occlusion causing lateral medullary and inferior cerebellar infarcts have a good prognosis for neurological recovery. However, sometimes thrombus extends distally into the basilar artery, leading to more extensive brainstem infarction.

The vertebral arteries join to form the basilar artery at the junction of the medulla and pons. The basilar artery lies on the ventral surface of the pons and divides into the left and right posterior cerebral arteries at the junction on the pons and midbrain. Along its course, the basilar artery gives off multiple small penetrating vessels that provide blood to the corticospinal and pontocerebellar tracts in the ventral pons. Isolated occlusion of one of these small vessels leads to a lacunar infarct, producing one of the following hemiparetic/hemiataxic syndromes: pure motor hemiparesis, clumsy-hand dysarthria, or ataxic hemiparesis. Several larger branches of the basilar artery, known as short and long circumferential arteries, provide blood to the central, lateral, and dorsal portions of the pons and midbrain. Occlusion of these vessels often creates crossed signs, for example, ipsilateral peripheral facial weakness, sixth nerve palsy, and contralateral arm and leg weakness. The combination of ipsilateral cranial nerve and contralateral long tract findings indicates a brainstem localization. Occlusion of these larger vessels is usually due to atherosclerosis of the circumferential vessel or the basilar artery at the ostia of the circumferential branches. A less common cause of circumferential branch occlusion is cardiac or artery-to-artery embolism. Two of the long circumferential branches have been given names – the anterior inferior and superior cerebellar arteries – and supply portions of the cerebellum and dorsolateral brainstem. Infarction of these areas typically causes ipsilateral ataxia, nystagmus, and vertigo.

Basilar artery occlusion commonly produces a dramatic presentation consisting of quadriparesis or quadriplegia, small pupils, loss of horizontal gaze with sparing of vertical gaze, decreased corneal re-flexes, bifacial paralysis, and anarthria (inability to speak). The patient can appear comatose; however, careful examination reveals the patient to be awake and able to communicate through vertical gaze, which is spared. This is the *locked-in syndrome.* The ischemic injury is in the pons, and because the midbrain typically is spared, the vertical eye movements remain intact. Typically, when basilar artery occlusion produces injury that extends into the central portion of the midbrain and thalamus, the patient is comatose.

The posterior cerebral artery (PCA) provides blood to the thalamus, inferior and medial temporal lobes, and occipital lobes. Small penetrating arteries arise from the first portion of the PCA and supply the thalamus. Occlusion of one of these small vessels produces a lacunar infarct that manifests as a pure sensory stroke affecting the contralateral face, arm, trunk, and leg. Posterior cerebral artery occlusion causes a contralateral homonymous hemianopia due to infarction of the occipital lobe. When the occlusion is proximal to be penetrating arteries of the thalamus (thalamogeniculate arteries), an accompanying contralateral hemisensory deficit is present. When both PCAs are occluded, binocular visual loss (cortical blindness) occurs. Occasionally, an embolus lodges in the distal basilar artery, occludes both PCAs, and produces cortical blindness of which the patient may be unaware (*Anton's syndrome*). Left PCA territory infarction affects the left occipital lobe and the posterior corpus callosum, and can produce a posterior disconnection syndrome known as "alexia without agraphia." In addition to having a right hemianopia, the patient is unable to read (alexia). All the visual information enters the right occipital cortex, which cannot communicate with the language areas in the left hemisphere due to infarction of the posterior corpus callosum. The ability to write (graphia) is preserved because the language areas and motor cortex in the left hemisphere are in the MCA territory and remain intact.

Intracerebral Hemorrhage: Anatomy and Pathophysiology

Nontraumatic ICH is most commonly due to long-standing hypertension. The basal ganglia (lentiform and caudate nuclei), internal capsule, thalamus, lobar white matter, brainstem, and cerebellum are the common sites of ICH, with the basal ganglia being the most frequent. The hemorrhages are caused by rupture of microscopic outpouchings, known as Charcot-Broussard aneurysms, that form on small arteries that penetrate the brain substance.

Another common cause of lobar ICH in the elderly (over 60 years of age) is cerebral amyloid angiopathy. Amyloid is deposited in the leptomeningeal blood vessels of elderly individuals and is found in almost 50% of people over 80 years of age at autopsy.[10] Presumably, amyloid makes the blood vessels weak and susceptible to rupture. Some, but not all, of the patients with ICH due to cerebral amyloid angiopathy have underlying Alzheimer's dementia.

ICH in younger patients is more likely to be due to a vascular malformation, either an arteriovenous malformation or cavernous angioma. The absence of a history of hypertension also makes these entities more likely.

The symptoms of ICH begin abruptly and typically worsen over a few hours. Reasons for worsening include edema surrounding the hematoma and expansion of the hematoma. The factors that arrest hematoma expansion remain unknown. Persistent elevation of blood pressure may be responsible for hematoma enlargement in patients with hypertensive ICH; however, this correlation has not been established.

Prognosis after ICH depends on several factors including level of consciousness, size and location of the hematoma, and underlying medical condition. Several studies have shown that patients with ICH who have impaired consciousness at the time of presentation have a poor prognosis. Similarly, the larger the ICH, the worse the prognosis. While some patients can survive and function after relatively small, deeply situated ICH, large hematomas within the brainstem or thalamus are usually devastating.

Large-volume ICH, usually more than 3 cm in diameter, can produce increased ICP and brain herniation. Initial signs of transtentorial herniation include worsening level of consciousness, a dilated and poorly reactive pupil (usually ipsilateral to the bleed), and altered breathing patterns. Ultimately, herniation can cause coma and death. Increased ICP can also cause a reduction in cerebral perfusion pressure (CPP) and lead to cerebral ischemia. CPP is the difference between mean arterial pressure (MAP) and ICP (normally, less than 15 mm Hg), when it drops below 50 mm Hg, irreversible ischemic injury occurs.

Subarachnoid Hemorrhage: Anatomy and Pathophysiology

Most intracranial aneurysms occur at the bifurcation of arteries located around the circle of Willis, on the undersurface of the brain. When an aneurysm ruptures, blood quickly leaks into the subarachnoid space, resulting in a sudden increase in ICP, irritation of the meninges, and stimulation of pain fibers. The corresponding symptoms include severe headache, often with nausea and vomiting, stiff neck, and loss of consciousness or death when the hemorrhage is severe. Seizures occur infrequently. Occasionally, focal neurological findings such as hemiparesis are present initially and are usually related to intraparenchymal blood. A third cranial nerve palsy indicates compression of the third cranial nerve by an aneurysm located at the junction of the internal carotid and posterior communicating arteries. Unilateral or bilateral sixth cranial nerve palsies can occur in association with increased ICP. Although physical exertion has frequently been reported to precipitate aneurysmal rupture, SAH can occur at any time, even during sleep. The complications of SAH are: rebleeding, vasospasm, hydrocephalus, increased ICP, cerebral herniation, cardiac arrhythmia, electrolyte imbalance, and seizure. After an aneurysm ruptures and the leak spontaneously seals, there is a significant risk of rerupture. Rebleeding occurs suddenly and can produce any of the symptoms associated with the initial rupture. The risk of rebleeding is highest during the first two weeks following the initial hemorrhage (20%). Surgical clipping of the neck of the aneurysm eliminates this risk. Cerebral vasospasm causing ischemia most commonly occurs 3–13 days after SAH. The clinical presentation usually consists of one or more of the following: decreased level of consciousness, increased headache, or focal motor deficits.

Other complications of SAH include acute hydrocephalus (which may require emergency ventricular drainage), subendocardial ischemia, myocytolysis, and arrhythmias. The cardiac abnormalities have been attributed to a sudden rise in sympathetic tone or electrolyte imbalance. Electrolyte imbalance, typically hyponatremia (inappropriate antidiuretic hormone release or true natriuresis from cerebral salt wasting) or hypernatremia (diabetes in-

---

Emergency Department Management and Disposition

1. Suspect acute stroke
2. Obtain chemstrip, BP reading, check cardiac rhythm
3. Do immediate non-contrast CT scan and labs (stat PT/PTT, platelets, hematocrit, chemistries, O_2 saturation)
4. Blood on CT? (epidural, subdural, SAH, ICH) If yes, go to 4a.
5. Suspect SAH? If yes and CT negative, go to 5a.
6. Candidate for t-PA? If yes, go to 6a.
7. Probable cardiac source; fluctuating or progressive neurologic signs/symptoms; suspected vertebrobasilar or carotid occlusive disease? If yes, go to 7a.
8. Administer 325 mg of aspirin or 250 mg of ticlopidine if no contraindications.

- -

4a. Consult neurosurgeon – END
5a. Perform LP; if positive for SAH, go to 4a – END
6a. Review inclusionary/exclusionary criteria (table 16.2), consider t-PA administration. Neurology consultation – END
7a. Consult neurologist and consider anticoagulation with IV heparin if no contraindications. END

FIGURE 16.2. Algorithm for the management of acute stroke in the emergency department.

sipidus), usually takes several days to develop and is not commonly seen in the emergency department. Seizures can also occur after SAH.

Emergency Department Management and Disposition

An outline for the management of patients with acute stroke in the emergency department is shown in Figure 16.2. After a focused history and examination, various laboratory tests are performed: chemistry profile, CBC, platelets, PT/PTT, O_2 saturation, and drug screen. Immediate neuroimaging is performed in most patients with suspected stroke. A noncontrast CT scan of the head is most effective for detecting ICH. CT scanning is virtually 100% sensitive for detecting acute ICH (Fig. 16.3). In contrast, patients with acute cerebral ischemia often have a normal CT scan. Findings depend on the time from symptom onset, the suspected size of the infarct, and the experience of the individual interpreting the CT scan. In patients with large hemispheric infarcts, the earliest CT findings of ischemia include blurring of the basal ganglia, sulcal effacement, or mild hypodensity in the MCA territory (Fig. 16.4

shows a CT scan of early ischemic changes). These findings are usually not present in the first 2–3 hours of ischemia and begin to appear 3–12 hours from symptom onset. After 24 hours, the CT scan abnormalities become much more obvious in patients with large ischemic strokes (Fig. 16.5).

Some MRI facilities have the ability to perform diffusion-weighted MRI (DWI). This new technique identifies cerebral ischemia within one hour of symptom onset, which is much earlier than CT or conventional MRI can achieve. Focal ischemia appears hyperintense and is relatively easy to identify. An accompanying apparent diffusion coefficient (ADC) map helps to differentiate acute from chronic lesions. This ultrafast MRI technique (one to two minutes) can help confirm the clinical impression of acute ischemic stroke when the CT scan is normal. In general, the decision to use thrombolytic therapy is not based on this technique; however, it can be useful in certain situations when an accurate diagnosis of acute ischemic stroke is not clear from the clinical evaluation alone. Further research is needed in this area before definite conclusions can be made about the utility of DWI in therapeutic decision making.

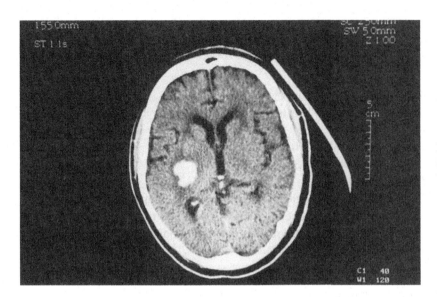

FIGURE 16.3. CT scan showing acute intracerebral hemorrhage in a patient with left hemisphere hemiplegia.

CT scanning is essential in patients with suspected acute SAH. A noncontrast CT scan detects SAH in 90–95% of cases when performed within 72 hours of symptom onset. The sensitivity is reduced to 80% after 5 days, and 50% at the end of the first week.[11] Figure 16.6 shows the typical appearance of SAH. LP is reserved for patients with a normal CT scan in whom the diagnosis is still suspected. It is essential to distinguish between a traumatic LP and hemorrhage, and the most reliable method is to centrifuge the cerebrospinal fluid and examine the supernatant for the presence of discoloration. Xan-

thochromia (yellow discoloration), caused by pigment released from degenerating red blood cells, is invariably present after 12 hours and usually remains for 2 weeks. The term *xanthochromia* is commonly used to describe either a pinkish (oxyhemoglobin) or yellowish (bilirubin) discoloration of the supernatant. The supernatant begins to turn pink 2–4 hours after the initial SAH and becomes yellowish after 10–12 hours. However, it can take as long as 12 hours for the supernatant to become discolored.[12] Spectrophotometry is more sensitive than direct visual inspection in identifying xanthochro-

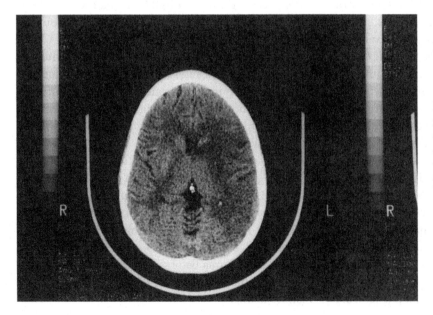

FIGURE 16.4. CT scan showing early ischemic changes in the left hemisphere (blurring of basal ganglia, sulcal effacement, mild hypodensity in the left hemisphere). CT scan done approximately 12 hours from symptom onset (right hemiplegia, global aphasia).

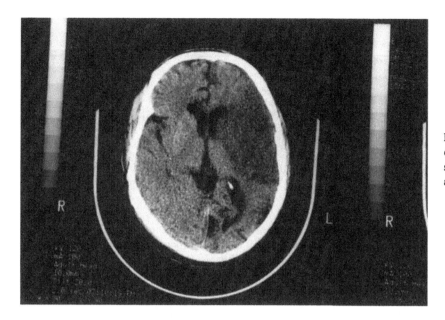

FIGURE 16.5. CT scan of left MCA distribution infarct 24 hours from symptom onset. (Not the same patient as in Fig. 16.4.)

mia and can be used to detect the presence of pigments in the supernatant.

LP is usually not performed in patients with acute ischemic stroke unless the patient is suspected of having bacterial, fungal, or tuberculous meningitis, syphilis, or CNS vasculitis. LP is not indicated in patients with acute ICH.

The risk of blood pressure reduction after acute stroke has been discussed in detail. The blood pressure level that requires reduction is variable. In general, blood pressure is lowered in the acute setting when accompanied by cardiovascular decompensation related to elevated afterload or aortic dissection, or when thrombolytic therapy is planned. The National Stroke Association has published guidelines recommending treatment of blood pressure when it is greater than 220/120 on repeated measurements over one hour for cerebral infarction or ICH.[13] When elevated blood pressure is treated, the patient is examined every five minutes while blood pressure is reduced. Any sign of worsening neurological function, such as increasing weakness or decreasing level of consciousness, indicates the need to discontinue intravenous antihypertensive medication immediately. When it is necessary to reduce blood pressure, labetalol is given intravenously because nitroprusside given intravenously can secondarily increase ICP. Sublingual nifedipine is not used because it can cause a precipitous and unpredictable drop in blood pressure that can be difficult to reverse.

Ischemic Stroke: Specific Treatment

Thrombolytic Therapy

The recently completed double blind study sponsored by the National Institute of Health (NIH) that compared intravenous tissue plasminogen activator (t-PA) to placebo for acute ischemic stroke provided the first convincing evidence of a beneficial effect of

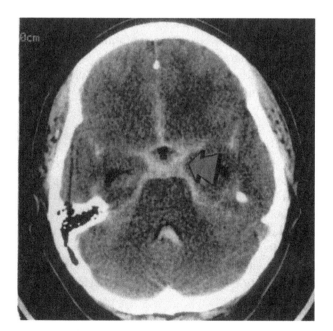

FIGURE 16.6. CT scan showing acute subarachnoid hemorrhage (arrow points to blood in the basal cisterns).

TABLE 16.2. Inclusion/Exclusion Criteria for the Use of t-PA for Ischemic Stroke

Inclusions:
- Ischemic stroke with clearly defined symptom onset
- Measurable deficit on the NIH Stroke Scale
- No evidence of intracranial blood on brain CT
- 180 minutes or less from the time of symptom onset to initiation of IV t-PA

Exclusions:
- Rapidly improving or minor stroke symptoms
- Stroke or serious head trauma within 3 months
- Major surgery within 14 days
- History of intracranial hemorrhage
- Systolic BP >185 mm Hg or diastolic blood pressure >110 mm Hg at the time of treatment initiation
- Aggressive BP treatment, i.e., use of continuous IV antihypertensive drip to achieve above goal; single or double doses of 10–20 mg of IV labetalol and/or 1–2 inches of nitropaste is acceptable
- Suspected subarachnoid hemorrhage despite a normal CT
- Gastrointestinal or urinary tract hemorrhage within 21 days
- Arterial puncture at a noncompressible site within 7 days
- Seizure at the onset of stroke
- Current use of oral anticoagulants
- Use of heparin within 48 hours and an elevated PTT
- PT >15 seconds, platelet count <100,000, glucose <50 or >400

thrombolytic therapy in this setting.[14] This multicenter study enrolled 624 patients and initiated treatment within 3 hours of symptom onset. After a focused history and examination, patients who met clinical criteria (Table 16.2) underwent a noncontrast CT of the head. Patients who met the criteria were treated with 0.9 mg/kg (no more than 90 mg) of t-PA or placebo. A 10% bolus was given intravenously over 1 minute, the remainder infused over 1 hour. Neurological evaluations were performed at 2 hours, 24 hours, 7–10 days, and 3 months, and repeat CT of the brain was done at 24 hours, 7–10 days, and 3 months. The primary outcome measurement was based on three separate scales of functional outcome and one scale measuring neurological deficit at 3 months. The number of patients with minimal or no disability at 3 months was compared between treatment groups.

The study showed that patients were 30–50% more likely to have minimal or no disability at 3 months when they were treated with t-PA (*P* value = 0.008, global test). This benefit occurred despite an increased incidence of symptomatic ICH (6.4% versus 0.6%). The effect of t-PA was independent of age, stroke subtype, and stroke severity, and there

was no difference in outcome between patients whose treatment began in less than 90 minutes and those in the 90–180-minute treatment group. This may mean that t-PA could be effective beyond 3 hours; however, this has not been established. Follow-up data at 1 year from treatment in this study showed sustained benefit for patients treated with t-PA as compared with placebo. In 1996, the Food and Drug Administration approved the use of t-PA for treatment of acute ischemic stroke.

Recently, additional data were reported from two series of consecutively treated patients in community settings and showed a similar rate of symptomatic ICH. The National Institute of Neurological Disorders and Stroke (NINDS) study utilized a rigorous protocol requiring careful patient selection and management. Similar results may not be seen in everyday practice unless the inclusion and exclusion criteria (Table 16.2), and principles of patient management (Tables 16.3 and 16.4) are adhered to closely. A few of these management principles are discussed further.

Every patient requires a noncontrast CT scan of the brain to exclude hemorrhage prior to treatment. Additionally, in the NINDS study, only 4% of the

TABLE 16.3. Patient Management after t-PA Administration

- No anticoagulants or antiplatelet agents for 24 hours
- Blood pressure monitoring for the first 24 hours: every 15 minutes for 2 hours after starting infusion, every 30 minutes for 6 hours, then every hour from the 8th hour until 24 hours after t-PA started
- Aggressive blood pressure management to maintain BP <180/105 mm Hg

624 baseline CT scans had evidence of early ischemic changes. Although patients with CT scans showing early ischemic changes were at increased risk of symptomatic ICH, this did not eliminate the potential for benefit with t-PA. The first step before deciding to use t-PA in patients with these CT findings is to requestion the patient, family, and witnesses about the exact time of symptom onset.

Time of symptom onset must be clearly established. Patients who awaken with neurological symptoms are not treated unless they were asleep briefly and were known to be "normal" within three hours. Patients with minor deficits such as isolated sensory symptoms should probably not be treated. Patients who are improving rapidly should not be treated in order to minimize the number of patients who are likely to have a TIA.

Blood pressure above 185/110 is a contraindication for treatment with t-PA because of the potential risk of ICH following t-PA therapy. For this reason, patients can be treated with t-PA when their blood pressure lowers spontaneously, or with nonaggressive treatment such as nitropaste or up to 20 mg of labetalol given intravenously. In the NINDS study,

aggressive treatment was considered to be the use of a continuous intravenous antihypertensive infusion. Once infusion with t-PA is initiated, blood pressure is monitored closely and kept below 180/105 mm Hg during the first 24 hours using intravenous labetalol or nitroprusside when necessary according to a specific algorithm (Table 16.4). Anticoagulants, antiplatelet agents, and volume expanders are not administered during the first 24 hours of treatment.

Aside from early ischemic changes on CT scanning, stroke severity is the only other baseline variable identified as an important predictor of symptomatic ICH. Patients with severe stroke symptoms, such as hemiplegia with aphasia or neglect, were at increased risk of bleeding; however, the benefit of t-PA was independent of stroke severity. More t-PA-treated patients achieved a normal or near normal recovery at three months in this subgroup than placebo-treated patients in the same subgroup. Thus, the use of t-PA for a patient with signs of a severe stroke on neurological examination or early ischemic changes on CT scanning is discussed carefully with the family because most of these patients

TABLE 16.4. Blood Pressure Treatment Algorithm after Initiating t-PA Infusion*

- When diastolic blood pressure >140 mm Hg, start an infusion of sodium nitroprusside (0.5–10 mg/kg/minute).
- When systolic blood pressure >230 mm Hg and/or diastolic blood pressure is 121–140 mm Hg, give labetalol, 10 mg IV, over 1–2 minutes. The dose may be repeated and/or doubled every 10 minutes up to 150 mg total. Continue blood pressure check every 15 minutes. When labetalol cannot be used or is ineffective, nitroprusside can be tried.
- When systolic blood pressure is >180–230 mm Hg and/or diastolic blood pressure is >105–200 mm Hg on two readings 5–10 minutes apart, give labetalol, 10 mg IV, over 1–2 minutes. The dose may be repeated or doubled every 10–20 minutes up to 150 mg total. When labetalol is contraindicated (e.g., congestive heart failure), use the lowest amount of nitroprusside to keep systolic blood pressure <180 mm Hg and diastolic blood pressure <105 mm Hg.

* Modified from NINDS t-PA stroke trial protocol.

are unable to provide consent. Given the high likelihood of severe disability or death due to the presence of severe stroke symptoms, most families opt for use of t-PA because of the possibility of improvement despite the increased risk of ICH.

Other randomized, multicenter stroke studies using intravenous thrombolytic therapy in the acute setting have not shown a benefit of thrombolytic agents.[15-17] The most likely reason for the discordant results of these studies and the NIH study is that the NIH study was the only study to enroll patients exclusively within three hours. Two other large randomized trials using streptokinase given intravenously were terminated prematurely due to excessive intracerebral bleeding.[16,17] The European trial[16] used a six-hour treatment window, and the Australian trial[17] used a four-hour window, suggesting that the risk of ICH probably increases beyond three hours. It is not known whether streptokinase given intravenously is safe and effective in the first three hours. Until evidence for benefit is established, streptokinase is not used in the treatment of acute ischemic stroke outside of carefully monitored clinical trials. Similarly, the use of any thrombolytic agent beyond three hours is considered experimental until efficacy is established.

The largest published trial of intra-arterial thrombolytic therapy (59 patients) using supraselective catheterization showed a high rate of vascular recanalization and suggests that this approach is technically feasible.[18] To date, the only randomized, placebo-controlled pilot study of 40 patients using intra-arterial thrombolysis showed acceptable rates of recanalization and safety with pro-urokinase, a precursor of urokinase. However, additional data are needed to demonstrate the safety and efficacy of intra-arterial thrombolytic therapy for treating acute ischemic stroke; the third phase of the study is under way, with final results expected by the end of 1998 or early 1999.

Anticoagulation

The only widely accepted indication for anticoagulation (heparin given intravenously) in the acute ischemic stroke setting is to present recurrent stroke in patients with an unequivocal cardiac source of embolus, for example, atrial fibrillation or dilated cardiomyopathy. In general, the low risk of hemorrhagic conversion of ischemic stroke with anticoagulation is offset by the 12% risk of reembolization in the first two weeks following cardioembolism.[19] However, patients with large embolic stroke (e.g., global aphasia or neglect with hemiplegia and gaze deviation) can be particularly vulnerable to symptomatic hemorrhagic transformation related to heparin given intravenously in the first few days. Therefore, many clinicians do not anticoagulate patients with large ischemic stroke during the first five days.[20] When heparin is used, the partial thromboplastin time is kept below twice control[21] and blood pressure is controlled.

Proof of efficacy of anticoagulation in treating acute stroke unrelated to cardioembolism is not established. The largest placebo controlled, randomized trial showed that low molecular heparin did not improve the outcome in more than 1000 treated patients. Although some subgroups of patients may experience benefit, such as those with large vessel stroke, the final analysis of these studies is not completed. However, despite a lack of conclusive data from clinical trials demonstrating efficacy, many clinicians use heparin to treat patients with unstable cerebral ischemia. These patients include those with fluctuating or progressive neurological symptoms or signs. Treatments that have been studied for acute ischemic stroke in large clinical trials include: steroids, calcium channel blockers, hemodilution, and volume expansion. None of these treatments has been shown to be effective.

Numerous trials of novel neuroprotective agents are being conducted to determine safety and efficacy in the treatment of acute ischemic stroke. To date, none has been shown to be effective. However, these agents may become part of the routine treatment of patients with acute ischemic stroke in the near future.

Intravascular Volume

Volume expansion therapy has not been demonstrated to be effective for treating ischemic stroke; however, some patients benefit from hydration. Many patients with acute stroke are volume-depleted, which exacerbates cerebral ischemia. Restoring a euvolemic state with an isotonic fluid such as normal saline is essential for minimizing the extent of ischemic damage.

Intracerebral Hemorrhage

Patients with cerebellar hematomas compressing the brainstem are likely to benefit from surgical evacuation of the hematoma. Although uncommon, this condition is a neurosurgical emergency. Evacuation of hematomas in other locations (lobar, putamen, thalamus, brainstem) remains controversial. There has not been a large randomized clinical trial comparing surgery with nonsurgical therapy in these patients. Several small trials of surgery versus medical therapy have not shown a clear benefit for surgery. Most neurosurgeons do not operate on spontaneous supratentorial ICH unless (1) the hematoma is in an easily accessible location, usually lobar, measures more than 3 cm in diameter, and has life-threatening mass effect, and (2) brain herniation appears imminent or is refractory to medical therapy. In these situations, surgery may decrease mortality but increase morbidity.

Although unproven, less invasive surgical treatments using stereotactic, CT-guided, percutaneous burr hole evacuation with or without installation of a thrombolytic agent into the hematoma cavity may provide a greater chance for improved neurological recovery.

Medical management of patients with ICH is primarily supportive. Corticosteroids are ineffective for treating patients with ICH. Mechanical ventilation may be required in the emergency department for patients with a severely depressed level of consciousness. A Glasgow Coma Scale score of less than 9 is a useful guide for determining when ventilatory support is necessary in these patients. Endotracheal intubation and 1 mg/kg of intravenous lidocaine given slowly over 1 minute helps to reduce the sudden increase in ICP that accompanies intubation. When increased ICP is suspected, hyperventilation to a $Paco_2$ of approximately 30 mm Hg, mannitol, and sedation are useful in the acute setting.

Monitoring of ICP is essential when making decisions about the use of osmotic therapy, antihypertensive medication, and fluid management. ICP monitors are most useful when placed ipsilateral to the ICH.

Hyperventilation and hyperosmotic therapy are effective in lowering ICP but can lead to reduced cerebral perfusion when not used carefully. Hyperventilation lowers ICP at the expense of cerebral blood flow. Hyperventilation is used acutely in patients who are suspected to have brain herniation or increased ICP; these patients are weaned to normocapnia when ICP is in the normal range. Osmotic agents, such as mannitol, cause water to go from the interstitial space into the intravascular space, thereby lowering ICP. Mannitol given intravenously (1 g/kg) can be used acutely when brain herniation is suspected or when ICP is profoundly elevated. Repeat doses of mannitol every three to four hours (0.25 g/kg) are used when there is persistently elevated ICP. The goal of managing increased ICP is to lower ICP to less than 20 mm Hg and to maintain CPP between 70 and 100 mm Hg.

Subarachnoid Hemorrhage

The emergency management of SAH is similar to that of ICH. Immediate neurosurgical consultation is necessary. Mechanical ventilation may be required, and the caveats listed above are important. Blood pressure management is less controversial than with other types of stroke. Poorly controlled blood pressure can precipitate rerupture of an aneurysm. Therefore, lowering blood pressure to normotensive levels is advised. However, because increased blood pressure can be secondary to elevated ICP, lowering blood pressure can reduce cerebral perfusion. Consequently, when increased ICP is suspected by the neurological examination or by CT scanning, lowering of the blood pressure is performed in consultation with a neurosurgeon or neurologist.

Definitive treatment of a ruptured cerebral aneurysm is surgical clipping of the aneurysmal neck. Many neurosurgeons operate as soon as possible (usually within 24–72 hours) after SAH in order to reduce the chances of rebleeding and to allow aggressive management of vasospasm. Although intravenous antifibrinolytic therapy reduces the risk of rebleeding in patients who have not had surgery, the benefit is offset by the attendant increase in vasospasm-induced cerebral infarction, thrombophlebitis, and pulmonary embolism. As a result, antifibrinolytic therapy is not recommended.

Once deterioration from vasospasm occurs, treatment focuses on increasing cerebral perfusion pressure. This is done by increasing the intravascular volume with use of normal saline, albumin, or dextran, and by raising the arterial blood pressure with a vasopressor such as dopamine.[7] Because vasospasm usually takes several days to develop after SAH, it is not frequently encountered in the emergency department.

Disposition

Patients with TIA, acute ischemic stroke, ICH, or SAH are admitted to the hospital. Some physicians discharge patients from the emergency department who have had a single TIA. However, patients with TIA are at high risk for stroke, which is maximal in the first few weeks after TIA. It is strongly recommended that these patients are hospitalized, a thorough diagnostic evaluation is instituted, and intravenous heparin therapy is considered when the suspected cause of the TIA is carotid artery disease, vertebral or basilar artery disease, or cardiac embolism.

Patients hospitalized with acute cerebral ischemia should be cared for primarily by physicians with experience and expertise in this area, that is, neurologists, or in close consultation with the admitting physician. A neurosurgeon should participate in the care of most patients with ICH and all patients with SAH.

PEARLS AND PITFALLS

- Elevated blood pressure after acute ischemic stroke is common. Aggressively lowering blood pressure in this setting can worsen the ischemia and cause greater neurological injury.
- Some strokes do not cause weakness. Common locations of stroke without paralysis include the occipital lobe (hemianopia), dominant temporal/parietal lobe (Wernicke's aphasia), nondominant temporal/parietal lobe (confusion, agitation, and hemianopia), and thalamus (confusion, somnolence, and hemianopia).
- A psychogenic neurological deficit (e.g., hysterical paralysis) is often difficult to differentiate from organic brain injury. In general, the diagnosis is not made without neurological consultation.

- A normal CT scan does not rule out SAH. Lumbar puncture is required in patients with normal imaging whose clinical presentation suggests SAH. After cerebrospinal is centrifuged, the supernatant may not become discolored for up to 12 hours after the onset of SAH.

REFERENCES

1. Feinberg WM, Albers GA, Barnett HJM, et al. Guidelines for the management of transient ischemic attacks. *Stroke.* 1994;25:1320–35.
2. Qureshi AI, Frankel MR. Recognition and management of subarachnoid hemorrhage. *Heart Dis Stroke.* 1994;270–4.
3. Hill MD, Hachinski V. Stroke Treatment: Time Is Brain. *Lancet* 1998;352:[supp. 3] 10–14.
4. Adams HP Jr, Jergenson DD, Kassell NF, Sahs AL. Pitfalls in the recognition of subarachnoid hemorrhage. *JAMA.* 1980;244:794–6.
5. Powers WJ. Acute hypertension after stroke: the scientific basis for treatment decisions. *Neurology.* 1993; 43:461–7.
6. Broderick JP, Brott TG, Tomsick T, Barsan W, Spilker J. Ultra-early evaluation of intracerebral hemorrhage. *J Neurosurg.* 1990;72:195–9.
7. Kopitnik TA, Samson DS. Management of subarachnoid hemorrhage. *J Neurol Neurosurg Psychiatry.* 1993;56:947–59.
8. Fisher CM. Lacunar strokes and infarcts: a review. *Neurology.* 1982;32:871–6.
9. Caplan LR. Large vessel occlusive disease of the posterior circulation. In: Caplan LR, *Stroke, a Clinical Approach.* 2nd ed. Boston, Mass: Butterworth-Heinemann; 1993:241–5.
10. Vinters HV, Gilbert JJ. Cerebral amyloid angiopathy: incidence and complications in the aging brain. *Stroke.* 1983;14:924–8.
11. Camarata PJ, Latchaw RE, Rufenacht DA, Heros RC. Intracranial aneurysms. *Invest Radiol.* 1993;28: 373–82.
12. Vermeulen M, van Gijn J. The diagnosis of subarachnoid hemorrhage. *J Neurol Neurosurg Psychiatry.* 1990;53:365–72.
13. National Stroke Association Consensus Statement. Stroke: the first six hours. Emergency evaluation and treatment. *Stroke Clin Updates.* 1993;4:3–12.
14. The National Institute of Neurological Disorders and Stroke rt-PA Stroke Study Group. Tissue plasminogen activator for acute ischemic stroke. *N Engl J Med.* 1995;333:1581–7.
15. Hacke W, Kaste M, Fieschi C, et al. Intravenous thrombolysis with recombinant tissue plasminogen activator for acute hemispheric stroke. *JAMA.* 1995;274: 1017–25.

16. Hommel M, Boissel JP, Cornu C, et al. Termination of trial of streptokinase in severe acute ischaemic stroke. *Lancet.* 1995;345:57.

17. Donnan GA, Hommel M, Davis SM, McNeil JJ. Streptokinase in acute ischemic stroke. *Lancet.* 1995;346:56.

18. Zeumer H, Freitag HJ, Zanella F, Thie A, Arning C. Local intra-arterial fibrinolytic therapy in patients with stroke: urokinase versus recombinant tissue plasminogen activator. *Neuroradiology.* 1993;35:159–62.

19. Cerebral Embolism Study Group. Immediate anticoagulation of embolic stroke: brain hemorrhage and management options. *Stroke.* 1984;15:779–89.

20. Sherman DG, Dyken ML, Gent M, Harrison JG, Hart RG, Mohr JP. Antithrombotic therapy for cerebrovascular disorders: an update. *Chest.* 1995;108:444S–56S.

21. Chamorro A, Vila N, Saiz A, Alday M, Tolosa E. Early anticoagulation after large cerebral embolic infarction: a safety study. *Neurology.* 1995;45:861–5.

22. Kay R, Wong KS, Yu YL, et al. Low-molecular weight heparin for the treatment of acute ischemic stroke. *N Engl J Med.* 1995;333:1588–93.

23. Adam HP Jr, Woolson RF, Clarke WR, et al. Design of the Trial of ORG 10172 in Acute Stroke Treatment (TOAST). *Control Clin Trials.* 1997;18:358–77.

17 Movement Disorders

SID M. SHAH AND ROGER L. ALBIN

SUMMARY Movement disorders encountered in the emergency department range from the familiar parkinsonism and drug-induced dystonias to rare disabling hemiballism secondary to a stroke. Movement disorders constitute the symptoms and signs of an underlying neurological or nonneurological disorder that manifests primarily as an abnormality of movement. In the emergency department, movement disorders are diagnosed on the basis of clinical evaluation, with relatively few contributions from laboratory and radiographic studies. Movement disorders are classified as hypokinetic disorders, hyperkinetic disorders, tremor, and myoclonus. Characteristics of various movement disorders are described and drug-induced movement disorders, which commonly present to the emergency department, are reviewed in detail.

Introduction

Movement disorders is the term used by neurologists to describe disorders of motor function *not* associated with primary dysfunction of the corticospinal tracts, cerebellum, sensory pathways, or peripheral nervous system. This term is often used as a synonym for basal ganglia disorders. However, some disorders classified as movement disorders, such as myoclonus and some forms of tremor, are not associated with basal ganglia pathology. A movement disorder is typically the symptoms and signs of an underlying neurological or nonneurological disorder, rather than a diagnosis itself. Movement disorders encountered in the emergency department range from familiar parkinsonism and drug-induced dystonias to rare disabling hemiballism secondary to acute stroke. Movement disorders can be associated with acute primary neurological disease such as a cerebrovascular event or focal neurological disease such as a neoplasm. Some movement disorders are a manifestation of underlying systemic illness such as hepatic or renal failure, or autoimmune disease. Movement disorders, dystonia in particular, are often misdiagnosed as being hysterical or psychiatric in origin. The primary task of the emergency physician in evaluating a patient with a suspected movement disorder is to identify the nature of the presenting complaint by obtaining a thorough history and by performing a focused neurological examination. This chapter concentrates on the diagnosis and management of movement disorders that require immediate intervention, and distinguishes conditions that allow safe discharge from the emergency department.

Prehospital Care

Movement disorders, especially acute dystonic reactions, can easily be confused with focal or generalized seizure activity. Prehospital care providers are advised against pursuing aggressive measures when the diagnosis of ongoing seizure is uncertain. It is important to differentiate generalized tonic-clonic status epilepticus from a movement disorder or other cause of involuntary movements. Generalized tonic-clonic status epilepticus is a medical emergency treated with medications that can cause serious adverse effects. For other conditions, supportive measures usually suffice as long as the airway is not compromised and vital signs are stable. Patients who fall are transported on a backboard with cervical spine immobilization. Information collected by prehospital care providers on conditions leading to falls or other acute events can be important in the emergency department evaluation of patients with suspected movement disorders. Drug ingestion, substance abuse, and exposure to environmental toxins such as carbon monoxide are associated with several different types of movement disorders. Prehospital care providers should investigate the scene and gather relevant clinical information for subsequent patient care.

Emergency Department Evaluation

Vital signs and the adequacy of the airway are assessed on arrival in the emergency department. A seizure disorder is distinguished from a movement disorder on presentation by obtaining a thorough history and by performing a focused physical examination.

Movement disorders are usually diagnosed on the basis of clinical evaluation, with little additional information provided by laboratory and radiographic studies. The emergency department evaluation of a movement disorder is guided by a suspected or known underlying disease process, history taking, and neurological examination. Important features of the history include the manner and temporal nature of symptom onset, the location of symptoms and body parts most affected, and mitigating and exacerbating factors. The patient is asked if the symptoms are present at rest, with sustained posture, with movement, or only during the execution of specific tasks. Possible association to environmental factors, toxins, or medication use is determined. Family, social, and psychiatric history are reviewed. In a pediatric patient, evidence of premature birth, perinatal injury, or behavioral problems is sought. Use of psychotropic medications or antiemetics is questioned. A careful physical examination can reveal signs of metabolic or endocrine derangements, or toxic exposures.

A careful neurological examination with accurate characterization of the abnormalities is the basis of evaluating movement disorders. The character of the involuntary movement(s) or movement problem is first assessed by observation of the patient's head, trunk, and limbs. Eye movements (saccadic and pursuit movements), tone (resistance of muscles/joints to passive manipulation), gait (casual, toe, heel, and tandem), and fine coordination (rapid finger tapping, alternating pronation and supination of the hands) are tested. Detection of neurological abnormalities other than the movement disorder is essential in neuroanatomical localization of pathology and assists in generating a focused differential diagnosis. Incoordination does not indicate the presence of a movement disorder, because it can result from injury to the corticospinal tracts, cerebellum, sensory pathways, or basal ganglia.

Laboratory evaluation guided by results of the history, and physical examination can include basic serum chemistries, drug levels, and toxicological studies. Urine can be tested for illicit substances.

The role of neuroimaging studies in the evaluation of movement disorders is limited. Some movement disorders occur acutely from focal structural lesions such as stroke. Typically, they are present in a localized body area or follow a "hemi-distribution," as in hemidystonia or hemiballism. Urgent brain imaging can be helpful following the acute onset of symptoms with a focal distribution of findings.

Classification of Movement Disorders

Movement disorders can be classified into four broad categories based on phenomenological features, clinical pharmacology, and neuropathology: (1) hypokinetic disorders, which are identical with the syndrome of parkinsonism; (2) hyperkinetic/choreic movement disorders; (3) tremors; and (4) myoclonus (Table 17.1).

The initial step in the diagnosis of a movement disorder is the description and classification of the abnormal movement. This is established by observing the abnormality and by conducting further neurological examination. Descriptive features of individual movement disorders are summarized in Table 17.2. In some cases, differentiating movement disorders can be difficult and at times unnecessary – for example, distinguishing mild myoclonus from chorea. Chorea, athetosis, and ballism are appropriately viewed as part of a spectrum of involuntary movements with a common pathophysiology.

Table 17.1. Classification of Movement Disorders

Hypokinetic Movement Disorders/Parkinsonism	Hyperkinetic/Choreic Movement Disorders
Parkinson's disease	Chorea
Drug-induced parkinsonism	Athetosis
Parkinsonism syndromes	Ballism (Hemiballism is more common)
	Dystonia
	Tics

Tremors	Myoclonus
Resting tremors	Generalized
Postural tremors	Segmental
Kinetic tremors	Focal
Task-related tremors	

Parkinsonism

Parkinsonism is a syndrome associated with deficient dopamine innervation or dopamine effect within the striatum (caudate and putamen). Any process interfering with striatal dopaminergic function can cause parkinsonism. The clinical picture is characteristic and composed of a related set of clinical features. The cardinal features are: (1) bradykinesia, slowness of movement with a paucity of normal spontaneous movements such as arm swing when walking; (2) rigidity, a form of increased resistance to passive manipulation in which the increased tone has a "plastic" (constant resistance to passive manipulation) quality or "cogwheel" rigidity (in which resistance has a ratchetlike characteristic); (3) tremor, typically a 4–6-Hz resting tremor of the hands/arms, legs, or chin that improves with use of the affected body part; and (4) impairment of postural reflexes, frequently manifested by falls or near falls, and by difficulty in maintaining a stable stance when displaced gently backward on examination. Symptoms and findings are often asymmetrical,

with onset on one side of the body. Patients commonly complain of incoordination, notably with fine motor tasks. Family members may note loss of facial expression (hypomimia or masked facies) or loss of voice amplitude (hypophonia). Historical features often useful in establishing a diagnosis are: difficulty with initiating or halting movement, especially getting in or out of chairs, and a history of micrographia, the tendency for letter size to become progressively smaller during handwriting. Examination reveals stooped posture, masked facies, saccadic pursuit eye movements, low-volume voice, reduced blinking rates, and generalized slowing of movement. Rapid, rhythmic movements such as finger tapping are reduced in speed and amplitude. Gait is often slow and shuffling, with loss of associated arm swing and the need to take several steps to turn. Tone is increased, with plastic (increased resistance throughout range of motion independent of velocity) or cogwheel (ratchetlike) quality. Patients can find it difficult to arise from a chair without use of their arms, and exhibit generalized problems with starting and stopping movement. Typically, postural reflexes are impaired. A characteristic resting tremor is often present in the hands, legs, or chin.

The primary differential diagnosis of this constellation of symptoms and findings is idiopathic Parkinson's disease, drug-induced parkinsonism, and rarer neurodegenerative disorders involving the basal ganglia. Medication history and exposure to antipsychotics, antiemetics, and some antihypertensives that can interfere with dopaminergic neurotransmissions are documented. In the absence of exposure to agents that block the effect of or deplete dopamine, a diagnosis of Parkinson's disease is most likely. A useful confirmatory diagnostic maneuver is treatment with carbidopa/L-dopa or alternative therapy for Parkinson's disease. Failure to respond significantly to an adequate trial of therapy suggests the presence of one of the neurodegenerative disorders that can affect the basal ganglia, which are heterogeneous and numerous but individually rare. A final and important point of differential diagnosis is to exclude essential tremor, a common cause of tremor in the elderly that lacks the other features of parkinsonism.

Parkinson's disease is the most common cause of parkinsonism, with several hundred thousand affected individuals in the United States. The inci-

TABLE 17.2. Phenomenology of Movement Disorders

Movement Disorder	Features	Areas of Involvement	Anatomical Localization
Parkinsonism	Bradykinesia, rigidity, often resting tremor, often postural instability, stooped posture, masked facies, hypophonia	Often asymmetrical at onset but can be generalized	Basal ganglia – interruption of or interference with nigrostriatal dopaminergic neurotransmission
Dystonia	Sustained, spasmodic, repetitive contractions causing involuntary abnormal postures	Any voluntary muscle can be affected; usually head, neck, face, and limbs	Presumed to be basal ganglia – associated with putamen lesions in some cases
Tremor	Involuntary, rhythmic, and roughly sinusoidal movements; some are action-induced	Head, hands, limbs, and voice	In parkinsonian resting tremor – basal ganglia. Most other tremors may involve cerebellar dysfunction
Chorea	Involuntary, irregular, rapid, jerky movements without a rhythmic pattern; dancelike	Generally limbs, but any body part can be affected	Basal ganglia – striatum or subthalamic nucleus
Athetosis	Akin to chorea but distinct "writhing" movements	Limbs, but any body part can be involved	Identical with chorea
Myoclonus	Brief, rapid, shocklike jerks	Generally involves very small muscles	Can result from dysfunction at any level of the central nervous system
Tics	Intermittent, brief, sudden, repetitive, stereotyped movements or sounds	Any body part can be affected; phonation sounds	Presumed to be basal ganglia
Hemiballism	Uncontrollable, rapid, large-amplitude flinging movements of a limb	Generally a limb	Basal ganglia – subthalamic nucleus striatum

dence increases with age, resulting in high prevalence in the elderly. Parkinson's disease usually has an insidious onset and is slowly progressive. Patients rarely present to the emergency department for initial evaluation, but some complications of Parkinson's disease and its treatment can result in problems requiring urgent attention. For example, falls are common in Parkinson's disease due to impaired postural reflexes and inability to respond rapidly to minor perturbations of balance. Significant trauma can result, leading to a need for urgent medical/orthopedic intervention.

Modern medical therapy with dopamine replacement and/or dopamine agonists provides excellent symptomatic relief for several years. Many patients experience progression of disease that results in poor response to medication or difficult-to-manage side effects. Many patients develop marked fluctuations in response to therapy, with periods of complex involuntary movements (dyskinesias). These dyskinesias have features of both dystonia and chorea occurring in close temporal association with periods of severe bradykinesia and rigidity. These fluctuations are difficult to manage and often require judicious manipulation of medications and dosage schedules over a long period of time for optimal control of symptoms. Choreic dyskinesias tend to occur at times when the effect of dopamine replacement therapy is at its peak. Choreic dyskinesias can be improved by decreasing medication doses or lengthening the dosing interval.

Nausea is another common problem associated with use of carbidopa/L-dopa or dopamine agonists. Nausea can be reduced by taking medications at the end of a meal to slow their absorption. For patients taking carbidopa/L-dopa, an adequate amount of carbidopa must be taken to block the peripheral effects of L-dopa and reduce nausea. For an average-size person, 75 mg of carbidopa is usually sufficient to reduce peripheral side effects. Other peripheral side effects include flushing and orthostatic hypotension. Orthostatic hypotension is especially troublesome, and some patients with Parkinson's disease can have autonomic insufficiency independent of drug treatment. Orthostatic hypotension can lead to syncope and falls, with their attendant consequences.

All medications used in the treatment of Parkinson's disease can cause altered mental status. Hallucinations are a relatively common side effect of carbidopa/L-dopa and dopamine agonists, and can occur with use of anticholinergics and amantadine. These hallucinations are usually visual, typically nonthreatening in character, and commonly occur in the absence of other features of delirium. However, typical delirium can also occur. Hallucinations, delirium, and other mental status changes occur most frequently in the many patients with Parkinson's disease who develop dementia. As with other demented patients, they are susceptible to the behavior-altering effects of many medications, not only dopamine replacement therapies. Frequent falls are a cause of minor, sometimes unnoticed, head trauma. In patients with Parkinson's disease who present with worsening mental status, subdural hematoma is an important diagnostic consideration.

Many patients with Parkinson's disease can manifest varied pain symptoms such as muscle spasms, cramps, and burning paresthesias.[1-4] These painful symptoms have several causes. Painful muscle spasms are common in patients with Parkinson's disease. Many patients with complex dyskinesias have a dystonic component to their involuntary movements that is painful. Patients with Parkinson's disease have uncomfortable paresthesias of uncertain cause. Severe localized limb pain, chest pain, or abdominal pain in the patient with Parkinson's disease can be difficult to diagnose in the emergency department.

Discontinuation of dopamine replacement therapy can cause the neuroleptic malignant syndrome, which is a medical emergency (see Chapter 40, "Neurotoxicology").

Hyperkinetic Movement Disorders

The hallmark of hyperkinetic movement disorders is the intrusion of involuntary movements into the normal flow of motor acts. Hyperkinetic movement disorders include dystonia, chorea, hemiballism, and tics. Distinguishing features of these movement disorders are presented in Table 17.2. A specific hyperkinetic movement disorder may not be present at all times in its standard form, and overlap of some of these disorders is common.

Dystonia. Dystonia is characterized by sustained (tonic), spasmodic (rapid or clonic), patterned or repetitive muscular contractions that frequently result in a wide range of involuntary twisting, repetitive movements, or abnormal postures. Abnormal postures such as neck torsion, forced jaw opening, or inversion and dorsiflexion of the foot are characteristic of dystonia. Dystonia can affect any voluntary muscle in the body, but some muscle groups are more commonly involved than others. Dystonia can be classified by the area of the body involved or by its etiology.

Some patients describe dystonia elicited by specific tasks or postures. For example, dystonia can be elicited by writing (writer's cramp) but not by other fine coordinated movements. Some patients with spasmodic dysphonia, a laryngeal dystonia, report difficulty with speaking but not with singing. Commonly, patients discover postures or maneuvers that reduce dystonia. The most frequently used "sensory trick" is gentle stimulation of one side of the face to reduce torticollis. Dystonia is one of the most frequently misdiagnosed neurological conditions.[5] It can be misinterpreted as a psychiatric or a hysterical condition because of (1) the patient's bizarre movements and postures, (2) the finding of "action-induced dystonia" (the exacerbation of symptoms with stress and improvement with relaxation), (3) diurnal fluctuations, and (4) frequent effectiveness of various sensory tricks.

TABLE 17.3. Classification of Dystonia Based on Distribution

Focal: involves a single body part
Blepharospasm: involves muscles of facial expression including orbicularis oculi
Torticollis: involves cervical muscles
Oromandibular dystonia: involves muscles of the jaw, tongue, and oropharynx
Spasmodic dysphonia: involves vocal cords
Occupational cramps (writer's cramp): involves hand
Multifocal: two or more noncontiguous body parts
Segmental cranial dystonia: two or more cranial and/or neck muscles
Segmental brachial dystonia: one arm plus axial muscles or both arms without or with axial muscles
Segmental axial dystonia: neck or trunk
Segmental crural dystonia: one leg plus trunk or two legs without or with trunk
Hemidystonia: arm and leg on the same side
Generalized: thigh or leg plus any other segment

Dystonia is commonly primary neurological disorder or a prominent manifestation of a neurological disorder due to metabolic derangement as occurs in Wilson's disease, Lesch-Nyhan syndrome, and mitochondrial cytopathies, or is secondary to structural central nervous system (CNS) injury (see Table 17.3). It is unlikely for a patient known to have one of these neurological disorders to present to the emergency department with dystonia as the primary concern. Patients with acute dystonic reactions associated with the use of certain medications typically present to the emergency department. A list of etiologies of selected dystonias is presented in Table 17.4.

Specific Dystonias

- *Idiopathic torsion dystonia (dystonia musculorum deformans):* Most common among Ashkenazi Jews, this is usually an autosomal dominant trait with variable penetrance.[6] This is the most common childhood-onset primary dystonia. In the early stages, the abnormal movements are characterized by "action dystonia" and commonly start in one leg. With progression of the disease, dystonia often becomes generalized and

is present at rest. The phenomenon of "overflow" can occur in generalized dystonia. "Overflow" refers to the activation of dystonia by action in some other area of the body, such as torticollis made worse by handwriting.

- *Focal dystonia:* Focal dystonia refers to the involvement of a specific part of the body. A primary dystonia that begins in adulthood is usually focal, for example, spasmodic torticollis. Torticollis can mimic a variety of orthopedic and neurological disorders that are important to recognize in the emergency department (Table 17.5).
- *Blepharospasm:* Blepharospasm is the second most common focal dystonia, either isolated or associated with oromandibular dystonia. It occurs more frequently in women than in men and is characterized by an increased frequency of blinking that progresses to clonic and then tonic closure of the eyelids. Blepharospasm can respond to sensory stimulation that occurs in talking, singing, and yawning. Approximately 15% of patients with blepharospasm cannot keep their eyes open and are functionally blind.[7]
- *Oromandibular dystonia:* Oromandibular dystonia is characterized by forced mouth opening, occasionally with tongue protrusion, or involuntary jaw clenching that can result in mutilation of the lips and teeth. Blepharospasm-oromandibular dystonia syndrome is commonly referred to as *Meige syndrome.*
- *Spasmodic dysphonia:* Spasmodic dysphonia is a form of laryngeal dystonia that causes spasm of the vocal cords. Patients are generally asymptomatic except for abnormalities of voice.
- *Writer's cramp:* Writer's cramp is a focal action dystonia described as task-specific. As suggested by the name, there is dystonia of the hand and arm when the patient attempts to write. A change in handwriting can be the presenting complaint. Pain can be prominent, but most patients complain of aching, dystonic spasms of the forearm musculature. Analogous task-specific dystonias involving other skilled hand tasks occur – for example, telegraphist's cramp, which was well described in the nineteenth century.
- *Dopa-responsive dystonia:* Dopa-responsive dystonia is a rare, treatable childhood-onset dystonia. This disorder is caused by a deficiency in guano-

TABLE 17.4. Etiologies of Selected Dystonias

Dystonia Due to Degenerative Disorders of CNS	Dystonia Due to Nondegenerative Disorders of CNS
Parkinson's disease	Traumatic brain injury
Huntington's disease	History of perinatal anoxia
Progressive supranuclear palsy	Kernicterus
Other degenerative disorders of the basal ganglia and midbrain	Stroke (cerebral infarction)
Wilson's disease	Arteriovenous malformation
Storage diseases	Encephalitis
GTP cyclohydrolase deficiency	Toxins (e.g., manganese)
Lesch-Nyhan disease	Brain tumors
Mitochondrial disorders	Multiple sclerosis
Leigh's syndrome	Drugs
	Peripheral trauma

sine triphosphate (GTP) cyclohydrolase activity that results in inadequate dopamine synthesis. It is readily treated by carbidopa/L-dopa. A family history and marked diurnal fluctuations in the intensity of this generalized dystonia suggest its presence. A trial of carbidopa/L-dopa is indicated.

- *Secondary dystonias:* Secondary dystonias are a consequence of underlying metabolic disorders, degenerative processes, or structural lesions. There are no distinguishing clinical features of secondary dystonia. However, sudden onset, presence of dystonia at rest, rapid progression, or an unusual distribution such as hemidystonia in an adult suggests secondary dystonia. A thorough neurological examination usually reveals dysfunction of other parts of the CNS, including the cranial nerves, pyramidal system, cerebellar system, or the higher cortical functions. Hemidystonia suggests a focal lesion such as a mass, infarction, or hemorrhage of the basal ganglia. Secondary dystonia can have delayed onset of weeks to years following a cerebral injury such as stroke. The most frequent causes of delayed-onset dystonia are perinatal trauma or hypoxia.
- *Torticollis:* Torticollis refers to dystonia-producing abnormal neck postures. Specifically, torticollis is rotation of the neck with anterocollis (flexion), retrocollis (extension), or laterocollis (lateral flexion). Causes of torticollis other than

dystonia are given in Table 17.5. Direct or indirect trauma to the neck suggests atlantoaxial subluxation. Gradually progressive extremity paresthesias and weakness suggest a herniated cervical disc. Visual disturbance and headaches can be caused by a posterior fossa tumor. Cervical adenopathy can cause torticollis in children. Associated neck dystonia with an impaired level of consciousness or other symptoms suggests the possibility of seizures. Dystonic torticollis can produce neurological complications such as cervical myelopathy or radiculopathy due to persistent abnormal neck postures.

EMERGENCY DEPARTMENT EVALUATION AND MANAGEMENT OF DYSTONIA. A comprehensive history and physical examination is directed toward distinguishing primary idiopathic dystonia from secondary dystonia due to a treatable cause. Presentation of primary dystonia in the emergency department is unlikely. However, it is important to distinguish dystonia from focal seizures. Recent-onset twisting and repetitive abnormal movements in an adult may respond to sensory stimuli or may be suppressed voluntarily.

Evaluation and management of drug-induced acute dystonic reactions is reviewed in a later section on drug-induced movement disorders. The patient with torticollis due to orthopedic or neurosur-

TABLE 17.5. Disorders Simulating Dystonic Torticollis (Cervical Dystonia)

Neurological disorders:
  Posterior fossa tumor
  Focal seizures
  Bobble-head syndrome (third ventricular cyst)
  Syringomyelia
  Congenital nystagmus
  Extraocular muscle palsies
  Arnold-Chiari malformation
Musculoskeletal/structural:
  Herniated cervical disc
  Rotational atlantoaxial subluxation
  Congenital muscular or ligamentous absence, laxity, or injury
  Bony spinal abnormalities: degenerative neoplastic infectious
  Cervical soft tissue lesions: adenitis, pharyngitis
  Labyrinthine disease
  Abnormal posture in utero

Source: Adapted from Weiner W, and Lang A. *Movement Disorders: A Comprehensive Survey.* Futura Publishing Company, Mount Kisco, New York (1989).

gically treatable disorders is referred to the appropriate specialist. Management of most dystonias is difficult, and generally symptomatic therapy is prescribed. Anticholinergic medications are frequently successful in ameliorating dystonia, but the high doses required are frequently better tolerated in children than in adults. For some secondary dystonias, treatment can be directed toward the few causes for which specific drug therapy is available, for example, Parkinson's disease and Wilson's disease. Management of neuroleptic-induced tardive dystonia requires reassessment of medication use. Botulinum toxin is an effective therapy for treating focal dystonias such as blepharospasm, oromandibular dystonia (especially jaw closing), spasmodic torticollis, spasmodic dysphonia, and cases of focal limb dystonia.

Chorea. *Chorea,* the Greek term for dance, consists of involuntary irregular, rapid, jerky movements without a rhythmic pattern, randomly distributed with a flowing "dancelike" quality that involves multiple body parts. Athetosis (writhing movement) and ballism are part of the spectrum of chorea, and appear to share a common pathophysiology, usually involving the striatum or subthalamic nucleus. Unlike primary dystonia, chorea/athetosis/ballism are regarded as symptoms of an underlying neurological disorder.

EMERGENCY DEPARTMENT EVALUATION AND DIFFERENTIAL DIAGNOSIS. Chorea can be a presenting symptom of a variety of neurological and nonneurological disorders (Table 17.6).[8] Chorea can be a manifestation of immunological, infectious, metabolic, degenerative, and drug- and toxin-induced disorders. It is important to recognize chorea as a distinct movement disorder and consider the possibility of an underlying cause that is amenable to therapy.

L-dopa-induced chorea in patients with parkinsonism is the "chorea" commonly encountered in the emergency department. When indicated, titration of L-dopa dosing can minimize the abnormal movements.

Systemic lupus erythematosus (SLE) and primary antiphospholipid antibody syndromes are the most frequent autoimmune causes of chorea. SLE is the systemic disorder most commonly associated with chorea, although only approximately 2% of patients with SLE have chorea. Chorea can be the only neurological finding that occurs before the diagnosis of SLE is made.[9] The chorea can last from days to years, and can be episodic and recurrent. The choreiform movements usually affect one side of the body (hemidistribution), although generalized chorea can occur. Other neurological symptoms or findings in SLE include migraine, stroke, seizures, cognitive impairment, peripheral neuropathy, and transient ischemic attacks.

Antiphospholipid antibody syndrome is associated with recurrent vascular thrombosis, recurrent spontaneous abortions, and stroke. An antiphospholipid antibody titer is obtained in cases of chorea associated with these clinical situations. The presence of antiphospholipid antibodies can cause false-positive Venereal Disease Research Laboratory (VDRL) test, or for anticardiolipin antibodies, or the lupus anticoagulant.[10] The mechanism of development of chorea in SLE is not known. Imaging studies are typically normal, and autoimmune-mediated injury to the basal ganglia has been postulated. Treatment with corticosteroids can be beneficial.[11]

TABLE 17.6. Differential Diagnosis of Chorea

Hereditary choreas
  Huntington's disease (classic choreiform movement)
  Neuroacanthocytosis
  Wilson's disease
  Benign familial chorea
  Inborn errors of metabolism
  Porphyria
  Ataxia-telangiectasia
  Tuberous sclerosis
Metabolic choreas
  Hyper- and hypothyroidism
  Hyper- and hypoparathyroidism
  Hypocalcemia
  Hyper- and hyponatremia
  Hypomagnesemia
  Hepatic encephalopathy
  Renal encephalopathy
Infectious or immunological choreas
  Sydenham's chorea (postrheumatic fever)
  Chorea gravidarum
  Systemic lupus erythematosus
  Polycythemia vera
  Multiple sclerosis
  Sarcoidosis
  Viral encephalitis
  Tuberous meningitis
Cerebrovascular choreas
  Basal ganglia infarction
  Arteriovenous malformation
  Venous angiomata
  Polycythemia
Structural choreas
  Posttraumatic
  Subdural and epidural hematoma
  Tumor (primary CNS or metastatic)
Drugs/medications
  Phenytoin, phenothiazines, lithium,
  Amphetamines, oral contraceptives, levodopa
Toxins
  Mercury, carbon monoxide
Infections
  Neurosyphilis
  Lyme disease
  Subacute sclerosing panencephalitis

There are case reports of transient chorea due to multiple sclerosis; sustained choreoathetosis is infrequent.[12–15]

Chorea that results from neuropathological lesions of basal ganglia caused by abscess can occur. Viral, bacterial, and tubercular meningitis are other rare infectious causes of chorea.

Structural lesions from cerebral infarctions involving the basal ganglia and thalamus can produce chorea. Stroke is likely the most common cause of hemichorea-hemiballismus.[16–18] Other causes include arteriovenous malformations, venous angiomas, metastatic tumors, or primary CNS neoplasms.

Chorea is rarely associated with hyperthyroidism or hypothyroidism. The pathophysiology of chorea in hyperthyroidism is not well understood but is likely due to altered function of the basal ganglia, particularly the striatum. Exaggerated physiological tremor is more common in hyperthyroidism; distinguishing this "toxic" tremor from chorea is straightforward. Although chorea is estimated to occur in approximately 2% of patients with hyperthyroidism,[19] the actual frequency may be less. Choreiform movements in patients with hyperthyroidism can be ameliorated by neuroleptic medication such as haloperidol.

Chorea associated with polycythemia rubra vera occurs in less than 1% of patients and is usually seen in older individuals. Other metabolic and endocrine causes of chorea are listed in Table 17.6.

Chorea gravidarum refers to choreiform movements associated with pregnancy (see Chapter 39, "Neurological Emergencies of Pregnancy") which is more common in patients who have a history of Sydenham's chorea. Approximately one-third of patients with chorea gravidarum have had Sydenham's chorea, suggesting that previous injury to the basal ganglia predisposes to chorea when estrogens and progesterone levels are elevated.[20,21] The use of oral contraceptives in women is associated with the development of chorea, especially in patients with a history of Sydenham's chorea.

Sydenham's chorea is a form of autoimmune chorea preceded by group A streptococcus infection, typically rheumatic fever. Unlike other manifestations of rheumatic fever, Sydenham's chorea occurs several months after the onset of acute streptococcal infection and usually affects patients between 5 and 15 years of age, girls more frequently than boys.[22] There appears to be a familial prevalence, suggesting hereditary susceptibility. It tends to occur abruptly, worsens over two to four weeks, and usually resolves spontaneously in three to six weeks. Although it occurs more commonly in children of developing countries who lack appropriate antibiotic care, outbreaks of Sydenham's chorea occur in the United States and other developed countries as well. Measurement of antistreptolysin-O titers can help physicians to detect recent streptococcal infection. However, Sydenham's chorea can occur six months after the streptococcal infection, and measurements of antistreptolysin-O and antistreptokinase antibody concentrations obtained later may not be helpful.

Chorea can be caused by a toxic effect of numerous drugs (see Table 17.6).

HEREDITARY AND DEGENERATIVE CAUSES OF CHOREA. *Huntington's disease* (*HD*) is an autosomal dominant, completely penetrant neurodegenerative disorder characterized by chorea, incoordination, dementia, and numerous psychiatric problems. HD is the most common choreiform neurodegenerative disorder. Athetosis and dystonia are common in HD. Neurobehavioral disturbances such as personality changes, agitation, apathy, depression, obsessive-compulsive disorders, social withdrawal, and sometimes features of psychosis can precede choreiform movements. Symptoms and signs of HD begin at any age but commonly present in the fourth and fifth decades. Life expectancy is approximately 15–20 years after diagnosis. Approximately 5% of all cases of HD begin in childhood. These patients tend to have parkinsonian features, rigidity, and dystonia rather than chorea. Along with rapid clinical progression, seizures frequently occur in these juvenile-onset cases.

Patients with HD are rarely diagnosed in the emergency department but are evaluated for complications for their disease that can require immediate care. Swallowing dysfunction can lead to poor nutrition and/or aspiration pneumonia, and sometimes asphyxia. Poor balance and coordination cause frequent falls. Because of cerebral atrophy, these patients are prone to subdural hematomas. Severe dysarthria, dysphagia, dementia, and loss of ambulation occur in the final stages of the disease, and these patients are prone to complications that accompany immobility. Psychiatric disorders are common in patients with HD and are the major cause of

difficulties in the earlier phases of the disease. Affective disorders are frequent and are associated with a high rate of suicide. Conventional treatment with antidepressants is frequently very successful. Many patients have obsessive-compulsive features, and treatment with serotonin selective reuptake inhibitors is frequently useful. Psychosis is rare and is treated conventionally. Other common behavioral problems include irritability, impulsivity, and generalized disinhibition. Other neurodegenerative disorders can exhibit chorea (see Table 17.6). Of these, Wilson's disease, which usually manifests a prominent dystonia, is the most important to consider in the differential diagnosis because it is the only treatable disorder.

MANAGEMENT. Chorea rarely requires treatment. Attention is focused on assessing the underlying cause of chorea. In some patients, chorea can be so violent as to become disabling. Medications that reduce dopaminergic neurotransmission can lessen the severity of chorea. The dopamine receptor antagonist haloperidol is the medication most frequently used to achieve this effect. Dopamine-depleting agents such as reserpine or tetrabenazine can also be effective. Chorea is not treated unless it interferes with function. In many patients, impairments of coordination or mentation result from the doses of dopamine antagonists needed to reduce chorea significantly.

Hemiballism

CHARACTERISTICS. This movement disorder is characterized by uncontrollable, rapid, large-amplitude proximal flinging movements of a limb. Unilateral involvement is termed *hemiballism*, whereas rare bilateral involvement is called *biballism*. Typically, the face is not affected. Hemiballism is an extreme form of hemichorea and is part of a spectrum that includes chorea and athetosis.[16] Formerly, hemiballism was attributed solely to lesions of subthalamic nucleus. It is now known that hemiballism can occur from lesions in other parts of the basal ganglia and the thalamus.

EMERGENCY DEPARTMENT EVALUATION AND MANAGEMENT. The most common cause of hemiballism is stroke, generally a lacunar infarct in the subthalamic nucleus. Hemiballism occurs most frequently in individuals over 60 years of age with risk factors for stroke. Other causes of hemiballism are listed in

TABLE 17.7. Causes of Hemiballism

Cerebrovascular events:	ischemic, hemorrhagic arteriovenous malformation, subarachnoid hemorrhage
Space-occupying lesions:	metastatic cancer, subthalamic nucleus cyst
Infections:	tuberculous meningitis
Cerebral trauma	
Metabolic disorders:	nonketotic hyperosmolar state
Multiple sclerosis	
Drugs:	phenytoin toxicity oral contraceptives and estrogens levodopa
Complications of stereotactic surgery	

Source: Adapted from Weiner W J. and Lang L., *Movement Disorders: A Comprehensive Survey.* Futura Publishing Company. Mount Kisco, 1989.

Table 17.7. Common predisposing factors include hypertension, diabetes, thrombocytosis, or vasculitis.

Appropriate measures are taken to prevent injuries caused by violent hemiballistic movements. Disabling hemiballism requires immediate symptomatic relief even when the cause is not known. Neuroleptic medication such as haloperidol is most effective. Following a focused history and physical examination, ancillary tests are directed at diagnosing metabolic disorders, particularly a nonketotic hyperosmolar state. A history of medication use including estrogens, oral contraceptives, phenytoin toxicity, and levodopa is sought. CT of the brain may reveal evidence of a stroke.

Tics

CHARACTERISTICS. Tics are the most common movement disorders. They are characterized by intermittent, sudden, repetitive, stereotyped movements (motor tics) or sounds (vocal tics). Tics can be abrupt and fast, or slow and sustained. Tics can result from contraction of only one group of muscles, causing *simple tics,* which are brief, jerklike movements or single, meaningless sounds. *Complex tics* result from a coordinated sequence of movements

TABLE 17.8. Classification of Tics

Simple Motor Tics

eye blinking, eyebrow raising, nose flaring, grimacing, mouth opening, tongue protrusion, platysma contraction, head jerking, shoulder shrugging or abduction, neck stretching, arm jerks, fist clenching, abdominal tensing, pelvic thrusting, buttock or sphincter tightening, hip flexion or abduction, kicking, knee extension, foot dorsiflexion, toe curling

Simple phonic tics

sniffing, grunting, throat clearing, shrieking, yelping, barking, growling, squealing, snorting, coughing, hissing, clicking, humming, moaning

Complex motor tics

head shaking, teeth gnashing, wrist shaking, finger cracking, touching, hitting, jumping, skipping, stamping, squatting, kicking, smelling hands/objects, rubbing, finger twiddling, echopraxia, copropraxia, spitting, exaggerated startle

Complex vocal tics

coprolalia (wide variety, including shortened words), unintelligible words, whistling, "Bronx cheer," panting, belching, hiccough, stuttering, stammering, echolalia, palilalia

(see Table 17.8). Complex vocal tics can include linguistically meaningful utterances. Sustained tics, also known as *dystonic tics,* are commonly associated with premonitory feelings that are relieved by performance of a particular "tic." Sensory tics are patterns of uncomfortable, somatic sensations such as pressure, tickle, or temperature change localized to a specific part of the body that result in dysphoric feelings.[23] Patients often admit that the tic occurs as an unavoidable but purposeful performance of the movement or sound. Tics can be suppressed temporarily, and often wax and wane in type, frequency, and severity.

EMERGENCY DEPARTMENT EVALUATION AND DIFFERENTIAL DIAGNOSIS OF TICS. Tics rarely present as an emergency. They represent a continuum from a mild, transient form to a potentially devastating neurobehavioral disorder. Several neurological and nonneurological disorders are associated with tics (see Table 17.9). Simple tics are common and are exhibited by much of the population. Tics can be associated with stroke, head trauma, encephalitis, pos-

TABLE 17.9. Etiological Classification of Tics

Primary tic disorders
  Tourette's syndrome
  Various chronic tic disorders
Secondary tic disorders
  Inherited: Huntington's disease
         Neuroacanthocytosis
         Torsion dystonia
         Chromosomal abnormalities
  Acquired: *Drugs* – neuroleptics, stimulants,
         anticonvulsants, levodopa
         Trauma
         Infections – encephalitis, Creutzfeldt-Jakob
         disease, Sydenham's chorea
         Developmental – mental retardation, static
         encephalopathy, autism, pervasive
         developmental disorder
         Stroke
         Degenerative – parkinsonism, progressive
         supranuclear palsy
         Toxic – carbon monoxide poisoning

Source: Adapted with permission from Kurlan Roger (ed), *Treatment of Movement Disorders*, J.B. Lippincott Company, Philadelphia, 1995.

tencephalitic syndrome of encephalitis lethargica, brain tumors, and carbon monoxide poisoning. They can occur as a result of long-term neuroleptic use (tardive tics).

The most well-known tic disorder is Gilles de la Tourette's syndrome. *Tourette's syndrome (TS)* is a disorder characterized by childhood onset of motor and vocal tics. Obsessive-compulsive disorder (OCD) and attention deficit hyperactivity disorder (ADHD) are strongly associated with TS. The established criteria for diagnosis of TS are: onset before age 21 years; multiple motor tics; one or more vocal tics; and a fluctuating course and presence of tics longer than one year. Males are affected more frequently than females, and there is a substantial genetic component.[24] Nongenetic factors such as maternal life stressors during pregnancy, gender of the child, and severe hyperemesis gravidarum are known to influence the form and severity of TS. The precise neuroanatomical location of a pathological

lesion in TS is not known, although striatal abnormalities are possible. The biochemical basis of TS is likely an increased activity of the dopaminergic system. TS frequently has a variable course, with waxing and waning of tics over several years. Tics tend to worsen in adolescence and abate in adulthood.

Tic disorders that are present in childhood for less than one year are categorized as transient tic disorder (TTD) and are common among school-aged children, with an estimated prevalence of 5–24%. It is important not to confuse TTD with TS. Inappropriate assignment of a diagnosis of TS can be distressing to parents and children.

MANAGEMENT. Dopamine receptor antagonists (neuroleptics) are most effective in controlling tics. Haloperidol is used in doses ranging from 0.25–2.5 mg per day. Higher doses can be used acutely. Clonidine, an alpha$_2$-adrenergic receptor agonist, can be useful in treating TS. Selective serotonin reuptake inhibitors such as fluoxetine are widely used to treat OCD, which is frequently associated with TS. Because of the possibilities of developing a tardive movement disorder and other complications of neuroleptic use, these agents are reserved for disabling tics. Initial treatment with clonidine is preferred. A comprehensive assessment of a patient with TS is performed by a team of professionals, including a psychiatrist, social worker, and neurologist, and a pediatrician when indicated.

Tremors

CHARACTERISTICS. *Tremors* are defined as involuntary, rhythmic, and roughly sinusoidal movements.[25] It is useful to characterize tremor as resting, postural, kinetic, or task-related. *Resting tremor* refers to tremor while a body part is relaxed without the influence of gravity. *Postural tremor* occurs during maintenance of steady body posture against gravity. This is usually assessed by asking patients to extend their arms in front of them. *Kinetic tremor* occurs during goal-directed movements such as finger-to-nose testing. *Task*-related tremors occur only during the performance of a specific task, for example, a primary writing tremor. *Intention tremor* is an imprecise term generally used to describe wide oscillations that occur when a limb approaches a precise destination. Tremor, with its regular and stereotyped quality, is differentiated from dysmetria,

TABLE 17.10. Conditions that Can Enhance Physiological Tremor

Mental state: anger, anxiety, stress, fatigue, excitement
Metabolic: fever, thyrotoxicosis, pheochromocytoma, hypoglycemia
Drugs and toxins: (see Table 17.11)
Miscellaneous: caffeinated beverages, monosodium glutamate, nicotine

Source: Adapted from Weiner W. and Lang A. *Movement Disorders: A Comprehensive Survey.* Futura Publishing Company, Mount Kisco, (1989).

TABLE 17.11. Well-Known Causes of Tremor

Physiological
Pathological
 Essential tremor
 Parkinson's disease
 Wilson's disease
 Midbrain tremor
 Peripheral neuropathy
 Multiple sclerosis
 Cerebellar infarction
 Cerebellar degenerative disorders
Drugs and toxins
 Neuroleptics
 Lithium
 Adrenocorticosteroids
 Beta-adrenergic receptor agonists
 Theophylline
 Ethanol
 Calcium channel blockers
 Valproic acid
 Thyroid hormone
 Caffeine
 Nicotine
 Tricyclic antidepressants
Psychogenic

which is irregular and involves inaccuracy of directed movement.

EMERGENCY DEPARTMENT EVALUATION. Isolated tremors are not medical emergencies unless accompanied by other focal neurological findings resulting from various causes such as cerebral infarction, hemorrhage, or demyelination.

CLASSIFICATION AND CLINICAL FEATURES OF TREMORS. As with other movement disorders, a descriptive characterization of tremor is most important.

- *Physiological tremor* is a normal phenomenon due to the viscoelastic properties of joints and limbs. It can worsen because of anxiety, fatigue, or stress (Table 17.10). Hypoglycemia, hyperthyroidism, and pheochromocytoma can enhance physiological tremors. Normal physiological and enhanced physiological tremors are minimal at rest, present with posture, and worse with use of the affected limb. Endocrine disorders are included in the differential diagnosis of new-onset tremor (Tables 17.10 and 17.11). Since thyrotoxicosis can cause tremor, thyroid function tests are obtained. Many medications can cause tremor (Tables 17.10 and 17.11), likely by exacerbating physiological tremor.
- *Essential tremor (ET)* is a distinct neurological syndrome characterized by postural and kinetic tremor of the hands, isolated head tremor, and voice tremor with no identifiable cause such as drugs or toxins, or other focal neurological findings. ET can begin at any age; however, its incidence rises markedly with advancing years, mak-

ing it common in the elderly. ET is differentiated from parkinsonism. The tremor of parkinsonism is usually a resting tremor, and patients with ET do not have other features of parkinsonism. ET is a slowly progressive disorder with variable clinical expression. Patients typically complain of difficulty with eating, writing, and drinking, and ET can cause significant disability. A useful diagnostic maneuver is to have patients drink a cup of water. Affected individuals will usually have a marked exacerbation of tremor while holding the cup, which worsens as the cup approaches the mouth. In approximately 50% of patients, there is an affected first-degree relative (benign familial tremor), although many cases are thought to be sporadic (benign essential tremor). Findings that support the diagnosis of ET include improvement with the use of alcohol, propranolol, or primidone. ET can be exacerbated by emotional stress, anxiety, thyrotoxicosis, caffeine, and other stimulants. Hereditary and acquired demyelinating neuropathies are associated with an ET-like tremor. Common variants of ET are head tremor and voice tremor. Head tremor is often rotatory to nodding in quality and is virtually unique to ET. It is important to distinguish chin or jaw tremor, which is more frequent in parkinsonism, and to recognize that torticollis has a low-frequency rotatory head tremor, possibly the result of habitual attempts to correct neck position. The pathophysiology of ET is unknown but is likely due to alterations in cerebellar function.

Propranolol in a dose of 240–320 mg per day is a widely accepted treatment for ET. Other medications that treat ET with variable success include primidone, benzodiazepines, and other sedative-hypnotic medications.

- *Task-related tremors* occur during specific motor tasks. The most commonly occurring is primary writing tremor. Benzodiazepines can be useful in treating these unusual tremors.
- *Orthostatic tremor* is a rare but frequently misdiagnosed condition. It occurs more frequently in women, and the onset is typically in the sixth decade. It manifests as tremor of the legs triggered by standing.[26] Although clinically unreliable, evaluation of orthostatic blood pressures is a common practice in the emergency department. Orthostatic tremor is distinguished from ataxia and is unrelated to orthostasis.
- *Cerebellar tremor* is a common consequence of injury to the cerebellum or its outflow pathways. This type of tremor is called a rubral tremor because it can be seen after injury to the region of the red nucleus. However, the tremor likely results from injury to closely situated efferent cerebellar projections. This type of tremor can have resting, postural, and kinetic components. It is commonly described as affecting proximal muscles and is invariably associated with ataxia, dysmetria, and other signs of cerebellar dysfunction.
- *Psychogenic tremor* is the typical hysterical movement disorder. Careful observation of the patient with psychogenic tremor reveals marked fluctuation of the tremor. Patients demonstrate marked tremor that improves significantly when they are distracted. Other signs of functional illness are nonphysiological sensory deficits, tunnel vision, and bizarre gait disturbance (Table 17.12).

TABLE 17.12. Features of Psychogenic Tremor

1. History of many undiagnosed conditions
2. History of multiple somatizations
3. Absence of significant finding on physical examination or imaging study
4. Presence of secondary gain (pending compensation or litigation)
5. Spontaneous remissions and exacerbations
6. Employment in the health care delivery field
7. History of psychiatric illness

Myoclonus

CHARACTERISTICS. Myoclonus is defined as brief, very rapid, sudden, and shocklike jerks that involve very small muscles or the entire body. These movements can be caused by active muscle contractions (positive myoclonus) or lapses in posture or muscle contractions (negative myoclonus or asterixis). Each jerk or sudden movement is a discrete, separate movement, in contrast to chorea, where dancelike, continual flow of movement occurs from one body part to another without interruption. Myoclonus differs from "tic syndromes" in that tics are stereotypic in quality and anatomical distribution, and can generally be suppressed with conscious effort by the patient. A good example of physiological myoclonus is hiccup, which is called *diaphragmatic myoclonus*. Myoclonus is a descriptive term and not a diagnosis. Myoclonus does not indicate a specific etiology and is not useful in neuroanatomical localization of disease processes.[27] Myoclonus can arise from several sites within the neuraxis.[28,29]

CLASSIFICATION AND CLINICAL FEATURES. The four broad categories of myoclonus are: (1) physiological, (2) essential or idiopathic, (3) epileptic, and (4) symptomatic.

1. *Physiological myoclonus* occurs in normal people and includes sleep (hypnic) jerks, anxiety-induced myoclonus, exercise-induced myoclonus, and hiccup.
2. *Essential myoclonus* is likely an autosomal dominant hereditary disorder which begins at a young age and generally has a benign course. EEG and neurological examinations are essentially nor-

mal. This syndrome is rare. Essential myoclonus is idiopathic and progresses slowly or not at all.

3. *Epileptic myoclonus,* as the term suggests, occurs in the setting of a chronic seizure disorder, and is a component of several different epileptic syndromes. Myoclonus can occur as a component of a seizure or as the sole manifestation of a seizure.

4. *Symptomatic myoclonus* refers to myoclonic syndromes associated with an identifiable underlying neurological or nonneurological disorder. This is the most common cause of myoclonus. Associated neurological deficits include encephalopathy, dementia, ataxia, and pyramidal or extrapyramidal signs as dominant features of the illness. When recognized, clinical disorders responsible for this group of myoclonus may be treatable.

Posthypoxic myoclonus resulting from global cerebral hypoxia from any cause is an established clinical entity that occurs in two forms. Transient rhythmic myoclonic jerks can appear immediately following the hypoxic injury, while the patient is comatose. This signifies a very poor prognosis.[31,32] The second clinical form is delayed posthypoxic myoclonus, known as Lance-Adams syndrome, which is observed in patients during recovery from coma following cerebral hypoxic injury. This form of myoclonus characteristically demonstrates myoclonic jerks that are aggravated or precipitated by attempted movement. This is associated with anesthesia-related cerebral hypoxia, myocardial infarction, drug overdose, and airway obstruction.[33,34] The pathological basis of posthypoxic myoclonus is related to inhibition of serotonergic neurons.

Symptomatic myoclonus resulting from metabolic derangements such as uremia, hepatic coma, hypercapnia, and hypoglycemia usually produce multifocal, arrhythmic myoclonic jerks predominantly affecting the face and proximal musculature. Changes in mental status are characteristic. Generalized myoclonic activity can be prominent in the illness. The myoclonus resolves as the encephalopathy is corrected. No specific therapeutic measure is required.

Segmental myoclonus is a form of symptomatic myoclonus that refers to arrhythmic or rhythmic, involuntary, and repetitive contractions of muscles supplied by one or a few contiguous segments of the spinal cord or brainstem.[35] Common causes are inflammatory, demyelinating, posttraumatic, vascular, and neoplastic in origin (Table 17.13). Focal cortical lesions due to various causes can result in focal myoclonus.[31,36]

Asterixis, or *negative myoclonus,* was described originally in patients with hepatic encephalopathy but occurs in other metabolic or toxic disorders (Table 17.13). Asterixis can occur in the recovery phase of general anesthesia, with sedative or anticonvulsant drug administration, and in normal drowsy individuals.[37,38]

EMERGENCY DEPARTMENT EVALUATION. Immediate control of myoclonus may be required in certain cases of intractable myoclonus. Although rare, intractable myoclonus (as in viral encephalitis) can cause hyperthermia, hyperkalemia, hyperuricemia, systemic hypotension, and renal failure secondary to rhabdomyolysis.[30] Myoclonus can be a manifestation of serious underlying disease processes such as toxic or metabolic encephalopathies, or chronic epileptic disorders requiring urgent medical attention (see Table 17.12).

The focus of the examination in the emergency department is to determine the pathological basis of the underlying illness. Serum glucose levels, electrolytes, hepatic and renal function tests, and drug and toxin screens, brain imaging, and urgent EEG can assist in determining most common metabolic and neurological derangements. Advanced studies such as evoked potentials, determination of enzyme activities (for storage disorders), DNA tests, tissue biopsy (for storage disorders and mitochondrial disease), or copper studies (for Wilson's disease) require referral to a neurologist.

Management of myoclonic movements in the emergency department is directed to specific management of the underlying illness in cases of symptomatic myoclonus. In certain situations, valproic acid and clonazepam are effective in treating symptomatic myoclonus.[39,40] Physiological myoclonus does not require specific treatment. Reassuring the patient is helpful. Standard antiepileptic drug therapy is used for myoclonus that is a component of an epileptic syndrome.

Movement Disorders Caused by Commonly Used Drugs

Numerous movement disorders are attributed to the use of various medications. The cause-and-

TABLE 17.13. Differential Diagnoses of Myoclonus

Physiological myoclonus:
  Hypnic jerks (jerks induced during sleep)
  Anxiety-induced myoclonus
  Hiccup (singultus)
  Exercise-induced myoclonus
  Benign infantile myoclonus during feeding
*Essential myoclonus (no known cause and no other
neurological deficit)*
  Hereditary (autosomal dominant)
  Sporadic
Epileptic myoclonus (seizures are the dominant feature)
*Symptomatic myoclonus (progressive or static
encephalopathy dominates):*
  Storage diseases:
    Lafora body disease
    Ceroid lipofuscinosis (Batten disease)
    Lipidoses – gangliosidoses, Tay-Sachs disease, and
    others
  Ataxic syndromes (mostly spinocerebellar
  degenerations):
    Friedreich ataxia
    Ataxia-telangiectasia
  Basal ganglia degenerations:
    Wilson's disease
    Huntington's disease
    Torsion dystonia
    Parkinson's disease
    Progressive supranuclear palsy
  Dementias:
    Alzheimer's disease
    Creutzfeldt-Jakob disease
  Viral encephalopathies:
    Herpes simplex encephalitis
    Arbovirus encephalitis
    Human immunodeficiency virus (HIV)
    Encephalitis lethargica

Postinfectious encephalitis
Subacute sclerosing panencephalitis
Metabolic entities:
  Hepatic failure
  Renal failure
  Hyponatremia
  Hypoglycemia
  Nonketotic hyperglycemia
  Dialysis syndrome
Toxic and drug-induced syndromes:
  Heavy metal intoxications
  Psychiatric medications: Cyclic antidepressants
    selective serotonin uptake inhibitors
    monoamine oxidase inhibitors
    lithium, buspirone, clozapine
  Antibiotics: penicillin, carbenicillin, ticarcillin,
    isoniazid, piperazine, acyclovir,
    monolactam, vidarabine, cefmetazole
  Narcotics
  Anticonvulsants: phenytoin, valproic acid,
  carbamazepine
  Anesthetics: etomidate, isoflurane, tetracaine,
  midazolam, enflurane
  Contrast media
  Cardiac medications: calcium channel blockers
    antiarrhythmics – flecainide
  Antineoplastics: chlorambucil, prednimustine
  Miscellaneous medications: levodopa,
  metoclopramide, physostigmine, bromocriptine
Physical encephalopathies:
  Posthypoxia (Lance-Adams syndrome)
  Posttraumatic
  Heat stroke
  Electrical shock
  Decompression injury

Source: Adapted from Fahn S, Marsden CD, Van Woert MH. Definition and classification for myoclonus. *Adv Neurol.* 1986;
43:1–5.

effect relationship between the drug and the movement disorder is poorly understood, but preexisting CNS pathology likely predisposes to the development of movement disorders. Many movement disorders improve after the offending medication is discontinued. Severe disability may require immediate intervention, as in the case of an acute dystonic reaction. Commonly prescribed medications that result in movement disorders include the following groups: antiepileptics; neuroleptics, stimulants, oral contraceptives, calcium channel blockers, antihistaminics and anticholinergics, and antidepressants.

Antiepileptics. Cerebellar signs including nystagmus, dysarthria, and ataxia are commonly associated with toxic levels of antiepileptics, most typically phenytoin and carbamazepine. Asterixis and spontaneous myoclonic jerks are common in the toxicity of phenytoin, phenobarbital, primidone, and carbamazepine. Chorea and dystonia can be observed with antiepileptic drug use.[41,42] Chorea is generally associated with the chronic use of multiple antiepileptics. Initial use rarely results in chorea or dystonia, which can occur with intravenous administration of phenytoin for status epilepticus.[43] This effect resolves gradually as the peak drug levels decrease.

Postural tremor, similar to benign essential tremor or enhanced physiological tremor, is observed in approximately 20–25% of patients taking valproate.[44] Severity of tremor does not directly correlate with serum drug levels of valproate, but symptoms subside with decreasing drug levels.

Neuroleptics. The literal meaning of neuroleptic is "that which grips the nerve." There are five major categories of movement disorders associated with the use of neuroleptic medications: (1) acute dystonic reaction (ADR); (2) akathisia; (3) parkinsonism; (4) neuroleptic malignant syndrome (NMS); and (5) tardive disorders. Tardive disorders occur with prolonged use of neuroleptics. ADR, akathisia, and parkinsonism can occur early in the treatment, and NMS can occur at any time. The dopamine-blocking effects of neuroleptic medications are likely the pharmacological basis for the development of these movement disorders.

Acute dystonic reaction usually occurs at the initiation of neuroleptic therapy; 95% of episodes of ADR occur within 96 hours of initiation of therapy.[45] ADR has a familial incidence and is more common in children, and young males, and in relatives of patients with idiopathic torsion dystonia (ITD). Females between the ages of 12 and 19 years are more prone to metoclopramide (Reglan) induced ADR.[46] A history of ADR with neuroleptic therapy is an indicator for future risk.[47] Cocaine abuse increases the risk of neuroleptic-induced ADR.[48]

ADR typically involves cranial or truncal musculature. Children tend to have more generalized involvement, particularly the trunk and extremities. Adults have a more restricted involvement of cranial, neck, and upper limb musculature. ADR is the most common cause of oculogyric crisis, which consists of forced conjugate eye deviation upward or laterally, often accompanied by extension or lateral

movements of the neck, mouth opening, and tongue protrusion. Blepharospasm, grimacing, trismus, forceful jaw opening, and tongue twisting are examples of involvement of other cranial musculature. Milder forms of muscle involvement can present as muscle cramps or tightness of jaw and tongue, leading to difficulty chewing, swallowing, and speaking. Respiratory stridor with resultant cyanosis can occur in patients with severe ADR.[49] ADR can result in extremely disabling dysarthria, dysphagia, jaw dislocation, compromised extremity function, and abnormal gait. ADR typically follows a varied course, with symptoms lasting from minutes to hours. ADR can be difficult to diagnose in the emergency department because abnormal movements can subside or fluctuate spontaneously, and can improve with reassurance of the patient.

The risk of developing ADR increases with the potency of the neuroleptic and occurs more frequently with parental neuroleptics than with oral medications.

ADR resolves spontaneously when the offending drug is withheld. The duration of symptoms depends on the half-life of the drug. Symptoms of ADR can be controlled quickly by parenteral administration of anticholinergics such as benztropine (cogentin) or biperiden. The initial dose of benztropine is 2 mg given intravenously, with a maintenance dose of 1–2 mg orally twice daily for 7–14 days to prevent recurrence. Alternatively, diphenhydramine, which has antihistaminic and anticholinergic properties, can be given in a dose of 25–50 mg parenterally for rapid control of symptoms, and a maintenance dose of 25–50 mg orally three to four times daily for a few days. Some neurologists prescribe prophylactic use of amantadine for young males requiring neuroleptic therapy.

Tardive disorders (TD) occurs following prolonged use of neuroleptic medications in about 20% of patients treated with these drugs.[50] TD is often precipitated or worsened when the dose of the neuroleptic is reduced or the drug is withdrawn. Increasing age increases the risk for developing tardive dyskinesia,[51] and the probability of spontaneous remission declines with advancing age.

Involuntary stereotypical movements involving orofacial, neck, trunk, and axial muscles constitute the typical tardive dyskinesia. Patients commonly demonstrate pursing, smacking, chewing with frequent tongue protrusion, or pushing the tongue into the inner cheek. Twiddling movements of the hands, pelvic thrusting, or rocking of the legs is also common. Some patients have true "akathisia" or restlessness with the constellation of abnormal movements. Other forms of TD include *tardive dystonia,* where dystonic movements predominate, and *tardive Tourettism,* where tics dominate the clinical picture. Tardive chorea can occur.

Neuroleptic medication is given in reduced dose or discontinued with the earliest signs of TD. This typically causes the underlying psychiatric condition to worsen. Hence, the need for continued neuroleptic therapy is weighed against the morbidity caused by TD. The antipsychotic medication clozapine can reduce the incidence of TD and improve TD in up to 44% of patients.[52] Clozapine is associated with significant adverse effects. Dopamine-depleting agents such as reserpine or tetrabenazine can be used successfully, and anticholinergics can be used for tardive dystonia.

Drug-induced parkinsonism (DIP) can be caused by several different medications. In addition to neuroleptic medications, calcium channel blockers (cinnarizine and flunarizine), antinausea medication (metoclopramide), and antihypertensive agents (reserpine) can cause DIP. The features of DIP are generally indistinguishable from those of idiopathic parkinsonism. A rhythmic, perioral, and perinasal tremor mimicking a rabbit chewing, termed *rabbit syndrome,* is typical of DIP.[53] The risk of developing DIP is higher in females than in males. Other risk factors include the dose and potency of neuroleptic medications. Anticholinergics and amantadine are frequently used to treat DIP, with variable success.

Akathisia is a subjective sensation of restlessness commonly associated with the inability to remain seated.[54] Abnormal limb sensation, inner restlessness, dysphoria, and anxiety are the commonly described symptoms associated with akathisia. This disabling condition can be mistaken for psychiatric illness such as agitation, hyperactivity, or anxiety in patients with agitated depression or schizophrenia.[55] Symptoms abate when the responsible medication is withheld, but management of this disorder is often very difficult.

Stimulants. Dextroamphetamine, methylphenidate (Ritalin), pemoline, and cocaine are all stimulant (dopaminomimetic) drugs with peripheral and central actions. Commonly associated movement disorders with acute and chronic use of these drugs include chorea, orofacial dyskinesia, stereotyped movements, dystonia, and tics. Of these, the most common are stereotyped movements – comprising compulsive and complex activities that can occupy a person for hours. These movement disorders can manifest without evidence of "other" stimulant effects such as postural tremor, psychosis, or insomnia. Development or enhancement of certain ticlike behaviors such as nail biting is associated with the use of stimulants.

Oral Contraceptives. Chorea is the most frequently experienced movement disorder caused by the use of oral contraceptives in otherwise healthy young females. It typically develops in a nulliparous woman who has been taking the contraceptive for nine weeks.[21] A unilateral distribution of chorea suggests the possibility of preexisting basal ganglia pathology. Symptoms generally abate within a few weeks following discontinuation of the contraceptive.

Calcium Channel Blockers. The calcium channel blockers most frequently responsible for movement disorders are flunarizine and cinnarizine, which are sometimes used for migraine prophylaxis and the treatment of vertigo. The features of the movement disorder most often mimic those of drug-induced parkinsonism, although acute dystonic reactions, akathisia, orofacial tremor, and tardive dyskinesia can occur. Females are at greater risk, as are the elderly. The incidence of movement disorders with the use of other calcium channel blockers is low, which supports the role of dopaminergic system involvement unique to cinnarizine and flunarizine.[56,57]

Antihistaminics and Anticholinergics. The use of chlorpheniramine, brompheniramine, phenindamine, and mebhydroline is associated with the development of orofacial dyskinesia, blepharospasm, ticlike movements, dystonia, and involuntary, semipurposeful movements of the hands.[43] Acute dystonic reaction with the use of diphenhydramine (Benadryl) has occurred.[57] The H_2 receptor blockers cimetidine and ranitidine are associated with the development of postural and action tremor, dystonic reactions, parkinsonism, confusion, and cerebellar dysfunction.[58] The movement abnormalities induced by these agents are generally short-lived and resolve after the responsible medication is discontinued.

Antidepressants. The use of monoamine oxidase (MAO) inhibitors is associated with tremors and less often with myoclonic jerks.[59] Tricyclic antidepressants such as amitriptyline, imipramine, and nortriptyline cause choreiform movements infrequently, particularly orofacial dyskinesia.[60,61] The anticholinergic effects of tricyclic antidepressants are likely partially responsible for the development of chorea. As with MAO inhibitors, an overdose of tricyclic antidepressants is associated with myoclonus.

PEARLS AND PITFALLS

- Movement disorders resulting from an acute event such as a stroke are rare but are commonly manifested in a localized body area or follow a "hemidistribution," as in hemidystonia or hemiballism.
- An emergency imaging study is most likely to yield positive results following the acute onset of focal, abnormal movements.
- Falls due to impaired postural reflexes in a patient with Parkinson's disease can result in significant trauma.
- Prescribed medications are the most common cause of mental status change in a patient with Parkinson's disease.
- Many patients with Parkinson's disease manifest varied pain symptoms such as painful muscle spasms, cramps, and burning paresthesias. Localized limb pain, chest pain, and abdominal pain can be difficult to diagnose in the emergency department.
- Torticollis is a focal dystonia producing abnormal neck postures that can be due to orthopedic and other neurological conditions.
- Neuroleptic medications and phenothiazines are responsible for most of the acute dystonic reactions evaluated in the emergency department.

- Although chorea can be a manifestation of immunological, infectious, metabolic, degenerative, or drug- and toxin-induced disorders, the most common "chorea" evaluated in the emergency department is L-dopa-induced chorea in a patient with Parkinson's disease.
- Chorea can be associated with the chronic use of numerous antiepileptic drugs.
- Transient tic disorder is common in children, with an estimated prevalence of 5–24% in school-age children. Conditions such as chronic cough or behavioral disorders can mimic this disorder in the emergency department.
- Asterixis, or "negative myoclonus," was described originally in patients with hepatic encephalopathy but occurs in toxic and metabolic derangements including those related to drugs.
- Many movement disorders commonly evaluated in clinical practice are due to medication use.

REFERENCES

1. Quinn NP, Koller WC, Lang AE, Marsden CD. Painful Parkinson's Disease. *Lancet.* 1986;1:1366.
2. Goetz CG, Lance CM, Levy M, et al. Pain in idiopathic Parkinson's disease. *Mov Disord* 1986;1:45.
3. Koller WC. Sensory symptoms in Parkinson's disease. *Neurology.* 1984;34:957.
4. Snider SR, Fahn S, Isgreen WP, et al. Primary sensory symptoms in Parkinsonism. *Neurology.* 1976;26:423.
5. Fahn S. The varied clinical expressions of dystonia. *Neurol Clin.* 1984;2:541–54.
6. Zeman W, Dyken P. Dystonia musculorum deformans. Clinical, genetic and pathoanatomical studies. *Psychiatria, Neurologia, Neurochirurgia.* 1967;70:77–121.
7. Jankovic J, Orman J. Blepharospasm. Demographic and clinical survey of 250 patients. *Ann Ophthalmol.* 1984;16:371.
8. Shoulson I. On Chorea. *Clin Neuropharmacol.* 1986;9:585.
9. Bruyn GW, Padberg G. Chorea and systemic lupus erythematosus – a critical review. *Eur Neurol.* 1984;23:278–90.
10. Hughes GRV. Thrombosis, abortion, cerebral disease and the lupus anticoagulant. *Br Med J.* 1983;297:1088.
11. Lahat E, Eschal G, Azizi E, et al. Chorea associated with systemic lupus erythematosus in children. A case report. *Isr J Med Sci.* 1989;25:568.
12. Agarwal BL, Foa RP. Collagen vascular disease appearing as chorea gravidarum. *Arch Neurol.* 1982;39:192.
13. Sarkari NBS. Involuntary movements in multiple sclerosis. *Br Med J.* 1968;2:738.

14. Taff I, Sabato UC, Lehrer G. Choreoathetosis in multiple sclerosis. *Clin Neurol Neurosurg.* 1985;87:41.

15. Bachman DS, Lao-Velez G, Estanol B. Dystonia and choreathetosis in multiple sclerosis. *Arch Neurol.* 1976;33:590.

16. Dewey RB, Jankovic J. Hemiballism-hemichorea. Clinical and pharmacologic findings in 21 patients. *Arch Neurol.* 1989;46:862.

17. Klawans HL, Moses H, Nausieda PS, et al. Treatment and prognosis of hemiballism. *N Engl J Med.* 1976; 295:1348.

18. Johnson WG, Fahn S. Treatment of vascular hemiballism and hemichorea. *Neurology.* 1977;27:634.

19. Logothetic L. Neurologic and muscular manifestations of hyperthyroidism. *Arch Neurol.* 1961;5:533–44.

20. Nausieda PS, Bieliauskas LS, Bacon L, et al. Chronic dopaminergic sensitivity after Sydenham's chorea. *Neurology.* 1983;31:750.

21. Nausieda PA, Koller WC, Weiner WJ, et al. Chorea induced by oral contraceptives. *Neurology.* 1979;29: 1605.

22. Riley D, Lang A. Movement disorders. In: Bradley W, Daroff R, Fenichel A, Marsden CD, eds. *Neurology in Clinical Practice.* Boston, Mass: Butterworth-Heinemann; 1991.

23. Kurlan R, Lichter D, Hewitt D. Sensory tics in Tourette's syndrome. *Neurology.* 1989;39:731.

24. Pauls DL, Leckman JF. The inheritance of Gilles de la Tourette's syndrome and associated behaviors. Evidence for autosomal dominant transmission. *N Eng J Med.* 1986;315:993.

25. Elbe RJ, Koller WC. *Tremor.* Baltimore, Md: Johns Hopkins University Press; 1990.

26. Fitzgerald PM, Jankovic J. Orthostatic tremor: an association with essential tremor. *Mov Disord.* 1991;6:60.

27. Caviness J. Myclonus. *Mayo Clin Proc.* 1996;71: 679–88.

28. Marsden CD, Obeso JA, Traub MM, Rothwell JC, Kranz LT, LaCruz F. Muscle spasms associated with Sudek's atrophy after injury. *Br Med J.* 1984;288:173–6.

29. Banks G, Nielsen VK, Short MP, Kowel CD. Brachial plexus myoclonus. *J Neurol Neurosurg Psychiatry.* 1985;48:582–4.

30. Langston JW, Ricci DR, Portlock C. Nonhypoxemic hazards of prolonged myoclonus. *Neurology.* 1977;27:542.

31. Swanson PD, Luttrell CN, Magladery JW. Myoclonus – a report of 67 cases and review of literature. *Medicine (Baltimore).* 1962;41:339.

32. Wolf P. Periodic synchronous and stereotyped myoclonus with postanoxic coma. *J Neurol.* 1977;215:39.

33. Fahn S. Posthypoxic action myoclonus: review of the literature and report of two new cases with response to valproate and estrogen. *Adv Neurol.* 1979;26:49.

34. Fahn S. Posthypoxic action myoclonus: literature review update. *Adv Neurol.* 1986;43:157.

35. Marsden CD, Hallett M, Fahn S. The nosology and pathophysiology of myoclonus. In: Marsden CD, Fahn S, eds. *Movement Disorders.* London: Butterworth; 1982.

36. Kuzniecky R, Berkovic S, Anderman F, Melanson D, Olivier A, Robitaille Y. Focal cortical myoclonus and rolandic cortical dysplasia: clarification by magnetic resonance imaging. *Ann Neurol.* 1988;23:317–25.

37. Young RR, Shahani BT. Asterixis: one type of negative myoclonus. *Adv Neurol.* 1986;43:137.

38. Young RR, Shahani BT. Anticonvulsant asterixis. *Electroencephalogr Clin Neurophysiol.* 1973;34:760a.

39. Meldrum BS. Drugs acting on aminoacid neurotransmitters. *Adv Neurol.* 1986;43:687–706.

40. Pranzatelli MR, Snodgrass SR. The pharmacology of myoclonus. *Clin Neuropharmacol.* 1985;8:99–130.

41. Harrison MB, Lyons GR, Landow ER. Phenytoin and dyskinesias: a report of two cases and a review of the literature. *Mov Disord.* 1993;8:19.

42. Bimpong-Buta K, Froescher W. Carbamazepine-induced choreoathetotic dyskinesia. *J Neurol Neurosurg Psychiatry.* 1982;45:560.

43. Miyasaki JM, Lang AE. Treatment of drug induced movement disorders. In: Kurlan R, ed. *Treatment of Movement Disorders.* Philadelphia, Pa: JB Lippincott Co., 1995.

44. Karas BJ, Wilder BJ, Hammond EJ, et al. Valproate tremors. *Neurology.* 1982;32:428–32.

45. Keepers GA, Clappison VJ, Casey DE. Initial anticholinergic prophylaxis for neuroleptic-induced extrapyramidal syndromes. *Arch Gen Psychiatry.* 1983; 40:113.

46. Bateman DN, Rawlins MD, Simpson JM. Extrapyramidal reactions with metoclopramide. *Br Med J.* 1985;291:930.

47. Keepers GA, Casey DE. Use of neuroleptic-induced extrapyramidal symptoms to predict future vulnerability to side effects. *Am J Psychiatry.* 1991;148:85.

48. Cardoso FEC, Jankovic J. Cocaine-related movement disorders. *Mov Disord* 1993;8:175.

49. Marsden CD, Tarsy D, Baldessarini RJ. Spontaneous and drug induced movement disorders in psychotic patients. In: Benson DF, Blumer D, eds. *Psychiatric Aspects of Neurological Disease.* New York, NY: Grune & Stratton; 1975.

50. Kane JM, Smith JM. Tardive dyskinesia: prevalence and risk factors, 1959–1979. *Arch Gen Psychiatry.* 1982;39:473.

51. Kane JM, Woerner M, Lieberman J. Tardive dyskinesia: prevalence, incidence and risk factors. *J Clin Psychopharmacol.* 1988;8(suppl):52.

52. Casey DE. Clozapine: neuroleptic-induced EPS and tardive dyskinesia. *Psychopharmacol.* 1989;99:547.

53. Villeneuve A. The rabbit syndrome: a peculiar extrapyramidal reaction. *Can Psychiatr Assoc J.* 1972;17 (suppl):SS69.

54. Lang AE. Akathisia and the restless leg syndrome. In: Jankovic J, Tolosa E, eds. *Parkinson's disease and other movement disorders.* Baltimore, Md: Urban and Schwarzenberg; 1987.

SID M. SHAH, ROGER L. ALBIN

55. Weiner WJ, Lang AE. *Movement Disorders: A Comprehensive Survey.* Mount Kisco, NY: Futura Publishing Co; 1989.

56. Micheli FE, Fernandez Pardal MM, Giannaula R. Movement disorders and depression due to flunarizine and cinnarizine. *Mov Disord.* 1989;4:139–46.

57. Lavenstein BL, Cantor FK. Acute dystonia. An unusual reaction to diphenhydramine. *JAMA.* 1976;236:291.

58. Handler CE, Besse CP, Wilson AO. Extrapyramidal and cerebellar syndrome with encephalopathy associated with cimetidine. *Postgrad Med J.* 1982;58:527.

59. Lieberman JA, Kane JM, Reife R. Neuromuscular effects of monoamine oxidase inhibitors. *Adv Neurol.* 1986;43:231.

60. Fann WE, Sullivan JL, Richman BW. Tardive dyskinesia associated with tricyclic antidepressants. *Br J Psychiatry.* 1976;128:490–3.

61. Woogen S, Graham J, Angrist B. A tardive dyskinesia-like syndrome after amitryptaline treatment. *J Clin Psychopharmacol.* 1981;1:34–6.

62. Kurlan R, ed. *Treatment of Movement Disorders.* Philadelphia, Pa: JB Lippincott Co; 1995.

63. Fahn S, Marsden CD, VanWoert MH. Definition and classification for myoclonus. *Adv Neurol.* 1986;43:1–5.

18 Neuromuscular Disorders

JOHN J. WALD AND JAMES W. ALBERS

SUMMARY The hallmarks of neuromuscular diseases are weakness or numbness. Patients with neuromuscular diseases are seen in the emergency department when (1) there is rapid progression of disease, (2) the disease process is associated with pain, and (3) speech, swallowing, or breathing are involved. Understanding the underlying disease mechanisms and the typical course of these disorders directs testing, diagnosis, treatment, and disposition. Certain neuromuscular diseases and their management require special attention during treatment of unrelated conditions.

Introduction

The emergency physician frequently has contact with patients who have peripheral nervous system (PNS) disorders. Most of these patients have chronic illness, not emergency conditions. When the muscles of speech, swallowing, or ventilation become involved, even chronic conditions can become life-threatening emergencies. Several conditions of the peripheral nerves and their roots, the neuromuscular junction, or muscles require emergency treatment, most commonly when progressing rapidly or involving swallowing or respiratory function. The role of the emergency physician is to recognize symptoms suggesting neurological involvement, identify neurological impairment, and determine whether unstable situations requiring emergency treatment or neurological consultation exist.

The PNS includes:

1. Nerve roots (dorsal or sensory, ventral or motor) exiting the brainstem or spinal cord
2. Mixed nerves (formed by the dorsal and ventral roots) exiting the skull or spinal column
3. Brachial plexus and lumbosacral plexus (in the subclavicular and retroperitoneal areas, respectively)
4. Peripheral nerves, traveling from the plexus to end organs, including afferent (sensory), efferent (motor), and autonomic nerve fibers
5. Neuromuscular junction, transducing motor-nerve depolarization to muscle contraction
6. Muscle, the end organ producing contraction and movement

Knowledge of the neuroanatomy of the PNS and the neurological examination are necessary for appropriate "localization" of PNS-involved structures in diseases. Certain diseases that primarily involve the PNS also affect the central nervous system (CNS), for example, amyotrophic lateral sclerosis (ALS).

The temporal course of PNS disorders, neuroanatomical localization by a focused neurological examination, associated conditions, and confirmation of the diagnosis by appropriate testing leads to treatment and disposition. Typical features of the most frequently encountered PNS diseases, including examination findings and treatments, are reviewed. Conditions affecting the PNS that can alter the presentation in the emergency department or treatment of other conditions are discussed.

Prehospital Management

The most important factors in prehospital management involve ventilation and swallowing function. There can be a rapid transition from unlabored breathing to decompensation and hypoventilation because of muscular fatigue (e.g., myasthenia gravis), or with aspiration of oral secretions in patients with marginal ventilatory function (e.g., ALS). As decompensation can occur abruptly, respiratory rate can provide false reassurance. It is important to ask patients if they are tiring and to note increasing anxiety. Increased ventilatory effort can produce sweating across the brow.[1] A rapid screening test of ventilatory function is to assess the patient's cough. A forceful cough indicates respiratory muscle reserve and protection from aspiration in the short term.[2]

Other factors requiring prehospital consideration include autonomic nervous system involvement in peripheral nerve disorders that can lead to cardiac arrhythmias and volatile blood pressure changes, and consequences of acute muscle destruction. Rhabdomyolysis occurs after muscle injury due to trauma, overexertion, prolonged excessive external pressure (e.g., unconscious or obtunded patient) or internal pressure (e.g., compartment syndrome), alcohol, drug (prescribed or illicit) and toxin exposure, and infections.[3,4] Unprovoked rhabdomyolysis occurs with metabolic and mitochondrial muscle disorders. Treatment consists of hydration, which may begin in the field, and forced diuresis with alkalinization.[5]

Emergency Department Evaluation and Differential Diagnosis

Ventilation and swallowing function are evaluated promptly in the patient with potential neuromuscular disease. The forced vital capacity (FVC) and maximal negative inspiratory force (NIF) are useful quantitative measures of ventilatory muscle function. An FVC of less than 15 ml/kg or NIF of less than 15 mm Hg indicates the need for elective intubation when the procedure can be performed safely.[1,6,7] Aspiration can occur in the patient with dysphagia even with adequate ventilatory function, and requires tracheal intubation (with placement of nasogastric feeding tube) to protect the airway.[8] Historical factors suggesting aspiration include nasal regurgitation of liquids and frequent coughing while eating or drinking. Swallowing assessment ranges from observing the patient drinking water to viewing the mechanics of swallowing liquid barium or barium-coated cookies by fluoroscopy.[9]

History

Following adequate ventilation and airway protection, further evaluation begins by obtaining additional historical data. Determining the time course, type, and distribution of symptoms, discovering associated but seemingly unrelated symptoms, and reviewing the medical history, exposures, and family history often lead to a correct diagnosis. Symptoms also guide the subsequent neurological examination, suggesting the components that require examination in greater detail (e.g., a thorough mapping of sensory perception is less important in patients complaining of proximal weakness).

Information regarding underlying neuromuscular illness, whether controlled or quiescent, is important. Patients with neuromuscular junction, peripheral nerve, or muscle disorders are prone to unexpected "toxicities" after administration of certain agents. For example, questions often arise when choosing antibiotics for patients with myasthenia gravis, anticonvulsants for patients with porphyria, or cholesterol-lowering agents for patients with myopathies.

Neurological Examination

The goal of the neurological examination is to determine if, and where, the nervous system is functioning abnormally. Details of the complete examination are reviewed in Chapter 1, "Neurological Examination." When a patient with PNS disease is examined, symptoms suggest parts of the examination that are emphasized.

Strength Testing. *Weakness* indicates the need for strength testing. Strength testing is performed by assessing the power of several proximal and distal muscle groups, and by noting patterns of weakness and asymmetry. A screening examination includes shoulder abduction, elbow flexion/extension, wrist flexion/extension, hip flexion/extension, knee flexion/extension, and ankle plantar flexion/dorsiflexion. Symmetrical weakness that is diffuse and greatest proximally suggests myopathy. Weakness that is greatest distally suggests neuropathy. Asymmetri-

TABLE 18.1 Nerve Root Distribution Suggested by Pattern of Weakness and Reflex Change

Nerve Root	Weakness	Reflex Diminished or Absent
Upper extremity		
C5,6	Shoulder abduction, elbow flexion	Biceps, brachioradialis
C7	Elbow, wrist extension	Triceps
C8	Wrist, finger flexion	Triceps
T1	Finger, thumb abduction, adduction, opposition	
Lower extremity		
L2,3,4	Hip flexion, knee extension	Patellar
L5	Ankle dorsiflexion, inversion, eversion	Internal hamstring
S1	Ankle plantar flexion	Achilles

cal weakness in the distribution of one or several nerve root(s) or specific nerve(s) is consistent with localized disease such as a herniated disk causing radiculopathy, or local compression causing mononeuropathy. These findings require a more detailed and refined testing of strength (Table 18.1). Finally, weakness that is made worse by repeated testing suggests abnormal fatigability as seen in neuromuscular junction disorders. When weakness is variable or results are inconsistent, the patient's ability and desire to cooperate are considered. Patients experiencing pain often are unable to provide full effort. Weakness in some patients is feigned.

Sensory Testing. *Numbness* indicates the need for sensory testing to determine the patient's ability to perceive sensory stimuli. Painful stimuli are transduced and carried by small, unmyelinated nerve fibers. Pain is tested by gently touching the patient with a pin or other sharp object, inquiring whether the sensation produced is similar with side-to-side and proximal-to-distal comparisons. Sensation carried by the large nerve fibers is tested using a vibrating 256-Hz tuning fork. Sensory loss that is diffuse, symmetrical, and greatest distally suggests a peripheral polyneuropathy. Sensory loss that is asymmetrical or "focal" in the distribution of one or several nerve root(s) or specific nerve(s) is more consistent with localized disease and requires

more refined sensory testing to determine which dermatome (Fig. 18.1) or cutaneous nerve distribution (Fig. 18.2) is affected. Detailed sensory testing fatigues the patient and examiner, and except for observable responses (e.g., grimacing), the results of clinical sensory testing are subjective.

Reflexes. Testing of the deep tendon reflexes (DTRs) is important in patients with weakness or numbness, or focal pain. DTRs are complementary to the strength and sensory evaluations, and are relatively objective. The reflex arc begins with stretching the tendon as it is struck by the reflex hammer. An *afferent* volley of large fiber nerve depolarization travels through the nerves, plexus, and dorsal nerve root before synapsing in the spinal cord with interneurons, ultimately producing an *efferent* volley of depolarization in the anterior horn cells innervating the muscle that was stretched by tapping the tendon. This produces a brief muscle contraction, observed by the examiner as the "reflex." In general, the biceps, brachioradialis, triceps, patellar, and Achilles reflexes are evaluated. Upper motor neuron involvement (e.g., ALS, stroke) is suggested when the reflex is unexpectedly brisk; nerve root, plexus, or nerve involvement is suggested by a diminished reflex. Reflex loss or diminution that is diffuse, symmetrical, and greatest distally suggests polyneuropathy. DTR loss that is asymmetrical or

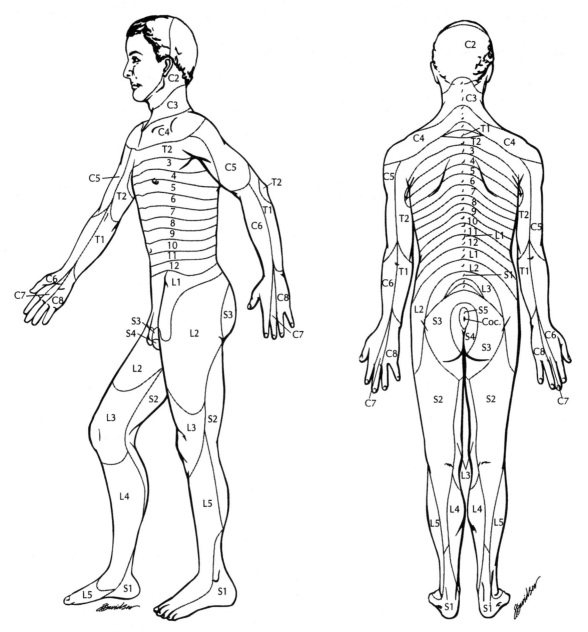

FIGURE 18.1. Diagram of dermatomes, anterior (A) and posterior (B) views.

"focal" in the distribution of one or several nerve root(s) or specific nerve(s) suggests localized disease (Table 18.1). Several cutaneous reflexes are tested. The Babinski response is the most familiar. It is tested by scratching the sole of the foot; great toe extension indicates upper motor neuron abnormality.

Cranial Nerves. The cranial nerve examination is important as an extension of the motor, sensory, and reflex examinations. Eye movements, facial movements, and phonation are affected by nerve, muscle, or neuromuscular junction disease. Extraocular eye movements are commonly abnormal early in myasthenia gravis.

The findings of the neurological examination are integrated into a neuroanatomical localization and differential diagnosis. Weakness in the distribution of a given nerve root that is accompanied by the appropriate sensory and DTR abnormalities is consis-

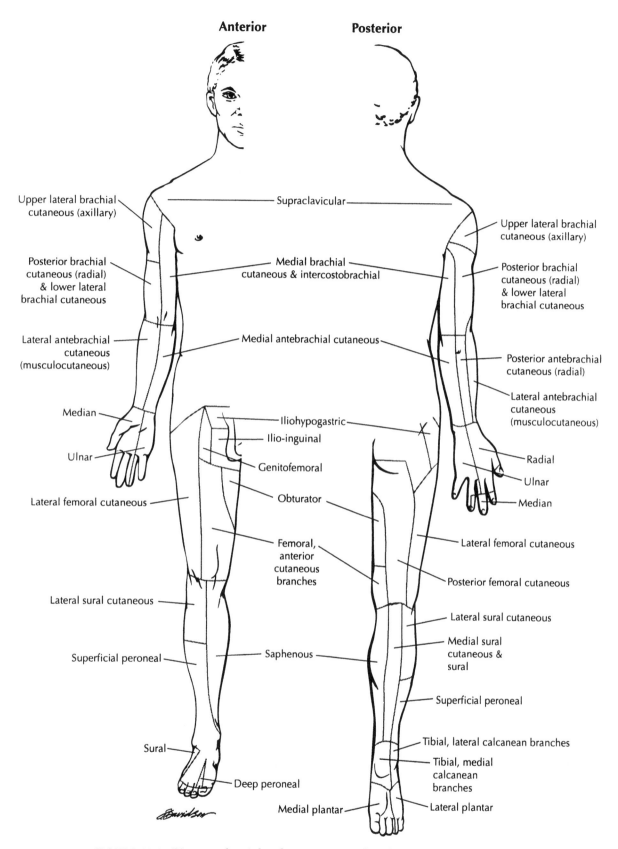

FIGURE 18.2. Diagram of peripheral nerve sensory distribution, anterior and posterior views.

257

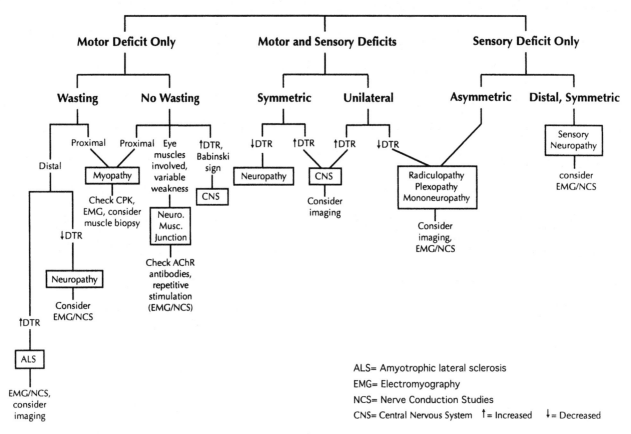

FIGURE 18.3. Diagram of neuromuscular evaluation.

tent with radiculopathy. Proximal weakness with normal sensation and normal DTRs is most likely due to myopathy (Fig. 18.3).

Emergency Department Management and Disposition

Specific anatomical and physiological changes, as well as diagnostic and management considerations, are grouped by disease entity, beginning with the nerve roots and proceeding peripherally.

Radiculopathy

Acute pain radiating into the dermatomal distribution of a given nerve root, with associated weakness, sensory loss, and diminished DTR (when available for the root in question), is the hallmark of compressive radiculopathy due to disk herniation or bony degenerative disease. The nerve roots can be involved in several other neuromuscular disor-

ders (Table 18.2). Pain is variable; however, a combination of weakness, sensory loss, and reflex diminution in the distribution of the involved roots allows localization. When imaging does not confirm a structural etiology, further evaluation with electromyography/nerve conduction studies (EMG/NCS) can confirm the localization, suggest etiology, and assist in prognosis. Cerebrospinal fluid (CSF) examination assists in excluding certain conditions (malignancy, infection). Evaluation of the CSF protein suggests nerve root inflammation with breakdown of the blood–nerve barrier (the equivalent of the blood–brain barrier).

The emergency physician must establish the time course of the disease, ensure no accompanying bladder dysfunction, and arrange further evaluation. Diffuse or progressive symptoms and signs require neurological consultation or hospital admission for documentation of progression, monitoring of ventilatory function, pain control, and expeditious evaluation.

TABLE 18.2 Etiologies of Radiculopathy

Etiology	Signs/Symptoms	Diagnostic Aids	Treatment
Trauma, spinal degenerative disease	Pain, weakness, numbness, diminished DTRs	Imaging, EMG	Bed rest, physical therapy, analgesia, surgery
Infectious (herpes zoster, CMV, HIV, Lyme)	Pain, weakness, numbness, diminished DTRs	Spinal fluid, skin change, evidence of systemic disease	Treat underlying infection
Inflammatory (GBS, CIDP)	Weakness, numbness, diminished DTRs, +/−pain	EMG/NCS, spinal fluid	See text
Metabolic (diabetes mellitus)	Anterior thigh pain, thoracic pain, +/−evidence of polyneuropathy	EMG/NCS, spinal fluid, evidence of diabetes	Analgesia, improved glucose control
Malignant invasion	Pain, weakness, numbness, diminished DTRs	EMG/NCS, spinal fluid, evidence of systemic malignancy	Analgesia, treatment of malignancy

Plexopathy

The brachial plexus and lumbosacral plexus are the regions distal to the nerve roots where the roots intermix to form specific nerves. Plexopathy is considered when muscle weakness or sensory loss is in a distribution greater than a single nerve root or peripheral nerve. Definitive diagnosis typically requires EMG evaluation. Multiple radiculopathies or mononeuropathies can mimic a plexopathy, often requiring extensive evaluation and imaging for precise localization. Historical features such as trauma, limb positioning, recent immunization, underlying medical conditions (malignancy, collagen vascular disease), and exposure to radiotherapy are helpful in diagnosis. The pattern of weakness can suggest the region of the plexus involved (Table 18.3).

Treatment of plexopathy consists of correcting underlying etiologies, pain control, and physical therapy. Evaluation by a physiatrist is important to direct therapy and prescribe assist devices as needed. In those without a traumatic etiology, neurological referral is important for confirmation of localization and initiation of evaluation.

Brachial Plexus. The most common etiologies of brachial plexopathy are traumatic injury, idiopathic (presumed to be inflammatory, occasionally preceded by immunization), and infiltration or compression by malignancies.[10] Radiation-induced injury can cause difficulty in determining the etiology in patients with malignancy who have undergone radiotherapy. Trauma is a common cause of brachial plexus injury. Forces causing downward shoulder movement (such as a forceful blow) injure the upper trunk, causing weakness of shoulder and proximal

TABLE 18.3 Distribution of Weakness in Brachial Plexopathy

Trunk	Clinical Findings
Upper	Weakness of arm abduction, elbow flexion; diminished biceps reflex
Middle	Weakness of elbow, wrist, and finger extension; diminished triceps reflex
Lower	Weakness of intrinsic hand muscles

arm muscles and proximal sensory loss. Upward shoulder displacement (reaching for a handhold when falling) injures the lower trunk causing hand muscle weakness and sensory loss along the ulnar (medial) side of the hand. Severe injuries can avulse nerve roots resulting in permanent deficits. Shoulder and neck trauma, as in contact sports, can cause transient burning or stinging of the shoulder, arms, or hands ("burners" or "stingers"), which are likely milder, transient forms of plexus injury. More complex trauma (shoulder trauma, stab and gunshot wounds) can cause mixed patterns of injury. In severely traumatized patients, the neurological impairment can be overlooked initially. Resultant weakness typically is accompanied by paresthesias or numbness. When nerve conduction block (suggesting myelin injury) is the prominent pathophysiology, recovery begins in weeks. The presence of axonal degeneration, requiring axonal regeneration and sprouting for recovery, leads to a worse prognosis and may require neurosurgical intervention. EMG and NCS are useful in determining the distribution and type (conduction block, axonal injury) of injury and determining prognosis (see Chapter 5, "Electromyography").

Idiopathic Brachial Plexopathy. Idiopathic brachial plexopathy, also called Parsonage-Turner syndrome or idiopathic brachial plexus neuritis, usually begins acutely with severe unilateral neck and shoulder pain.[11] Weakness develops within days, most prominent proximally, with only mild sensory impairment. Weeks later, atrophy becomes noticeable. Many patients have had an antecedent surgery, immunization, infection, or trauma, suggesting an autoimmune etiology similar to that in Guillain-Barré syndrome.

Diagnosis is based upon the clinical and electrodiagnostic distribution of impairment, the presence of an acute, painful onset, and the exclusion of local infection, hematoma, vascular occlusion, and neoplasm. Pain control is important, at times requiring narcotic analgesics during the acute phase. Most patients have good recovery of function; pain subsides in several weeks, and strength returns slowly, usually within 12 months, consistent with the rate of reinnervation.[11]

Lumbosacral Plexus. Lower extremity symptoms/signs involving the distribution of several nerves (e.g., sciatic and femoral) suggest lumbosacral plexus localization, although polyradiculopathy is also considered. Etiologies of *lumbosacral plexopathy* are similar to those of brachial plexopathy, but include retroperitoneal hemorrhage in patients receiving anticoagulant therapy and "diabetic amyotrophy" in diabetic patients. Traumatic lesions of the lumbosacral plexus are commonly associated with major pelvic trauma. The most common nontraumatic lumbosacral plexopathy is diabetic amyotrophy, presenting with proximal leg pain followed by weakness beginning days later. Weakness can involve muscles innervated by the femoral, obturator, or sciatic nerves, and can involve the other leg. It is believed that diabetic amyotrophy commonly involves the lumbar plexus, although some patients have the problem localized to dysfunction of anterior horn cells, nerve roots, or intramuscular branches of motor nerves.[12] The pathology is likely microangiopathic diabetic ischemia. Most patients have known diabetes and signs of an underlying polyneuropathy; however, amyotrophy can be the presenting sign of diabetes. Diagnosis requires exclusion of other causes of plexopathy and determination of the presence of diabetes. Treatment consists of pain control, physiotherapy, and glucose control. Prognosis is good, although recovery can be slow. Pain typically subsides in 4–6 weeks, and strength recovers over 12–24 months.[13]

The lumbosacral plexus can be injured by local compression (operative positioning, compression at the pelvic brim during childbirth) or stretch. Retroperitoneal hemorrhage is considered in new-onset lumbosacral plexopathy (Fig. 18.4). This occurs typically in hemophiliacs or patients receiving anticoagulant therapy and causes back and abdominal pain with weakness of hip flexion.[14] Most nondiabetic, nontraumatic amyotrophies are idiopathic. Some nontraumatic amyotrophies are associated with an autoimmune disorder and respond to immunosuppressive therapy.

Polyneuropathy

Polyneuropathy is common in the general population. The hallmarks of polyneuropathy are distal weakness and numbness. Examination findings are

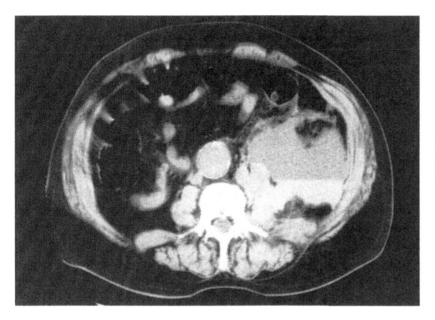

FIGURE 18.4. CT scan of large retro-peritoneal hematoma causing left lumbosacral plexopathy.

weakness, distal sensory loss, and hyporeflexia or areflexia. Rapid onset of symptoms including respiratory insufficiency rarely leads to presentation in the emergency department. The most common acute presentations are the acute or chronic inflammatory demyelinating polyneuropathies. These are acquired disorders of presumed immunological etiology that differ primarily in their onset and relapse rates. The patients with the acute form of inflammatory polyneuropathy (Guillain-Barré syndrome) typically develop respiratory failure, requiring ventilatory support, and clinically significant dysautonomia.

Guillain-Barré Syndrome. Guillain-Barré syndrome (BGS) is the most common disorder causing rapidly ascending numbness and weakness. It is preceded by a viral-like illness or other antecedent event in more than 75% of patients.[1,15,16] Symptoms include paresthesias or distal weakness, often in association with back and muscle pain, with progression of weakness over days in a distal to proximal fashion. Cranial nerves are commonly involved, producing facial weakness, difficulty chewing, and dysphagia. Facial weakness is easily recognized by incomplete eyelid closure. Extraocular muscles are involved rarely, and pupillary muscles are spared. Sensory loss consists of mild distal vibratory loss, and DTRs are absent or markedly reduced.[16-18] Bladder or bowel dysfunction is unusual.[18]

Chronic Inflammatory Demyelinating Polyneuropathy. Chronic inflammatory demyelinating polyneuropathy (CIDP) is a progressive or relapsing polyneuropathy that resembles GBS. The course of CIDP is prolonged; the interval from onset to peak impairment typically exceeds three months. Although GBS is almost always monophasic, 50% of patients with CIDP have a progressive illness, one-third experience relapse, and only one-sixth have a monophasic course.[19]

Diagnosis. Demyelinating neuropathy is suspected any time a patient notes rapidly progressive distal weakness and numbness. Diminished or absent DTRs confirm the peripheral nerve localization. Laboratory testing reveals CSF *albuminocytological dissociation* (CSF protein elevation without leukocytosis). Leukocyte counts greater than 40 cells/ml suggest alternative diagnoses, including HIV infection. Because diabetic neuropathy is common, diabetes should be excluded. Porphyric neuropathy is considered in patients with suspected GBS. Several events can precipitate an attack of GBS, including various medications, stress, pregnancy, fasting, and infection. Classification of the porphyrias involves identification of abnormal excretion of heme precursors, and requires analysis of the following: urine for δ-aminolevulinic acid, porphobilinogen, and uroporphyrin; stool for protoporphyrin and coproporphyrin; and blood cells for the specific enzyme deficiency.

EMG/NCS is required to confirm the diagnosis, revealing conduction velocity slowing, prolongation of distal latencies, conduction block with abnormal temporal dispersion of motor responses, and absent or prolonged F wave latencies.[6] Normal NCS early in the illness does not exclude the diagnosis of GBS. When symptoms and signs suggestive of GBS evolve rapidly, in-hospital monitoring is required to determine the rate of disease progression.

Treatment. When GBS is suspected, monitoring of autonomic dysfunction and possible ventilatory failure is considered. One-third of patients with GBS require ventilatory support, usually during the second or third week after onset; most deaths among individuals with GBS are associated with respiratory complications.[1,20] Ventilator assistance is less often required for patients with CIDP, but may be needed during severe exacerbations. Disposition of these patients depends upon the severity of weakness, rate of progression, and accompanying findings. Early in the clinical course, patients often require intensive care unit (ICU) monitoring of respiratory and autonomic functions. Abrupt respiratory failure suggests aspiration, cardiac dysrhythmia, or pulmonary embolism. FVC is monitored, although false low recordings can be obtained when mouth closure is poor. Arterial blood gas measurements are poor measures of respiratory function in patients with acute GBS. Hypercapnia, generally preceding hypoxia, is a late finding of ventilatory failure and as such is not a reliable criterion for ventilatory support.[6] The mortality rate of patients with GBS (approximately 2–5%) has improved considerably since the advent of ICUs.[1]

Dysautonomia commonly occurs in patients with GBS and can account for 50% of deaths.[1,21] Findings of autonomic dysfunction include bradycardia or other dysrhythmia, labile pulse, and fluctuating hypotension and hypertension. Although dysautonomia is not directly related to the extent of weakness, clinically significant dysrhythmia and blood pressure lability are unusual in patients with only mild impairment. Suspicion of autonomic instability requires monitoring in an ICU. Hypotension is managed with administration of fluids, and sympathomimetics are generally not required. Hypertension is treated with short-acting medications such as nitroprusside or beta blockers. Dysrhythmias occur in 20% of hospitalized patients and arrhythmias affecting blood pressure or requiring medication occur in 5% of patients.[6]

The syndrome of inappropriate antidiuretic hormone (SIADH) secretion is associated with GBS and can lead to hyponatremia.

Definitive treatment of the patient with GBS or CIDP begins after diagnosis and assurance of patient stability. Therapeutic plasma exchange (TPE) and IgG administered intravenously (IVIG) over weeks to months are effective treatments in patients with GBS and CIDP. Chronic corticosteroids or other immunosuppressants (e.g., azathioprine) are used in patients with CIDP.

GBS is typically a monophasic disorder, although residual numbness and weakness can remain. Recurrent symptoms require evaluation for other conditions. Commonly, symptoms of CIDP return, often in association with changes in immunosuppressive medication or recent infection. When evaluating a patient with CIDP, the emergency physician considers residual disability from previous "attacks" of polyneuropathy and possible iatrogenic immunosuppression.

Motor Neuron Disease

Motor neuron diseases involve diffuse, painless degeneration of the motor neurons without sensory involvement. The most common is ALS, also known as Lou Gehrig's disease. Motor neuron disease is rarely diagnosed in the emergency department, but respiratory distress or aspiration of gastric contents requires evaluation in the emergency department.

Clinical Features. ALS involves degeneration of the upper motor neurons (causing hyperreflexia, spasticity, pseudobulbar affect) and lower motor neurons (causing weakness, wasting, and fasciculations). The pattern of hyperreflexia in weak, wasted limbs is fairly specific for ALS, although diagnosis requires exclusion of conditions such as lymphoma, viral infection, and spinal degenerative disease (e.g., cervical spondylosis), which can mimic this disorder.

Weakness is the hallmark of ALS. When disease onset is bulbar, dysarthria and dysphagia are early symptoms. Upper motor neuron disorder presents with spasticity and hyperreflexia but there is no wasting, sensory change, or pain. The findings of hyperreflexia, muscle wasting, and fasciculations are most important in diagnosing this condition. EMG and NCS are helpful in excluding other conditions (myasthenia gravis, polyneuropathy) and in documenting the distribution and severity of disease. Thyroid and parathyroid function, serum calcium, serum protein electrophoresis, and measurement of anti-G_{M1} antibodies can exclude "mimicking" disorders. Magnetic resonance imaging (MRI) helps to exclude local pathology as an etiology of the upper and lower motor neuron degeneration. Practically, this is required when upper extremity wasting and weakness is combined with lower extremity hyperreflexia suggesting cervical radiculopathy and myelopathy. When there is evidence of more diffuse lower motor neuron involvement (wasting, or denervation documented with EMG), imaging is less important. Treatment is primarily symptomatic and supportive. Riluzole, a benzothiazole, is currently available for treatment of ALS and is typically prescribed by a neurologist. Its mechanism of action is unknown. Several other medications are under development for the treatment of ALS. Excessive emotional lability related to upper motor neuron and frontal lobe and involvement can be treated with tricyclic antidepressants. Excessive oral secretions are treated with anticholinergic medications. Cramps can be treated with quinine or phenytoin. Patients who have progressive bulbar dysfunction with aspiration and inadequate nutrition require a feeding gastrostomy tube. Although some patients elect to undergo tracheostomy and artificial ventilation, these decisions are best made before ventilatory compromise is imminent.

Mononeuropathy

Mononeuropathies produce abnormal motor or sensory function, usually both, in the distribution of a peripheral nerve. Etiologies are diverse, including acute trauma, repetitive minor trauma, and injury related to metabolic (diabetes) or vascular disease. Compressive or traumatic mononeuropathy can produce pain and nerve tenderness at the site of injury. Compressive injury commonly occurs during sleep or decreased consciousness. Features of several common mononeuropathies are described in Table 18.4.

Precise neuroanatomical localization is often possible with EMG/NCS. Because definite evidence of axonal loss may not be apparent until approximately one week after an acute injury, the greatest amount of information is gained when the electrodiagnostic studies are delayed, although an early study might be warranted to document preexisting conditions. When several mononeuropathies are present, mononeuritis multiplex, or "multiple mononeuropathies," is considered. This syndrome is associated with diabetes, malignancy, and collagen vascular disorders.

Facial. Facial nerve mononeuropathy (*Bell's palsy*) produces acute or subacute facial weakness. It is relatively common (incidence of 25 per 100,000 individuals) and is frequently encountered in the emergency department (because of the obvious nature of the weakness and patient/family member concerns regarding the possibility of stroke). For these reasons, it is discussed here in greater detail than the other mononeuropathies. The etiology and pathophysiology of Bell's palsy remain unknown, although compression or swelling of the nerve within the facial canal may play a role.[22] There can be associated pain behind the ear, hyperacusis, and altered taste sensation, depending on which area of the facial nerve is involved.

Evaluation in the emergency department is aimed primarily at localizing the abnormality to the distribution of only the facial nerve. Facial weakness due to facial nerve involvement (i.e., not due to CNS disease) involves the entire face, including muscles that furrow the brow. Involvement of other cranial nerves (true facial numbness, diplopia, speech/swallowing abnormalities) or more diffuse weakness suggests alternate diagnoses and requires more extensive evaluation.

TABLE 18.4 Selected Examples of Mononeuropathy

Nerve Involved	Common Sites of Compression, Entrapment	Distribution of Weakness	Distribution of Sensory Loss	Frequent Cause	Clinically Useful Muscle(s)
Facial	Stylomastoid foramen	Face	None	Idiopathic	Face
Median	Wrist	Thumb abduction, opposition	Digits 1 and 2	Wrist flexion/extension, compression at ventral wrist, diabetes	Abductor pollices brevis
Ulnar	Wrist, elbow	Hand, intrinsic muscles	Digits 4 and 5	Elbow trauma, compression from limb positioning	First dorsal interossei (abduct index finger)
Radial	Spiral groove (lower humerus)	Extensors of wrist and fingers	Dorsal arm and hand	Arm draped over back of chair, bed partner's head on outstretched arm, lead intoxication	Weak brachioradialis, wrist extensors normal triceps (innervated above spiral groove)
Femoral	Inguinal ligament, retroperitoneal space	Knee extension, hip flexion	Anterior thigh	Hip abduction, external rotation, direct compression, hemorrhage into the iliacus retroperitoneal tumors, or diabetes mellitus (diabetic amyotrophy)	Quadriceps
Sciatic		Leg flexor (hamstring), all muscles below the knee	Lower leg and foot	Fracture, dislocation, surgery (at hip) Compression in unconscious patient, IM injections, aneurysm, hematoma	
Peroneal	Fibular head (knee)	Foot dorsiflexion, eversion	Lateral leg, dorsum of foot	Prolonged squatting, bed rest, crossed legs	Ankle dorsiflexors

Treatment is controversial. Many advocate prednisone in doses of approximately 1 mg/kg followed by rapid taper.[23,24] Others suggest that the good prognosis without treatment (>80% with complete recovery) militates against steroid therapy. Acyclovir has been used in conjunction with steroid therapy. However, its effectiveness has not been fully established. All patients with facial weakness require corneal protection until eye closure returns. This is accomplished with moisturizing drops and ointment, or patching at night.

Defective Neuromuscular Transmission

Neuromuscular junctions transduce a nerve action potential into muscle membrane depolarization and subsequent muscle contraction. Defective function in this region of the nervous system leads to weakness without numbness or pain. When a patient with weakness is evaluated, neuromuscular junction disorders such as myasthenia gravis (MG), anticholinesterase toxicity, Lambert-Eaton myasthenic syndrome (LEMS), and botulism are considered.

Myasthenia Gravis. MG is one of the best understood autoimmune disorders. It is characterized by rapid fatigability and weakness of voluntary muscles. These symptoms of MG are related to the binding of antibodies to acetylcholine receptors (AChRs). The thymus gland has been implicated in the initiation of illness and is possibly the source of an AChR-like autoantigen. A decreased number of functioning postsynaptic AChRs leads to impaired neuromuscular transmission.[25,26]

The hallmark of MG is weakness, which varies in severity hour to hour and day to day, increasing with repetitive activity and improving with rest.[25,27] Weakness can affect ocular, bulbar, and limb muscles. Most patients have extraocular muscle involvement (ptosis and diplopia) at some time in their illness, and about one-third of patients develop dysarthria or dysphagia.[28] Respiratory distress is uncommon in isolation, but in individuals with generalized disease it can lead to presentation to the emergency department. The course of MG includes remissions and exacerbations, with some degree of stabilization after five to seven years. Exacerbations of MG can be associated with infection, surgery, emotional upset, immunization, increased body temperature, change in thyroid function, and other factors.[27]

Myasthenic crisis is commonly defined as acute weakening of bulbar and respiratory muscles, requiring ventilatory support.[25,29] It can be due to poor diaphragm contractility or frequent aspiration with bulbar dysfunction.

Cholinergic crisis is characterized by increased weakness after receiving cholinergic medications. It is uncommon and usually associated with cholinergic side effects (e.g., muscle cramping and fasciculations, abdominal cramping, diarrhea, palpitations, sweating, increased secretions, salivation, tearing, bradycardia, increased urinary frequency).

MG is diagnosed using a combination of clinical, pharmacological, immunological, and electrodiagnostic evaluations. The *Tensilon test* uses intravenous edrophonium (a short-acting anticholinesterase medication) to identify reversible weakness by prolonging the synaptic ACh availability.[30] Strength in weak muscles (particularly those easily tested, such as levator palpebrae, orbicularis oculi, extraocular muscles, or specific limb muscles) is documented prior to and after the administration of edrophonium. A test dose of 2 mg is followed by an additional 3 mg and 5 mg, given at 2-minute intervals. Patients are monitored for bradycardia during the testing. Edrophonium is effective within 60 seconds and lasts 2–10 minutes. Patients can be "masked" to the active drug by beginning with a placebo injection (saline), although the cholinergic effects of edrophonium preclude true blinding. Many patients with moderately severe generalized MG have a positive response to edrophonium, although its specificity is poor because weakness due to other conditions (denervation, myopathy) can improve as well. Edrophonium can be useful in diagnosing cholinergic crisis, but other cholinergic side effects suggest excessive cholinergic medication use. In patients with suspected cholinergic crisis, edrophonium is used cautiously (limit dose to 1 or 2 mg) because the additional anticholinesterase can cause respiratory failure.

Up to 90% of patients with MG have antibodies that bind to the AChR.[31,32] Laboratory testing screens for other autoimmune disorders and thyroid disease. Approximately 15% of patients with MG may develop thymoma. Computerized tomography (CT) and MRI are the most sensitive methods for identifying a mediastinal mass.

Suspected defective neuromuscular junction transmission can be confirmed by electrodiagnostic testing (see Chapter 5, "Electromyography"). Abnormalities noted by testing reflect a reduced "safety factor" in neuromuscular junction transmission and decreased probability of muscle fiber depolarization.

Treatment includes supportive care, symptomatic treatment, and treatment aimed specifically at the underlying disease mechanisms. Symptomatic treatment involves administration of anticholinesterase medications such as pyridostigmine (Mestinon). Improved strength occurs within 30 minutes of ingestion and peaks by 90–120 minutes, but lasts only 4 hours. The typical initial dose of Mestinon is 60 mg every 3–6 hours while the patient is awake. This can be increased, although higher doses can produce weakness. Dosage is individualized and often limited by muscarinic side effects such as abdominal cramping and diarrhea. Patients who are unable to take oral medications can be given pyridostigmine intravenously (approximately 1/30th of the oral dose). However, once the disease has become so severe that the patient's ability to swallow is affected, more definitive treatment is required.

Thymectomy is another treatment for patients with MG. Patients with *generalized* symptoms are likely candidates for thymectomy; uncontrolled studies report improvement in 50–80% of patients.[25,33] Thymectomy is indicated in all patients with thymoma, to prevent local spread to adjacent tissues.

TPE is used commonly to treat patients with myasthenic crisis.[34] TPE removes AChR antibodies from circulation, which is followed by improvement days to weeks later. This effect is short-lived, almost all patients undergoing TPE are started on another form of immunosuppressive treatment, usually corticosteroids. With long-term administration of corticosteroids, over 80% of patients note improvement or elimination of symptoms.[34,35] There can be clinical deterioration in the first weeks after administration of oral corticosteroids. Low-dose prednisone (10–20 mg per day) can be initiated and increased gradually to approximately 1 mg/kg per day.[36,37] Eventually, the corticosteroids are tapered to an alternate-day, low-dose schedule. The majority of patients require indefinite maintenance corticosteroid therapy, or the use of other immunosuppressants. High-dose intravenous methylprednisolone has been recommended for patients with life-threatening exacerbations of MG, with response reported in days,[38] and IVIG can be useful in treating patients with marked weakness.[39] Azathioprine and other cytotoxic agents are often recommended for long-term immunosuppression as corticosteroid-sparing agents.

Emergency Department Considerations. The emergency physician may suspect the diagnosis of MG in a weak patient. More commonly, the emergency physician is involved in caring for a patient with established MG who presents with worsening symptoms. The most important neuromuscular considerations relate to pulmonary and swallowing

TABLE 18.5 Commonly Used Medications Implicated in Worsening Weakness in MG

ACTH/corticosteroids
D-penicillamine
Intravenous contrast agents
Magnesium
Antiarrythmics
   Lidocaine
   Quinidine
   Procainamide
   Phenytoin
   Beta blockers
   Calcium channel blockers
Antibiotics
   Aminoglycosides
   Tetracyclines (some)
Muscle relaxants
Sedative/hypnotics, tranquilizers

functions. The best indicator of ventilatory function is the FVC. Patients with FVC of less than 1.5 l are monitored and treated aggressively; any deterioration in function can result in intubation. Similarly, patients with satisfactory ventilatory function but prominent dysphagia are at risk for recurrent aspiration, and require careful monitoring and aggressive treatment. A patient treated with chronic corticosteroids can require corticosteroid supplementation when injured or acutely ill.[40] Any medication is used with caution in patients with MG until it is certain that it will not worsen their weakness. Many commonly administered medications have neuromuscular blocking properties (Table 18.5). In general, the use of these medications is not absolutely contraindicated in the myasthenic patient, although alternatives should be considered. Stable patients with MG may tolerate these medications; however, in patients with borderline function, these medications are administered while the patient is observed closely, with special attention to respiratory depression.

When MG is suspected in a weak but otherwise stable patient, and weakness is not reported to be progressing rapidly, outpatient evaluation can be initiated. Serum is obtained for measurement of AChR antibodies, creatine kinase (CK), erythrocyte sedimentation rate (ESR), and thyroid function, and confirmatory electrodiagnostic studies are arranged. Because Mestinon can decrease the sensitivity of the electrodiagnostic studies, it is not used on the day of the test, when possible. Because of the chronic and variable course of MG, and the number of potential treatments available, most patients with this disease are cared for by neurologists.

Lambert-Eaton Myasthenic Syndrome. LEMS is another disease characterized by defective neuromuscular junction transmission, although this defect is associated with impaired release of ACh. LEMS is characterized by progressive weakness and autonomic features including dry mouth and impotence.[41,42] Patients with LEMS can resemble those with MG, although bulbar muscles are usually spared in the former. Brief exercise causes a dramatic increase in the release of ACh, which can result in *improved* strength or reflexes. LEMS is immune-mediated; the antibody binding site is the presynaptic calcium channel. Antibody binding is likely to result in decreased calcium entry during depolarization and decreased ACh release. Antineuronal calcium channel antibodies can be measured in LEMS patients.[43] Presynaptic neuromuscular junction dysfunction can be demonstrated electrodiagnostically when suspected. LEMS is often associated with small cell lung carcinoma or other malignancy.[44]

Treatment of patients with LEMS includes anticholinesterase medications (although they are less effective in patients with LEMS compared to the positive response in patients with MG), immunosuppression protocols similar to those used in MG, and 3,4-diaminopyridine (which improves presynaptic ACh release).[42,45–47] Any identified underlying disorder (such as a small cell carcinoma) is addressed, and treatment of these conditions can lead to significant improvement or resolution of the LEMS symptoms. In the emergency department, considerations of the patient with LEMS are similar to those of the patient with MG, with a few exceptions. The dysautonomia of LEMS (unlike the profound dysautonomia associated with GBS) is typically mild. When arranging electrodiagnostic studies to assess for suspected LEMS, it is important to recognize that facilitation can occur after muscles are exercised and that 50-Hz repetitive stimulation is painful, and not required for diagnosis.

Botulism. Botulinum toxin can produce acute, diffuse weakness associated with presynaptic neuromuscular junction dysfunction. Although rare, botulism is at times considered in the differential diagnosis of MG and GBS.[48] Exposure (in adults) usually occurs from improper home canning. Clinically, extraocular and pupillary muscle involvement is important in differentiating botulism intoxication from other causes of acute weakness. Electrodiagnostic testing can document impaired neuromuscular junction function. Definitive diagnosis requires identification of other affected individuals or measurement of toxin levels in food. Evaluation in the emergency department includes securing samples of any recently ingested canned foods. Treatment in the emergency department is usually supportive. Antibiotic and antitoxin therapies can be instituted following diagnosis.

Myopathy

Myopathies cause weakness and, at times, muscle discomfort (myalgia). Important factors in determining etiology include time course, recent trauma, medication or toxin exposure, underlying medical conditions, and recent infection. Patients typically have proximal muscle weakness; ventilation or swallowing is affected infrequently. Myopathies range from those present at birth that remain relatively static to acquired inflammatory myositis associated with other medical conditions.

Inflammatory Myopathy Inflammatory myopathy denotes three diseases: dermatomyositis (DM), polymyositis (PM), and inclusion body myositis (IBM). In these diseases primarily (but not exclusively) skeletal muscle invasion by inflammatory cells occurs. DM is a humoral autoimmune attack directed primarily against muscle blood vessels.[49] PM is a cell-mediated disease directed against muscle fibers.[50] IBM is a distinct form of inflammatory myopathy with "inclusions" apparent on muscle biopsy, although the role of autoimmunity is unknown.[51,52] Proximal muscle weakness is present in most patients with myopathy. Distal muscle weakness (in IBM) and skin changes (in DM) are differentiating factors. Dysphagia, esophageal dysmotility, and slowed gastric emptying occur occasionally. Cardiac muscle can be involved, resulting in cardiomegaly, congestive heart failure, or conduction abnormalities. Pharyngeal weakness can lead to aspiration pneumonia, and interstitial lung disease can affect up to 10% of patients.[53] Inflammatory myopathy, DM in particular, can be associated with malignancy, and is sometimes apparent before the muscle disease is discovered.[54] Serum CK and other cellular enzymes, for example, lactate dehydrogenase (LDH), are elevated in up to 90% of patients. A high ESR or the presence of autoantibodies suggests the presence of an associated collagen vascular disorder.

Corticosteroids, cytotoxic agents (azathioprine, cyclophosphamide, and methotrexate), and IVIG are commonly used treatments.[55,56] IBM usually does not respond to treatment, although immunosuppression is often attempted and the lack of response can help to differentiate it from PM.

Necrotizing Myopathy. Necrotizing myopathy, an acute or subacute onset of painful weakness with necrosis of muscle fibers, is commonly caused by myotoxins. Because these conditions are potentially reversible, their recognition is important. A broad range of medications has been implicated in causing necrotizing myopathy.[57–59] Lipid-lowering agents, including HMG-CoA-reductase inhibitors (particularly when given concurrently with cyclosporin or other immunosuppressants), nicotinic acid, and clofibrate have been associated with necrotizing myopathy. The mechanism of muscle damage is unknown; however, there is speculation that the HMG-CoA-reductase inhibitors can impair cellular metabolism. Other commonly encountered toxins producing necrotizing myopathy include substances of abuse such as cocaine, heroin, amphetamines, and alcohol.

Metabolic Myopathy. Metabolic myopathy implies muscle disease due to abnormal glycogen, lipid, or purine metabolism. There are many potential enzymatic defects, most of which are rare. Patients with metabolic myopathy can note exercise-induced muscle pain, exercise intolerance, or progressive weakness. Diagnosis depends on the clinical presentation and usually requires biopsy for histological and biochemical evaluation. Myoglobinuria is considered when metabolic muscle diseases are suspected. McArdle disease (due to myophosphorylase deficiency, one of many enzymes required for glycogen metabolism) causes intolerance of high-intensity exercise (such as sprinting), with attacks of muscle cramping, stiffness, and weakness that improve in some after a brief rest ("second-wind phenomenon"). Serum CK is often elevated between attacks, and there is the potential association with malignant hyperthermia. Lipid metabolism occurs within the mitochondria, requiring transport of fatty acids by carnitine and carnitine palmitoyl transferase (CPT). Carnitine deficiency (inherited or secondary to underlying conditions such as organic acidurias, liver failure, pregnancy, or medications (such as valproate acid) can cause progressive weakness or intermittent acidosis and Reye's syndrome–like attacks provoked by fasting, fever, or overexertion. Acute treatment consists of correcting the acidosis. CPT deficiency commonly presents after stressors such as infection, hypoglycemia, general anesthesia, or exercise. Associated myoglobinuria requires treatment.

Mitochondrial myopathy is a specific form of metabolic myopathy. Mitochondria are the site of the electron transport chain, generating adenosine triphosphate (ATP) through oxidative phosphorylation. Mitochondrial disorders can be inherited or acquired. Some mitochondrial proteins are encoded by mitochondrial deoxyribonucleic acid (DNA) (multiple copies present in each mitochondrion), while others are encoded by nuclear DNA. Mitochondrial DNA is present in the ovum at conception; thus nearly all mitochondrial genes are maternally inherited. Mitochondrial function requires nuclear DNA; therefore, dominant, recessive, and X-linked inheritance of mitochondrial disorders are possible. Organs with the greatest energy requirements (nervous system, muscles, gastrointestinal system) usually exhibit dysfunction related to impaired energy production with mitochondrial disease. Progressive external ophthalmoplegia (PEO) is a common finding in patients with mitochondrial muscle disease and can be associated with other systemic features that suggest a particular syndrome. There is significant overlap between many of the described syndromes. The Kearns-Sayre syndrome includes PEO, myopathy, retinal degeneration, and cardiac conduction block. Myoclonic epilepsy with ragged red fibers (MERRF) causes limb weakness, seizures, and myoclonus.[60] Another syndrome with strokelike episodes, not seizures, is mitochondrial myopathy, encephalopathy, lactic acidosis, and stroke-like episodes (MELAS). Acute treatment of patients with these disorders consists of supportive care, administration of anticonvulsants when required, treatment of other associated conditions, and treatment of acidosis when severe. Chronic treatment using cofactors such as coenzyme Q to improve mitochondrial function is occasionally effective.[61,62]

When a patient with an underlying metabolic or mitochondrial disorder is experiencing an exacerbation, symptoms such as worsening weakness, pain, or altered consciousness can lead to evaluation in the emergency department. Rapid determination of the blood glucose, lactic acid, pyruvate, and ammonia levels can lead to diagnosis and possibly direct further treatment (e.g., discovering hypoglycemia, a potential exacerbating factor, or lactic acidosis). Furthermore, obtaining urine organic acid screen and serum acyl-carnitine screen (which may be normal between attacks) can be helpful in diagnosis (however, these screens cannot assist with immediate diagnosis or treatment).

Dystrophy. Muscular dystrophies are inherited disorders causing progressive muscle weakness. Other organ systems are often involved. The best-understood dystrophy is Duchenne muscular dystrophy (DMD), an X-linked disorder of young males causing progressive weakness. As in most myopathies, DMD is characterized by elevated CK and proximal muscle weakness. Diagnosis is made by analysis for muscle dystrophin, a cytoskeletal protein that is absent in DMD. Joint contractures, scoliosis, intellectual impairment, and EKG abnormalities are common. Becker muscular dystrophy presents with less rapidly progressive weakness and is due to decreased or abnormal dystrophin.

Treatment of muscular dystrophies includes physical therapy, bracing, surgical release of contracture, and spinal stabilization. Respiratory support is required in the later stages of disease, when the FVC approaches 10% of predicted.[63] Decisions regarding respiratory support are best made before ventilatory compromise is imminent. Prednisone treatment can temporarily improve strength and function in DMD.[64]

There are many other muscular dystrophies, most of which are rare. Myotonic muscular dystrophy is the most common adult muscular dystrophy. It is a multisystem disorder characterized by limb weakness, facial muscle wasting, and weakness and frontal balding, producing a "hatchet face." Myotonia (sustained contraction related to repetitive muscle membrane depolarization) can be present clinically (produced by percussing muscle with a reflex hammer or noting slowed relaxation after sustained muscle contraction) and during EMG testing. Patients can have cardiac conduction abnormalities (including complete heart block) and arrhythmias. The cardiac conduction abnormalities can confound treatment of arrhythmias and are considered whenever medications are prescribed for patients with myotonic dystrophy.[65]

Periodic Paralysis. Occasionally, patients present to the emergency department with acute, severe weakness and a history of similar previous attacks following exercise or carbohydrate meals. Commonly, there is a family history of similar attacks. Several conditions associated with altered potassium levels or metabolism are likely to produce these attacks, and these periodic paralyses are commonly classified according to the potassium abnormality present with the acute weakness (hypo-, normo-, and hyperkalemic periodic paralysis).[66] Thyrotoxicosis, common in Asians, is related to a similar syndrome. There is considerable overlap between the hyperkalemic forms of periodic paralysis and rare myotonic conditions.

Respiratory muscle involvement is uncommon during attacks; cardiac arrhythmias are more common. During an episode of weakness, it is critical to obtain serial electrolyte measurements. In hypokalemic periodic paralysis, the potassium level is often less than 3.0 mEq/l, but can be "normal." Relative changes in the potassium concentration correlated with changes in the neurological examination are more significant than the actual potassium level. Electrocardiogram (EKG) abnormalities related to the potassium levels, including arrhythmia, can be anticipated. During the attacks, EMG findings are abnormal, with decreased nerve conduction response proportionate to the degree of weakness. Between attacks, the presence of myotonia can suggest a diagnosis, but EMG and nerve conduction studies are normal and are most useful in excluding other diagnoses. Provocative tests, such as manipulating the serum potassium level or body temperature, have been used in the diagnosis of periodic paralysis and myotonic disorders. However, genetic testing is becoming available for patients with many of these conditions.[67]

Treatment consists of normalizing the potassium level, either acutely during an attack of weakness or chronically to prevent attacks. In patients with hypokalemic paralysis, oral potassium (0.25 mEq/kg) is preferred, using parenteral replacement only when patients are vomiting or are unable to swallow. With any intravenous infusion of glucose, the serum potassium level decreases, worsening the weakness. In hyperkalemic paralysis, the usual methods to lower potassium levels are effective. A number of dietary and medical regimens have been used to normalize potassium levels chronically. Acetazolamide is effective in both hyper- and hypokalemic paralysis, although it has been reported to cause worsening in some patients diagnosed with the latter,[68] and severe weakness in patients with paramyotonia congenita.[69]

Management of patients with myotonic disorders and periodic paralyses requires consideration of the effects that altered potassium levels can have on the underlying condition and the increased frequency of cardiac conduction abnormalities. Any medication that can alter serum potassium levels or exacerbate conduction abnormalities or arrhythmias is used cautiously.

Systemic Conditions. Many underlying systemic conditions and their medical treatment can lead to myopathy. Hypo- or hyperthyroidism, hypo- or hyperkalemia, hypo- or hyperparathyroidism, hypo- or hypercalcemia, hypophosphatemia, hypomagnesemia, excess or insufficient adrenal function, and chronic renal insufficiency can be associated with underlying symptoms referable to muscle, including weakness. Appropriate laboratory testing is warranted when evaluating the weak patient, when other etiologies are not immediately apparent. Furthermore, medications, corticosteroids in particular, can cause myopathic weakness.

PEARLS AND PITFALLS

Nerve Disease

- Patients with normal Achilles reflexes rarely have a clinically significant polyneuropathy.
- It can take up to 7 days for NCS changes to become evident after nerve injury, unless the nerve can be stimulated proximal to the injury.
- It can take up to 21 days for needle EMG abnormalities (fibrillation potentials, positive waves) to develop after nerve injury.
- Diabetes is the most common cause of polyneuropathy in the United States.
- GBS is considered in patients with newly recognized ascending numbness, weakness, or reflex loss.

Motor Neuron Disease

- Motor neuron disease is considered in any patient with painless, progressive asymmetrical weakness.

Neuromuscular Junction Disease

- Rapid transition can occur from unlabored breathing to hypoventilation because of muscular fatigue (e.g., MG), or with aspiration of oral secretions. Normal blood gas measurements provide false reassurance.
- A forceful cough indicates respiratory muscle reserve and protection from aspiration in the short term.
- Consider potential neuromuscular blocking effects when prescribing *any* medication for a patient with MG.
- Any cause for elevated body temperature (infection, increased ambient temperature) worsens symptoms of MG.

Muscle Disease

- Proximal, painless, symmetrical, weakness suggests myopathy.

■ Exertional muscle pain suggests metabolic myopathy; serum CK, lactate, glucose, ammonia, and urine myoglobin should be measured.

■ Consider potassium-sensitive paralysis in patients with acute severe weakness and a history of similar attacks.

REFERENCES

1. Ropper AH. The Guillain-Barré syndrome. *N Engl J Med.* 1992;326:1130–6.
2. Ropper AH. Tips for neurologists who care for patients with mechanical respiratory failure. *Semin Neurol.* 1984;4:497.
3. Knochel JP. Rhabdomyolysis and myoglobinuria. *Ann Rev Med.* 1982;33:435–43.
4. Roth D, Alarcon FJ, Fernandez JA, Preston RA, Bourgoignie JJ. Acute rhabdomyolysis associated with cocaine intoxication. *N Engl J Med.* 1988;319:673–7.
5. Better OS, Stein JH. Early management of shock and prophylaxis of acute renal failure in traumatic rhabdomyolysis. *N Engl J Med.* 1990;322:825–9.
6. Albers JW, Kelly JJ Jr. Acquired inflammatory demyelinating polyneuropathies; clinical and electrodiagnostic features. *Muscle Nerve.* 1989;12:435–51.
7. Ropper AH, Kennedy SF. *Neurological and Neurosurgical Intensive Care.* Rockville, Md: Aspen Publishing, Inc; 1988.
8. Kennedy SK. Airway management and respiratory support. In: Ropper AH, Kennedy SK, eds. *Neurological and Neurosurgical Intensive Care.* Rockville, Md: Aspen Publishing, Inc; 1988:55–79.
9. Sorin R, Somers S, Austin W, Bester S. The influence of videofluoroscopy on the management of the dysphagic patient. *Dysphagia.* 1988;2:127–35.
10. England JD, Sumner AJ. Neuralgic amyotrophy: an increasingly diverse entity. *Muscle Nerve.* 1987;10:60–8.
11. Tsairis P, Dyck, PJ, Mulder DW. Natural history of brachial plexus neuropathy. Report on 99 patients. *Arch Neurol.* 1972;27:109–117.
12. Wilbourn AJ. The diabetic neuropathies. In: Brown WF, Bolton CF, eds. *Clinical Electromyography.* Boston, Mass: Butterworths; 1987:329–64.
13. Chokroverty S, Reyes MG, Rubino FA, Tonaki H. The syndrome of diabetic amyotrophy. *Ann Neurol.* 1977;2:181–94.
14. Cranberg L. Femoral neuropathy from iliac hematoma. Report of a case. *Neurology.* 1979;29:1071–2.
15. Kaslow RA, Sullivan Bolyai JZ, Holman RC, Hafkin B, Dicker RC, Schonberger LB. Risk factors for Guillain-Barré syndrome. *Neurology.* 1987;37:685–8.
16. Aranason BGW, Soliven B. Acute inflammatory demyelinating polyradiculopathy. In: Dyck PJ, Thomas PK, Griffin JW, Low PA, Podulso JF, eds. *Peripheral Neuropathy,* 3rd ed. Philadelphia, Pa: WB Saunders; 1993:1437–97.
17. Asbury AK, Arnason BGW, Karp HR, McFarlin DE. Criteria for diagnosis of Guillain-Barré syndrome. *Ann Neurol.* 1978;3:565–6.
18. Asbury AK. Diagnostic considerations in Guillain-Barré syndrome. *Ann Neurol.* 1981;9(suppl):1–5.
19. Dyck PJ, Lais AC, Ohta M, Bastron JA, Okazaki H, Groover RV. Chronic inflammatory polyradiculoneuropathy. *Mayo Clin Proc.* 1975;50:621–37.
20. Campbell WW, Swift TR. Differential diagnosis of acute weakness. *South Med J.* 1981;74:1371–5.
21. Arnason BGW. Acute inflammatory demyelinating polyradiculopathies. In: Dyck PJ, Thomas PK, Lambert EH, Bunge R, eds. *Peripheral Neuropathy.* Philadelphia, Pa: WB Saunders; 1984:2050–2100.
22. Katusic SK, Beard M, Wiederholt WC, Bergstralh EJ, Kurland LT. Incidence, clinical features, and prognosis in Bell's palsy, Rochester, Minnesota, 1968–1982. *Ann Neurol.* 1986;20:622–7.
23. Adour KK, Wingerd J, Bell DN, Manning JJ, Hurley JP. Prednisone treatment for idiopathic facial paralysis (Bell's palsy). *N Engl J Med.* 1972;287:1268–72.
24. Wolf SM, Wagner JH, Davidson S, Forsythe A. Treatment of Bell's palsy with prednisone: a prospective, randomized study. *Neurology.* 1978;28:158–61.
25. Drachman DB. Myasthenia gravis. *N Engl J Med.* 1994;330:1797–810.
26. Lindstrom JM. Pathophysiology of myasthenia gravis: the mechanisms behind the disease. *Adv Neuroimmunol.* 1994;1:3–8.
27. Oosterhuis HJGH. Clinical aspects. In: de Baets MH, Oosterhuis HJGH, eds. *Myasthenia Gravis.* Boca Raton, Fla: CRC Press; 1993:13–42.
28. Lisak RP, Barchi RL. Clinical considerations. In: Walton JN, ed. *Major Problems in Neurology, Myasthenia Gravis.* Philadelphia, Pa: WB Saunders Co; 1982;2:5–36.
29. Stricker RB, Kwiatkowska BJ, Habis JA, Kiprov DD. Myasthenic crisis. Response to plasmapheresis following failure of intravenous gamma-globulin. *Arch Neurol.* 1993;50:837–40.
30. Daroff RB. The office Tensilon test for ocular myasthenia gravis. *Arch Neurol.* 1986;43:843–4.
31. Kelly JJ Jr, Daube JR, Lennon VA, Howard FMJ, Younge BR. The laboratory diagnosis of mild myasthenia gravis. *Ann Neurol.* 1982;12:238–42.
32. Vincent A, Newsom-Davis J. Acetylcholine receptor antibody as a diagnostic test for myasthenia gravis: results in 153 validated cases and 2967 diagnostic assays. *J Neurol Neurosurg Psychiatry.* 1985;48:1246–52.
33. Lindberg C, Andersen O, Larsson S, Oden A. Remission rate after thymectomy in myasthenia gravis when the bias of immunosuppressive therapy is eliminated. *Acta Neurol Scand.* 1992;86:323–8.
34. Lewis RA, Selwa JF, Lisak RP. Myasthenia gravis: immunological mechanisms and immunotherapy. *Ann Neurol.* 1995;37:S51–S62.

35. Drachman DB. Present and future treatment of myasthenia gravis. *N Engl J Med.* 1987;316:743–5.

36. Seybold ME, Drachman DB. Gradually increasing doses of prednisone in myasthenia gravis. Reducing the hazards of treatment. *N Engl J Med.* 1974;290:81–4.

37. Miller RG, Milner-Brown HS, Mirka A. Prednisone-induced worsening of neuromuscular function in myasthenia gravis. *Neurology.* 1986;36:729–32.

38. Arsura E, Brunner NG, Namba T, Grob D. High dose methylprednisolone in myasthenia gravis. *Arch Neurol.* 1985;42:1149–53.

39. Dwyer, JM. Manipulating the immune system with immune globulin. *N Engl J Med.* 1992;326:107–16.

40. Napolitano LM, Chernow B. Guidelines for corticosteroid use in anesthetic and surgical stress. *Int Anesthesiol Clin.* 1988;26:226–32.

41. Lambert EH, Eaton LM, Rooke ED. Defect of neuromuscular transmission associated with malignant neoplasms. *Am J Physiol.* 1956;187:612–13.

42. McEvoy KM, Windebank AJ, Daube JR, Low PA. 3,4-diaminopyridine in the treatment of Eaton-Lambert syndrome. *N Engl J Med.* 1989;321:1567–71.

43. Lennon VA, Lambert EH. Autoantibodies bind solubilized calcium channel-Ω-conotoxin complexes from small cell lung carcinoma: a diagnostic aid for Lambert-Eaton myasthenic syndrome. *Mayo Clin Proc.* 1989;64:1498–1504.

44. Lambert EH, Rooke DE, Eaton LM. Myasthenic syndrome occasionally associated with bronchial neoplasm. In: Viets HR, ed. *Myasthenia Gravis.* Springfield, Ill: Charles C Thomas Publishers; 1961:362–410.

45. Takano H, Tanaka M, Koike R, Nagai H, Arakawa M, Tsuji S. Effect of intravenous immunoglobulin in Lambert-Eaton myasthenic syndrome with small-cell lung cancer: correlation with the titer of anti-voltage-gated calcium channel antibody. *Muscle Nerve.* 1994;17:1073–5.

46. Mendell J. Neuromuscular junction disorders: a guide to diagnosis and treatment. *Adv Neuroimmunol.* 1994;1:9–16.

47. McEvoy KM. Diagnosis and treatment of Lambert-Eaton myasthenic syndrome. *Neurol Clin.* 1994;12:387–99.

48. Rapoport S, Watkins PB. Descending paralysis resulting from occult wound botulism. *Ann Neurol.* 1984;16:359–61.

49. Griggs RC, Karpati G. The pathogenesis of dermatomyositis. *Arch Neurol.* 1991;48:21–2.

50. Arahata K, Engel AG. Monoclonal antibody analysis of mononuclear cells in myopathies, I: quantitation of subsets according to diagnosis and sites of accumulation and demonstration and counts of muscle fibers invaded by T cells. *Ann Neurol.* 1984;16:193–208.

51. Carpenter S, Karpati G. The pathological diagnosis of specific inflammatory myopathies. *Brain Pathol.* 1992;2:13–19.

52. Carpenter S, Karpati G, Heller I, Eisen A. Inclusion body myositis: a distinct variety of idiopathic inflammatory myopathy. *Neurology.* 1978;28:8–17.

53. Lakhanpal S, Lie JT, Conn DL, Martin WJ. Pulmonary disease in polymyositis/dermatomyositis: a clinicopathological analysis of 65 autopsy cases. *Ann Rheum Dis.* 1987;46:23–9.

54. Manchul LA, Jin A, Pritchard KI, et al. The frequency of malignant neoplasms in patients with polymyositis-dermatomyositis. A controlled study. *Arch Intern Med.* 1985;145:1835–9.

55. Dalakas MC. How to diagnose and treat the inflammatory myopathies. *Semin Neurol.* 1994;14:137–45.

56. Dalakas MC. Current treatment of the inflammatory myopathies. *Curr Opin Rheumatol.* 1994;6:595–601.

57. Langer T, Levy RI. Acute muscular syndrome associated with administration of clofibrate. *N Engl J Med.* 1968;279:856–8.

58. Corpier CL, Jones PH, Suki WN, et al. Rhabdomyolysis and renal injury with lovastatin use. Report of two cases in cardiac transplant recipients. *JAMA.* 1988;260:239–41.

59. Folkers K, Langsjoen P, Willis R, et al. Lovastatin decreases coenzyme Q levels in humans. *Proc Natl Acad Sci USA.* 1990;87:8931–4.

60. DiMauro S, Moraes CT. Mitochondrial encephalomyopathies. *Arch Neurol.* 1993;50:1197–208.

61. Folkers K, Simonsen R. Two successful double-blind trials with coenzyme Q10 (vitamin Q10) on muscular dystrophies and neurogenic atrophies. *Biochim Biophys Acta.* 1995;1271:281–6.

62. Peterson PL. The treatment of mitochondrial myopathies and encephalomyopathies. *Biochim Biophys Acta.* 1995;1271:275–80.

63. Fukunaga H, Okubo R, Moritoyo T, Kawashima N, Osame M. Long-term follow-up of patients with Duchenne muscular dystrophy receiving ventilatory support. *Muscle Nerve.* 1993;16:554–8.

64. Griggs RC, Moxley RT, Mendell JR, et al. Prednisone in Duchenne dystrophy. A randomized, controlled trial defining the time course and dose response. Clinical Investigation of Duchenne Dystrophy Group. *Arch Neurol.* 1991;48:383–8.

65. Motta J, Guilleminault C, Billingham M, Barry W, Mason J. Cardiac abnormalities in myotonic dystrophy. Electrophysiologic and histopathologic studies. *Am J Med.* 1979;67:467–73.

66. Griggs RC. Periodic paralysis. Neurology and Neurosurgery, Update Series. *CPEC.* 1983;4:1–8.

67. Ptacek LJ, Johnson KJ, Griggs RC. Genetics and physiology of the myotonic muscle disorders. *N Engl J Med.* 1993;328:482–9.

68. Torres CF, Griggs RC, Moxley RT, Bender AN. Hypokalemic periodic paralysis exacerbated by acetazolamide. *Neurology.* 1981;31:1423–8.

69. Riggs JE. The periodic paralyses. *Neurol Clin.* 1988;6:485–98.

19 Musculoskeletal and Neurogenic Pain

ROBERT G. KANIECKI AND L.R. SEARLS

SUMMARY This chapter provides information on the clinical presentation, pathophysiology, and emergency evaluation of musculoskeletal and neurogenic pain. Emphasis is placed on those disorders that are either most common or associated with significant morbidity and mortality. Organization of this chapter is grounded in the anatomical localization of various painful conditions. Once the disorder has been localized, the discussion continues with differential diagnosis, evaluation, and management steps. This chapter provides a concise, accessible outline of painful disorders affecting the musculoskeletal or nervous systems.

Introduction

Pain is the most common complaint voiced in acute care settings, yet it is frequently understated or ignored. Headaches, back pain, and other painful disorders account for billions of dollars in health care expenditures, millions of days of lost work or lowered productivity, and countless hours of human suffering. Physicians are generally poorly trained and uncomfortable concerning the treatment of patients who are in pain. One study established that over 50% of patients presenting to an emergency department with an acutely painful condition had no analgesics administered, while the majority of those treated waited over an hour for analgesic, often at suboptimal dosage.[1]

Pain is an unpleasant experience involving sensory and emotional distress, suggesting real or potential tissue injury. Acute pain can be defined as pain of recent onset, often accompanied by anxiety and signs of sympathetic hyperactivity, which is expected to resolve within a period of weeks. Chronic pain is that which persists or recurs beyond a period of six months. Chronic pain is often associated with the affective and vegetative symptoms of depression. Pain can also be distinguished as being *nociceptive* or *neuropathic*. Nociceptive pain, or "somatic pain," involves activation of the periph-

eral receptors of an intact nervous system, often as a result of tissue damage. Neuropathic pain arises from aberrant somatosensory processing in either the peripheral or central nervous system.

This classification of pain into nociceptive and neuropathic syndromes allows organized evaluation of patients presenting to the emergency department with pain and helps to establish a diagnosis. Following a thorough evaluation in the emergency department, a majority of patients lack a definitive diagnosis. However, this appears to have little negative impact on successful management.[1]

The purpose of this chapter is to discuss the presentation, pathophysiology, evaluation, and treatment of patients with painful disorders that are commonly seen in the emergency department. Emphasis is placed on those conditions associated with severe morbidity or death. For ease of reference, topics are presented along anatomical lines, and common drug therapies are outlined in Tables 19.1–19.4.

Prehospital Management

Prehospital management begins with the rapid assessment of vital signs and addressing any potential life-threatening conditions. Appropriate precau-

TABLE 19.1. Opioid Analgesics

Drug (Brands)	Oral-Parenteral Potency Ratio	Potency Relative to Equivalent Parenteral Morphine Dose	Dosing
Morphine (MSIR, MS Contin)	1.6	1.0	5–15 mg IM/SQ q4h
Propoxyphene (Darvocet)	NA	<0.1	50–100 mg PO q4h
Codeine (Tylenol #2–4)	1:1.5	0.1	30–60 mg PO/IM/SQ q4h
Meperidine (Demerol)	1:3	0.15	50–150 mg PO/IM/SQ q3h
Methadone (Dolophine)	1:2	1.0	5–15 mg PO q4–6h
Oxycodone (Percocet)	1:2	1.0	5 mg PO q6h
Hydrocodone (Lorcet, Vicodin)	NA	1.0	5–10 mg PO q6h
Butorphanol (Stadol)	NA	5.0	1–2 mg IM/nasal q3–6h
Hydromorphone (Dilaudid)	1:5	6.0	2 mg PO/IM/SQ q4h

Note: NA = not applicable.

TABLE 19.2. Nonsteroidal Anti-inflammatory Drugs

Chemical Class	Drug	Brand Names	Dose
Salicylates	Aspirin	Many	325–1000 mg q4h
	Diflusinal	Dolobid	500 mg q8–12h
Propionic acids	Ibuprofen	Many	200–800 mg q4–8h
	Flurbiprofen	Ansaid	50–100 mg q6–8h
	Ketoprofen	Orudis	25–75 mg q4–8h
	Naproxen	Naprosyn, Anaprox	250–550 mg q4–8h
Indoles	Etodolac	Lodine	300–400 mg q6–8h
	Indomethacin	Indocin	25–75 mg q6–8h
	Sulindac	Clinoril	200 mg q12h
	Tolmetin	Tolectin	400 mg q8h
Nonindole acetic acids	Diclofenac	Voltaren	50 mg q8–12h
		Toradol	30–60 mg IM q6h 10 mg PO q4–6h (max 3 days)
	Nabumetone	Relafen	1 g q12–24h
	Piroxicam	Feldene	20 mg 2–24h

TABLE 19.3. Adjuvant Analgesics

Chemical Classes	Drug	Brand Name	Daily Dose (Intervals)
Tricyclic antidepressants	Amitriptyline	Elavil	50–300 mg (qd–tid)
	Doxepin	Sinequan	50–300 mg (qd–tid)
	Nortriptyline	Pamelor	25–150 mg (qd–tid)
Other antidepressants	Fluoxetine	Prozac	5–80 mg (qd–bid)
	Paroxetine	Paxil	10–40 mg (qd–bid)
	Trazodone	Desyrel	150–400 mg (qd–bid)
Beta blockers	Propranolol	Inderal	60–320 mg (qd–tid)
	Atenolol	Tenormin	50–200 mg (qd–bid)
	Nadolol	Corgard	80–240 mg (bid–tid)
Calcium blockers	Verapamil	Calan	120–360 mg (qd–tid)
Serotonin antagonists	Methysergide	Sansert	4–12 mg (bid–tid)
Anticonvulsants	Carbamazepine	Tegretol	200–1800 mg (bid–qid)
	Phenytoin	Dilantin	200–500 mg (qd–tid)
	Gabapentin	Neurontin	300–4800 mg (bid–qid)
	Sodium Valproate	Depakote	500–2000 mg (bid–tid)
$GABA_B$ agonist	Baclofen	Lioresal	10–100 mg (qd–qid)
Neuroleptics	Fluphenazine	Prolixin	1–20 mg (qd–tid)
	Haloperidol	Haldol	6–40 mg (bid–tid)
Other	Tramadol	Ultram	200–400 mg (tid–qid)
	Clonidine	Catapres	0.1–0.9 mg (qd–tid)
	Corticosteroids	Prednisone	10–100 mg (qd–tid)
	Capsaicin	Zostrix	Topical application qid

tions in handling and transporting patients with back or neck pain are taken, because absence of trauma does not ensure a stable spine. Inappropriate use of stiff neck collars and back boards can cause further injury.[2,3] An unstable spine may also be injured by inappropriate airway maneuvers or transportation techniques. Painful peripheral joints are splinted in positions of comfort.

Prior to transportation, a secondary survey includes assessment of neurological symptoms and signs, including radiation of pain, areas of numbness or paresthesias, or focal weakness. Suspicion of head injury requires an adequate evaluation of level of consciousness and pupillary function. Further assessment addresses quality and symmetry of peripheral pulses, chest or abdominal pain, as well as presence of bruits or pulsatile abdominal masses.

Parenteral analgesics can be used judiciously when prolonged or rough travel is anticipated. Intravenous access is established for those patients who may require analgesia or are suspected of having a serious underlying illness. Frequent evaluation during transport for evidence of clinical deterioration is essential.

Emergency Department Evaluation and Management

Facial Pain

Overview. Facial pain can arise as a result of sinusitis, dental disease, facial trauma, or various neurological conditions (Table 19.5). Patients with acute facial pain commonly describe excruciating discomfort. Patients with chronic pain are often

TABLE 19.4. Muscle Relaxants

Drug	Brand Name	Dose
Carisoprodol	Soma	200–400 mg q6–8h
Chlorzoxazone	Parafon Forte	250–500 mg q6–8h
Cyclobenzaprine	Flexeril	10 mg q8h
Diazepam	Valium	2–10 mg q8–12h
Methocarbamol	Robaxin	1.5 mg q6–8h
Orphenadrine	Norflex	25–100 mg q8–12h

frustrated by the lack of explanation or relief. The history and physical examination direct the diagnosis. Radiographs and serum studies offer limited help.[4]

Nociceptive Syndromes. *Odontalgia* (toothache) is the most common cause of orofacial pain in adults. The dental pulp is the primary source of such pain, although inflammation of the periodontal ligament and adjoining structures may also cause discomfort. Inspection of the mouth, with digital palpation with a gloved hand, percussion or pressure with biting, and application of heat or cold stimuli often clarify the source of discomfort. Panorex® and sinus radiographs may assist in assessment. Analgesics are given to patients with isolated pain, with referral to dentistry. When intraoral swelling or low-grade fever are present, antibiotics (penicillin or erythromycin) are added, and referral

TABLE 19.5. Common Causes of Facial Pain

Nociceptive	Neuropathic
Sinusitis	Trigeminal neuralgia
TMJ syndrome	Herpetic neuralgia
Disorders of neck, salivary glands	Glossopharyngeal neuralgia
Eyes and ears	Geniculate neuralgia

to dentistry within 24 hours is made. Pronounced fever, or intraoral or extraoral swelling requires intravenous antibiotics, incision and drainage of abscesses, and immediate referral to dentistry or oral surgery.

Acute sinusitis is diagnosed by well-localized pain, nasal obstruction, purulent rhinorrhea, fever with leukocytosis, and abnormal radiographs. Blood tests and radiographs are not necessary in immunocompetent patients who appear to be healthy. Typically, patients with acute ethmoid or maxillary sinusitis are treated with decongestants and oral antibiotics. Acute sinusitis in the frontal or sphenoid sinuses is a medical emergency, due to the potential for intracranial spread of infection. Surgical drainage is indicated for those not responding quickly to intravenous antibiotics.

Temporomandibular joint dysfunction is a controversial, frequently diagnosed source of facial pain. Pain is localized at the joint and is associated with abnormal radiographic findings and two of the following four criteria: pain with joint movement; tenderness on joint palpitation; decreased joint range of motion; and crepitus during joint movement. Analgesics or muscle relaxants are the primary considerations in the emergency department.

Disorders of the neck, salivary glands, eyes, and ears can also be sources of facial pain.

Neuropathic Syndromes. *Trigeminal neuralgia* is the most common cranial neuralgia and one of the most stereotyped syndromes of facial pain. It is characterized by sudden paroxysms of lancinating pain lasting seconds to minutes, often recurring many times a day. It affects the second or third division of the trigeminal nerve in 95% of cases. Pain can occur spontaneously or be provoked by sensory stimulation of facial trigger points. Trigeminal neuralgia is more common in women, with peak prevalence in the sixth and seventh decades of life. The primary, or idiopathic form of trigeminal neuralgia implies a normal examination and no underlying anatomical lesion, although some believe such cases are due to compression of the trigeminal nerve root by a tortuous blood vessel.[5] Secondary forms of trigeminal neuralgia are associated with changes in facial sensation or the corneal reflex and anatomical pathology such as compressive or demyelinating disease. Magnetic resonance imaging (MRI) is the most helpful diagnostic procedure. Initial treatment is pharmacological; the antiepileptic agent carbamazepine is the drug of choice. Opiate analgesics are helpful adjuncts. Intravenous fluids may need to be considered for those at risk for dehydration due to inability to take fluids orally. Other antiepileptic drugs, antispasticity agents (baclofen), neuroleptics, or antidepressants may be effective in some patients. Referral to neurosurgery for chemical or radiofrequency rhizotomy or microvascular decompression is considered for refractory cases.

Acute herpetic neuralgia most often affects the first division of the trigeminal nerve. Symptoms are often controlled with the use of local heat or cold, soothing emollients, nonsteroidal or opioid analgesics, and antiviral drugs such as acyclovir or valacyclovir.

Postherpetic neuralgia is that pain which persists beyond one month. This affects 10% of all patients who have contracted shingles, particularly the elderly. Tricyclic antidepressant drugs provide the most benefit; antiepileptics, neuroleptics, opioid analgesics, and surgical procedures are relatively unproved and ineffective.[6] Topical agents such as local anesthetics or capsaicin provide modest results at best.

Glossopharyngeal and *geniculate neuralgia* are less common than trigeminal neuralgia and usually involve pain in the throat or ear. These syndromes are treated in a similar fashion to trigeminal neuralgia.[7]

Neck and Upper Extremity Pain

Overview. At any given time, 10% of individuals report some neck pain, and 35% of all adults have some recollection of an episode of significant neck discomfort. Although the most common sources of pain are musculoskeletal or neurogenic, ischemic processes and visceral sources of referred pain occur (Table 19.6). Pain-sensitive structures in or near the vertebral column include the annular fibers of the disc, the anterior and posterior longitudinal ligaments, the intraspinous and supraspinous ligaments, the posterior synovial joint, the vertebral endplates, and the paraspinal muscles.[7–12]

Nociceptive Syndromes. These syndromes are categorized as disorders of the cervical spine and disorders of the upper extremity. The cervical spine consists of seven vertebrae connected by numerous joints and ligaments, intervertebral discs, and the paraspinal musculature. Eight cervical roots exit the spinal cord through foraminal spaces to serve the head, neck, and upper extremities. Bony disorders generally result in examination findings of limited cervical range of motion and local tenderness. Plain radiographs help make the diagnosis of bony spinal conditions.

The most common cause of neck pain is *cervical strain,* which is characterized by transient cervical pain, stiffness, and posterior cervical muscle spasm. Local application of heat and anti-inflammatory analgesics are generally required for 72 hours. One of the most frequent and controversial sources of strain is the hyperextension-hyperflexion injury of the "whiplash" syndrome. In such cases, the pathophysiology appears to include stretching and disruption of muscles and ligaments, tearing of articular capsules, hemorrhage into paraspinal soft tissues, and damage to cervical roots or sympathetic nerves. Pain in the neck, head, and upper extremities; dizziness; anxiety; and depression may all be observed. The majority of patients recover quickly with heat and use of muscle relaxants and analgesics. One month following injury, 60% of patients are pain-free and 80% are working; six months following injury, 80% are pain-free and 90% are working. Approximately 10–15% of patients require management for indefinite periods.

Cervical osteoarthritis is the most common cause of neck pain in individuals over age 40, radiographic evidence of cervical osteoarthritis is present in over 70% of the elderly population.[4,13] Pain from the apophyseal joints typically is isolated to the neck and shoulders; further radiation into the upper

TABLE 19.6. Common Causes of Neck and Upper Extremity Pain

Nociceptive	Neuropathic
Disorders of cervical spine	Cervical radiculopathy
Cervical strain	
Cervical osteoarthritis	Brachial plexus disorders
Rheumatoid arthritis	Erb-Duchenne (upper plexus) palsy
Ankylosing spondylitis	Dejerine-Klumpke (lower plexus) palsy
Disorders of upper extremities	Radiation plexitis
(a) Inflammatory causes	
Septic arthritis	Idiopathic brachial plexitis
Noninfectious arthritides	Thoracic outlet syndrome
Tendinitis	Reflex sympathetic dystrophy
Bursitis	Suprascapular nerve palsy
Tenosynovitis	Radial nerve neuropathies
(b) Ischemic (vascular) causes	Ulnar nerve neuropathies
Acute arterial dissection	Median nerve neuropathies
Subclavian steal syndrome	
Reynaud's phenomenon	
(c) Traumatic causes	

extremity suggests root irritation. *Compression fractures* from osteoarthritis or osteoporosis rarely cause symptoms other than acute pain. Chronic pain is best managed with nonsteroidal anti-inflammatory drugs (NSAIDs); acute exacerbations of pain require narcotics.

Rheumatoid arthritis (RA) is an erosive, systemic polyarthritis primarily involving small joints, affecting 1–4% of the population. Following the hands, the cervical spine is the next most common area of involvement, with 30–86% of patients experiencing vertebral column disease, often limited to the cervical spine.[13,14] Dysfunction of the occipitoatlantoaxial unit is of utmost concern. Atlantoaxial subluxation, diagnosed by finding the predental space greater than 4 mm (space between dens and anterior mass of C1), can be asymptomatic or cause spastic quadriplegia and death from cord compression. Vertical subluxation of the odontoid into the foramen magnum, or basilar invagination, may result in cervico-occipital pain, C2 dermatomal sensory loss, myelopathy, and, in some patients with trauma, rapid quadriplegia and death.[15] Extreme

caution is necessary during endotracheal intubation in those patients with known advanced RA. Key diagnostic tests are the rheumatoid factor (80% sensitivity, 95% specificity) and careful routine, flexion, and extension plain radiographs. Treatment involves a combined program of surgical, rehabilitative, and medical services, the latter including NSAIDs, glucocorticoids, and disease-modifying drugs such as gold and methotrexate.

Ankylosing spondylitis (AS) is a spondyloarthropathy classified along with Reiter's syndrome, psoriatic arthritis, and the arthritis of inflammatory bowel disease. These disorders share the characteristics of spondylitis, sacroiliitis, tendon insertion inflammation, asymmetrical oligoarthritis, and often extraarticular manifestation such as uveitis, urethritis, and mucocutaneous lesions. An association with the HLA-B27 haplotype has been identified. Although cervical involvement may occur, dysfunction of the lower thoracic and lumbosacral regions is much more common. Pain and limited range of motion are frequent findings; spinal cord compression due to ossification or epidural hemorrhage is uncommon.[14] The diagnosis of AS is assisted by identification of annular or longitudinal ligament ossification or fusion of the facet joints via the typical "bamboo spine" appearance on plain radiographs. NSAIDs, most commonly indomethacin, and physical therapy remain the cornerstones of effective management.

Nociceptive pain in the upper extremity generally arises from inflammatory or ischemic causes. Local infection and disruption of arterial or venous circulation typically exhibit obvious findings and dictate acute therapy. Acute arterial dissection, subclavian steal syndrome, and Raynaud's disease are examples of such vascular disorders.

Nonbacterial *septic arthritis* (rubella, Epstein-Barr virus, hepatitis) generally is self-limited and responsive to immobilization and NSAIDs. The bacterial septic arthritides are commonly divided into gonococcal and nongonacoccal (staphylococcal or streptococcal species) groups, with both requiring joint fluid aspiration and examination and hospitalization for administration of intravenous antibiotics and analgesics. Surgical drainage is often necessary.

Noninfectious causes of inflammation in the articular or periarticular tissues may be diagnosed as *arthritis, tendinitis, tenosynovitis,* or *bursitis.* Common sites of inflammation include the shoulder (supraspinatus or bicipital head tendinitis), elbow (epicondylitis, or "tennis elbow"), and thumb (deQuervain's disease). Flares of systemic rheumatoid or osteoarthritic disease may cause local limb pain. Acute shoulder tendinitis can present with a dramatic onset of severe incapacitating pain over the anterolateral shoulder and aching in the deltoid and lateral arm. Motion of the shoulder, especially arm abduction, is exquisitely painful, and tenderness is noted at the insertion points of the biceps or supraspinatus tendons. The illness is self-limited but requires NSAIDs and possible immobilization of the shoulder in a sling for up to two weeks. Subsequent physical therapy or glucocorticoid injections may be necessary.

Neuropathic Syndromes. *Lesions of the cervical spinal cord* generally result in deep segmental pain that is poorly localized and infrequently influenced by positional changes or Valsalva maneuvers. Segmental weakness, sensory loss, and hyporeflexia are found in the upper extremities. The lower extremities may exhibit variable combinations of spasticity,

weakness, sensory loss, hyperreflexia, and a Babinski sign. Urinary or fecal incontinence may occur relatively late in the course. Extramedullary or intramedullary tumors, arteriovenous malformations, syringomyelia, central disc herniations, or severe cervical spondylosis and spinal stenosis may be visualized by magnetic resonance imaging (MRI) or computerized tomography (CT) myelography.

Cervical radiculopathy is most commonly caused by cervical spondylosis and cervical disc disease. *Cervical herniated nucleus pulposus* (HNP) may be traumatic[16] or occurs secondary to the process of disc degeneration.[14] Dehydration, collapse of disc height, deterioration and bulging in the annulus fibrosus, and eventual frank disc herniation are potential events in this process. Neck pain in such situations may be acute or chronic, and upper limb radiation of the pain in a segmental fashion is reported in most cases. Segmental sensory loss, motor weakness, and reflex changes can often be identified during a thorough neurological examination (Table 19.7). The lower cervical roots of C6–8 require the most thorough attention, because C6–7 ruptures account for 70% of all cases and C5–6 ruptures account for 20% of cases.[13,17] Additional information may be gained from the "chin-chest" maneuver, which involves provocation of pain with neck flexion.[17] The "head-tilt" maneuver generates discomfort upon lateral flexion toward the side of radiculopathy. Head compression (Spurling's maneuver) may worsen pain; manual cervical traction may alleviate pain by altering the diameter of foraminal spaces.[13,14,15] Many cases are investigated acutely via plain radiographs and managed conservatively with rest, heat, and analgesics. Significant sensory loss (seen in 25% of patients), weakness (seen in 75%), or intractable pain is addressed with outpatient referral for cervical MRI or CT myelography and surgical opinion. Signs of spinal cord compression require emergency neuroimaging and consultation with surgery when appropriate. CT scanning and electrophysiological studies – electromyography (EMG) and nerve conduction velocity (NCV) – are of little utility in a nontraumatic emergency setting.[17]

Brachial plexopathy is occasionally painless; however, when it is painful, the discomfort is centered at the shoulder and radiates to the neck and upper limb. Trauma to the brachial plexus may result in *Erb-Duchenne* (upper plexus) or *Dejerine-*

TABLE 19.7. Localization of Cervical Nerve Root Pathology

Disc Involved	Nerve Root Involved	Area of Pain	Area of Sensory Change	Motor	DTR
C3–4	C4	Shoulder	Variable	± Deltoid	None
C4–5	C5	Shoulder, lateral upper arm	Shoulder	Deltoid ± biceps	Biceps
C5–6	C6	Shoulder, upper arm, lateral forearm, thumb and index finger	Lateral forearm, thumb	Biceps, triceps, wrist extensors	Brachio-radialis and biceps
C6–7	C7	Postero-lateral upper arm, shoulder, neck	Index and middle fingers	Wrist flexors, finger extensors, triceps	Triceps
C7–T1	C8	Ulnar forearm and hand	Medial forearm, small finger	Hand intrinsics, finger flexors, wrist extensors	None

Klumpke (lower plexus) palsy and initially may require only analgesia and physical care. *Metastases* to the brachial plexus typically involve the lower plexus and are painful; *radiation plexopathy* is typically painless and predominant in the upper plexus.

Idiopathic brachial plexopathy, or brachial plexitis, arises as an acute painful process affecting previously healthy adults, with subsequent muscle weakness (pronator teres, pinch) and atrophy. Men are most often affected, and 30% of cases are bilateral. Initial management involves a course of corticosteroids lasting 7–14 days and immobilization in a sling. Physical therapy and analgesics are necessary subsequently during a course that may last 3–36 months.

Thoracic outlet syndrome is an uncommon condition observed most often in thin adult women with drooping shoulders. Compression of the lower trunk of the brachial plexus and subclavian vein or artery is observed in varying combinations, usually from a cervical or abnormal first thoracic rib, clavicle, fascia, or abnormal scalene muscle. Pain in the shoulder and arm, paresthesias in the median or ulnar nerve distributions, and weakness, atrophy, and vascular changes in the distal forearm and hand are the usual clinical manifestations. Diagnosis is as-

sisted via a number of clinical tests that may weaken the distal radial pulse. These include the Wright or "hold up" maneuver (abduct and externally rotate the arm 90 degrees, with the elbow flexed 90 degrees) and the Adson maneuver (extension and rotation of the head to the affected side while holding an inspiration).[9,10] Plain radiographs of the cervicothoracic area may demonstrate a cervical rib. Treatment includes analgesics, flexibility exercises, and postural and ergonomic changes.[9,10] Surgery is necessary occasionally.

Reflex sympathetic dystrophy (*RSD*) is another cause of neurologically mediated shoulder and arm pain characterized by vasomotor and dermal changes, musculoskeletal dysfunction, and premature osteoporosis. Also called *shoulder-hand syndrome,* or *Sudek's atrophy,* RSD is defined as an otherwise unexplained syndrome of ongoing pain that is not limited to a single nerve distribution, disproportionate to an initial noxious event, and associated with abnormal vascular or sudomotor (sweat gland) activity.[18]

Causalgia is an identical disorder arising as a result of direct nerve injury. Clinical findings include burning pain with hyperesthesia, dysesthesia, and edema with trophic changes in the hair, skin, and nails, and eventually muscle atrophy with limited joint motion. Urgent treatment involves exercise, which is the cornerstone of therapy and provides the greatest response, supplemented by nonsteroidal or opioid analgesics. Subsequent care may involve sympathetic ganglion blockade, oral sympatholytic agents, or regional or central neural blockade.

Numerous *entrapment syndromes* also affect nerves in the shoulder and upper extremity and result in pain.[8] The *suprascapular nerve* may be compressed between the suprascapular notch and the transverse scapular ligament, resulting in pain at the glenohumeral or acromioclavicular joints and weakness in abduction and external rotation at the shoulder. Radial nerve palsy may occur at the level of the spiral groove of the humerus (*Saturday night palsy*), the radial tunnel (*posterior interosseous syndrome*), or the wrist (*cheralgia paresthetica*). This results in varying levels of weakness involving the triceps and extensors at the wrist and digits, and possibly numbness in a radial nerve distribution. Pain is most commonly noted with radial tunnel compression.[9,13,17] Ulnar neuropathy may be reflected as pain at the elbow when compressed in the cubital tunnel, or pain at the wrist when impingement occurs in Guyon's canal. Both may cause pain, paresthesias, and numbness in the ulnar half of the ring finger and the entire small finger. Weakness may be noted in metacarpophalangeal flexion, finger abduction and adduction.[9,13] Median nerve compression may become symptomatic as the *pronator teres syndrome,* which results in proximal arm pain on pronation and both weakness and sensory loss in the hand, or the *anterior intraosseous syndrome,* which results in similar weakness but spares sensation and is generally painless. *Carpal tunnel syndrome* is the most common nerve entrapment, affecting 0.1% of individuals and occasionally arising from systemic conditions including rheumatoid arthritis, hypothyroidism, and pregnancy. A more common precipitant is overuse from repetitive hand and wrist movements. Symptoms include pain, paresthesias, and weakness involving the palmar aspect of the thumb, entire index and long fingers, and radial half of the ring finger. Often these symptoms are more bothersome at night or with sustained use of the hand. Sensory examination may be normal or may elicit a two-point tactile discrimination deficit. Muscle atrophy is a late finding. Physi-

TABLE 19.8. Thoracic and Truncal Pain

Nociceptive	Neuropathic
Tumors of the spine Diffuse idiopathic skeletal hyperostosis (DISH)	Tumors of the spine (spinal cord compression) Thoracic disc disease (HNP) Herpetic neuralgia Epidural abscess Transverse myelitis Spinal cord infarction

cal examination may also provoke paresthesias on Tinel's maneuver (percussion of the volar aspect of the wrist overlying the median nerve) or Phalen's maneuver (maintenance of wrist hyperflexion at 90 degrees for 60 seconds). Acute treatment involves wrist splinting with "cock-up" devices and NSAIDs. Patients with chronic nerve entrapments may also respond to antidepressant or anticonvulsant medication. Referral for surgical release is made in refractory cases.

Thoracic and Truncal Pain

Nociceptive Syndromes. *Tumors of the axial skeleton* are commonly metastatic in origin, and the thoracic spine is the most common location of spinal metastatic deposits (Table 19.8). Breast, lung, prostate, and colon carcinomas and multiple myeloma provide the bulk of cases, usually in patients over 50 years of age.[19–22] Benign tumors occasionally causing pain include hemangioma, osteoid osteoma, and giant cell tumors. Lymphoma, Ewing's sarcoma, and chordoma are less common. Presentation includes slowly progressive back pain, which is often worst when the patient is supine, localized tenderness to percussion, and, in patients with malignancy, weight loss, malaise, and fevers or night sweats. Plain radiographs are commonly normal because 30% of bone mass must be lost before typical pedicle destruction is seen.[14,20] When neurological deficits are identified, urgent MRI or myelography is performed.

Diffuse idiopathic skeletal hyperostosis (DISH) is a disorder characterized by ectopic bone formation in the spine and extremities. Anterolateral spurring in the lower thoracic spine is the most common finding. It may be asymptomatic, associated with thoracic spine stiffness, or, in rare circumstances, result in myelopathy.[14] It is more prevalent in older adults and males, and 40% have diabetes.[23]

Disorders of the heart and pericardium, lungs and pleura, esophagus, gallbladder, and rib cage can also present as thoracic pain.

Neuropathic Syndromes. The thoracic region is the most common spinal location for metastatic disease; 70% of spinal cord compression cases arise from thoracic cord involvement.[12] See Chapter 23, "Brain Tumors and Other Neuro-oncological Emergencies" for evaluation and management.

Thoracic disc disease or herniated nucleus puplosus is uncommon, probably due at least in part to the lack of mobility at this level.[17] Vague back pain with or without radiation along one or more of the intercostal nerves is the typical presentation. Tenderness and local sensory deficit may be present, and respiratory excursion may worsen the pain. T9–12 are the levels most commonly affected.[17] MRI is the test of choice for imaging this area.

The thoracic region is also a common location of *acute herpetic* or *postherpetic neuralgias*. The discomfort follows dermatomal patterns and occasionally precedes the rash. Other clinical features and treatment recommendations were discussed previously, in the section on facial pain.

Epidural abscess is most commonly seen at the thoracic level, typically involving an average of four vertebral levels and intervertebral disc spaces. Two-thirds of patients present acutely, with fever, leukocytosis, and back pain progressive over hours to days. One-third presents with chronic pain developing over weeks, often without fever or leukocytosis. Signs of myelopathy can be present; MRI is the imaging test of choice. Treatment requires intravenous administration of antibiotics and surgical drainage.

Transverse myelitis is another source of back pain and myelopathy, discussed in Chapter 21, "Multiple Sclerosis."

Spinal cord infarction is a rare event, presenting as acute partial (anterior) myelopathy (sparing vibratory and proprioceptive sensation associated with posterior column function) with chest, abdominal, or back pain.[12] It is commonly accompanied by limb ischemia or diminution of peripheral pulses, with aortic dissection as an underlying cause.[12,24] Atheroembolic disease, fibrocartilaginous emboli from disc herniation, vasculitis, sepsis, and complication of vascular catheterizations or epidural anesthesia are other etiologies.[12,25,26]

Low Back and Lower Extremity Pain

Overview. Low back pain is the most common complaint voiced to physicians, affecting over 80% of adults in the United States.[13,19,27] Forty percent of adults experience sciatica, and in one year, 5% of the population experience an attack of acute low back pain requiring medical attention. The annual costs are $10 billion for disability from back pain and $20 billion in overall medical expenditures.[21,28] Accurate diagnosis of lumbosacral and lower limb pain requires an organized assessment of those tissues containing pain fibers, which are the bony periosteum, ligaments and joint capsules, muscles and tendons, meninges, and the nerves themselves (Table 19.9).

Nociceptive Syndromes. These syndromes are categorized as disorders of the lumbar spine and disorders of the lower extremity. *Lumbar strain* or *sprain* is the most common source of simple "backache." The history may suggest acute or subacute pain with the first attack, but often there is a pattern of acute recurrent attacks superimposed on chronic discomfort. The pain may radiate, but rarely below the knee, thus distinguishing it from radiculopathy of discogenic pain. Physical examination reveals reproducible tenderness and spasm in the paraspinal muscles with restricted range of motion, and the hands of a skilled examiner may detect rotation of the transverse and spinous processes. Plain radiographs of the lumbosacral region are typically negative; their routine use is discouraged. Bed rest, application of cold and heat, and liberal use of NSAIDs and muscle relaxants result in improvement over several days. A recent study indicated patients who resumed normal activities recovered more quickly than those treated with extended bed rest or physical therapy.[29] Overall, more than 90% of patients return to their baseline condition within

TABLE 19.9. Common Causes of Low Back and Lower Extremity Pain

Nociceptive	Neuropathic
Disorders of the lumbar spine	Disorders of the lumbar spine
Lumbosacral strain	Conus medullaris syndrome
Trauma	Cauda equina syndrome
Discogenic disease	Spinal stenosis
Systemic arthritides (RA,AS)	Lumbar HNP
Cogenital spinal diseases	
Degenerative spinal disorders	
Spinal stenosis	
Vertebral osteomyelitis	
Sacroliliitis	
Tumors	
Abdominal aortic aneurysm	
Peptic ulcer disease	
Disorders of the kidneys	
Disorders of female reproductive tract	
Prostatitis	
Diverticulitis	
Hemoglobinopathies	
Psychogenic	
Disorders of the lower extremities	Disorders of the lower extremities
Vascular (ischemic): acute arterial occlusion	Lateral femoral cutaneous neuropathy
Deep venous thrombosis	Peroneal neuropathy
Systemic and septic arthritides	Joplin's neuroma
Acute gout	Morton's neuroma
Tendinitis, bursitis, and tenosynovitis	

two to eight weeks.[21,28] Some patients continue to have chronic low back pain. Pain continuing beyond three weeks is evaluated by neuroimaging studies such as CT or MRI. Sources of such pain are discussed most practically with reference to the age at presentation. *Children and adolescents* are most likely to have congenital malformations (*spina bifida, spondylolisthesis*), postural abnormalities (*scoliosis, kyphosis*), or other conditions such as *osteochondritis* (Scheuermann's disease). *Young adults* are prone to *lumbosacral strains* or direct *trauma, discogenic disease,* or systemic disorders such as *rheumatoid arthritis, ankylosing spondylitis,* and *Reiter's syndrome. Older adults* are most likely to experience *osteoarthritis* with spondylitic changes, spinal stenosis, and *vertebral metastases.* The inflammatory and malignant etiologies have

been discussed in the sections on cervical and thoracic pain.

Vertebral osteomyelitis presents as subacute pain progressing over weeks to months, worsening with activity, and not disappearing with rest.[13] Comorbid conditions include diabetes, intravenous drug use, and, commonly, recent infection of the skin, urinary tract, or lungs. Involvement of the first and second lumbar vertebrae is most common, and the likely pathogens include staphylococcus and pseudomonas species. Infection may also primarily involve the disc as *acute discitis,* with the postsurgical state providing a major risk factor. Organisms most frequently cultured are the staphylococcal species. Physical examination reveals exquisite local tenderness with muscle spasm and restricted range of motion. Radiculopathy can be present. Plain radiographs can show erosion of vertebral endplates or loss of disc-space height, and the erythrocyte sedimentation rate (ESR) and white blood cell (WBC) counts can be elevated. MRI is the most sensitive imaging procedure.[21] Treatment involves bed rest, opioid analgesics, intravenous antibiotics, and surgical consultation.

Sacroiliitis may present as back, buttock, or leg pain. In young adults this may reflect the onset of ankylosing spondylitis; in older adults it generally arises from nonspecific inflammation. Local tenderness and stress on the joint when the patient is prone or supine are helpful diagnostic points. Treatment programs generally use NSAIDs and physical therapy.

Lumbar pain may have additional causes such as abdominal aortic aneurysm, peptic ulcer disease, pancreatitis, disorders of the kidneys or female reproductive tract, prostatitis, or diverticulitis. Hemoglobinopathies, such as sickle cell disease and the thalassemias, may also present as back pain. *Psychogenic pain* is a diagnosis of exclusion.[19,30,31]

As stated for the upper extremity, nociceptive pain in the lower limb most often has vascular or inflammatory origins. Acute arterial occlusion is more common in the leg than arm, as is deep venous thrombosis. Septic arthritis has been discussed in the section on cervical and upper limb pain, as were the systemic arthritides.

Tenditinitis, tenosynovitis, and bursitis can affect the hip, knee, or ankle joints, as well as the foot. *Bursitis* is most common, and trochanteric bursitis at the hip, prepatellar bursitis at the knee, and calcaneal bursitis at the heel are the most common sites of involvement. Joint rest and NSAIDs are essential. A local injection of 10–40 mg of triamcinolone plus 1 ml of 1% lidocaine often provides immediate relief.

Acute gouty arthritis typically presents as an attack of excruciating pain in the foot or ankle. A history of gout may be present, and attacks can be precipitated by stress, excess food or alcohol intake, surgery, or dehydration. Prompt diagnosis is made by clinical findings and elevation of uric acid level, observed in 70% of patients. Initiation of high-dose, rapid-acting NSAIDs may abort the attack within hours. Indomethacin is considered a drug of choice, and colchicine is also useful early in the course of the disease. Allopurinol should not be given during

an acute attack but can be instituted as maintenance therapy.

Neuropathic Syndromes. Because the spinal cord ends at the L1–2 level, myelopathies are rarely seen in disorders of the lumbosacral spine. However, compression or dysfunction at the level of the conus medullaris or cauda equina may result in back pain and neurological compromise requiring emergency attention. The *conus medullaris syndrome* is usually acute, painless, and primarily symptomatic as early bowel and bladder dysfunction with bilateral sensory loss in a "saddle" distribution. Motor weakness is generally mild, but hyperreflexia and Babinski sign may be seen. The *cauda equina syndrome* is subacute and painful, and involves unilateral sensory and motor dysfunction in the limb ipsilateral to the pain. Sphincter changes occur later in the course of the syndrome. Compression from tumor, disc, hemorrhage, fracture, infection, or spondylolisthesis is a potential cause. Immediate imaging with MRI or CT myelography is indicated, and dexamethasone (a 10-mg bolus given intravenously, followed by 4 mg given intravenously every four hours) with surgical consultation is required.

Spinal stenosis is defined as narrowing of the spinal canal diameter. Patients may remain asymptomatic or can experience low back pain. Patients may complain of unilateral or bilateral pain in the extremities with activity; the classic *pseudoclaudication* presentation involves provocation of thigh or calf pain upon standing or ambulating.[21] Improvement in pain on spinal flexion distinguishes stenosis from discogenic pain, and the "bicycle sign" (absence of pain when riding a bicycle or leaning over a shopping cart) helps to distinguish it from ischemic claudication. Most individuals with spinal stenosis are adult males, with the L3–5 levels most frequently affected. Plain radiographs, CT, or MRI may help confirm the diagnosis. Treatment involves analgesics, adjuvant analgesics (antidepressants or antiepileptics), physical therapy, and surgery in appropriate cases.[21]

Lumbar HNP may present as back, buttock, or leg pain, and when nerve root compression occurs, pain radiates below the level of the knee.[13,14] Pain is generally relieved to some extent when the patient is in the supine position. Positional changes, the

TABLE 19.10. Localization of Lumbar Nerve Root Pathology

Disc Involved	Nerve Root Involved	Area of Pain	Area of Sensory Change	Motor	DTR
L3–4	L4	Posterolateral hip and thigh	Anterior thigh	Knee extensors	Patellar
L4–5	L5	Posterolateral thigh and leg, dorsal foot	Lateral calf, dorsum of foot, great toe	Ankle and great toe dorsiflexors	None
L5–S1	S1	Posterior thigh, lateral calf and foot, heel and lateral toes	Lateral calf, foot, and toes	Plantar flexion	Achilles

upright posture, and Valsalva maneuvers such as coughing, sneezing, and defecation all increase pain by increasing intradiscal pressure. Numbness, paresthesias, and weakness may follow or precede the development of pain in the lower extremity. The examination is tailored to focus on areas felt to be abnormal based on information from the history, although the entirety of the lumbosacral area and lower extremities is investigated with the patient in the standing, seated, and supine positions. Spinal alignment, heel-and-toe walking, spinal percussion, and special emphasis on segmental sensory, motor, and reflex testing provide a sound basis for evaluation (Table 19.10). Straight leg raising stretches the L5 and S1 nerve roots and produces radicular pain as a Lasegue sign; extending the hip while prone may stretch the L2–4 nerve roots and produce a "reverse Lasegue" sign. Pain during the *rotation test,* which involves rotation of the torso as a unit at the hips, or the *axial loading test,* which involves compression of the head downward, suggests nonneurogenic dysfunction or malingering. Uncomplicated presentations require no particular studies, and conservative management includes bed rest, nonsteroidal analgesics, and muscle relaxants. Plain radiographs and blood work are reserved for patients under 15 and over 50 years of age, patients with a history of malignancy or trauma, and those individuals with systemic symptoms (Table 19.11). MRI and CT myelography may help in complicated cases. Urgent surgical referrals are indicated in cases of rapidly progressive neurological impairment and conus medullaris or cauda equina syndrome.

Nerves in the lower extremities are subject to compression at the various levels. *Lateral femoral cutaneous neuropathy,* or *meralgia paresthetica,* involves a pure sensory neuropathy presenting as burning pain, paresthesias, and hypesthesia in the

TABLE 19.11. Indications for Plain Radiographs in Back Pain

1. Unable to assess the patient clinically
2. History of significant trauma
3. Suspected pathological lesions (carcinoma)
   a. Age > 50 (a relative indication)
   b. History of cancer with suspected metastasis to bone
4. Suspected infection
   a. Immunocompromised patients
   b. Patients on dialysis
   c. Patients with recent spine surgery
   d. Intravenous drug users
   e. Children (age < 15) (a relative indication)
5. Neurological deficit
6. Suspected ankylosing spondylitis (sclerosis of sacroiliac joints).

anterolateral thigh. Entrapment at the inguinal ligament may be caused by pregnancy, obesity, or tight-fitting garments, and confirmed by provocation of symptoms upon percussion of this area. Motor and reflex examinations and electrophysiological studies are normal. Treatment involves analgesics, adjuvant antidepressants, and correction of any underlying etiology. *Peroneal neuropathy* generally arises from compression of the nerve at the fibular head due to leg crossing, repetitive trauma, or extended bed rest. Pain below the knee, paresthesias, and numbness in the first web space on the foot, and weakness of foot eversion and dorsiflexion may be detected. *Joplin's neuroma* causes pain and paresthesias over the first metatarsophalangeal joint with radiation to the toes. It arises from perineural fibrosis of the plantar digital nerve. *Morton's neuroma* typically causes pain between the third and fourth tarsals, which worsens with weight bearing. This pain arises from entrapment of the interdigital nerve by the transverse metatarsal ligament. Both neuromas can be managed by NSAIDs and surgical referral.

- Cervical spondylosis is the most common cause of cervical radiculopathy, and disc herniation is the most common cause of lumbar radiculopathy.
- In radiculopathies from either cervical or lumbar disc disease, the root affected generally carries the same number as the vertebral body inferior to the disc; that is, the C6–7 disc affects the C7 root, the L4–5 disc affects te L5 root.
- Ninety percent of cervical radiculopathies affect the C6 or C7, and 95% of all lumbar radiculopathies affect the L5 or S1 nerve root.
- Neurogenic claudication differs from ischemic claudication in that the former produces pain when the patient is standing still.
- The gonadal dose of a typical five-view lumbosacral series of radiographs is equal to that of a one-view chest radiograph daily for six years.
- An ipsilateral straight-leg-raise sign is 95% sensitive, but a contralateral or "crossed" straight-leg-raise sign is more specific.
- The C1 nerve root is the only segmental nerve root lacking a sensory dermatome.

PEARLS AND PITFALLS

- The typical patient with chronic facial pain sees an average of 7.5 health professionals.
- The fifth, ninth, and tenth cranial nerves all provide sensory innervation to the external ear – explaining referral of otalgia to the head or throat.
- The physician searches for indicators of multiple sclerosis in any patient under age 40 with trigeminal neuralgia.
- Pain in the stylomastoid foramen is characteristic of Bell's palsy.
- Be aware of cervical spine instability in patient with Down's syndrome or rheumatoid arthritis.
- Brachial plexopathy from metastatic disease is characteristically painful and involves the lower plexus. Radiation plexopathy is painless and typically involves the upper plexus.
- Pain is the most common symptom of malignant spinal cord compression, and is present in 96% of patients at diagnosis.

REFERENCES

1. Wilson JE, Pendleton JM. Oligoanalgesia in the Emergency Department. *Am J Emerg Med.* 1989;7620–3.
2. Chan D, Goldberg R, Tuscone A, et.al. The effects of spinal immobilization on healthy volunteers. *Ann Emerg Med.* 1994;(23)1:48–51.
3. Cordell WH, Hollingsworth JC, Olinger ML, et.al. Pain and tissue interface pressures during spine board immobilization. *Ann Emerg Med.* 1995;(26)1:31–36.
4. Solomon S, Lipton RB. Facial Pain. *Neurol Clin.* 1990;8:9–13–928.
5. Hanes SJ, Jannetta PJ, Zorub DS. Microvascular relations of the trigeminal nerve. An anatomical study with clinical correlation. *J Neurosurg.* 1980;52:381–8.
6. Watson CP. The treatment of postherpetic neuralgia. *Neurology.* 1995;45(suppl 8):558–60.
7. Dalessio DJ. Diagnosis and treatment of cranial neuralgias. *Med Clin North Am.* 1991;75:606–15.
8. Mementhaler M, Schliach H. *Peripheral Nerve Lesions. Diagnosis and Therapy.* New York, NY: Thieme Medical Publishers; 1991.
9. Wall PD, Melzack R (eds). *Textbook of Pain.* 3rd ed. New York: Churchill, 1994.
10. Cailliet R. *Neck and Arm Pain.* 3rd ed. Philadelphia: FA Davis Co., 1991.

11. Ashbury AK, McKhamm GM, McDonald WI, (eds). *Diseases of the Nervous System - Clinical Neurobiology.* Philadelphia: WB Saunders Co., 1986.
12. Woosley RM, Young RR, eds. Disorders of the spinal canal. *Neurol Clin North Am.* 1991;9:3.
13. Lian MH (ed). Musculoskeletal pain syndromes. *Primary Care Clinics and Office Practice.* 1988;15:4.
14. Esses SI. *Textbook of Spinal Disorders.* Philadelphia: JB Lippincott & Co., 1995.
15. Breedveld SC, Algra PR, Vielvoye CJ, et al. Magnetic resonance imaging in the evaluation of patients with rheumatoid arthritis and subluxations of the cervical spine. *Arth Rheum.* 1987;30:624–629.
16. Smith MD. Cervical radiculopathy: Causes and surgical treatment. *Minnesota Medicine.* Vol. 78, 1995; Apr:28–45.
17. Weiderhold WC. *Neurology for the Non-Neurologist.* 3rd ed. Philadelphia: WB Saunders, 1995.
18. Merskey H, Bogduk N. *Classification of Chronic Pain. Descriptions of Chronic Pain Syndromes and Definitions of Pain Terms.* Seattle: IASP Press; 1994.
19. Deyo RA. Re-thinking strategies for acute low back pain. *Emerg Med.* 1995:38–56.
20. Flotre M. Evaluation and management of oncologic emergencies. *Emerg Med Reports.* 1991;12:11–20.
21. Wiens DA. Acute low back pain: Differential diagnosis, targeted assessment, and theraupeutic controversies. *Emerg Med Reports.* 1995;16(14):129–140.
22. Brown MD, Rydevik BL (eds). Causes and cure of low back pain and sciatica. *Orthoped Cl N Am.* 1991; 22:2.
23. Gillette RD. A practical approach to a patient with back pain. *Am Family Physicians.* 1996(53)2:670–676.
24. DeBakey ME, McCollum CH, Crawford ES. Dissection and dissecting aneurysm of the aorta: Follow-up of 527 patients treated surgically. *Surg.* 1982;92: 1118.
25. Mikulis DJ, Ogilvy CS, McKee A, et.al. Spinal cord infarction and fibrocartilagenous emboli. *Am J Neuro Radiology.* 1992;13:155–160.
26. Ackerman WE, Mushtague MJ, Knapp RK. Maternal paraparesis after epidural anesthesia and cesarean section. *Southern Med J.* 1990;83:695–697.
27. Nachemson A. The lumber spine - An orthopedic challenge. *Spine.* 1976;1:59.
28. Mauer TG, Mooney D, Gatchel RJ (eds). *Contemporary conservative care for painful spinal disorders.* Philadelphia: Lea & Febiger, 1991.
29. Malmivaara A, Hakkinen U, Aro T, et.al. The treatment of acute low back pain – bedrest, exercises or ordinary activity? *N Engl J Med.* 1995;332:351–5.
30. Henry GL, Little N. *Neurologic Emergencies – A symptom oriented approach.* New York: McGraw-Hill, 1985.
31. Weintraub MI. (ed) Malingering and conversion reaction. *Neurol Cl.* 1995;13:2. Philadelphia: WB Saunders.

20 Neuro-ophthalmology

ERIC R. EGGENBERGER AND TIM HODGE

SUMMARY Diplopia and visual loss are common neuro-ophthalmological symptoms in patients presenting to the emergency department. Binocular diplopia results from ocular misalignment and can be produced by lesions of cranial nerve III, IV, or VI, or dysfunction of the extraocular muscles, the neuromuscular junction, or internuclear connections. Visual loss categorized by monocular or binocular presentation can further help localize the lesion to the prechiasmal, chiasmal, or postchiasmal region. Pupillary abnormalities are commonly observed in the emergency department. The finding of pupillary dysfunction or asymmetry can be approached in a systematic fashion.

Introduction

Neuro-ophthalmological disorders can be divided into eye movement disorders (efferent diseases), visual loss (afferent diseases), and pupillary dysfunction. Acute intervention necessary to treat each neuro-ophthalmic disease depends on the underlying condition. Immediate neuro-ophthalmologic evaluation is rarely required in the emergency department. Neuro-ophthalmological consultation is recommended for unexplained diplopia, visual loss, or pupillary abnormalities.

Prehospital Evaluation

Most neuro-ophthalmological conditions presenting to the ED require a detailed evaluation. Prehospital evaluation of these conditions usually consists of describing the abnormalities unless they are associated with other medical emergencies, such as trauma or stroke, for which prehospital care is directed.

Emergency Evaluation

General History

The medical history and the list of medications are essential aspects of evaluation, and serve to highlight predisposing conditions for neuro-ophthalmic diseases. Family history can provide critical information for patients with hereditary or genetic diseases. Aspects of the patient's social history such as alcohol, tobacco, and caffeine use provide clues to specific diagnoses.

Efferent Disease: Diplopia

When evaluating a patient with diplopia, the physician establishes whether the symptoms are monocular or binocular (when diplopia resolves when either eye is covered, the patient has binocular diplopia; when diplopia is present in only one eye, the patient has monocular diplopia); and whether images are separated vertically, obliquely, or horizontally. Monocular diplopia (see Fig. 20.1) generally does not indicate neurological dysfunction or ocular

Sid M. Shah and Kevin M. Kelly, eds., *Emergency Neurology: Principles and Practice.* Copyright ©
1999 Cambridge University Press. All rights reserved.

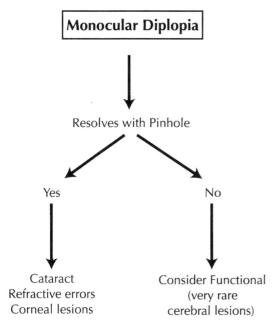

FIGURE 20.1. Evaluation of monocular diplopia

misalignment; it results from cornea, lens, or retinal pathology (refractive error and cataract are the most common causes). Binocular diplopia (see Fig. 20.2) results from misalignment of the eyes. This can result from disease of cranial nerve III, IV, or VI (see Fig. 20.3) (or their connections, i.e., internuclear ophthalmoplegia), disorders of the extraocular muscles (e.g., thyroid disease, orbital trauma, or tumor), or disorders of the neuromuscular junction (e.g., myasthenia gravis). Occasionally patients interpret subtle binocular diplopia as "blur," especially when the two images overlap; blur that resolves with closure of either eye has the same significance and differential diagnosis as binocular diplopia.

Afferent Disease: Visual Loss

When there is sensory visual dysfunction (visual loss), the examiner establishes whether symptoms are present in one or both eyes and whether symptoms are worse with near or distance vision. There are six pathophysiologies of monocular visual dysfunction: (1) refractive error; (2) lens/cornea/ocular media opacity; (3) retina/macula dysfunction; (4) optic nerve disease; (5) amblyopia; and (6) functional visual loss. The onset, pace, and associated symptoms of visual dysfunction are important considerations. Acute visual loss without pain can be caused by vascular occlusion or retinal detachment. Painful loss of vision is more characteristic of an inflammatory condition (such as optic neuritis) or acute angle closure glaucoma. Slow, progressive, painless visual loss typically characterizes compressive optic neuropathies. Difficulty with only near or distance vision implies refractive error.

Neuro-ophthalmological Examination

Visual Acuity. The measurement of visual acuity is one of the most important aspects of the emergency eye examination. Visual acuity is tested in each eye separately with the patient's corrective lens by using a Snellen chart or a near card. When optimal correction is not available, pinhole testing is used. Pinhole testing uses an occluder with multiple small holes (approximately 16–18 gauge size) placed over the patient's eye while he or she reads the visual chart.

When a formal chart is not available, newsprint, which corresponds to approximately 20/80 isotype, can be used to measure acuity. Patients with vision less than 20/400 are quantified according to their ability to count fingers, detect hand movements (specify distance and quadrant), or perceive light.

Pupils. When evaluating pupillary dysfunction, the size of the pupil under conditions of light and dark, and reactivity in response to light and near stimuli are considered. When the pupil fails to respond normally to light, a near target is used to assess reactivity. Near-light dissociation (NLD) exists when the pupil reacts to a near target, but not to light. The differential diagnosis for NLD is discussed in the later section on pupils. The swinging flashlight test is used to check for apparent "paradoxical" pupillary dilation in response to light (relative afferent pupillary defect, or RAPD, also referred to as the Marcus Gunn pupil). This test is the only objective confirmation of monocular anterior visual dysfunction. This test is performed in a dark room by shining a bright light in one of the patient's eyes for one to two seconds, then swinging the light to stimulate the other eye. A normal response is initial constriction with light stimulation in each eye. Pupil dilation that occurs when the light is presented indicates an afferent (sensory) visual lesion (most commonly an optic neuropathy).

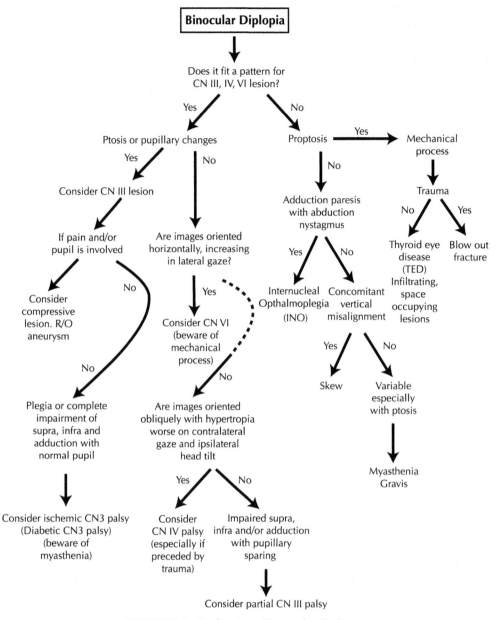

FIGURE 20.2. Evaluation of binocular diplopia

Visual Fields. In an emergency department neurological examination, monocular confrontational testing of visual fields is one of the most important aspects of the neurological examination for localizing abnormalities. Prechiasmal lesions cause monocular visual field defects. Bitemporal hemianopsia results from a lesion at the optic chiasm. Homonymous hemianopsia results from postchiasmal lesions of the optic tract, optic radiation, or occipital cortex. Associated symptoms and signs, and neuroimaging help distinguish the various locations of abnormal-ity. Formal visual field testing with either Goldmann or Humphrey perimetry may be required to detect or quantify visual field defects accurately.

Motility. Neuro-ophthalmological examination of the patient with binocular diplopia emphasizes ocular alignment and movement of the eyes through the nine cardinal positions of gaze. *Ductions* refer to the excursion of each eye separately; *versions* refer to conjugate eye movements (e.g., leftward or upward). Occasionally, especially in patients with

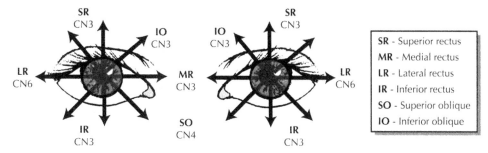

FIGURE 20.3. Depicts extraocular muscle innervation by cranial nerves III, IV, VI, and the direction of eye movements that result with contraction of the different extraocular muscles.

complete nerve lesions, the eye is unable to move in a characteristic direction (see Fig. 20.3). Other patients with diplopia have only subtle misalignment in a particular position of gaze, and general assessment in the positions of gaze is unrewarding. In such patients, formal measurements of ductions and ocular alignment are valuable.

Ductions can be measured according to the extent of movement limitation, either as a percent of normal, or in millimeters of "scleral show" remaining at the end of the ocular movement. *Ocular alignment* refers to the angle of deviation of one eye in relationship to the other eye. Exotropia (XT) indicates an outward deviation of the eye ("wall-eyed"); esotropia (ET) is the inward turning of the eye ("cross-eyed"). Hypertropia refers to one eye that is higher than the other eye. Techniques to dissociate the eyes, such as alternate cover or red Maddox rod testing, are required to quantify the amount of ocular misalignment. Alternate cover testing is performed with the patient fixing on an accommodative target (such as a particular letter on the Snellen chart). One of the patient's eyes is covered with an occluder while he or she views the target. The occluder is then shifted to cover the other eye, thus forcing the patient to fix the target with the previously covered eye. When ocular misalignment is present, the eyes move to take up fixation when uncovered. An esotropic eye deviates inward toward the nose under the occluder, and moves outward to fixate when the other eye is covered. A hypertropic eye deviates upward under the cover, and moves downward to fixate when the occluder is removed. The pattern of misalignment can assist in diagnosis; an ET increasing in right gaze can indicate a limitation of

abduction in the right eye due to a right sixth nerve palsy.

The red Maddox rod is another dissociative method to measure ocular alignment (see Fig. 20.4). The red Maddox rod is a panel of adjacent red cylinders. A bright, point source of light is used as the target. The Maddox rod is always placed over the patient's right eye by convention and creates the appearance of a red line from the light source. The patient perceives the point source of light with the left eye (the "white light"), while the right eye with the Maddox rod views a red line (the "red line"). When the Maddox rod has created a horizontal line, the patient is asked whether the white light is above, below, or through the red line, and measurement of the vertical alignment is made with prisms. When the light is above the line, a right hypertropia exists. With the line oriented vertically, the patient is asked if the line is to the right or left of the light, and the horizontal alignment is assessed. When the line is to the right of the light, an esotropia exists; when the line appears to the left of the light there is an exotropia ("crossed" for exotropia, with the red line from the Maddox rod over the *right* eye appearing displaced to the *left*). The line from the Maddox rod can be displaced with prisms until it dissects the light and thus quantifies the amount and direction of deviation in all positions of gaze. The red Maddox rod has several advantages in that it is inexpensive, quick, accurate, and relatively easy to use.

Lids and External Examination. Ptosis can result from disorders of the nerve (cranial nerve III or sympathetics – Horner's syndrome), neuromuscular junction (e.g., myasthenia gravis), or muscle (e.g., dehiscence of the levator palpebrae muscle from its

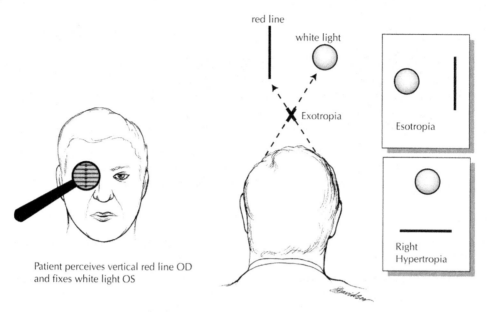

FIGURE 20.4. Use of the red Maddox rod (RMR) to determine ocular alignment. See text for details. OD (right eye); OS (left eye).

tendon, mitochondrial myopathy or muscular dystrophies). Lid retraction is typically a symptom of thyroid eye disease; however, certain medications or hydrocephalus (as part of Parinaud's syndrome) can also produce this sign. Proptosis can result from either traumatic (orbital hemorrhage, bony displacement, or carotid-cavernous fistula) or nontraumatic mechanisms (infection, tumor, carotid-cavernous fistula, thyroid eye disease, or other myopathy).

Fundus. The optic disc is examined for distinctness of margins, and color. Disc edema can result from several pathophysiologies; papilledema refers to disc edema due to increased intracranial pressure (ICP) and is a neurological emergency. In the early stages of disc edema, the margins of the nerve head appear indistinct due to disc elevation (the direct ophthalmoscope resolves in only two dimensions and therefore cannot provide elevation details).[1] In advanced cases of disc edema, the retinal vessels are obscured as they pass over the disc margin, and splinter hemorrhages can be observed.

Disc edema can be unilateral or bilateral. Papilledema is typically bilateral and associated with normal visual acuity. Monocular disc edema resulting from ischemic, inflammatory, demyelinating, compressive, or infiltrating pathophysiologies is generally associated with decreased visual function.

Pupillary dilation is required for complete retinal evaluation, and mydriatics such as phenylephrine and tropicamide are used. Dilation with these agents temporarily hinders pupillary assessment for four to six hours, which can be critical in some patients with neurological disease, and also carries a small risk of precipitating acute angle closure glaucoma. Optimal treatment of angle closure glaucoma involves laser iridotomy, and administration of 1% pilocarpine is often used as acute therapy.

Ocular Motility Problems: Diplopia

Overview. The ocular motor system is divided into supranuclear, nuclear, infranuclear and internuclear components. The supranuclear neurons are located diffusely in the cerebral hemispheres. The saccadic system is crossed; the right frontal eye fields give rise to fibers that cross the midline on their way to the left paramedian pontine reticular formation (PPRF), or horizontal gaze center, which controls gaze to the left. The pursuit system is primarily uncrossed, with principal fibers originating in the parieto-occipital lobes, which descend ipsilaterally to the PPRF. Most supranuclear lesions result in gaze palsies or preferences (skew deviation is a notable exception). The most common supranuclear hemispheric lesion is a frontoparietal stroke with resultant gaze preference; a large right fron-

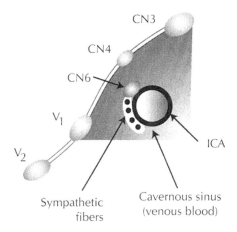

FIGURE 20.5. Diagram of the cavernous sinus depicting the anatomical relationships of neural and vascular structures. ICA (internal carotid artery).

toparietal cortical infarction can produce conjugate deviation of the eyes to the right (a right gaze preference). The eye deviation of a gaze preference can be overcome with reflexes such as the oculocephalic maneuver. Gaze preferences typically are observed acutely, and resolve within days.

Nuclear or infranuclear lesions cannot be overcome by reflex movements such as the oculocephalic maneuver, because the final common pathway for eye movement is involved in the lesion. Pontine lesions affecting the PPRF produce gaze palsies; a left PPRF lesion results in conjugate deviation of the eyes to the right (a left gaze palsy).

The cerebellum plays a crucial part in pursuit and saccadic accuracy as well as the vestibular ocular reflex. Abnormalities of the cerebellum or its connections lead to nystagmus, eye movement inaccuracies, and skew deviation.

Cranial Neuropathies

I. OCULOMOTOR NERVE: CRANIAL NERVE III. The oculomotor nerve emanates from a single joined midline nucleus in the dorsal midbrain, and its fascicles traverse the red nucleus and cerebral peduncle. The nerve lies in close proximity to the posterior communicating artery within the subarachnoid space before entering the cavernous sinus (see Fig. 20.5). The fibers are located in the lateral wall within the cavernous sinus and enter the orbit via the superior orbital fissure.

The presentation of third nerve palsies varies depending on the location and degree of involvement,

producing combinations of ptosis, mydriasis, and vertical, horizontal, or oblique diplopia. Third nerve fibers are vulnerable to lesions anywhere along their course, and associated symptoms and signs help distinguish among midbrain, subarachnoid space, cavernous sinus, or orbital lesions.

Cranial nerve III can be thought of as the "vasculopathic" cranial nerve due to the ischemic third nerve palsies commonly seen in diabetic patients, and its vulnerability to compression by an aneurysm. Aneurysmal third nerve palsy, commonly related to posterior communicating artery aneurysm compression, is a neurological emergency. Approximately 35% of all aneurysms occur in this location. The history of pain and progression and a detailed examination of the pupil help in evaluating third nerve palsies. In most compressive third cranial nerve palsies, the *pupil is involved* (poorly reactive and larger compared to the contralateral eye). Any patient with findings consistent with a pupil-involved third nerve palsy with *pain* is considered to have posterior communicating aneurysm until angiography proves otherwise. These patients require emergency evaluation so that life-threatening aneurysmal rupture and subarachnoid hemorrhage can be either avoided or treated. Uncal herniation due to a space-occupying lesion can also produce a compressive third nerve palsy with pupillary involvement; however, this is almost universally associated with other symptoms and signs of increased ICP (see Chapter 26 "Increased Intracranial Pressure").

VASCULOPATHIC OR "DIABETIC" THIRD NERVE PALSY. Frequently a pupil-sparing third nerve palsy results from microvascular (ischemic or "diabetic") pathophysiology. Diplopia caused by third nerve dysfunction and initial pain referred to the eye commonly are present. Typically, these patients have vascular risk factors such as diabetes, hypertension, hyperlipidemia, tobacco use, and age greater than 45 years. Pupillary sparing is almost always observed in these "ischemic" third nerve palsies. A compressive cause (e.g. aneurysm) of the third cranial nerve palsy is not a consideration when the pupil is normal and ocular motility is completely affected (eye is "down and out" with no adduction, supraduction, or infraduction) along with complete ptosis. Pupillomotor fibers travel on the outside of the third nerve fascicle, and are therefore selectively vulnerable to compression while being resistant to ischemia, which preferentially affects the interior of the nerve. Third nerve palsies resulting from oculomotor nerve ischemia mechanism generally resolve within three months without sequelae.

Several other pathological conditions can affect the third nerve fascicle along its course from the midbrain.[2] Accurate diagnosis of these conditions is dependent on associated symptoms and signs. Weber's syndrome consists of an ipsilateral third nerve palsy with contralateral hemiparesis indicating a midbrain lesion involving the cerebral peduncle, which typically results from infarction. When third nerve palsy is associated with an ipsilateral Horner's syndrome or cranial nerve IV, V, or VI dysfunction, localization in the cavernous sinus or superior orbital fissure is suggested. However, myasthenia gravis can cause painless, pupillary abnormalities and virtually any pattern of ocular dysmotility.

TROCHLEAR NERVE: CRANIAL NERVE IV. The trochlear nucleus is located in the dorsal midbrain. The trochlear nerve is the only cranial nerve to exit from the dorsal surface of the brain. The fourth nerve fibers cross in the dorsal perimesencephalic subarachnoid space, then course around the midbrain to enter the cavernous sinus before innervating the superior oblique muscle. The superior oblique muscle acts to depress and intort (incyclotort, or turn the superior pole of the eye toward the nose) the eye. Trochlear neuropathies result in oblique diplopia with a slight tilt to one of the images without ptosis. Frequently, no obvious impairment of ductions is visible when observing the eyes through the nine cardinal positions of gaze. A hypertropia is present that increases in contralateral gaze and ipsilateral head tilt (e.g., a right fourth nerve palsy results in a right hypertropia, which increases in left gaze and right head tilt). The relative excyclotorsion can be demonstrated by a simple technique using a straight horizontal line. A pointer, or other straight edge is held horizontally and viewed by the patient. The patient with a CN IV palsy perceives two lines, vertically displaced but also intersecting, with the resulting "arrow" pointing toward the side of the palsy.

Cranial nerve IV can be thought of as the "trauma" cranial nerve, because trauma is the most common cause of fourth nerve palsies.[2,3] Head injury with loss of consciousness often produces a tor-

sional movement of the hemispheres around the brainstem; the long subarachnoid course of the nerve, coursing around the midbrain and adjacent to the tentorial edge, contributes to its vulnerability to trauma. Diplopia (with no ptosis or pupillary abnormalities) in the traumatic brain-injured patient is often associated with trochlear neuropathies, especially when mechanical orbital process such as muscle entrapment from "blowout" fractures can be excluded. Microvasculopathic processes associated with diabetes and hypertension can produce fourth nerve palsies that typically follow the same course as vasculopathic or "diabetic" third nerve palsies, improving within three months.

ABDUCENS NERVE: CRANIAL NERVE VI. The abducens nerve emanates from nuclei in the dorsal pons, course through the brainstem to exit ventrally at the pontomedullary junction before ascending along the dorsal aspect of the clivus to enter the cavernous sinus, where it lies in close proximity to the carotid artery. The nerve enters the orbit through the superior orbital fissure to innervate the lateral rectus muscle.

Sixth nerve palsies produce binocular horizontal diplopia that worsens with gaze toward the side of the lesion. The nerve can be affected anywhere along its course in the brainstem, subarachnoid space, cavernous sinus, or orbit; accurate localization depends on associated symptoms and signs. Increased ICP from any cause can produce a "false localizing" sixth nerve palsy. Accordingly, cranial nerve VI can be thought of as the "tumor" nerve. The nerve can be affected by direct compression due to mass lesions, but also through the indirect effects of increased ICP related to space-occupying lesions distant from the nerve.[2] Space-occupying lesions or other causes of intracranial hypertension are considered in the differential diagnosis of sixth nerve palsies, especially when papilledema or other symptoms or signs of elevated ICP exists.

Cranial nerve VI can also be affected by ischemia ("diabetic" or microvasculopathic cause). Typically, this occurs in patients with risk factors for vascular disease such as hypertension, hyperlipidemia, and diabetes. Nerve palsies of this type typically follow the same clinical course as "diabetic" third nerve palsies, improving over approximately three months.

Multiple Cranial Neuropathies and Other Causes of Diplopia.

Patients with multiple cranial neuropathies can present with symptoms and signs that are confusing. The movements of each of the patient's eyes are evaluated separately in the horizontal and vertical planes. Combinations of cranial nerve palsies are extremely helpful in localizing the abnormality. Combinations of cranial nerves III, IV, and VI commonly are the result of cavernous sinus lesions (see Fig. 20.5), especially when no upper motor neuron signs (e.g., weakness or numbness of a limb) are present; such a combination *with* optic nerve dysfunction points to the orbital apex. This localization has particular importance when imaging such patients, as coronal sections on imaging studies are required to best visualize the cavernous sinus.

1. MYASTHENIA GRAVIS. Myasthenia gravis (MG) occurs in either generalized or ocular forms. Ocular involvement often produces diplopia and ptosis. MG is considered in any patient with painless, pupil-sparing, binocular diplopia of virtually any pattern, especially when ptosis is present. Variability of symptoms is the hallmark of MG; a history of worsening symptoms as the day progresses suggests the diagnosis. MG can be diagnosed clinically, but ancillary testing – such as acetylcholine receptor antibody assay, electromyography (EMG) with repetitive stimulation, and Tensilon (edrophonium) – help confirm the diagnosis.

It is important to consider the diagnosis of MG because ocular involvement can occur prior to progression to generalized disease (see Chapter 18 "Neuromuscular Disorders"). The treatment of ocular MG parallels therapy of generalized disease, which includes the use of acetylcholinesterase inhibitors, or immune modulation with use of steroids, plasmapheresis, or thymectomy.

GUILLAIN-BARRÉ AND MILLER FISHER SYNDROMES. Guillain-Barré syndrome (GBS) (see also Chapter 18) is an immune-mediated, monophasic, primarily *motor* neuropathy that produces progressive weakness over hours to days. The examination is notable for weakness and generalized areflexia associated with minimal or no sensory change. Severe GBS often affects the extraocular muscles and eyelids, resulting in diplopia and ptosis, respectively.[4] The importance of diagnosing GBS in the emergency department is the recognition of the potential for se-

vere generalized weakness, including respiratory failure. The Miller Fisher syndrome (MFS) is a variant of GBS characterized by ophthalmoplegia, ataxia, and areflexia *without* extremity weakness. GBS and MFS share several features, including relative sparing of sensation, CSF abnormalities, and available therapeutic options. CSF analysis in patients with either disease is characterized by protein elevation without cells; the peak protein level of this *albumino cytological dissociation* typically occurs at least one week after disease onset. The differential diagnosis commonly includes MG and botulism.

INTERNUCLEAR OPHTHALMOPLEGIA. Internuclear ophthalmoplegia (INO) is a common pattern of ocular misalignment that indicates medial longitudinal fasciculus (MLF) dysfunction.[3] The MLF serves to connect the abducens nucleus innervating the lateral rectus muscle with the contralateral third nerve nucleus innervating the medial rectus muscle resulting in coordinated horizontal eye movements. Lesions of this pathway result in impaired ipsilateral adduction, with contralateral abducting nystagmus, and can be associated with a skew deviation of the eyes. INO localizes to the dorsal pontomesencephalic region, and can result from several pathological processes. INO in younger patients is typically associated with the demyelination of multiple sclerosis; brainstem infarction is a more common cause in older patients. INO is distinguished from third nerve disease by the lack of other oculomotor dysfunction – that is, absence of ptosis, pupillary abnormality, infraduction, or supraduction weakness. A "pseudo-INO" can result from peripheral causes of ophthalmoparesis such as MG.

Skew deviation is a vertical misalignment of the eyes resulting from a supranuclear lesion within the brainstem involving the otolith or vestibular pathways.[3] The majority of patients with skew deviation have nystagmus acutely (especially downbeat nystagmus, best observed in down and lateral gaze). Specific localization of the lesion within the brainstem depends on other symptoms and signs. Patients present with binocular vertical diplopia without ptosis and there is a full range of extraocular movements. Although skew deviation can result from numerous causes, infarction in older patients with risk factors for vascular disease is the most common. Skew deviation can be observed in association with the dorsal midbrain (Parinaud's syndrome). Parinaud's syndrome also includes impaired vertical gaze, near-light dissociation of the pupils (greater reactivity to a near target than to light stimulation), lid retraction, and convergence-retraction nystagmus (CRN). CRN is best observed while the patient views an optokinetic drum or other repeating pattern (such as a tape measure) rotated slowly in a downward direction.

BOTULISM. A neurotoxin produced by the bacteria *Clostridium botulinum* causes botulism. This disease occurs from ingestion of improperly cooked or canned food. The toxin affects the presynaptic portion of the neuromuscular junction to inhibit the release of acetylcholine, which results in a purely motor pattern of dysfunction.[4] Typically, symptoms occur within 48 hours of the ingestion of contaminated food. The most common early neurological complaints are diplopia and weakness. Ocular signs include ptosis, extraocular muscle weakness, and pupillary mydriasis. Gastrointestinal symptoms are also associated with botulism. EMG is often helpful in diagnosis. Early treatment with botulinum antitoxin is considered; however, this is commonly associated with serious side effects. Supportive care typically results in full recovery that occurs in several months.

ORBITAL (MECHANICAL) PATHOLOGIES. Orbital tumors can produce diplopia, visual loss, or proptosis. Visual loss is typically slowly progressive as a consequence of tumor growth. Ocular motility defects often involve more than one cranial nerve.

Thyroid eye disease is the most common cause of proptosis in adults. The three most common complications of thyroid orbitopathy (TO) include corneal disease, extraocular muscle disease with diplopia, and optic nerve dysfunction with loss of vision. The findings of TO or Graves' disease can include exophthalmos, lid retraction, lag, or edema, limitation of ocular motility, or conjunctival injection.[4,5] Thyroid eye disease is typically painless unless corneal decompensation is present. Severe pain strongly suggests a diagnosis other than that of TO. The orbital process of TO follows a separate and distinct course from that of thyroid disease and can occur in hyper-, hypo-, or euthyroid patients (hyperthyroid status is most common). The medial and inferior rectus muscles are most commonly in-

volved, and restriction of these swollen muscles produces diplopia that increases with upward or lateral gaze; esotropic and hypertropic patterns are the most common. The most serious sequelae of TO is optic neuropathy with optic nerve compression by the swollen extraocular muscles. Compressive optic neuropathy related to thyroid disease is an emergency. Treatment options include steroids, radiation therapy, and surgical decompression.

Trauma can produce diplopia from neuropathy or myopathy, resulting in mechanical dysfunction of the extraocular muscles. Entrapment of extraocular muscle by bony orbital injury produces ocular misalignment that generally does not conform to patterns of single cranial nerve abnormalities. Inferior orbital blowout fractures with entrapment or injury of the inferior rectus muscle is the most common pattern. Examination typically reveals impaired supraduction of the involved eye with proptosis or enophthalmos. Trauma can also cause trochlear nerve palsies (less commonly abducens or oculomotor nerve involvement) or carotid-cavernous fistulas. Diagnostic imaging includes magnetic resonance imaging (MRI) or computerized tomography (CT) scans. MRI has the advantage of multiple imaging planes and greater soft tissue resolution; CT performed in both the axial and coronal planes is faster and provides excellent detail of bony structures.

WERNICKE'S ENCEPHALOPATHY. Wernicke's encephalopathy results from thiamine deficiency; in the United States, it is most often seen in alcoholics.[6] The characteristic triad includes ophthalmoplegia, ataxia, and alteration in mental status. Lesions of the brainstem nuclei can cause diverse patterns of ocular muscle weakness. Untreated Wernicke's disease results in irreversible neurological dysfunction with pathological lesions observed in several locations within the brainstem including the mammillary bodies; the permanent cognitive difficulties associated with prominent amnesia constitute Korsakoff's psychosis. Acute ophthalmoparesis can be reversed quickly by the intravenous administration of thiamine, indicating that a biochemical deficiency can be treated for a period of time before an irreversible abnormality is established. The disease rarely presents as the typical triad of symptoms described. Accordingly, suspected Wernicke's disease is treated with thiamine.[1]

ORBITAL PSEUDOTUMOR AND TOLOSA-HUNT SYNDROMES. Orbital pseudotumor and Tolosa-Hunt syndromes are idiopathic inflammatory processes in the orbit and cavernous sinus, respectively, and share histopathological features and treatment strategies.[4] Orbital pseudotumor syndrome presents with *painful* ophthalmoplegia due to combined myopathic and neuropathic mechanisms, often with proptosis. Visual loss can be associated when inflammation affects the optic nerve. Tolosa-Hunt syndrome produces painful ophthalmoplegia in a neuropathic pattern (i.e., combinations of third, fourth, or sixth nerve palsies) and other evidence of cavernous sinus dysfunction, such as trigeminal nerve involvement or Horner's syndrome, without proptosis. Orbital pseudotumor and Tolosa-Hunt syndromes are diagnoses of exclusion. Similar presentations can be produced by other pathological processes, such as infection (e.g., mucormycosis or other fungal infection) or neoplasm (e.g., lymphoma, especially if painless). MRI is helpful in establishing the diagnosis. Treatment of orbital pseudotumor or Tolosa-Hunt syndrome includes immunosuppressive therapy. Typically, there is prompt relief of pain following administration of steroids.

Ocular Oscillations and Nystagmus. Nystagmus results from dysfunction of any of several mechanisms that control the eyes during movement. Vestibular nystagmus results from either peripheral (labyrinth and vestibular nerve) or central lesions (brainstem or cerebellum). This is typically small-amplitude, fine nystagmus that increases upon gaze in direction of the fast phase (see Chapter 6, "Electronystagmography," and Chapter 11, "Dizziness"). Commonly, peripheral vestibular nystagmus is suppressible with fixation (i.e., viewing an object), and is associated with autonomic symptoms such as nausea and vomiting. Peripheral vestibular nystagmus has a mixed torsional – vertical and horizontal direction; central vestibular nystagmus includes pure vertical forms that fail to suppress with fixation and that are typically associated with minimal autonomic disturbance. Downbeat nystagmus is the most common pattern of central vestibular nystagmus, and is caused by dysfunction of central vestibular pathways in the brainstem or cerebellum, es-

pecially in the cervicomedullary junction. Gaze-evoked or end-point nystagmus is generally coarser and of larger amplitude than vestibular nystagmus, and occurs in extremes of gaze. It can be normal when it is unsustained and symmetrical. Symmetrical and sustained horizontal gaze-evoked nystagmus commonly results from toxic or metabolic factors (e.g., antiseizure medications or sedatives). Asymmetrical, sustained gaze-evoked nystagmus suggests a focal lesion and can result from lesion involving the ipsilateral cerebellum or its connections.

Afferent Disease – Visual Loss

OPTIC NERVE (CRANIAL NERVE II). The photoreceptors in the retina synapse on intermediary cells forming the nerve fiber layer, and ultimately provide input to the optic nerve, which forms at the optic disc. The optic nerve head or papilla is unique and preferentially affected by several disease processes. The optic nerve traverses the orbit and exits at the optic foramen prior to joining the contralateral optic nerve, forming the optic chiasm. The optic tracts, emanating from the chiasm, synapse in the lateral geniculate body. Prior (or anterior) to formation of the optic chiasm, visual representation is monocular, whereas posterior to the chiasm, visual information is separated in left and right, binocularly. Accordingly, monocular visual loss indicates a lesion anterior to the chiasm; lesions posterior to the chiasm result in binocular visual field loss, but generally without diminution of visual acuity or color perception.

ANTERIOR ISCHEMIC OPTIC NEUROPATHY: GIANT CELL ARTERITIS AND NONARTERITIC FORMS OF ISCHEMIC OPTIC NEUROPATHY. Ischemia is a common cause of optic nerve dysfunction, and almost exclusively affects the optic nerve head, or anterior portion of the nerve. The two varieties of anterior ischemic optic neuropathy (AION) are: the arteritic form (associated with giant cell arteritis), and the more common nonarteritic form. Nonarteritic anterior ischemic optic neuropathy (NAION) is the most common cause of sudden visual loss in the elderly. The typical presentation of a patient with NAION is sudden, painless, monocular visual loss. Examination acutely reveals decreased acuity and color, visual field defects (often altitudinal), a relative afferent pupillary defect (signs typical of any optic neuropathy), and a swollen optic nerve. Approximately 50% of patients with NAION have a history of hypertension; 25% have diabetes.[7] Additionally, the optic nerve configuration appears to influence the risk of NAION, and anomalous nerve heads with a small crowded appearance and a small or absent optic cup are at higher risk. Almost 50% of patients with NAION recover three lines or more of visual acuity over time. Patients with NAION appear to have a 10–15% probability of involvement of the other eye. Aspirin is considered to help reduce the chances of contralateral eye involvement. The important aspect of emergency department evaluation of these patients is the exclusion of an arteritic pathology (giant cell, or temporal arteritis).

Giant cell arteritis (GCA) is a medical emergency. GCA is a systemic, inflammatory disease of large and medium-size arteries, typically affecting individuals over 55 years of age. Untreated disease can result in blindness, stroke, myocardial infarction, and aortic dissection. Visual symptoms are present in about one-third of patients, and can include blurred vision, diplopia, or amaurosis fugax. The diagnosis of GCA is based on history, laboratory data erythrocyte sedimentation rate (ESR), and temporal artery biopsy. History of headache, jaw or tongue claudication, scalp tenderness, myalgias, anorexia and weight loss, fatigue, or fever provides the most helpful clues to the diagnosis. ESR is typically elevated and serves as a valuable diagnostic clue when present; however, a normal ESR does not rule out GCA.[4] The histological features of GCA are present in the majority of cases even days to weeks after the institution of steroids; accordingly, treatment is never withheld pending biopsy results. Ocular findings in association with visual loss often include optic disc edema, retinal artery occlusion, and tender or prominent temporal arteries. Approximately 5–10% of patients with GCA present with diplopia related to extraocular muscle or cranial nerve ischemia. High-dose steroids are the treatment of choice. Initial treatment with intravenous methylprednisolone (500–1500 mg per day), followed by conversion to oral prednisone and a slow taper as directed by the patient's symptoms and ESR, is recommended. Once visual loss has occurred, it is rarely recovered regardless of treatment.

OPTIC NEURITIS. Optic neuritis is a common cause of visual dysfunction, especially among patients between 18 and 45 years of age. Optic neuritis presents with painful monocular visual blur. Ocular pain or soreness, present in 92% of patients, typically increases with eye movements.[8] Visual blur typically progresses over the initial week to reach a nadir by 7–10 days. Examination reveals findings typical of all optic neuropathies, including diminished visual acuity and color perception, visual field defects, and an afferent pupillary defect. Approximately two-thirds of patients have a normal-appearing optic disc at presentation, while one-third exhibit disc edema (papillitis). Optic neuritis can be idiopathic; the most commonly associated neurological disease is multiple sclerosis (MS). Treatment of patients with optic neuritis is individualized and dependent upon issues concerning both visual recovery and potential development of MS based on findings of the neurological examination and MRI. Oral prednisone alone is *contraindicated* in the treatment of patients with optic neuritis due to an increased rate of optic neuritis recurrence following treatment. Intravenous methylprednisolone administered according to the Optic Neuritis Treatment Trial (ONTT) protocol (250 mg every 6 hours for 3 days, followed by prednisone, 1 mg/kg orally for 11 days) is known to hasten visual recovery but does not influence ultimate visual status. This regimen is associated with a decreased rate of development of MS over the subsequent 2 years posttreatment in high-risk patients (as predicted by the presence of three or more lesions on MRI).[9,10] Treatment issues in these patients must be individualized, ideally with the benefit of MRI data.

COMPRESSIVE OPTIC NEUROPATHIES. Typically, compressive optic neuropathies (e.g., caused by meningiomas, pituitary adenomas, aneurysms, etc.) do not present suddenly, but rather with gradually declining visual function in one eye. Neuroimaging of the appropriate area with MRI or CT is required to establish the diagnosis. An exception to this rule is *pituitary apoplexy*. This results from hemorrhage or infarction within a pituitary tumor with resultant rapid expansion and edema. Pituitary apoplexy can produce sudden visual loss (monocular or binocular with diminished pupillary reaction), diplopia, headache, and altered level of consciousness. Although the optic chiasm and sella are best imaged with MRI, emergency imaging more often utilizes

CT scans. The CT scan is obtained with attention to the parasellar region, and should include coronal sections through this area in order to demonstrate the lesion. Pituitary apoplexy requires emergency attention to endocrine status (especially cortisol levels) and neurosurgical evaluation with prompt decompression.

TRAUMATIC OPTIC NEUROPATHY. Traumatic optic neuropathy results from contusion or compression of the optic nerve, often at or within the bony optic nerve canal. Signs common to all optic neuropathies are evident, such as decreased visual acuity, and color, visual field defects, and a relative afferent pupillary defect (RAPD). Symptoms depend upon the overall neurological status and the ability to demonstrate and detect visual dysfunction. This highlights the importance of the RAPD, because it can be the only sign of optic nerve injury in the comatose patient. Treatment is controversial and includes surgical decompression, high-dose steroids (i.e., spinal cord injury protocol), and observation, depending on the clinical circumstances.

RETINAL CAUSES OF VISUAL LOSS. Central retinal artery or vein occlusions (CRVO or CRAO) present with sudden, painless monocular visual loss. Early retinal findings in the patient with CRAO are often subtle, such as retinal edema and a macular cherry red spot. CRAO can result from carotid artery disease or giant cell arteritis (GCA), or it can occur in the setting of common risk factors for vascular disease. CRVO has a typical retinal appearance when fully developed, including diffuse and scattered retinal hemorrhages known as "blood and thunder." Both CRAO and CRVO commonly result from vascular disease or coagulopathy-induced thrombosis, and require ophthalmologic (retinal) and medical or neuro-ophthalmologic management.

TRANSIENT MONOCULAR BLINDNESS AND AMAUROSIS FUGAX. Patients with transient visual disturbances are commonly observed in clinical practice. The differential diagnosis includes ischemia (amaurosis fugax), migraine, or transient visual obscurations related to disc edema. Ischemic symptoms are important to recognize because they can represent progressive cerebrovascular disease. Ischemic visual events are typically short-lived, lasting less than 1–2 minutes, and rapidly appear and disappear. They produce "negative" symptoms characterized by complete or partial visual loss *without* color, movement, shapes, or dynamic change in regions of visual loss. These episodes are managed as transient ischemic attacks (TIAs) and carotid Doppler studies, coagulation profile, and cardiac evaluation are used to evaluate the patient. In contrast, migrainous phenomena generally produce "positive" phenomena characterized by slow buildup of visual effects including color and movement or shimmer.[4] Migraine visual phenomena typically last 10–30 minutes and often migrate over parts of the visual field with time. These phenomena can be observed with the patient's eyes closed, and are often stereotyped over time. Some patients experience migraine headache following these episodes; in other patients, visual phenomena are painless. Migraine visual phenomena are typically benign events and often respond to the same prophylactic treatments for migraine headache. The primary importance of these events is distinguishing them from TIAs or transient visual obscurations. Transient visual obscurations are episodes of bilateral (occasionally, unilateral) visual loss or graying, lasting seconds and occurring in the context of optic disc edema or papilledema. They are often precipitated by postural changes, such as bending over, or Valsalva maneuver, and are typically benign. Treatment is directed at the optic disc edema or papilledema as indicated by the underlying problem.

VISUAL HALLUCINATIONS. Visual hallucinations are either formed (objects or people), or unformed (flashes of light or geometric shapes). These occur in the context of encephalopathies or severe visual loss (generally worse than 20/100 vision in each eye), regardless of etiology. Visual hallucinations can also occur secondary to seizure, usually in association with the more typical manifestations of epileptic activity. Isolated visual hallucinations alone are rarely psychiatric in origin.

VISUAL FIELD DEFECTS. Visual field defects have localizing value, but can result from several etiologies such as stroke, tumor, or trauma. Identification of the cause depends on other symptoms and signs and ancillary testing (imaging). Monocular visual loss implies a lesion anterior to the optic chiasm; a bitemporal field loss is associated with chiasmal disease. Patients are typically unaware of bitemporal hemianoptic defects because overlapping field

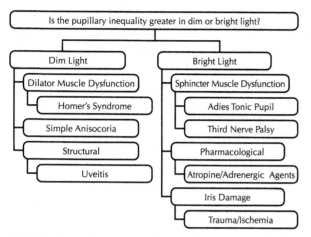

FIGURE 20.6. Anisocoria: The first step in evaluation of anisocoria is the pupillary measurement in light and dark illumination. The muscles of dilation are innervated by the sympathetic nervous system, and dysfunction of these nerves results in a Horner's syndrome. The pupillary sphincter muscles are innervated by the parasympathetic nerves; third nerve palsies and Adie's pupil are common manifestations of parasympathetic dysfunction.

points from each eye provide nearly full binocular peripheral vision; accordingly, these defects must be assessed carefully in each eye *individually.* Homonymous hemianopia refers to complete loss of right- or left-sided vision in both eyes, and results from lesions anywhere in the postchiasmal visual pathways. More accurate localization of homonymous defects from the optic tract to the occipital lobe depends upon the associated symptoms, signs, and findings with neuroimaging. Patients with such a defect retain 20/20 visual acuity unless other visual structures are also affected.

Pupils. Pupils are evaluated for size in light and dark, and for reactivity.[11] Anisocoria of 0.5 mm or less, consistent in both light and dark, can be physiological when the pupils react normally and there are no other associated symptoms or signs. Physiological (or "simple") anisocoria is present in approximately 20% of the population and has no clinical significance. The flow diagram in Figure 20.6 can be helpful in determining the cause of anisocoria.

SYMPATHETIC SYSTEM AND HORNER'S SYNDROME. The sympathetic nervous system control of pupillary function involves three neurons and a very circumferential course, beginning in the posterolateral hypothalamus, and traversing the ipsilateral brainstem to synapse on second-order neurons within the ciliospinal center of Budge-Waller (C8–T2). Fibers ascend via the sympathetic chain to synapse on the third-order neuron in the superior cervical ganglion. The third-order sympathetic fibers ascend with the carotid artery to enter the cavernous sinus. The fibers enter the orbit via the superior orbital fissure to innervate dilators of the iris and Müller's muscle (partial lid elevator) (see Fig. 20.7).

Horner's syndrome consists of miosis, minimal ptosis (1–2 mm), and anhydrosis. The extensive course of the sympathetic fibers suggests that a lesion at several locations can produce a Horner's syndrome. Associated symptoms and signs and pharmacological testing of the pupils are required for accurate localization to the first-, second-, or third-order segments of the nerve.

Third-order Horner's syndrome can result from carotid dissection, cavernous sinus, or orbital diseases. Second-order Horner's syndrome can result from carotid dissection, C8–T1 radiculopathy, brachial plexus lesions, or apical lung mass. First-order Horner's syndrome can result from lateral medullary infarction (Wallenberg's syndrome) or other lesions within the brain.

Wallenberg's syndrome, also known as the lateral medullary syndrome or the posterior inferior cerebellar artery (PICA) syndrome, is perhaps the most common brainstem stroke syndrome. It does not produce weakness; consequently, stroke may not be considered on initial evaluation. The complete constellation of signs resulting from disruption of lateral medullary structures include ipsilateral facial numbness (descending tract of the trigeminal), ipsilateral Horner's syndrome (sympathetic nerves), dysphagia and dysarthria (cranial nerves IX and X), ipsilateral limb ataxia (inferior cerebellar peduncle), contralateral body numbness (ascending spinothalamic tracts, which have crossed the midline in the spinal cord), and vertigo (vestibular nucleus).[6] Occasionally, patients with Wallenberg's syndrome develop diplopia due to skew deviation. Hiccups and a 90–180-degree tilt of the perceived world can occur. Most patients exhibit several but not all of the above features. This syndrome usually results from infarction due to vertebral artery occlusion, although PICA occlusion can occur.

PARASYMPATHETIC SYSTEM. The oculomotor nerve (cranial nerve III) innervates the pupillary

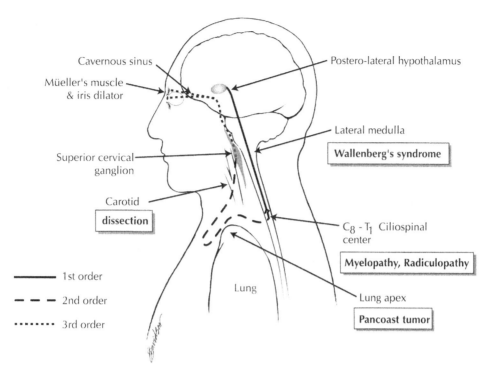

FIGURE 20.7. Diagram of the anatomical course of fibers of the sympathetic nervous system involved in the control of pupillary function. Different pathological conditions are indicated that can alter the normal function of the sympathetic fibers at various sites along their course from the hypothalamus to the pupil.

constrictors via fibers emanating from the Edinger-Westphal nucleus. Pupillary involvement is a point of special importance when evaluating the patient with a third nerve palsy; however, *isolated* pupillary dysfunction is rarely indicative of a third nerve palsy. The dilated pupil due to third nerve dysfunction is typically midposition (not maximally dilated), poorly reactive, and accompanied by other symptoms and signs of oculomotor palsy. Adie's tonic pupil is a more common cause of an isolated light-fixed pupil. Adie's pupil results from postganglionic parasympathetic denervation, and produces mydriasis with poor light reactivity but retained pupillary reactivity to a near target (convergence, accommodation, and miosis). Unilateral Adie's pupil is usually idiopathic, or can result from orbital trauma such as surgery. An isolated unilateral tonic pupil is typically a benign condition. Adie's syndrome refers to Adie's pupil plus generalized areflexia. Bilateral Adie's pupils or Adie's syndrome can result from viral or syphilitic infection, or can be associated with more widespread autonomic dysfunction. Adie's pupil can be confirmed with in-

stillation of dilute pilocarpine solution, and should be evaluated on a nonemergency basis by a neuro-ophthalmologist. Adie's pupil is one of several syndromes resulting in near-light dissociation (NLD) (greater reaction to near than to light stimuli). The differential diagnosis for NLD includes Parinaud's syndrome, tonic pupils (e.g., Adie's), Argyll Robertson pupils (syphilis), diabetic or other peripheral neuropathies, anterior visual pathway injury, or aberrant regeneration of the oculomotor nerve.

PHARMACOLOGICAL CAUSES OF ANISOCORIA. Inadvertent or deliberate instillation of several drugs can produce a widely dilated and unreactive pupil. Atropine-like agents such as scopolamine (used for motion sickness) are a common cause of pharmacologically dilated pupils. The pharmacologically dilated pupil is maximally dilated; other aspects of the examination, including motility and eyelid function, are normal (with the exception of diminished near vision in the affected eye). Proof of pharmacological instillation may be obtained through the use of 1% pilocarpine. This agent constricts most other causes of a widely dilated pupil, with the exception of pharmacological blockade or a mechanical iris damage (e.g., iris scar or trauma).

STRUCTURAL ANISOCORIA. Iris trauma or scar can produce a poorly reactive pupil. Typically, this pupil dilates *and* constricts incompletely, and interruption or thinning of sections of the iris can be visible under slit lamp microscopy. Previous iritis can also result in synechiae that inhibit pupillary reaction.

PHYSIOLOGICAL ANISOCORIA. A significant percent of the population has minimal anisocoria without pathology, termed *physiological* or *simple anisocoria*.[12] This is generally less than or equal to 0.5 mm, and the amount of anisocoria remains essentially the same in light and dark (or is slightly greater in dark). The side of the larger eye can change over time in some patients. Old photographs such as a driver's license viewed with a magnifying glass can be helpful in establishing the date of onset of the anisocoria. The remainder of the examination is normal in patients with physiological anisocoria. Only physiological anisocoria or Horner's syndrome produce anisocoria with normally reactive pupils; the associated ptosis and lack of response to cocaine ophthalmic drops in the latter is helpful diagnostically.

PEARLS AND PITFALLS

- Lesion localization of abnormality is the goal of neuro-ophthalmic evaluation.
- Binocular diplopia can result from nerve, muscle, neuromuscular junction, or internuclear or supranuclear (skew) dysfunction.
- Important historical features of diplopia include monocular or binocular characteristics, and vertical, horizontal, or oblique separation of images.
- Visual acuity is one of the most important measures in patients with blurred vision.
- Transient visual loss due to ischemia (amaurosis fugax) rarely lasts more than seconds to minutes.

- Visual field examination has important localization value.
- The keys to pupillary evaluation are reactivity and the degree of anisocoria in light and dark.
- Isolated pupillary dysfunction rarely is caused by a third nerve palsy.

REFERENCES

1. Frisén L. Swelling of the optic nerve head: a staging scheme. *J Neurol Neurosurg Psych.* 1982;45:13–18.
2. Rush JA, Younge BR. Paralysis of cranial nerves III, IV, and VI, causes and prognosis in 1000 cases. *Arch Ophthalmol.* 1981;99:76–9.
3. Leigh RJ, Zee DS. *The Neurology of Eye Movements.* 2nd ed. Philadelphia: Davis; 1991.
4. Miller NR, Newman NJ. *Walsh and Hoyt's Clinical Neuro-Ophthalmology.* 5th ed. Baltimore; Williams & Wilkins; 1998.
5. Glaser JS. *Neuro-ophthalmology.* 2nd ed. Philadelphia: JB Lippincott Co., 1990.
6. Adams RD, Victor M, Ropper AH. *Principles of Neurology,* 6th ed. New York: McGraw-Hill, 1997.
7. The Ischemic Optic Neuropathy Decompression Trial Research Group. Optic nerve decompression surgery for nonarteritic anterior ischemic optic neuropathy (NAION) is not effective and may be harmful. *JAMA.* 1995;273:625–32.
8. Beck RW, Cleary PA, Trobe JD, et al. The effect of corticosteroids for acute optic neuritis on the subsequent development of multiple sclerosis. *N Engl J Med.* 1993;329:1764–9.
9. The LONS Study Group. The five year risk of multiple sclerosis after optic neuritis: experience of the Optic Neuritis Treatment Trial. *Neurol.* 1997;49: 1404–13.
10. The LONS Study Group. Visual function five years after optic neuritis: experience of the Optic Neuritis Treatment Trial. *Arch Ophthalmol.* 1997;115:1545–52.
11. Thompson HS, Kardon RH. Clinical importance of pupillary inequality. *American Academy of Ophthalmology: Focal Points.* 1992;10:1–10.
12. Loewenfeld IE. *The Pupil, Anatomy, Physiology, and Clinical Applications.* Vol. 1. Detroit, MI: Wayne State University Press, 1993.

21 Multiple Sclerosis

THOMAS F. SCOTT AND DANIELLE RAY

SUMMARY Multiple sclerosis (MS) is a difficult diagnosis to make either in the emergency department or at the office of a neurologist. The diagnosis of MS is based on clinical information and is supported by magnetic resonance neuroimaging. The diagnosis of MS is generally made not at the time of initial evaluation but over time as symptoms and signs evolve and information is gathered from diagnostic tests. Patients with established relapsing – remitting MS present to the emergency department with acute exacerbations of their illness, sometimes requiring immediate attention for new symptoms. Patients with chronic progressive MS present to the emergency department with commonly occurring problems associated with their illness.

Introduction

Multiple sclerosis (MS) is a common disorder, characterized by inflammatory lesions of the brain and spinal cord, affecting approximately 0.1% of the population in the United States.[1] The disease has a peak incidence in the second and third decades of life, typically presenting in this age group as relapsing-remitting disease (RRMS).[2] At least 60% of patients with MS have RRMS at the onset, and a significant percentage of these patients have a benign long-term course.[3] Patients tend to have a higher rate of attack frequency in the first several years of the disease. Good recovery from attacks is seen typically following the initial attacks. Attack frequency decreases with time, but many patients begin to accumulate permanent disability. In patients over 50 years of age, the disease most commonly presents as a slow chronic progressive illness (CPMS). Approximately 10–15% of patients have CPMS. Some exhibit slow progression with occasional exacerbations. Approximately one-third of all patients with MS progress to being wheelchair-dependent.

In predominantly temperate climates, MS primarily affects persons of European descent. Female patients outnumber male patients 1.7 to 1. The prevalence of MS is known to increase with distance from the equator. Studies comparing prevalence rates of MS in genetically distinct populations within the same geographic areas have shown definite increases in certain ethnic subgroups such as in Palestinian Arabs compared with Kuwaiti Arabs,[4] and the Parsees compared with the Hindus in Bombay.[5] There is evidence of increased incidence of MS with certain HLA antigens. Migration studies have shown that individuals who migrate before puberty have the same prevalence rate of MS as those born in the place they are migrating to, whereas individuals who migrate after puberty retain the prevalence rate of their place of origin. Thus unknown environmental influences seem to be of some importance. A history of trauma does not appear to be an important environmental risk factor, although this issue remains controversial.[6] A slightly decreased attack rate is observed during pregnancy, but a slightly increased attack rate is observed in the first six months following pregnancy. The reason for the observed change in attack rate during and briefly following pregnancy is unclear but is presumed to be hormonally mediated. The only other known environmental or acquired risk factor is viral infections in patients with known disease, because the relapse rate is slightly increased following viral illness.

MS is diagnosed primarily from clinical data. The criteria developed by the Schumacher panel in 1965 are the most widely used clinical guidelines for the diagnosis of MS.[7] According to these guidelines, a patient (age 10 years to 50 years) must exhibit neurological abnormalities attributable to the central nervous system (CNS) involving two or more areas (primarily white matter), and that two or more episodes of associated dysfunction must occur, each lasting more than 24 hours. Alternatively, a stepwise progression of neurological disability over a 6-month period or more can qualify a patient for the diagnosis. However, patients over 50 years of age can develop MS, usually the CPMS variety. Several diagnostic tests are used to help establish the diagnosis of MS. These include cerebrospinal fluid testing, evoked potential studies, and magnetic resonance imaging (MRI). In 1983, Poser and colleagues set forth a new set of diagnostic criteria, including the use of these tests and characterizing patients as having either probable or definite MS.[8]

Pathophysiology

The primary pathological event in MS lesion development is an immune-mediated destruction of the neuronal myelin sheath.[20] The earliest recognizable event appears to be infiltration of the perivenular brain parenchyma by autoreactive T lymphocytes. Once in the parenchyma, these cells are of critical importance in a chain of immunological events. A central step is the formation of a trimolecular complex that includes the major histocompatibility complex (MHC) type II molecule, the antigen (presumed to be myelin basic protein in most cases, although evidence exists for other important antigens such as proteolipid protein), and the T-cell receptor. After recognizing these appropriate signals, the T cell then produces disease-mediating cytokines. Important cytokines appear to be tumor necrosis factor, transforming growth factor beta, and the interferons. Some scattered remyelination takes place, but this is probably of minor importance following MS attacks. Resolution of edema and restoration of the blood–brain barrier are important early events, and scar tissue for-

mation in the wake of inflammatory lesions appears to be important for long-term functioning of nervous tissue. Immune therapies have been aimed at disrupting the formation of this presumed autoimmune bimolecular complex, as well as disrupting cytokine-mediated inflammatory events, which appear to result from autoreactive T-cell stimulation.

Lesions of MS may be present throughout the white matter of the CNS, but they have a predilection for certain areas. Prominent areas of involvement include the optic nerve, periventricular white matter, spinal cord, and brainstem. Occasionally, the spinal cord alone may be affected. Based on pathological or immunological criteria, it is difficult to differentiate between lesions of MS and other demyelinating diseases such as Devic's disease (neuromyelitis optica), acute transverse myelitis (ATM), and encephalomyelitis. Differentiation between MS and these entities is achieved primarily on a clinical, not a histopathological, basis.

Prehospital Care

Prehospital care for patients with known MS is largely supportive in nature. Patients may experience an exacerbation of MS or have worsening of commonly occurring problems associated with their illness. Most presenting symptoms necessitate only a general evaluation prior to transport. In some cases, MS can present as a strokelike illness with confounding symptoms and signs that require stabilization and immediate transport to the emergency department.

Emergency Department Evaluation

The inflammatory lesions of MS can affect any part of the CNS and optic nerves, resulting in a wide variety of presenting symptoms. The first symptoms of MS in a study of 937 patients were weakness (48%), paresthesias (31%), visual loss (25%), incoordination (15%), vertigo (6%), and sphincter impairment (6%).[9] Onset of symptoms occurs most typically over days, but strokelike onset may evolve over minutes to hours. Clinical features often allow localization of the area of involvement to either the cerebral hemispheres, brainstem, or spinal cord. For example, hemifacial spasm or trigeminal neuralgia can be presenting symptoms of MS referable to the brainstem. Symptoms referable to MS involving the spinal cord commonly present in an asymmetrical fashion (i.e., *partial transverse myelitis*). Lhermitte's sign (electriclike sensations radiating up and down the spine, often exacerbated by neck flexion) is commonly observed. A "sensory-level" or hemi–spinal cord (Brown-Sequard) syndrome may also be observed. Other presenting symptoms include speech disturbance, a wide variety of pain syndromes (including radicular pain), and transient acute nonpositional vertigo. Psychiatric manifestations of MS include depressive illness, manic-depression (observed much less frequently), and psychosis (observed rarely).

Neurological Examination

The neurological examination of patients with MS may be normal, minimally abnormal, or markedly abnormal. Focused testing of cranial nerve function, strength, coordination, gait, and sensation, and an evaluation for pathological reflexes are important.

It is best to record corrected visual acuity with a Snellen chart and to determine whether optic nerve head pallor exists. Assessment for red desaturation is carried out by asking the patient to view a red object with each eye in an alternating fashion and indicate any subjective change in depth of color. A decrease in perceived redness in one eye suggests impairment of vision in that eye. The typical visual field loss in optic neuritis is a central scotoma. Occasionally, a junctional defect (a small temporal area of field loss opposite a more severe and generalized field loss) may be observed. Rarely, altitudinal defects, arcuate defects, or peripheral visual loss are noted. Disc swelling is present in about 10–50% of patients with MS, and sometimes optic disc pallor from an old asymptomatic injury is observed. Hemorrhages are rare and typically linear. An afferent pupillary defect (Marcus Gunn pupil) is often found. In the majority of patients, prognosis is good for return of vision to near normal or normal. Internuclear ophthalmoplegia (INO) is a classic finding in patients with MS and results from a lesion in the medial longitudinal fasciculus. Adduction is lost ipsilateral to the lesion and is easily demonstrated on extraocular movement testing.

The findings of distinct lower motor neuron signs, such as fasciculations and loss of reflexes, do not support a diagnosis of MS. A "stocking" distribution of numbness, usually indicating a peripheral neuropathy, can be observed in early cases of MS. Acute onset of numbness from the waist down with findings of a distinct thoracic sensory level, associated with bilateral lower extremity weakness, decreased reflexes, and bladder dysfunction, suggests a diagnosis of ATM and not MS. Hyperreflexia and extensor plantar responses develop days to weeks after an acute paresis, or slowly as more subacute symptoms evolve.

Common Presentations and Differential Diagnosis

Optic Neuritis

The onset of MS is heralded by a bout of optic neuritis in about 20% of patients; in most of these patients, other symptoms or signs associated with MS are absent. Relatively few patients presenting with optic neuritis develop MS within a few years; however, more than 50% eventually develop the disease.[10,11] MRI can usually identify those at increased risk. Typically, optic neuritis is associated with pain either preceding, during, or following the onset of visual loss. The pain is often accentuated with eye movement, and the eye may be tender. The onset of visual loss can be sudden or occur upon awakening, and most patients can identify the day of the onset of decreased vision. Visual problems are described initially as blurred vision or a sensation of looking into a fog. This is often followed by a steady progression of visual loss over a three- to seven-day period. Visual loss may be severe, but complete blindness is very rare. Few patients are aware of a distinct visual field defect.

The differential diagnosis for optic neuritis primarily includes anterior ischemic optic neuropathy (see Chap. 20, "Neuro-ophthalmology"), viral papillitis, and central retinal artery occlusion (see Table 21.1). Anterior ischemic optic neuropathy is unlikely to occur in young patients, and is associated with risk factors for arterial disease. A swollen disc is a nonspecific sign and can be observed in any of the above-mentioned conditions. Sectoral swelling can be observed in anterior ischemic optic neuropathy, whereas more diffuse swelling is observed in viral papillitis and in some cases of optic neuritis. "Retro bulbar" optic neuritis is not associated with disc swelling because the inflammatory lesion is more

TABLE 21.1. Differential Diagnosis for New-Onset MS Categorized by Neuroanatomical Presentation

Hemispheric or brainstem focal lesion
  Mass lesion
  Cerebrovascular event
    Ischemic stroke
    Intracerebral hemorrhage
Hemispheric or brainstem multiple lesions
  Neoplastic (multifocal primary or metastatic)
  Infectious (abscess)
  Cerebrovascular
    Cardioembolic (consider subacute bacterial
      endocarditis and atrial lesions)
    Coagulopathies (often resulting in cardiac emboli)
    Vasculitis/connective tissue diseases
    Moya-moya disease
Spinal cord lesion
  Acute transverse myelitis (acute transverse myelopathy)
  Ischemic injury/vascular malformation
  Mass lesion
  Connective tissue disease/sarcoidosis/vasculitis
Ocular onset
  Amaurosis fugax/vascular
  Papilledema
  Viral papillitis
Spinal cord and ocular combined
  Devic's disease (neuromyelitis optica)
  Vasculitis/sarcoidosis/connective tissue disease
  Metastatic disease
Spinal cord and brain
  Encephalomyelitis
  Vasculitis/sarcoidosis/connective tissue disease
  Metastatic disease

proximal. Exudates, or "cottonwool patches," are not related to MS, but suggest connective tissue diseases or viral conditions. Central retinal artery occlusion is generally a disorder of the elderly, and is associated with a pale retina and a cherry-red spot in the macula. Central retinal artery branch occlusion can rarely occur in young patients at risk for thromboembolic disease, such as patients with heart defects, carotid artery disease, or coagulopathy. Typically this occurs as a sudden, painless, monocular, central visual loss resulting in amaurosis fugax when the occlusion is transient. Disc swelling is unusual in central retinal artery occlu-

sions due to emboli but can occur in a sectoral fashion when a branch occlusion occurs in the posterior ciliary arteries.

Stroke-like Syndromes

The most important and difficult diagnostic decisions made in the emergency department involve distinguishing the acute onset of RRMS from symptoms due to CNS ischemia. Although several episodic or multifocal CNS disease processes can resemble MS, stroke is the most common cause of acute focal or multifocal neurological dysfunction in young people, approaching the incidence of MS. An apoplectic onset of MS is rare, and this is the most important historical feature distinguishing the two processes. Clinical features suggesting a single lesion in the CNS favor a diagnosis of stroke in the acute setting. The presence of risk factors associated with stroke, including a history of smoking or use of oral contraceptives, is sought, as is a complete review of systems to assess for features of connective tissue disease or coagulopathy.

A history of migraine or "complicated" migraine is sought in patients with acute or rapidly evolving deficits, because complicated migraine can mimic a transient ischemic attack (TIA) or acute MS symptoms. However, a prominent headache component is unusual in MS and is more commonly associated with complicated migraine or stroke.

CPMS presents a different set of differential diagnoses than RRMS. It occurs primarily in patients over 40 years of age, and is the most common form of MS observed in patients over 55 years of age. Patients are affected primarily in the lower extremities with weakness and spasticity, and occasionally signs of cerebellar dysfunction are also observed. These patients are typically evaluated in an outpatient setting and rarely present to the emergency department for their initial evaluation. Spinocerebellar degenerative syndromes are the most difficult to distinguish from this form of MS.[12] Insidious spinal cord compression due to cervical stenosis is also an important condition to consider in the differential diagnosis. Slow-growing tumors are more likely to present with prominent sensory findings, as are conditions resulting from vitamin B_{12} deficiency. Initial evaluation in these cases typically consists of an MRI study of the cervical and thoracic cord. HTLV-1 myelopathy is endemic in the tropics and southeastern United States and is a strong consideration in patients infected with human immunodeficiency virus (HIV) or those with risk factors such as blood transfusion or a history of intravenous drug abuse.

Myelopathy

An urgent evaluation for spinal cord compression by a mass lesion is necessary when signs of acute or subacute spinal cord dysfunction are present. Acute spinal cord dysfunction may cause symmetrical or asymmetrical motor weakness, a sensory deficit level, sphincter disturbance, and variable abnormalities of deep tendon reflexes. Deep tendon reflexes are usually lost in hyperacute spinal cord injuries. If a compressive lesion is not found by MRI or myelography, ATM and MS are considered as possible causes of myelopathy. These conditions are often identified by the increased signal observed in the spinal cord on T2-weighted MRI. MS presenting as a spinal cord lesion is much more likely to be associated with asymmetrical motor and sensory signs. In ATM, a sensory level is almost always present, motor findings are symmetrical, and sphincter dysfunction is also usually present. Urinary retention requiring bladder catheterization is commonly present. ATM is a syndrome often related to postinfectious immune dysregulation and may involve antecedent viral infections or vaccination. ATM is also observed in association with connective tissue diseases such as systemic lupus erythematosus and Sjögren's disease. Some cases appear to be paraneoplastic. It is usually a monophasic disorder, and improvement is the rule rather than an exception. The overall prognosis for the patient with ATM is likely to be better than for the patient with MS. Patients with ATM rarely develop MS. Treatment includes the use of high doses of corticosteroids.

Fatigue Syndromes

Fatigue is a very common symptom in patients with MS. Symptoms associated with fatigue are often mistaken for depression in patients with MS. Because many patients who have MS also have anxiety, an initial misdiagnosis of a hysterical condition or depression is common. Some patients with fatigue of unclear etiology also complain of paresthesias. Most patients with persistent fatigue and paresthesias do not have MS; however, these complaints should prompt a detailed neurological evaluation. When an antecedent viral illness is reported, the possibility of postviral fatigue is considered. When evaluating patients with fatigue, consideration is given to thyroid function, electrolyte imbalance, hematological abnormalities, and connective tissue disease.

Other Conditions

In the emergency department, new-onset MS is most often suspected in young patients (second and third decades of life) with acute or subacute neurological dysfunction. The differential diagnosis includes causes of stroke in young patients, which include cardiac emboli, coagulopathies (e.g., antiphospholipid antibody syndrome), and connective tissue diseases (e.g., vasculitis and other vasculopathies associated with systemic lupus erythematosus, periarteritis nodosa, etc.).[13,14] Encephalomyelitis is a monophasic, often postinfectious disorder resembling MS in its histopathology and MRI findings, and is considered in the differential diagnosis of MS (see Table 21.1). This disorder usually occurs in children and may be associated with antecedent or concurrent febrile illness and altered mental status. Seizures are observed occasionally. Severe permanent neurological injury can occur, and the mortality rate is much higher than in patients with acute bouts of MS. The extreme similarity of this disorder to MS underscores the necessity of two documented episodes of neurological dysfunction as criteria for the diagnosis of MS.

Lyme disease is also a consideration in the differential diagnosis of MS, especially in endemic areas. However, patients with Lyme disease who present with neurological symptoms mimicking MS but lacking other features suggestive of Lyme disease (no history of rash, meningitis, neuropathies) is exceedingly uncommon.

Sarcoidosis involving the CNS can be exceedingly difficult to distinguish from MS when systemic signs are absent; however, the prevalence of CNS sarcoidosis is very low. A family history of autoimmune illness is important to seek because familial cases of sarcoidosis and antiphospholipid

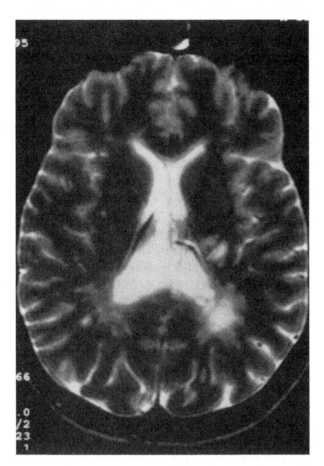 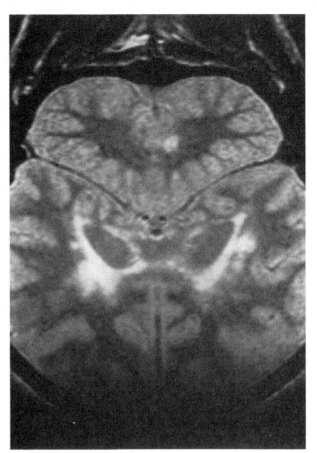

FIGURE 21.1. T2-weighted MRI scan showing (A) typical globular periventricular white matter lesions primarily in the posterior white matter, axial view. (B) Coronal view using proton density imaging showing periventricular white matter lesions and a lesion in the cerebellar white matter.

antibody syndrome are common. Persons with a first-degree relative with MS have approximately a 10-fold risk of developing MS.

Ancillary Tests

MRI or computerized tomography (CT) of the brain (without and with contrast), when available, provides the most comprehensive assessment in the emergency department. Neuroimaging assists in differentiating MS from mass lesions, infections, or strokes. MRI is a sensitive test for demonstrating lesions due to MS and is fairly specific for diagnosing MS in young patients (see Fig. 21.1). MRI is more sensitive in detecting MS than is CT scanning, cerebrospinal fluid (CSF) analysis, and evoked potential studies.[18] MRI is also used to monitor disease activity and has become an important tool for evaluating

clinical outcome trials (e.g., beta interferon for MS). MRI with gadolinium allows distinction between the chronic plaques[19] and acute lesions of MS, which are associated with transient abnormalities of the blood–brain barrier. MRI greatly increases the ability to visualize plaques within the spinal cord.

A concise battery of rheumatological screening tests including antinuclear antibody testing, erythrocyte sedimentation rate, Lyme titers, angiotensin-converting enzyme level (sarcoidosis), and SS-A and SS-B autoantibody titers (Sjögren's disease) is considered when the patient's history suggests the possibility of a rheumatological or a collagen vascular condition. A complete blood count including platelets and a coagulation profile are important in assessing possible hematological or coagulation defects.

Lumbar puncture is considered but is rarely required in the emergency setting for suspected MS.

CSF findings in acute phases of MS include a slightly increased protein level, a mild lymphocytosis, and a normal glucose level. Test results for oligoclonal bands and other abnormalities of CSF immunoglobulins are not immediately available in the emergency department. Oligoclonal IgG bands are present in the CSF but not in the plasma in up to 95% of patients with MS.[17] The finding of oligoclonal bands is nonspecific and present in many inflammatory conditions of the CNS.

Evoked potential studies (visual evoked potentials, brainstem auditory evoked potentials, and somatosensory evoked potentials) are elective tests that are performed in an electrophysiology laboratory. They measure the delay of central conduction velocity through injured white matter tracts. CSF

examination and evoked potential studies are performed much less commonly for the diagnosis of MS since the advent of MRI.

Management

Patients with RRMS who experience an acute exacerbation of their illness present with either recurrence or worsening of old symptoms, or entirely new neurological symptoms (Fig. 21.2). Although the role of intravenous or oral corticosteroids is controversial in the treatment of acute relapses, many patients are "steroid-responsive," and the use of corticosteroids should be strongly considered in this group of patients. The role of corticosteroids in the treatment of chronic MS remains even more

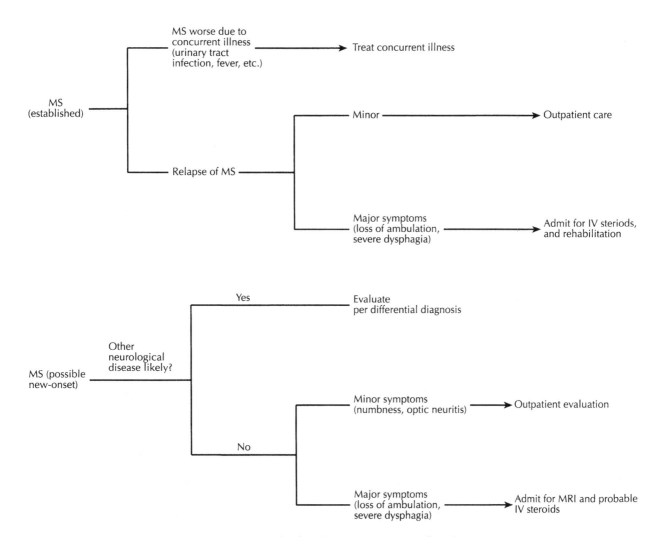

FIGURE 21.2. Multiple sclerosis management flowchart.

controversial. However, corticosteroids are widely used and given either intravenously at high doses over a period of several days or orally in moderate doses over variable periods of time. Decisions about the use and dosage of corticosteroids therapy is made in conjunction with a neurologist. Immunosuppressive therapy with cyclophosphamide, azathioprine, or methotrexate in special situations is also considered, although the efficacy of these agents remains inconclusive.[21,22]

The first medication clearly shown to reduce the attack frequency in RRMS was interferon beta-1b.[23,24] More recently approved, interferon beta-1a and Copolymer-1 also appear to decrease the frequency of exacerbations of MS.

Disposition

Patients with new neurological symptoms or signs referable to one or more areas of the CNS by history and examination are considered for admission to the hospital for a comprehensive diagnostic evaluation. Inpatient evaluation is based on the severity of symptoms and the overall clinical condition. Patients with mild symptoms such as paresthesias and numbness can be considered for outpatient evaluation. Clinical experience indicates that many patients with numbness of an extremity of uncertain etiology never achieve a specific neurological diagnosis and the etiology of numbness is usually a benign process. However, due to the difficulty of distinguishing between central and peripheral numbness in some patients, electromyography (EMG) with nerve conduction studies is advocated in these patients.

Many patients with an established diagnosis of MS require hospital admission due to acute loss of ambulation, deterioration of swallowing function, or other disabling effects of an acute exacerbation. Many patients require initiation or adjustment of medications for management of specific symptoms such as spasticity, bladder dysfunction, or psychiatric disturbance. Acute severe flexor spasms of the lower extremities occur occasionally and may be managed effectively with benzodiazepines or baclofen. Urinary tract infections are common in patients with moderately advanced MS and may be associated with lethargy and exacerbation of weakness or spasticity. Bladder catheterization for urinary retention is commonly required. An urgent psychiatric consultation is prudent in cases of suicidal depression or psychosis. A search for coexisting diseases is undertaken, especially in patients with a recurrence of previous neurological symptoms; underlying infections often are responsible for this condition even in the absence of new CNS inflammation due to MS. Silent aspiration and subsequent pneumonia occur in some patients with bulbar dysfunction.

PEARLS AND PITFALLS

- Patients must have two bouts of neurological dysfunction referable to the CNS to be considered for the diagnosis of RRMS.
- Patients should have experienced at least six months of progressive or stepwise neurological dysfunction to be considered for the diagnosis of CPMS.
- Emergency physicians should attempt to review briefly the neurological history of patients presenting with established MS before treating new or acute problems. Causes of neurological dysfunction other than MS must be considered.[24,5]
- In patients with poorly documented history, minimal neurological findings, or other equivocal factors in their past diagnosis of MS, documentation of an MRI scan consistent with the diagnosis of MS is the single most helpful factor.

REFERENCES

1. Hader WJ, Elliot M, Ebers GC. Epidemiology of multiple sclerosis in London and Middlesex County, Ontario, Canada. *Neurology.* 1988;38:617–21.
2. Matthews WB, ed. *McAlpine's Multiple Sclerosis.* New York, NY: Churchill Livingstone, 1991:43–71.
3. Weinsheker BG. *Natural History of Multiple Sclerosis. Ann Neurol.* 1994;36(suppl):S6–11.
4. Al Din AS, Khogali M, Poser CM, et al. Epidemiology of multiple sclerosis in Arabs in Kuwait: a comparative study between Kuwaitis and Palestinians. *J Neurol Sci.* 1990;100:137–41.
5. Wadia NH, Bhatia K. Multiple sclerosis is prevalent in the Zoroastrians (Parsis) of India. *Ann Neurol.* 1990; 28:177–8.

6. Siva A, Radhakrishnan K, Kurland LT, O'Brien PC, Swanson JW, Rodriguez M. Trauma and multiple sclerosis: a population-based cohort study from Olmsted County, Minnesota. *Neurology.* 1993;43:1878–82.

7. Schumacher GA, Beebe G, Kibler RF, et al. Problems with experimental therapy in multiple sclerosis: report by the panel on evaluation of experimental trials of therapy in multiple sclerosis. *Ann NY Acad Sci.* 1965;122:552–68.

8. Poser CM, Paty DW, Scheinberg L, et al. New diagnostic criteria for multiple sclerosis. Guidelines for research protocols. *Ann Neurol.* 1983;13:227–31.

9. Poser C, Presthus J, Horstal O. Clinical characteristics of autopsy-proved multiple sclerosis. *Neurology.* 1966; 16:791.

10. Cohen MM, Lessell S, Wolf PA. A prospective study of the risk of developing multiple sclerosis in uncomplicated optic neuritis. *Neurology.* 1979;29:208–13.

11. Rodriguez M, Siva A, Cross SA, O'Brien PC, Kurland LT. Optic neuritis: a population based study in Olmsted County, Minnesota. *Neurology.* 1995;45:244–50.

12. Rudick RA, Schiffer RB, Schwetz KM, Herndon RM. Multiple sclerosis; the problem of incorrect diagnosis. *Arch Neurol.* 1986;43:578–83.

13. Scott TF, Weikers N, Hospodar M, Wapenski J. Acute transverse myelitis. *Can J Neurol Sci.* 1994;21:133–6.

14. Scott TF. Diseases that mimic multiple sclerosis. *Postgrad Med.* 1991;89:187–91.

15. Bradley WG, Whitty CW. Acute optic neuritis: its clinical features and their relation to prognosis for recovery of vision. *J Neurol Neurosurg Psychiatry.* 1967; 30:531–8.

16. Isayama Y, Takahashi T, Shimoyoma T, Yamadori A. Acute optic neuritis and sclerosis. *Neurology.* 1982; 32:73–6.

17. Olsson T. Cerebrospinal fluid. *Ann Neurol.* 1994; 36(suppl):S100–2.

18. Gebarski SS, Gabrielsen TO, Gilman S, et al. The initial diagnosis of multiple sclerosis: clinical impact of magnetic resonance imaging. *Ann Neurol.* 1985;17:469–74.

19. Grossman RI, Braffman BH, Brorson JR, Goldverg HI, Silberberg DH, Gonzalez-Scarano F. Multiple sclerosis: serial study of gadolinium-enhanced MR imaging. *Radiology.* 1988;169:117–22.

20. Raine CS. The Dale E. McFarlin memorial lecture: the immunology of the multiple sclerosis lesion. *Ann Neurol.* 1994;36(suppl):S61–72.

21. Yudkin PL, Ellison GW, Ghezzi A, et al. Overview of azathioprine treatment in multiple sclerosis. *Lancet.* 1991;338:1051–5.

22. The Multiple Sclerosis Study Group. Efficacy and toxicity of cyclosporine in chronic progressive multiple sclerosis: a randomized double-blinded, placebo-controlled clinical trial. *Ann Neurol.* 1990;27:591–605.

23. Paty Dw, Li kB, UBC MS/MRI Study Group, et al. Interferon beta-IB is effective in relapsing-remitting multiple sclerosis, II: MRI analysis results of a multicenter, randomized, double-blind, placebo-controlled trial. *Neurology.* 1993;43:662–7.

24. INFB Multiple Sclerosis Study Group. Interferon beta-Ib is effective in relapsing-remitting multiple sclerosis, I: clinical results of a multicenter, randomized, double-blind, placebo-controlled trial. *Neurology.* 1993;43:655–61.

22 Dementia

JUDITH L. HEIDEBRINK AND NORMAN L. FOSTER

SUMMARY Dementia is a problem commonly observed in the emergency department and must be distinguished from other cognitive disorders. Unrecognized dementia has important implications, and particular attention should be focused on high-risk groups. Neurological consultation is recommended when dementia is rapidly progressive or when it is associated with new-onset seizures, an unexplained focal neurological deficit, or an unexplained gait disturbance. Unless there is a superimposed acute illness, the majority of patients with dementia can be managed on an outpatient basis. After testing is initiated to evaluate the cause of dementia, follow-up should be arranged at a multidisciplinary dementia clinic.

Introduction

Emergency departments commonly provide medical care to patients with dementia. Although many patients are residents of chronic care facilities and their dementia is obvious, most live in the community and their dementia may not have been recognized previously. The prevalence of dementia is high. It is most common in the elderly. Approximately 6% of community dwellers aged 65 or older and nearly 30% of all adults aged 85 or older have at least mild dementia.[1,2] These individuals may utilize the emergency department repeatedly for problems associated with dementia that is unrecognized or unaddressed. Proper evaluation and disposition of these patients by emergency physicians facilitates appropriate diagnosis and use of health care resources. It is the emergency physician's responsibility to recognize dementia, initiate an appropriate evaluation and treatment, and arrange for proper disposition.

Prehospital Management

Emergency medical service (EMS) is rarely needed for assessment and treatment of patients with un-complicated dementia. EMS is called usually for acute medical problems in patients with dementia, or for severe behavioral disturbances that occur in public or that family and caregivers can not control. In these cases, EMS personnel obtain medical information from caregivers and other witnesses, because the patient cannot provide a reliable history. Caregivers are encouraged to accompany the patient in transport, and provide any medical records that are available. Provisions for adequate medical information are equally important for institutionalized patients. Dementia is frequently not addressed in the medical record of chronic care facilities. Discussion with the staff is often necessary in order to judge whether changes in the patient's mental status have occurred and, if so, how rapidly.

When a behavioral disturbance is the major concern, the arrival of EMS personnel can sometimes calm matters and at other times exacerbate them. When a severe behavioral disturbance precludes transportation by EMS, pharmacological treatment may be required on site. Several people may be needed to restrain the patient carefully, and the assistance of law enforcement officers may be necessary. Once physical restraint is achieved, a neuroleptic, such as haloperidol, can be given safely as an intramuscular injection in progressively higher doses beginning at 1 mg. This will rapidly control acute agitation, is less likely to cause significant sedation and disorientation than a benzodiazepine, and does not have the risk of respiratory compromise. Thioridazine is not used because of its tendency to cause postural hypotension in the elderly. Long-acting (decanoate) forms of neuroleptics cannot be individually titrated and are not to be used in the setting of acute behavioral disturbances.

Emergency Department Evaluation and Differential Diagnosis

Common Presentations of Patients with Dementia

The emergency physician encounters patients with dementia under a variety of circumstances. One common presentation is "Granny dumping," in which a patient with Alzheimer's disease or another progressive dementia is left unaccompanied in the emergency department when he or she can no longer be cared for by family members. This action typically arises not from a family's disinterest in the patient's care, but from extreme caregiver frustration, inability to know where to turn for help, or financial crisis. Patients may be bewildered or agitated by this family crisis, and need calm and comforting support while social agencies are called upon to arrange disposition and mend social supports that already have collapsed due to extreme stress. Prompt recognition and evaluation of dementia can avert "Granny dumping" by addressing caregiver needs and providing appropriate social interventions.

Acute behavioral changes, such as agitation or increased disorientation, may also prompt an evaluation in the emergency department. The time course of behavioral changes is critical to determine whether a psychiatric or social work referral is sufficient. When symptoms have developed recently or become increasingly severe, evidence of an acute medical illness is sought. Patients occasionally can relate symptoms that direct the subsequent investigation. In other cases, the patient is uncooperative or unreliable, and the evaluator must rely on physical signs and laboratory studies.

On occasion, the emergency department is the site of the patient's first evaluation for symptoms of dementia. This is particularly true when a startling or unexpected "cardinal" event has occurred, such as driving the wrong way down a street, being unable to recognize familiar surroundings or people, or being found disoriented and lost. Given this variety of circumstances, ranging from an established etiology to a new cognitive complaint, patients with dementia must be recognized and evaluated adequately.

Definition of Dementia

Dementia is a decline in intellectual ability from a previous level of performance causing an altered pattern of activity in a setting of unimpaired consciousness. There are several key points in this definition. First, dementia represents a decline in ability. In order to determine whether there has been a decline, it is necessary to know what previous abilities had been attained. In some cases, dementia is so severe that previous independent living is no longer conceivable, and it is clear that there has been a significant change in a previously competent and independent person. Alternatively, in patients with mild dementia or patients with baseline mental retardation, mental illness, or other cognitive impairments, the extent of decline is more difficult to judge. In patients with mild dementia, previous occupation and education can help in determining whether a change has occurred, and information from family members and other informants may be critical. In individuals who were previously dependent or incompetent, serial observations are usually necessary to document a decline consistent with dementia. Second, the definition of dementia specifies that changes from prior performance levels cause an alteration in daily activities such as employment, independence, or socialization. A patient or family complaint of memory loss or change in ability is insufficient. Historical evidence of the consequences of intellectual decline is therefore important.

Third, dementia is an impairment in overall "intellectual ability," simultaneously involving multiple areas that contribute to intellect, such as memory, judgment, language, planning, and visuospatial skills. When all symptoms can be explained by deficits in a single ability, then more specific terms such as *aphasia* (language deficits) or *amnesia* (memory deficits) are applied and a regionally circumscribed and localizable neurological lesion is sought. This distinction is not simple but can be adequately addressed by a mental status examination that probes several facets of intellect. Finally, a diagnosis of dementia can be made only when the patient's consciousness is unimpaired. An altered level of consciousness suggests delirium, not dementia (see the section on differential diagnosis below and also Chapter 8, "Altered Level of Consciousness"). A determination of whether dementia is present is deferred until the patient is fully awake and stable.

Despite its precise definition, dementia is a syndrome, not a specific diagnosis. There are more than 70 recognized disorders that cause dementia.[3] Depending on the population studied, contributory conditions that are potentially reversible may be identified in more than 40% of patients with intellectual impairment.[4] Determining the precise cause of dementia is not the goal of an emergency department evaluation. Referral is made to a specialized clinic that provides a multidisciplinary approach to the evaluation and management of patients with dementia.

Dementia Recognition as Standard Emergency Care

Recognition of a patient's dementia is important in the emergency department. When dementia is present but not recognized, time and effort are wasted in trying to obtain a history from an incompetent patient. An inaccurate history can result in incorrect or delayed diagnoses, and treatment errors. Failure to consider dementia can also prevent the success of treatments in the emergency department. Patients with dementia are more susceptible to cognitive side effects of medications. Medical instructions at discharge will not be carried out when they cannot be remembered. Therefore, dementia must be recognized and steps taken to ensure compliance with the recommended treatment. Instructions are communicated directly to both patients and caregivers, and written down explicitly for their later reference.

Efforts to recognize dementia focus on those at greatest risk, that is, the elderly and those with chronic debilitating disease or delirium. It is especially critical that dementia is considered when its presence can alter medical management. For example, dementia in a patient with lung cancer would

prompt an evaluation for intracranial metastases; dementia in a chronic alcoholic could signify a subdural hematoma; and dementia in an intravenous drug abuser could indicate a brain abscess. Several etiologies are considered in the patient with acquired immunodeficiency syndrome (AIDS) who develops dementia, including neoplasms, opportunistic infections, or the dementia associated with human immunodeficiency virus (HIV) itself. Delirium is common among patients with underlying dementia;[5] therefore, an assessment for dementia is needed in all such patients once the delirium has resolved.

Guidelines for Cognitive Testing

Dementia encompasses a spectrum of disability. When severely affected, the patient is dependent on others for daily care, and significant cognitive deficits are evident even during limited interactions with the patient. Clues to less severe cognitive impairment may surface during a routine history or general physical examination. For example, the patient may fail to recall medications or significant medical history or be unable to follow multistep commands. These difficulties are frequently attributed to the patient being a "poor informant" or "uncooperative." Mild dementia, however, may not be apparent during the evaluation in the emergency department unless mentation is formally assessed. Patients with dementia may not complain of memory loss, and socially appropriate behavior can mask significant cognitive deficits. Therefore, even in the absence of specific symptoms or clues during usual interactions, cognition is formally assessed.

Mere documentation of level of orientation does not suffice for cognitive assessment. In fact, disorientation to time or date can be misleading as an indication of dementia; more than 20% of normal community-dwelling adults of all ages could not correctly identify specific date or time when surveyed.[6] Alternatively, significant memory impairment can exist in patients with Alzheimer's disease before orientation is affected. Hence, memory is tested specifically. This includes recall of general information such as current events, geography, and historical dates. In addition, short-term memory is assessed by having the patient repeat and then recall three items after a delay of five minutes. Assumptions about a patient's expected level of performance should not be made (for example, "He's not educated enough to know that."). Any difficulty with these tasks suggests the need for further investigation, including questioning the patient and family members about symptoms of cognitive decline that support a diagnosis of dementia. Family members' characterization that the patient's behavior is a "normal part of aging" are not automatically accepted. Age-related changes in cognition do not significantly impair everyday activities such as driving to and from a familiar destination.

In addition to memory, it is important to assess several other areas of cognition. This can be best accomplished with a careful mental status examination; however, some find it easier to assure that several cognitive domains are assessed by using a standard battery of screening questions. Perhaps the most widely used clinical battery for this purpose is the mini mental status examination (MMSE). This 30-point scale assesses orientation, memory, calculations, language, and visuospatial ability.[7] In most cases, scores of less than 26 reflect impairment in cognition, whether due to dementia or other causes.[8] This battery, like others, is not perfect. It has limited sensitivity and is disproportionately weighted for verbal abilities.[9] Education also has a large influence on the result.[10] Therefore, standard batteries cannot substitute for a careful history and examination. Nevertheless, the score on the MMSE reflects severity of impairment and can also be an effective means of describing to other physicians the performance of a patient.

Differential Diagnosis in Patients with a Cognitive Complaint

Dementia is only one possible explanation for cognitive deficits. Other disorders that cause impaired cognition include transient global amnesia, delirium, acute psychosis, aphasia, and depression (Table 22.1). Dementia can be distinguished with a careful history and examination, but all these conditions except transient global amnesia also can occur as a complication of dementia. As a result, considerable clinical judgment is required to assess the presence or interaction of each.

Transient Global Amnesia. Transient global amnesia (TGA) is a unique but poorly understood entity characterized by abrupt, temporary inability to form new memories (anterograde amnesia). Although it is uncommon, it is a very dramatic event

TABLE 22.1. Conditions Commonly Confused with Dementia

Transient global amnesia
Delirium
Acute psychosis
Aphasia
Depression

and almost always leads to an evaluation in the emergency department. Clinical recognition of this benign syndrome can avoid unnecessary, expensive investigations and treatments. Familiarity with TGA enables the emergency physician to distinguish it from dementia.

TGA represents a sudden change in memory function, which often is linked in onset to an identifiable stressor. The anterograde amnesia is associated with variable impairment of recent and remote memory (retrograde amnesia). The entire episode typically persists for 1–8 hours, rarely lasting more than 12 hours. TGA is a condition of later life, affecting individuals in the sixth to eighth decades of life, with a slight male predominance. A patient with TGA has preservation of nonmemory functions, such as language and visuospatial skills, unlike the patient with dementia. Level of consciousness and personal identity are maintained, distinguishing TGA from delirium and psychogenic amnesia. Epileptic features such as aura manifestations, automatisms, or a period of postictal sedation are notably absent in TGA. Any focal neurological signs (ataxia, hemiparesis, visual field deficit) exclude a diagnosis of TGA and warrant evaluation for posterior circulation ischemia. The etiology of TGA is controversial, yet observational studies of patients with strictly defined episodes of TGA have not demonstrated an increase in subsequent risk for vascular events or dementia.[11-13] However, patients with recurrent, brief (less than 1 hour) episodes may develop epilepsy.[14]

Emergency department evaluation of patients with suspected TGA hinges on confirmation of the diagnosis by careful history and examination. Ideally this includes evaluation by a neurologist while the patient is symptomatic. No other diagnostic testing, for example, computerized tomography (CT) scan of the head, is routinely recommended for typical patients with TGA, in whom symptoms resolve within 24 hours.[14] These patients can be reassured about the benign nature of TGA and the relatively low likelihood of recurrence (10–20%). Some neurologists choose to treat patients with daily aspirin for ischemic prophylaxis, although this is not a universal recommendation in the absence of a known increased risk for future vascular events. Patients whose memory deficits persist following assessment in the emergency department are not discharged; they require short-term admission or extended observation, with consideration of a CT scan of the head and/or electroencephalogram (EEG) when symptoms have not substantially improved within 24 hours after onset.

Delirium. Delirium is an acute, fluctuating disorder of attention that causes an altered level of consciousness, disturbance of perception, altered psychomotor activity, disorientation, and memory impairment. Like dementia, it is especially common among the elderly and in hospitalized patients. Like dementia, delirium is a syndrome, not a disease, and has many potential etiologies including medications, infections, electrolyte disturbances, and stroke. Although patients with dementia are more susceptible to delirium, it is crucial that the cognitive impairment from delirium not be attributed to dementia, because failure to evaluate delirium

would neglect many potentially life-threatening conditions.

Key features that distinguish delirium from dementia are summarized in Table 22.2. The onset of delirium occurs over hours to days, as compared to the more insidious course of most dementias. Rapid fluctuation in symptoms is a hallmark of delirium. The delirious patient may exhibit extreme variations in symptoms over 24 hours, especially in the level of consciousness, which can change from an alert, hypervigilant state to stupor or even coma. Sustained attention is difficult, because the delirious patient is easily distracted by irrelevant stimuli. This is in contrast to the patient with dementia, whose level of consciousness is unimpaired and attention generally maintained, until the dementia is quite severe. Hallucinations and delusions are more common in delirium, as are alterations in psychomotor activity, ranging from sluggish behavior to extreme agitation. Asterixis indicates a metabolic derangement contributing to delirium. Both delirium and dementia produce alterations in speech. The delirious patient speaks at an altered rate and is often incoherent. The speech of a demented patient is of normal pace, but with pauses for word finding. Identification of delirium mandates a detailed etiological evaluation (as reviewed in Chapter 8, "Altered Level of Consciousness").

Acute Psychosis. Patients with dementia may have severe behavioral disturbances, giving the im-

TABLE 22.2. Clinical Features Helpful in Distinguishing Dementia from Delirium and Acute Psychosis

Characteristic	Delirium	Dementia	Acute Psychosis
Onset	Acute	*Usually* insidious	Acute
Course over 24 hours	Marked fluctuations	Stable	Stable
Consciousness	Reduced	Normal	Normal
Attention	Usually impaired	Normal, unless dementia severe	May be disturbed
Cognition	Impaired	Impaired	Unimpaired if cooperative
Hallucinations	Visual, ±auditory	Often absent	Predominantly auditory
Psychomotor activity	Increased or reduced, shifts unpredictably	Often normal	Increased or reduced, but not rapidly shifting
Speech	Incoherent, slow, or rapid	Word finding, normal pace	Normal, slow, or rapid

pression that they have acute psychosis, not dementia. Distinguishing features are listed in Table 22.2. Unlike most dementias, acute psychosis develops over days. It is similar to dementia in that consciousness is preserved and fluctuations are not typically observed over a 24-hour interval. Establishing a history of cognitive decline is critical in distinguishing dementia from acute psychosis. Cognition itself is preserved in an acute psychosis that is not superimposed on dementia, although it may be very difficult to assess cognition in the inattentive, uncooperative psychotic patient who has systematized delusions. Auditory hallucinations are common in patients with acute psychosis, but they are rare in the early stages of dementia. Whereas dementia is common in the elderly, the onset of schizophrenia in late life is unusual and controversial;[15] however, up to 10% of geriatric psychiatry admissions are for patients with psychotic disorders unassociated with dementia or affective disorders.[16]

Aphasia. Aphasia is an acquired disturbance of language due to a cerebral insult. In contrast to dementia, aphasia refers to impairment of a single element of cognition, with sparing of other aspects. This distinction can be difficult, particularly when the aphasia involves the patient's ability to comprehend. Most examiners rely primarily on verbal communication during a patient evaluation, and the presence of aphasia necessitates use of nonverbal communication in assessing a patient's thinking abilities. Aphasia, like dementia, has many underlying causes. The time course of the aphasia is helpful in distinguishing acute etiologies (stroke, trauma) from subacute (neoplasm, infection) or chronic (neurodegenerative disorders, e.g., Alzheimer's disease) etiologies. Therefore, an abrupt change in language abilities in a patient with Alzheimer's disease would not be expected as part of the dementia, and an evaluation for stroke or other acute etiology is warranted.

Depression. Depression is a common contributor to cognitive impairment and should be considered in any evaluation for dementia. In the absence of a major depressive disorder, however, depression is unlikely to be the sole cause of memory loss.[17] Loss of interest in activities, not an actual loss of abilities, is a marker of depression. Depression rarely leads to frank disorientation, but patients may exhibit a sense of hopelessness and reduced effort when examined, quickly answering, "I don't know" when cognition is assessed. As always, vegetative symptoms and depressed mood are helpful in determining whether depression is present. Specific patterns of performance on formal neuropsychological testing are also useful in distinguishing depression from dementia. When depression is suspected, the emergency physician initiates an appropriate referral for evaluation and treatment. Long-term follow-up is necessary to assess for cognitive deficits that may remain despite resolution of the depression.

Relevant Neuroanatomy and Physiology

Dementia involves multiple components of cognition, and thus reflects involvement of multiple areas of the cerebral cortex. In most individuals, memory is maintained if either hemisphere is functioning, and therefore the memory impairment observed in patients with dementia implies bihemispheric injury. Although dementia has historically been classified as a "diffuse" disorder of brain function, it is more accurately described as bihemispheric and multifocal, with the specific anatomical alterations dependent on the precise diagnosis. Alzheimer's disease, the most common cause of dementia, is marked by pathological changes that are most prominent in (1) the multimodal association cortex of temporal, parietal, and anterior frontal regions; (2) the entorhinal cortex; and (3) the CA1 and dentate portions of the hippocampus. Other cortical areas, such as primary motor and visual cortex, are much less affected.[18] Histologically, Alzheimer's disease is confirmed by the presence of synaptic and neuronal loss, particularly of large neurons, with abundant neurofibrillary tangles and neuritic plaques. The most consistent and severe neurochemical change in Alzheimer's disease is the loss of the neurotransmitter acetylcholine, though several other neurotransmitters are also reduced. Vascular dementia is the second most common etiology, and pathological correlates include either multiple discrete areas of infarction (multi-infarct dementia) or more confluent periventricular demyelination with microvascular changes. No matter what the cause of the dementia, the areas of greatest pathological damage influence the types of symptoms the patients experience. Consequently, the diversity of symptoms and signs in dementing disorders reflects the variety of pathophysiological derangements. Further details are available in several recent, comprehensive texts.[19–20]

Emergency Department Management and Disposition

Special Considerations

When dementia is suspected, several steps can enhance emergency care. First, the adequacy of the patient's history is rapidly assessed before too much time is spent recording unreliable information. A collateral history, including information about prior level of functioning, and any recent changes in medications, environment, and health status are obtained from caregivers. Family members can be helpful, both for providing a collateral history and for reassuring the patient in the unfamiliar emergency department environment. Unattended patients with disorientation are at risk for wandering and need additional supervision. Emergency personnel introduce themselves and explain any tests that are ordered. The explanations are simple and concrete and may require multiple repetitions. Patient compliance with the physical examination can also be enhanced by "warning" patients in advance of the examiner's requests. For example, a request for the patient to lift his or her left leg can include a "warning" phrase: "Look at this leg" is followed by, "Please lift it." Finally, medications with central nervous system actions, for example, narcotics or sedatives, are avoided when possible. Anticholinergic agents may cause cognitive deficits even in healthy, young adults and are therefore contraindicated in dementia. When medications are necessary for the treatment of extreme agitation, haloperidol or another neuroleptic is preferable.

Unknown Etiology

Implications of Dementia of Unknown Cause. The emergency physician routinely sees nursing home patients whose charts document "dementia," "organic brain syndrome," or "senility" without a specific etiological diagnosis. An evaluation for reversible conditions may not have been performed, and inappropriate management of cognitive and be-

havioral disturbances may occur. For example, a neuroleptic may be prescribed for hallucinations without identification or correction of an underlying vitamin B_{12} deficiency. Similarly, use of a specific label such as "Alzheimer's disease" is also unjustified when an appropriate evaluation has not been performed. Alzheimer's disease has an expected clinical course and prognosis that is different from that of a patient whose dementia is due to a subdural hematoma. Alternatively, an accurate, specific diagnosis permits proper treatment with currently available therapies and participation in applicable research protocols. Diagnostic accuracy also permits a reliable prognosis, which is essential to future planning. The emergency physician facilitates diagnostic accuracy by referring patients with dementia for a comprehensive evaluation.

Neurological Consultation in the Emergency Department. The diagnostic evaluation of dementia is best done in the outpatient setting. The altered environment of an inpatient ward (with new caregivers, disrupted sleep conditions, medication changes) or an active medical problem can invalidate assessment of cognitive performance. The diagnostic tests involved are available to outpatients and often cannot be coordinated efficiently on an inpatient basis. Nonetheless, there are clear circumstances in which neurological consultation in the emergency department is warranted. These are listed in Table 22.3, along with the recommendations for CT scan of the head or lumbar puncture, and consist of the following: (1) the new occurrence of a seizure, (2) an unexplained focal neurological deficit, (3) an unexplained gait disturbance, and (4) an acute or subacute (less than three months) onset of dementia. In addition, behavioral disturbances occasionally are so severe that inpatient psychiatric care is required.

The combination of dementia and new-onset seizures has many potential causes, including subdural hematoma, stroke, and neoplasm. An emergency CT scan of the head is required; when negative, lumbar puncture is performed to assess the possibility of meningitis. A focal neurological finding (hemiparesis, visual field deficit) is also evaluated with a CT scan of the head for cerebrovascular disease or other focal pathology. Dementia and gait disturbance coexist in several disorders, such

TABLE 22.3. Indications for Emergency Department Neurological Consultation and Procedures in Patients with Dementia

Feature	Head CT*	Lumbar Puncture*
New-onset seizure	+	±
Focal neurological deficit	+	−
Gait disturbance	±	±
Subacute onset (less than 3-month duration)	+	+

Note:+: recommended procedure; ±: often recommended depending on clinical circumstances; −: not recommended.

as strokes, Parkinson's disease, chronic alcoholism, vitamin B_{12} deficiency, neurosyphilis, and normal pressure hydrocephalus (NPH). A specific diagnosis is often suggested by the pattern of gait disturbance. When gait disturbance is unexplained, a neurological consultation in the emergency department is advisable for consideration of additional testing (for example, a CT scan of the head to detect normal pressure hydrocephalus or cerebrospinal fluid (CSF) analysis for neurosyphilis), or treatment.

The rapid development of progressive dementia over a few months warrants urgent attention. Clinical deterioration over days or weeks is atypical in patients with neurodegenerative disorders and raises several other etiological possibilities, as listed in Table 22.4. Timely diagnosis can lead to successful reversal of many of these causes, and delay can mean permanent deficits or death. In the emergency department CT scan of the head should be followed by lumbar puncture, unless a mass lesion is identified. CSF testing includes cytology, cryptococcal antigen, and bacterial, fungal, and tuberculosis cultures. Polymerase chain reaction (PCR) testing for viral antigens is obtained, when indicated. Unless an inaccurate history or delirium is found to account for the rapid course, most patients need admission for additional diagnostic testing such as serial EEG's and MRI; angiography, functional imaging (position emission tomography or

TABLE 22.4. Differential Diagnosis of Rapidly Progressive Dementia

Creutzfeldt-Jakob disease
Meningitis/encephalitis (including tuberculosis, herpes, fungal, cryptococcal, carcinomatous, paraneoplastic)
Vasculitis
Primary or metastatic tumors, including central nervous system lymphoma
Subdural hematoma
Normal pressure hydrocephalus
Multi-infarct dementia (occasionally)
Alzheimer's disease (rarely)

single photon emission computed tomography) and cerebral biopsy are obtained in selected cases.

Creutzfeldt-Jakob Disease: Emergency Department Precautions. Of the disorders listed in Table 22.4, Creutzfeldt-Jakob disease (CJD) merits special mention because of its transmissibility. CJD is a prion disease, caused by a *proteinaceous, infectious* agent (prion). Prions have not been found in saliva, urine, or feces, and transmission does not occur with casual contact or routine nursing care. Universal precautions are sufficient in the emergency department, except for lumbar puncture. Prions are found in CSF and extra precautions are needed, as prions are not killed by alcohol or formaldehyde. Emergency department precautions with regard to CJD are summarized in Table 22.5. CJD is rare, but is

TABLE 22.5. Emergency Department Precautions for Creutzfeldt-Jakob Disease

Use universal precautions.
If accidental expsoure to blood or CSF occurs, cleanse wound with 0.5% bleach.
Use 5% bleach or phenol solution for surface contamination.
Autoclave instruments for ≥1 hour at ≥121°C and ≥15 psi.
Autoclave blood, brain tissue, and CSF before discarding. Immerse spinal fluid counting chambers in 5% bleach or phenol solution for at least 1 hour.

considered in all rapidly progressive dementias. Therefore, these specific precautions are established, documented, and readily available so that the occasional patient with a rapidly progressive dementia can be managed appropriately without undue concern.

Clinically, CJD produces rapidly progressive dementia, often with focal features such as ataxia, visual disturbances, and rigidity. Onset is in the mid fifth to seventh decades of life, and both sporadic and familial forms are observed. Late in the course of the disease there is commonly a striking myoclonic startle response to sudden noises. Death occurs within one year of symptom onset in the majority of cases. Sporadic cases have characteristic EEG findings of periodic high-voltage sharp wave complexes, but CSF and head CT are generally normal.

Initiation of Outpatient Evaluation and Referral. Patients are referred for outpatient evaluation and management to a multidisciplinary clinic with expertise in cognitive disorders, where a community-based management plan can be initiated with social services and caregiver education and support. The diagnostic evaluation and provisions for long-term management may be available through the patient's primary physician, although a referral to a dementia clinic is often necessary. Diagnostic evaluation includes a series of laboratory studies focusing on reversible causes of dementia[22] and an imaging study of the brain to look for structural abnormalities. When these tests have not been performed previously, the emergency physician can facilitate this evaluation by ordering the laboratory studies listed in Table 22.6 and arranging for an outpatient MRI scan of the brain.

Known Etiology

Expected Clinical Course. When a specific etiology of a patient's dementia has been established, the emergency physician confirms that the patient's current presentation is consistent with the expected clinical course. Each dementing disorder has a unique course, and deviation from this course suggests either a misdiagnosis or a superimposed condition. A brief review of the natural history of the two most common dementing diseases, Alzheimer's disease and multi-infarct dementia, follows.

TABLE 22.6. Laboratory Evaluation for Dementia

Serum chemistries: electrolytes, glucose, renal and liver function tests
Complete blood count
Urinalysis
Thyroid-stimulating hormone
Treponemal antibody test (nontreponemal tests are less sensitive for neurosyphilis)
Erythrocyte sedimentation rate
Vitamin B_{12} and folate levels
HIV testing (when indicated)

Alzheimer's disease is characterized by insidiously progressive cognitive decline, and its typical clinical course is depicted in Figure 22.1. Usually, deficits are noted by patients or others for at least one year before a diagnosis can be made reliably. Alzheimer's disease is no longer a "diagnosis of exclusion," because specific diagnostic criteria have been validated pathologically.[23] Impairment of short-term memory, mild naming difficulties, and visuospatial deficits (as can be assessed by three-dimensional drawings) arise early in the course of the disease. Personality changes at this stage are typically mild, such as occasional irritability, and the patient is still independent in activities of daily living. Therefore, with early referral a diagnosis can be made at a time when patients retain decision-making capacity and can direct future planning. In addition, symptomatic treatment of cognitive impairment is more likely to be successful in patients who are in the earlier stages of Alzheimer's disease. Despite treatment, there is progressive impairment in language, orientation, and judgment that eventually necessitates patient supervision. As a guide, scores on the MMSE will fall by roughly three points per year,[24] unless modified by treatment. Alterations in personality and behavior become more prominent and range from agitation and hallucinations to passivity and social withdrawal. By eight years after onset, more than 60% of patients with Alzheimer's disease reside in nursing homes.[25] This landmark is also modifiable, both by treating cognitive and behavioral impairments and by strengthening social supports.

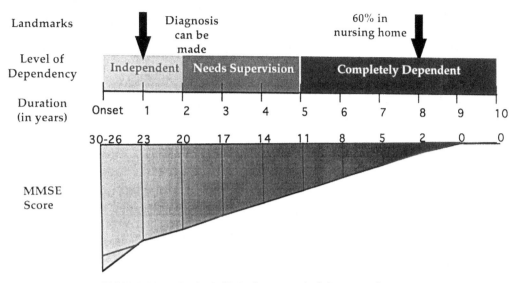

FIGURE 22.1. Typical clinical course of Alzheimer's disease.

Unexpected clinical changes in Alzheimer's disease require additional evaluation. In patients with mild to moderate cognitive symptoms, incontinence is unexpected and prompts an evaluation for cystitis, prostatic hypertrophy, or consideration of other causes of the dementia. Gait impairment is uncommon until late in the disease, when extrapyramidal symptoms develop in approximately 30% of patients.[26] Seizures suggest the presence of a superimposed illness, although they commonly occur in patients with Down's syndrome who develop Alzheimer's disease and can occur in others late in the course of the disease.[27–29] Alzheimer's disease cannot explain focal weakness or sensory loss; such symptoms therefore require further evaluation even when a diagnosis of Alzheimer's disease has been established.

Multi-infarct dementia (MID), in contrast to Alzheimer's disease, has an abrupt onset with stepwise decline, often in the setting of a known series of clinical strokes. Focal symptoms and signs (hemiparesis, spasticity) are present, reflecting localized injury from cerebral ischemia. Ischemic brain may serve as a focus for seizures, which are often observed early in the course of multi-infarct dementia. Other typical features include emotional lability and somatic complaints. Cognitive impairment may remain remarkably stable in the absence of further ischemic episodes.[30] Unlike patients with Alzheimer's disease, patients with MID commonly experi-

ence incontinence, even early in the disease. Although focal motor or sensory symptoms are expected at the time of diagnosis of MID, the subsequent development of new, focal symptoms reflects a failure of therapy to prevent further strokes and may require additional evaluation or treatment modification.

Medical Complications and Exacerbation of Cognitive Deficits. Complications common to all demented patients include falls, malnutrition, and pneumonia. Dementia associated with a gait disorder (e.g., MID, Parkinson's disease, NPH, and later stages of Alzheimer's disease) presents the highest risk for falls. Nutritional status deteriorates when the patient's swallowing function is compromised, as often occurs in patients with Huntington's disease or Parkinson's disease. Pneumonia is a common cause of death, related to aspiration or reduced mobility. Iatrogenic complications include urinary tract infection from chronic catheterization.

Any medical complication has the potential to exacerbate preexisting cognitive deficits. Patients may not be able to complain of dysuria or dyspnea, and elderly patients typically do not exhibit fever or leukocytosis. Thus, even when specific symptoms are lacking, common medical complications, such as pneumonia and urinary tract infection, are considered in any patient with dementia who has a precipitous decline in cognition. Medications with central nervous system actions, particularly sedatives and narcotics, are another frequent reason for decline from baseline. Agitation or worsening cognition may also occur acutely due to changes in environment, for example, when the patient travels away from home or when a new caregiver is present. Similar fluctuations also can occur on a daily basis and are termed "sundowning," which appears to be due to psychosocial factors.[31] When no changes in the environment or provision of care can be identified to explain the acute agitation or worsening cognition, a superimposed medical illness is considered. Impaired consciousness is not attributable to dementia and prompts further medical evaluation (see Chapter 8, "Altered Level of Consciousness").

Diagnosis-Specific Treatments and Potential Complications. Although there are many potentially reversible etiologies of dementia, they are the sole cause of dementia in only a small minority of cases. Most dementing illnesses are progressive. Nevertheless, all patients with dementia benefit from medical treatment, and much can be done to maximize the function of patients and relieve the burden of caregivers.[4] These nonspecific treatments for dementia are extremely important in improving quality of life and minimizing the need for institutional care. They include treatment of complicating medical and psychiatric conditions, maintenance of nutrition, physical therapy, and judicious use of psychoactive medications. These treatments, health education, and referral to social services should not be overlooked in the emergency department; however, they rely primarily on follow-up care and multidisciplinary efforts in outpatient clinics.

As knowledge about the pathophysiology of dementing disorders increases, both symptomatic and potentially curative specific therapies are becoming available. Currently, cognitive impairment in patients with Alzheimer's disease is treated symptomatically with acetylcholinesterase inhibitors, which increase cerebral acetylcholine levels. Tacrine (Cognex) and donepezil (Aricept) are presently available, and several other cholinergic agents are being investigated.

Principal side effects are gastrointestinal, including nausea, anorexia, and diarrhea. Tacrine requires careful dose titration and laboratory monitoring. Elevated liver transaminases are common, and discontinuation of tacrine therapy is recommended for an alanine aminotransferase greater than three times the normal upper limits. Donepezil has a lower incidence of gastrointestinal side effects and no hepatotoxicity. Cognitive benefits of either medication are only modest, and neither prevents disease progression. Initiation of anticholinesterase therapy requires thoughtful discussion and is not appropriate in the emergency department; it is best left to the patient's outpatient physician. Nevertheless, emergency physicians should be aware of potential complications of this therapy. Table 22.7 summarizes indications and adverse effects of commonly used medications in patients with Alzheimer's disease.

Specific management of MID depends on identification and modification of vascular risk factors. Treatment is identical to that appropriate for stroke under other circumstances (see Chapter 16, "Cerebrovascular Disease"). MID is a potentially preventable disorder, and early identification and specific treatment are the most likely to minimize disability and dependency. Extrapyramidal symptoms observed in patients with Parkinson's disease or Alzheimer's disease can be treated with dopaminergic agents such as levodopa (see Chapter 17, "Movement Disorders"). Neither AIDS dementia nor CJD has effective, specific, long-term treatments.

Management of Behavioral Disturbances. Behavioral disturbances in patients with Alzheimer's disease or other neurodegenerative disorders usually do not require hospitalization. For some patients, environmental or activity modifications suffice. For example, wandering behavior may resolve when frequently sought items are kept in a prominent location or when meaningful activities can occupy the patient's daytime hours. Use of night-lights or contrasting colors helps patients identify the bathroom correctly at night, and timed toileting will reduce incontinence in those who cannot express a need to void. Agitation is lessened by providing a stable environment

TABLE 22.7. Pharmacological Treatment of Alzheimer's Disease

Class/Name	Indication	Adverse Effects
Cholinesterase inhibitors	Cognitive impairment	
Tacrine (Cognex)		Hepatoxicity, nausea, diarrhea
Donepezil (Aricept)		Rare nausea, diarrhea
Dopaminergic agents	Extrapyramidal symptoms	
Levodopa (Sinemet)		Nausea, hallucinations, orthostasis
Neuroleptics (high potency)	Hallucinations, paranoia	
Haloperidol (Haldol)		Extrapyramidal symptoms, sedation
Risperidone (Risperdal)		Extrapyramidal symptoms
Olanzapine (Zyprexa)		Rare extrapyramidal symptoms
Anxiolytics	Anxiety, agitation	
Buspirone (Buspar)		Sedation
Anticonvulsants	Agitation, aggression	
Valproic acid (Depakote)		Nausea, thrombocytopenia
Carbamazepine (Tegretol)		Sedation, neutropenia
Antidepressants (serotinergic)	Agitation, depression	
Trazodone (Desyrel)		Sedation, orthostasis
SSRIs (Prozac, Zoloft)		Anxiety, insomnia

and correcting sensory impairments such as hearing or visual loss.

When behavioral modification techniques fail, pharmacological intervention is frequently necessary for management of behavior or mood disturbances. Agents with little or no anticholinergic activity are preferred in order to avoid worsening of cognitive deficits. Neuroleptics traditionally have been the mainstay of treatment for patients experiencing agitation or hallucinations. However, the high-potency neuroleptics (which have the least anticholinergic activity) may exacerbate or precipitate extrapyramidal symptoms. Newer agents, including risperidone (Risperdal) and olanzapine (Zyprexa), are less often accompanied by extrapyramidal side effects and are useful when haloperidol (Haldol) is not tolerated. Alternatives to neuroleptics include anxiolytics (buspirone), anticonvulsants (carbamazepine or valproic acid), and antidepressants (trazodone, fluoxetine). Discussion with a neurologist or psychiatrist is advised to select an appropriate agent and confirm arrangements for long-term care. When the patient can no longer be safely managed

on an outpatient basis due to severe agitation or aggression, hospitalization is pursued. Ideally, this entails admission to a neurology or psychiatry unit specializing in behavioral management, which may be available at a tertiary center.

Disposition and Medical-Legal Issues

Consultation and Placement from the Emergency Department. As previously discussed, consultation and/or hospitalization are indicated in cases of severe behavioral disturbances or when specific features of a dementia (new-onset seizures, unexplained focal neurological deficit or gait disturbance, or subacute onset of cognitive impairment) require further evaluation. Otherwise, outpatient management is appropriate. In fact, the majority of patients with dementia receive care at home for many years. Nonetheless, issues of patient safety, supervision, or medical care often eventually result in nursing home placement. Wait times for placement can be lengthy, and hospitalization solely for placement is not reimbursed. Thus, nursing home placement should be anticipated before the need arises. For these reasons, it is especially important that the care of patients with dementia be managed at a center where social work services are available. All patients with dementia and their caregivers should be referred to community-based support services such as the Alzheimer's Association and Area Agency on Aging. Interim assistance may be provided by emergency department social work staff, when available.

Social work services are also invaluable in facilitating reduction of caregiver burden and stress. This facilitation includes utilization of home care services, ranging from visiting nurse associations to community resources such as Meals on Wheels. Adult day care programs allow for both structured patient activities and caregiver respite. Many support groups, such as those run by local chapters of the Alzheimer's Association, are of immeasurable benefit. A comprehensive program of caregiver counseling, education, and support significantly increases the length of time a family member with Alzheimer's disease can be cared for at home.[32]

Medical-Legal Issues. Several medical-legal issues are considered prior to discharging a patient with dementia from the emergency department, including driving restrictions, elder abuse, and patient competency. Dementia clearly has the potential to alter driving skills, although the extent of this alteration may be difficult to predict on an individual basis. Patients are informed not to drive until their dementia has been assessed and until this issue has been addressed in the context of a comprehensive evaluation. Patients with cognitive impairment are also at increased risk for physical abuse by family members or other caregivers. Any suspicion of abuse must be reported to adult protective services. Demented patients may be the target of financial scams or mismanagement. For financial security and personal self-determination, a durable power of attorney for financial and medical decision-making is recommended as soon as dementia is recognized. When the patient is no longer competent to make decisions, guardianship is pursued, both to protect the caregiver and the health provider. Commonly, it is necessary for significant medical decisions to be made during the patient's illness, and establishing a responsible person to

make decisions can prevent unnecessary anguish and the need for legal recourse on an urgent basis. In all cases, discharge instruction should be explicit and reiterated in writing as well as with available family members.

PEARLS AND PITFALLS

- Memory is specifically tested in patients at risk for dementia.
- Identifying the specific cause of dementia is necessary to guide appropriate management.
- Treating patients with dementia can enhance cognition, improve associated medical and psychiatric conditions, and reduce caregiver burden.
- Infectious precautions are required when evaluating patients with rapidly progressive dementia.
- Abrupt changes in cognition may signify a superimposed medical complication, not a worsening of the underlying dementia.
- Neuroleptics are preferable to benzodiazepines for acute management of severe agitation in patients with dementia.
- Dementia may go undetected on casual observation.
- Not all patients with dementia complain of memory loss.
- Many patients with dementia *do* complain of memory loss.
- Age-related changes in cognition do not significantly impair everyday activities.
- Level of orientation does not adequately test cognition.
- Impaired, fluctuating consciousness is an indicator of delirium, not dementia.
- Not all patients with dementia have Alzheimer's disease.
- Alzheimer's disease is *not* a diagnosis of exclusion; specific diagnostic criteria exist.
- Nonspecific terms such as *senility* and *organic brain syndrome* are inaccurate and useless.

REFERENCES

1. Beard CM, Kokmen E, O'Brien PC, Kurland LT. The prevalence of dementia is changing over time in Rochester, Minnesota. *Neurology.* 1995;45:75–9.

2. Ebly EM, Parhad IM, Hogan DM, Fung TS. Prevalence and type of dementia in the very old: results from the Canadian Study of Health and Aging. *Neurology.* 1994;44:1593–1600.

3. Katzman R. Diagnosis and management of dementia. In: Katzman R, Rowe JW, eds. *Principles of Geriatric Neurology.* Philadelphia: FA Davis Co; 1992:170.

4. Larson EB, Reifler BV, Featherstone HJ, English DR. Dementia in elderly outpatients: a prospective study. *Ann Intern Med.* 1984;100:417–23.

5. Erkinjuntti T, Wikstrom J, Palo J, Autio L. Dementia among medical inpatients: evaluation of 2000 consecutive admissions. *Arch Intern Med.* 1986;146:1923–6.

6. Natelson BH, Haupt EJ, Fleischer EJ, Grey L. Temporal orientation and education: a direct relationship in normal people. *Arch Neurol.* 1979;36:444–6.

7. Folstein MF, Folstein SE, McHugh PR. Mini-mental state: a practical method for grading the cognitive state of patients for the clinician. *J Psychiatr Res.* 1975;12:189–98.

8. Roper BL, Bieliauskas LA, Peterson MR. Validity of the Mini-Mental State Examination and the Neurobehavioral Cognitive Status Examination in cognitive screening. *Neuropsychiatry Neuropsychol Behav Neurol.* 1996;9:54–7.

9. Tombaugh TN, McIntyre NJ. The mini-mental state examination: a comprehensive review. *J Am Geriatr Soc.* 1992;40:922–35.

10. Murden RA, McRae TD, Kaner S, Bucknam ME. Minimental state exam scores vary with education in blacks and whites. *J Am Geriatr Soc.* 1991;39:149–55.

11. Nausieda PA, Sherman IC. Long-term prognosis in transient global amnesia. *JAMA.* 1979;241:392–3.

12. Miller JW, Petersen RC, Metter EJ, Millikan CH, Yanagihara T. Transient global amnesia: clinical characteristics and prognosis. *Neurology.* 1987;37:733–7.

13. Hodges JR, Warlow CP. The aetiology of transient global amnesia: a case-control study of 114 cases with prospective follow-up. *Brain.* 1990;113:639–57.

14. Hodges JR. *Transient Amnesia: Clinical and Neuropsychological Aspects.* Philadelphia, PA: WB Saunders Co; 1991:25–48, 60.

15. Rabins PV, Pearlson GD, Strauss ME. Cognitive impairment in psychiatric syndromes. In: Whitehouse PJ, ed. *Dementia.* Philadelphia, PA: FA Davis Co; 1993:366.

16. Christison C, Blazer D. Clinical assessment of psychiatric symptoms. In: Albert MS, Moss MB, eds. *Geriatric Neuropsychology.* New York, NY: The Guilford Press; 1988:95.

17. Bieliauskus L. Depressed or not depressed? That is the question. *J Clin Exp Neuropsychol.* 1993;15:119–34.

18. Brun A, Englund E. Regional pattern of degeneration in Alzheimer's disease: neuronal loss and histopathological grading. *Histopathology.* 1981;5:549–64.

19. Terry RD, Katzman R, Bick KL. *Alzheimer Disease.* New York, NY: Raven Press, Ltd; 1994.

20. Calne D. *Neurodegenerative Diseases.* Philadelphia, Pa: WB Saunders Co; 1994.

21. Cummings JL, Benson DF. *Dementia: A Clinical Approach.* Boston, Mass.: Butterworth-Heinemann; 1993.

22. Corey-Bloom J, Thal LJ, Galasko D, et al. Diagnosis and evaluation of dementia. *Neurology.* 1995;45:211–18.

23. McKhann G, Drachman D, Folstein M, Katzman R, Price D, Stadlan EM. Clinical diagnosis of Alzheimer's disease: report of the NINCDS-ADRDA Work Group under the auspices of Department of Health and Human Services Task Force on Alzheimer's Disease. *Neurology.* 1984;34:939–44.

24. Salmon DP, Thal LJ, Butters N, Heindel WC. Longitudinal evaluation of dementia of the Alzheimer type: a comparison of 3 standardized mental status examinations. *Neurology.* 1990;40:1225–30.

25. Heyman A, Wilkinson WE, Hurwitz BJ, et al. Early onset Alzheimer's disease: clinical predictors of institutionalization and death. *Neurology.* 1987;37:980–4.

26. Mayeux R, Stern Y, Spanton S. Heterogeneity in dementia of the Alzheimer type: evidence of subgroups. *Neurology.* 1985;35:453–61.

27. Evenhuis HM. The natural history of dementia in Down's syndrome. *Arch Neurol.* 1990;47:263–7.

28. Lai F, Williams RS. A prospective study of Alzheimer disease in Down syndrome. *Arch Neurol.* 1989;46:849–53.

29. Romanelli MF, Morris JC, Ashkin K, Coben LA. Advanced Alzheimer's disease is a risk factor for late-onset seizures. *Arch Neurol.* 1990;47:847–50.

30. Tatemichi TK, Paik M, Bagiella E, et al. Risk of dementia after stroke in a hospitalized cohort: results of a longitudinal study. *Neurology.* 1994;44:1885–91.

31. Evans LK. Sundown syndrome in institutionalized elderly. *J Am Geriatr Soc.* 1987;35:101–8.

32. Mittelman MS, Ferris SH, Shulman E, Steinberg G, Levin B. A family intervention to delay nursing home placement of patients with Alzheimer's disease: a randomized controlled trial. *JAMA.* 1996;276:1725–31.

23 Brain Tumors and Other Neuro-Oncological Emergencies

HERBERT B. NEWTON

SUMMARY Neuro-oncological emergencies are a diverse group of disorders that occur commonly in patients with brain tumors and other types of cancer. Typically, they are caused by direct effects of tumor on the nervous system, but they can also develop as a result of treatment, infection, metabolic disturbances, medication side effects, and other mechanisms. Alteration of mental status is the most common type of neuro-oncological emergency, typically caused by toxicity from various medications, as well as other factors. Seizure activity, cerebrovascular disorders, focal neurological deficits, and compression of the spinal cord are the other neuro-oncological emergencies discussed in this chapter. Knowledge of the pathophysiology and differential diagnosis of the various neuro-oncological emergencies is required for a focused evaluation and rapid initiation of therapy so that neurological morbidity and mortality is minimized.

Introduction

In the United States, more than 150,000 new patients develop brain tumors each year (see Table 23.1). Of this number, approximately 15,000–18,000 cases represent primary brain tumors, primarily gliomas and meningiomas.[1,2] The majority of these tumors occur in adults; 1500–2000 children develop brain tumors.[2,3] Metastases to the brain occur more commonly than primary tumors and are estimated to affect 95,000–150,000 patients each year.[4,6] Brain metastases can arise in cancer patients of any age, but primarily they occur in adults. Primary and metastatic spinal cord tumors are less common than tumors of the brain (see Table 23.2).[7] The incidence of primary spinal cord tumors is 25% that of primary brain tumors. Metastatic tumors to the spine develop in 5% of patients who die of cancer each year. Approximately 20,000 patients have metastatic tumor in the epidural space and are at risk for spinal cord or cauda equina compression.[8,9]

Neurological emergencies are common in patients with primary and metastatic tumors of the central nervous system (CNS), which can affect any level of the neuraxis.[10] These patients seek emergency care because of the profound morbidity associated with neuro-oncological disease and its treatment. Many patients with neuro-oncological disorders present to the emergency department repeatedly before they have received a specific diagnosis. Often, the presenting complaint is part of a constellation of neurological symptoms and signs that have arisen recently and progressed over several weeks to months. In contrast, patients with an existing systemic or neuro-oncological condition (e.g., glioma, spinal metastasis, lymphoma) may present because of a new symptom. In patients with primary and metastatic brain tumors, the most common symptoms include headache, seizure, changes

TABLE 23.1. Common Primary and Metastatic Brain Tumors

Primary Tumors	Metastatic Tumors
Adults	
Glioblastoma multiforme (35–40%)	Lung (64%)
Astrocytoma grades I–III (18–20%)	Breast (14%)
Meningioma (18%)	Unknown primary (8%)
Pituitary adenoma (9%)	Melanoma (4%)
Oligodendroglioma (5%)	Colorectal (3%)
Schwannoma (3–5%)	Hypernephroma (2%)
Ependymoma (2%)	
Children	
Astrocytoma, low-grade (15–30%)	Wilms' tumor (18.6%)
Astrocytoma, high-grade (8–15%)	Rhabdomyosarcoma (18.6%)
Medulloblastoma (18–25%)	Osteogenic sarcoma (16.3%)
Brainstem glioma (6–15%)	Germ cell tumors (16.3%)
Ependymoma (6–13%)	Ewing's sarcoma (9.3%)
Craniopharyngioma (6–9%)	Neuroblastoma (4.6%)
Pineal region (2–5%)	Hepatocellular carcinoma (4.6%)

Source: From Newton;[2] Pollock;[3] Patchell;[4] Sawaya and Bindal;[5] and Allen.[6]

in personality and cognition, and focal weakness.[2,4] Typically, spinal cord tumors cause back pain, lower extremity weakness and loss of sensation, and urinary incontinence.[7,8]

Alterations of Mental Status in Patients with Cancer

Alterations of mental status are common in patients with brain tumors and other types of cancer.[1–5,10] Mental status changes can be caused by structural abnormalities within the CNS (e.g., tumor, abscess, hydrocephalus), new or treatment-related infections, seizures, metabolic or treatment-related encephalopathies, and other diagnostic considerations (see Table 23.3).

The changes in mental status can range from slight lethargy or confusion to encephalopathy or coma. Because of the extensive differential diagnosis for these patients, a focused search for diagnostic clues within a widely divergent group of potential disorders is undertaken. In many cases, the patient

can experience severe neurological injury when diagnosis and stabilization do not occur promptly, for example, when intracranial pressure (ICP) is increased and the patient is at risk for brain herniation.

Prehospital Management

The focus of prehospital management is supportive care until an etiology can be determined and treatment initiated. A succinct history is obtained by emergency medical services personnel from family members, focusing on the alteration of the patient's mental status, including its onset, severity, and associated symptoms. A history of brain tumor or cancer and all prescribed medications (e.g., antiepileptic drugs, dexamethasone, chemotherapy) are reported to the emergency physician. Physical examination includes an assessment of airway patency, breathing, and circulation. During transport of the patient to the hospital, a baseline neurological evaluation is documented. Intravenous access is established and infusion of normal saline begun

TABLE 23.2. Common Primary and Metastatic Spinal Cord Tumors

Primary Tumors	Metastatic Tumors
Extramedullary 89%	Breast (22%)
Neurofibroma (29%)	Lung (15%)
Meningioma (25%)	Prostate (10%)
Sarcoma (12%)	Lymphoma (10%)
Other (10–15%)	Sarcoma (9%)
Dermoid	Kidney (7%)
Epidermoid	Gastrointestinal tract (5%)
	Melanoma (4%)
Intramedullary 11%	Unknown primary (4%)
Ependymoma (55%)	Head and neck (3%)
Astrocytoma (31%)	
Vascular tumors (4%)	
Other (5–10%)	
Mixed glioma	
Oligodendroglioma	

Source: Newton, Newton, Gatens, Hebert, and Pack;[7] Byrne,[8] and Klein, Sanford, and Muhlbauer.[9]

when intravenous fluids are indicated. To minimize free water administration (which can exacerbate preexisting cerebral edema), lactated Ringer's and D5W solutions are not used.

Emergency Evaluation and Differential Diagnosis

The extensive differential diagnosis of alterations of mental status in patients with cancer include structural changes within the parenchyma of the brain, infections, toxic encephalopathies, metabolic encephalopathies, treatment-related encephalopathies, and seizure activity (see Table 23.3). Many of these disorders can increase ICP, which further contributes to alterations of mental status. The presence of primary or metastatic brain tumors is the most commonly encountered structural change that causes mental status changes (see Table 23.1). Depending on the location of the tumor (or tumors), the alterations in mental status range from subtle personality changes to lethargy and confusion, to coma.[1–5] The pace of alteration in mental status is usually gradual when it is caused by tumor growth and associated edema formation, and rapid in the

TABLE 23.3. Disorders Associated with Alterations of Mental Status in Cancer Patients

Structural Disease	*Toxic encephalopathy*
Primary/metastatic brain tumors	Sedative hypnotics
Elevated intracranial pressure	Narcotics
Hydrocephalus	Antidepressants
Intratumoral or parenchymal hemorrhage	Anticonvulsants
Leptomeningeal metastases	Neuroleptics
Cerebrovascular disorders	Antiemetics
Abscess	Steroids
Metabolic encephalopathy	*Infection*
Fluid/electrolyte disturbances	Neutropenic sepsis
Hypoxia	Meningitis
Renal failure/uremia	Encephalitis
Liver failure/hyperammonemia	Aspiration pneumonia
Endocrine disorders	
Wernicke's encephalopathy	
Treatment-related encephalopathy	*Seizure disorder*
Radiation therapy	Postictal state
Chemotherapeutic agents	Subclinical status epilepticus

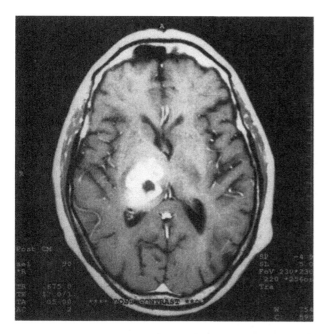

FIGURE 23.1. A 65-year-old man noted the gradual onset of ataxia and gait disturbance. (A) A gadolinium-enhanced T1-weighted MRI demonstrated the presence of a large, enhancing mass in the region of the right thalamus with associated ipsilateral ventricular compression. (B) Several days later, the patient had deteriorated acutely, becoming mute and unresponsive. A nonenhanced cerebral CT demonstrated the presence of a large hemorrhage within the tumor with more severe compression of the ventricular system.

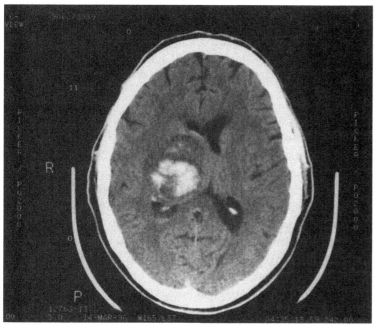

presence of intracranial hemorrhage (see the section on cerebrovascular emergencies and Fig. 23.1) or hydrocephalus.[10] Patients with hydrocephalus typically have symptoms suggestive of increased ICP (e.g., headache, nausea, vomiting) prior to the onset of mental status changes.[10] Hydrocephalus is caused by leptomeningeal tumor, infection, and intracranial hemorrhage. Other cerebrovascular disorders can cause alterations of mental status because of structural injury unrelated to hydrocephalus (see

the section on cerebrovascular emergencies and Fig. 23.2).[11–13] Leptomeningeal tumor frequently causes mild mental status changes (e.g., lethargy, confusion), headache, weakness, gait disturbance, pain, and other symptoms.[14,15]

A gradual deterioration of mental status is observed in patients with brain abscess formation. Sepsis caused by treatment-related neutropenia (e.g., chemotherapy, radiation) is often associated with mental status changes, which precede the fever

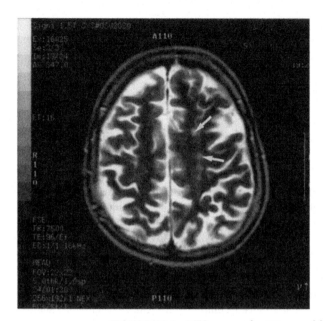 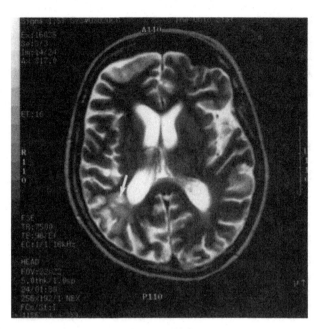

FIGURE 23.2. MRI scans of a 57-year-old woman with a history of non-Hodgkin's lymphoma who developed neurological symptoms and signs consistent with impaired short-term memory, dyscalculia, and other cognitive abilities. (A) and (B) On T2-weighted MRI, there are multifocal regions of high signal consistent with embolic infarct or leptomeningeal tumor involvement (white arrows). Lumbar punctures were unrevealing. Transesophageal echocardiography revealed vegetations on the mitral and aortic valves consistent with NBTE.

spike by 12–24 hours in some patients.[10] Meningitis from fungus, mycobacteria, and listeria, common in immunocompromised patients with cancer, presents with lethargy, confusion, seizures, meningismus, and cranial neuropathies.[10,16] Patients with viral encephalitis can present with seizures, confusion, encephalopathy, fever, and headache, and typically is caused by herpes simplex, herpes zoster, and cytomegalovirus.[10,16] In patients with brain tumor, head and neck cancer, or leptomeningeal tumor, aspiration pneumonia can result from an unrecognized dysphagia.[17]

Encephalopathic states can result from therapeutic interventions, medications, or metabolic disturbances. Radiation therapy can cause an acute encephalopathy (especially in the setting of a brain tumor with edema and mass effect) by further increasing ICP. Several chemotherapeutic agents can cause encephalopathy, including 5-fluorouracil, ifosfamide, high-dose or intrathecal methotrexate, cytosine arabinoside, alphainterferon, and interleukin-2.[10,18] A toxic encephalopathy caused by excessive concentrations of certain medications is the most common cause of mental status alteration in patients with cancer (see Table 23.3).[10] Metabolic encephalopathy, common in patients with electrolyte disturbances (e.g., hyponatremia), is also noted in patients with uremia, hyperammonemia, and Wernicke's encephalopathy.[10] Patients with Wernicke's encephalopathy have mental status changes, nystagmus, ophthalmoplegia, and ataxia; however, manifestation of only a part of the syndrome is more common.

A detailed history of mental status changes obtained from the patient (when possible) and family members includes the time of onset, severity, and rapidity of evolution. Associated symptoms such as headache, nausea, emesis, pain, weakness, fever, and focal deficits are reviewed. The patient's history of cancer is discussed, including past and current treatments. A complete list of medications is reviewed.

The general physical examination is directed toward gathering evidence of systemic disease that can contribute to the mental status alterations. Fever, evidence of infection or sepsis, meningismus, and bilateral asterixis or myoclonus are noted. A detailed neurological examination is necessary to evaluate specific alterations in mental status, to document any focal neurological findings, and to differentiate structural from metabolic causes of alterations of mental status.[19,20] Patients with focal, structural brain disease (e.g., tumor, hemorrhage, stroke) typically have localizing signs such as hemiparesis, facial weakness, sensory loss, or visual field defect. Neuro-ophthalmological findings are often critical in the examination of ill patients.[19,20] In patients with a structural brain lesion and increased ICP, pupils are symmetrical and reactive but sluggish early in the course of the disease. As the disease progresses and the patient becomes more obtunded or comatose, the pupils become more sluggish and can develop asymmetrical responsiveness with herniation of the brain. The pupils do not become asymmetrical or unreactive in patients with nonstructural brain lesions and therefore are relatively unaffected by metabolic disturbances.[19] Extraocular movements are tested carefully. In obtunded or comatose patients, oculocephalic or caloric testing may be needed to assess the integrity of the brainstem connections that mediate extraocular movements. Asymmetrical or dysconjugate pupillary responses suggest structural injury of the brainstem. Decorticate (arm flexion with leg extension) or decerebrate (arm and leg extension) posturing is commonly due to structural injury of the diencephalon or the midbrain and indicates poor clinical outcome.[10,19]

Ancillary Tests

Laboratory tests include complete blood counts (CBCs), electrolyte levels, renal and hepatic function studies (including ammonia level), blood cultures, blood gases, glucose levels, thyroid screen, coagulation profile (see the section on cerebrovascular emergencies), and serum levels of lactate, vitamin B_{12}, folate, thiamine, and medications (e.g., antiepileptic drugs, digoxin). An enhanced computerized tomography (CT) or magnetic resonance imaging (MRI) scan can evaluate for enlargement or progression of primary or metastatic brain tumors in patients with known disease. In patients with cancer who do not have CNS disease, neuroimaging serves to screen for structural lesions such as brain tumor, stroke, hemorrhage, brain abscess, and hydrocephalus.[20] MRI is superior to CT in detecting abnormalities that can cause alterations in mental status, particularly when the lesions affect the brainstem, diencephalon, or limbic structures.[20]

Lumbar puncture is necessary for cerebrospinal fluid (CSF) analysis when leptomeningeal metastases and CNS infection are suspected. CSF is analyzed for cytology and tumor markers when leptomeningeal metastases is considered in the differential diagnosis. An electroencephalogram (EEG) identifies patients with subclinical status epilepticus and helps distinguish patients with encephalopathy from those with dementia.

Neuroanatomy and Pathophysiology

Mental status changes in patients with structural or metabolic diseases are caused by bilateral cortical dysfunction, depression of the reticular activating system (RAS) structures within the brainstem and diencephalon, or both.[10,19] Encephalopathy from medications, metabolic disturbances, and chemotherapy is caused by a combination of neuronal dysfunction and neurotransmitter abnormalities within the cerebral cortex, and brainstem RAS. Brain tumors and other focal, structural lesions (e.g., stroke, abscess, hemorrhage) affect mental status through several mechanisms, including localized destruction and compression of neural structures and impingement of the brainstem RAS. Lesions that evolve rapidly or are large can cause increased ICP, which can further depress mental status by lowering the cerebral blood flow. ICP can be elevated in "diffuse" disorders such as leptomeningeal disease, subarachnoid hemorrhage, hyperammonemia, and meningitis.

Emergency Department Management and Disposition

Patients with increased ICP require rapid stabilization to prevent further clinical deterioration. Severely obtunded or comatose patients require tracheal intubation and ventilatory support. Brief periods of hyperventilation may be required to treat patients with increased ICP[21] (see Chapter 26, "Increased Intracranial Pressure"). Hyperventilation provides the most rapid reduction of ICP, although the effect is short-lived (i.e., hours). The use of osmotic diuretics can further reduce ICP.[21] Body temperature is carefully controlled, because hyperthermia can exacerbate ICP. Intravenous dexamethasone (a bolus of 10–20 mg, followed by 4–6 mg every four to six hours) is administered to patients with brain tumors or other masses that are associated with interstitial edema (e.g., abscess, hemorrhage). Dexamethasone is not recommended for the control of ICP in patients with stroke, leptomeningeal tumor, infection, and other diseases not associated with interstitial edema.[21]

Metabolic causes of mental status changes (see Table 23.3) are corrected. Seizure activity is controlled as outlined in the section on seizures and status epilepticus. Patients suspected of having CNS infection receive antibiotic therapy after appropriate cultures are obtained. Neutropenic patients receive hematological support with granulocyte colony–stimulating growth factor (Neupogen, 5 µg/kg per day given by subcutaneous injection), which helps increase the white blood cell and absolute neutrophil counts. Patients with toxic encephalopathy (see Table 23.3) require reduction in dosage or discontinuation of the responsible medication.

Patients with cancer and mental status alterations are hospitalized for further treatment and stabilization. Many patients need further management of increased ICP in an intensive care unit.[21] Patients with an advancing structural lesion, such as a brain tumor, may require a "debulking" neurosurgical procedure, radiation therapy, or chemotherapy.[2,5] Patients with hydrocephalus may require temporary drainage of CSF while awaiting a permanent CSF diversionary shunting procedure. Leptomeningeal disease is treated with radiation therapy and intrathecal chemotherapy.[14] In patients with cerebrovascular disorders (see the section on cerebrovascular emergencies), anticoagulation with heparin can be beneficial. Typically, patients with mental status changes caused by radiation-induced exacerbation of ICP respond to the administration of dexamethasone.

Seizures and Status Epilepticus in Patients with Cancer

Seizure is the initial manifestation of a brain tumor in 54% of patients with a primary brain tumor and in 15–20% of patients with metastatic brain tumors.[2,5] The frequency of seizure activity typically increases with tumor growth, due to irritation and injury of the surrounding brain. In patients with metastatic brain tumors, seizures are more likely to occur with multiple brain lesions or with certain histological types of cancer (i.e., melanoma, colon). Simple motor or sensory partial seizures can localize tumor location (e.g., face, arm, leg). They are more common than complex partial (temporal lobe) or generalized (tonic-clonic or absence) seizures. Status epilepticus is rare in patients with brain tumor. Although seizures can be the first sign of a brain tumor, they are more common among patients with an established diagnosis of cancer or idiopathic epilepsy. Oncology patients without brain tumors are at risk for seizures from disease-related metabolic disturbances, infections, and effects of treatment.

Prehospital Management

Seizure activity usually has stopped by the time prehospital care providers arrive at the scene, unless the patient is in status epilepticus. A concise history is obtained from family members or bystanders regarding the ictal event, history of seizures or head trauma, and medical history (including medications). Evaluation consists of assessment of vital signs, signs of trauma sustained during the ictus, and baseline neurological condition. The patient is protected from further injury; however, a patient experiencing a seizure is not restrained. Intravenous administration of benzodiazepines is required to treat patients with intractable seizures (see Chapter 12, "Seizures").

Emergency Department Evaluation and Differential Diagnosis

In patients with a known brain tumor, the most common cause of seizure activity requiring evaluation in the emergency department is inadequate antiepileptic drug dosing. Less often, the seizure occurs as the first symptom of an intracranial lesion in a patient without history of cancer. A thorough history includes past and recent medical illnesses, medications, and a description of the ictal event including aura, duration, typical pattern of seizures, focal or generalized seizure activity, incontinence, and tongue biting. Preictal symptoms such as fever, headache, nuchal rigidity, somnolence, or confusion are reviewed. The neurological examination typically is normal or reveals only established neurological deficits after the postictal period resolves. New focal neurological findings can represent

Todd's postictal paralysis, tumor progression, or seizure-related ischemia. Todd's paralysis is usually transient, resolving within hours to days. Other causes of seizures include metabolic disorders such as uremia, hyponatremia, hypoglycemia, hypoxia, hypocalcemia, and hypomagnesemia. Cerebral hemorrhage, infarction, infection (bacterial, viral, fungal, parasitic), or leptomeningeal metastasis can also induce seizures. Aspects of cancer treatment that can cause seizures include brain radiation, chemotherapy (e.g., methotrexate, cisplatin, L-asparaginase, ifosfamide, interferon), and the use of antiemetics (e.g., phenothiazines) and analgesics (e.g., meperidine).

Emergency Department Management and Disposition

Antiepileptic drug levels, CBC, platelets, blood urea nitrogen (BUN), creatinine, electrolyte (including calcium and magnesium), and glucose levels are checked. Arterial blood gases are obtained when hypoxia or metabolic derangements are suspected. Lumbar puncture is performed for CSF analysis when CNS infection or leptomeningeal metastases are suspected. Patients with brain tumors who have alterations in their baseline neurological status require CT or MRI to evaluate for tumor progression, hemorrhage, or hydrocephalus.

Patients with subtherapeutic antiepileptic drug levels require additional medication and possible adjustment of the daily dosage. Compliance issues are discussed. Metabolic causes of seizure activity require correction of the abnormality. Correction of the metabolic abnormality is definitive therapy, and antiepileptic drugs are not necessary in most cases. New-onset seizures in patients with a history of cancer require a screening CT or MRI scan and CSF analysis, especially when metabolic screening tests are inconclusive. Patients with status epilepticus, a prolonged postictal state, or neurological deterioration are hospitalized for evaluation and treatment.

Cerebrovascular Emergencies in Patients with Cancer

Cerebrovascular disorders are common in patients with cancer and occur commonly in patients with brain tumors. Autopsy studies reveal cerebrovascular lesions in approximately 15% of all patients with cancer.[10–12] The predisposing factors for cerebrovascular disease in patients with cancer are direct effects of tumors on blood vessels (e.g., brain tumor encroachment, leptomeningeal tumor invasion, hemorrhage), tumor-induced coagulation disorders (hemorrhagic and thrombotic), and treatment-related injury to blood vessels.[11,12] Risk factors for cerebrovascular disease in the general population, such as age, hypertension, coronary artery disease, and diabetes mellitus, are not as significant in patients with cancer. Although large vessel atherosclerotic thromboembolic disease is common in these patients at autopsy, it accounts for only a small percentage of cerebrovascular events in life.[12]

Cerebrovascular emergencies have a variable presentation. Some patients present with transient ischemic attack (TIA) or stroke, and others display symptoms and signs associated with a confusional state or encephalopathy.

Emergency Department Evaluation and Differential Diagnosis

The extensive differential diagnosis of cerebrovascular disorders includes tumor-related disorders, coagulation disorders, and treatment-related disorders (see Table 23.4).[10–12] Tumor-related disorders occur with either primary brain tumors or metastatic disease (parenchymal or leptomeningeal). TIA or stroke from intratumoral hemorrhage or ischemia is common.[1–6,11,12,14,15] Coagulation disorders can lead to intracranial vessel thrombosis, ischemia, or hemorrhage (intraparenchymal, subdural, or subarachnoid) (see Fig. 23.1).[10–12] Nonbacterial thrombotic endocarditis (NBTE) is characterized by sterile fibrin vegetations on one or more cardiac valves.[11–13] Patients with NBTE present with focal symptoms indicating either TIA or stroke in 50–60% of cases. Encephalopathy or confusion, as a manifestation of NBTE occurs in 20–30% of patients (see Fig. 23.2).[10–13] Approximately 25% of strokes in patients with cancer are caused by NBTE.

A thorough history is obtained from the patient (when possible) and family about the development of new neurological symptoms, including the time of onset, severity, and pace of evolution. Associated systemic symptoms, such as fever, rash, bruising, and regions of swelling or pain, are investigated.

TABLE 23.4. Cerebrovascular Disorders with Associated Tumor Types and Symptoms

Cerebrovascular Disease	Tumor Types	Symptoms
Tumor-related		
Intratumoral parenchymal hemorrhage	CPP, Pit. Ad., oligo., mal. astro., melanoma, chorio., renal, germ	HA, obtundation, SZ, focal signs
Superior sagittal sinus occlusion	Neuroblastoma, CA, lymph	HA, focal signs, Sz, confusion
Subdural hemorrhage	Carcinoma, leukemia, lymph	Confusion, lethargy, focal signs
Ruptured neoplastic aneurysm	Chorio., lung CA, cardiac myx.	HA, obtundation, Sz, focal signs, meningismus
Coagulation disorders		
DIC, thrombocytopenia	Leukemia	Confusion, disorientation, focal signs, ?HA, ?Sz
NBTE	Mucin-producing CA	Focal signs, encephalopathy, Sz
Cerebral intravascular coagulation	Lymph, breast CA, leukemia	Encephalopathy, focal signs
Superior sagittal sinus occlusion	CA, leukemia, lymph	Sz, encephalopathy, focal signs
Treatment-related		
L-asparaginase (infarction or hemorrhage)	Leukemia	Focal signs, ?HA, obtundation
RT-induced carotid occlusion	Head and neck tumors, lymph	Focal signs
Carotid rupture	Head and neck tumors, RT	Focal signs, obtundation
Mitomycin (hemolytic uremic syndrome)	Solid tumors	HA, focal signs, obtundation

Note: Abbreviations: DIC – disseminated intravascular coagulation; NBTE – nonbacterial thrombotic endocarditis; RT – radiation therapy; CPP – choroid plexus papilloma; Pit. Ad. – pituitary adenoma; oligo – oligodendroglioma; mal. astro. – malignant astrocytoma; chorio. – choriocarcinoma; HA – headache; Sz – seizure; germ – germ cell tumor; CA – carcinoma; lymph – lymphoma; myx. – myxoma.
Source: From Newton;[2] Sawaya and Bindal;[5] Forman;[10] Rogers;[11] Graus, Rogers, and Posner;[12] Rogers, Cho, Kempin, and Posner.[13]

The status of the patient's recent or ongoing cancer treatment is discussed. Prescribed medications, including chemotherapeutic agents, is noted.

The general physical examination is performed to assess the condition of the patient and determine possible causes of the cerebrovascular event. The patient is evaluated for petechiae, heart murmur, nail bed splinter hemorrhages, or new swelling in the neck. There are no neurological findings specific to cerebrovascular events in patients with cancer. The neurological deficits are variable and result from the vascular distribution affected within the CNS. Patients with confusion or encephalopathy are assessed for conditions that can cause bilateral cortical or subcortical dysfunction including cranial

intravascular coagulation, NBTE, sinus thrombosis, and subarachnoid hemorrhage.

Neuroanatomy and Pathophysiology

The cause of ischemic cerebrovascular symptoms in patients with brain tumors remains unclear. These symptoms are probably caused by encasement and stenosis of vessels by neoplasm, arterial "steal" effects in the distribution of vessels feeding the tumor, or a combination of these mechanisms. Typically, intratumoral hemorrhage occurs in regions of necrosis or as a result of structurally injured blood vessels within the tumor. Leptomeningeal tumor invades blood vessels within the subarachnoid or Virchow-Robin spaces, causing stenosis and thrombosis.[14] Subdural hemorrhage typically follows the rupture of vessels within dural metastases or dural capillaries that are dilated from tumor blockage, or as a result of coagulopathy. Sinus occlusion occurs as a direct effect of tumor encroachment; sinus thrombosis develops from tumor-induced hypercoagulable states. The coagulation disorders occur during a state of intravascular fibrinolysis, with production of fibrin-platelet clots. This process can lead to the production of emboli, hemorrhage, or thrombosis of the vessels. It is thought that the chemotherapeutic agent L-asparaginase causes hemorrhage or thrombosis by inducing a state of fibrinolysis and depleting levels of antithrombin III.[11] Radiation-induced carotid artery occlusion or rupture is caused by accelerated atherosclerosis within the vessel wall.

Ancillary Testing

Laboratory evaluation includes CBC with platelet count, coagulation factors (prothrombin time/partial thromboplastin time), and diffuse intravascular coagulation (DIC) panel (quantitative fibrinogen, thrombin time, fibrin degradation products, protamine sulfate gelation, and mixing studies). Cultures of blood, urine, and sputum are collected when infection is suspected.[10-13]

Transesophageal echocardiography can provide a diagnosis of NBTE. CT scan screens for intratumoral, parenchymal, subdural, and cerebral infarction–related hemorrhage (see Fig. 23.1). MRI is sensitive to the presence of hemorrhage. Although neither CT scan nor MRI easily detects cerebral ischemia or infarction soon after the event, MRI is superior to CT imaging in discerning regions of ischemia and infarction several days after the initial event has occurred (see Fig. 23.2).

Emergency Department Management and Disposition

Initial treatment of coagulopathy includes administration of vitamin K, fresh frozen plasma, and platelets. Heparinization is considered in patients with DIC and NBTE.[11] The use of anticoagulants is less well defined for other coagulation disorders. Patients with an intracranial hemorrhage and significant associated edema and mass effect receive intravenous corticosteroids such as dexamethasone.

Focal Neurological Deficits in Patients with Cancer

Focal neurological findings are common in patients with brain tumors, spinal cord tumors, and other forms of neuro-oncological disease. Greater than 50% of patients with primary brain tumors present with hemiparesis, cranial nerve palsies, and papilledema;[2] 25–30% have hemisensory deficits or abnormalities of speech and language. Seventy-three percent of patients exhibit extremity weakness, 62% have reflex abnormalities, and 56% have sensory alterations at the time of initial presentation with spinal cord tumors.[7] Metastatic tumors to the brain or spine are likely to have associated focal neurological findings.[4-6,8,22] Focal neurological deficits are commonly observed in patients who have experienced cerebrovascular events (see the section on cerebrovascular emergencies), leptomeningeal metastases, and treatment-related toxicities.[10,14,15] Established focal neurological signs can become worse with tumor progression or recurrence and with metabolic derangement.

Neuroanatomy and Pathophysiology

The pathophysiology underlying focal neurological deficits depends on the neuro-oncological process causing the deficit. In primary and metastatic neoplasms of the brain and spine, as the tumor and associated edema expands, the surrounding regions of the CNS become compressed, irritated, and ultimately destroyed. Leptomeningeal tumor usually causes focal signs by infiltrating blood vessels, with subsequent thrombosis and ischemia, and by directly invading the neural tissues.[14,15] Metabolic disturbances can exacerbate fixed neurological deficits by further altering neuronal function and neural transmission in the regions of injury.

Emergency Department Evaluation and Differential Diagnosis

A detailed patient history includes the time of onset, severity, and pace of evolution of focal neurological deficits. The patient's current history of cancer is explored in detail. A review of associated symptoms includes the presence of fever, rash, bruising, or erythema. The neurological examination is directed toward the site of neuraxis involvement.

In patients with a known brain tumor, CT of the brain with and without contrast helps determine the presence of tumor enlargement, tumor spread, exacerbation of edema, or intratumoral hemorrhage. MRI is the study of choice in patients with a known spinal cord tumor.

In patients with an established diagnosis of brain tumor, the differential diagnosis of focal neurological findings includes tumor progression, exacerbation of existing cerebral edema without tumor enlargement, intracranial or intratumoral hemorrhage, leptomeningeal metastases, infection, and metabolic derangements. Progression of neurological deficits due to tumor progression, exacerbation of edema, or hemorrhage is typically accompanied by signs of increased ICP, such as headache, nausea, emesis, and lethargy.[2] Leptomeningeal spread of tumor can present with myelopathy, radicular pain, sensory loss, or a cauda equina syndrome.[14,15] Metabolic alterations such as medication toxicity, hyponatremia, hypoglycemia, dehydration, and hyperammonemia can cause exacerbation of fixed neurological deficits. In a patient with a known brain tumor, focal neurological deficits can be caused by cerebrovascular accidents (see the section on cerebrovascular emergencies), new brain metastases, leptomeningeal tumor, spinal metastases (see the section on back pain and spinal cord compression), infection, or neurotoxicity from cancer therapy (see the sections on alterations of mental status and cerebrovascular emergencies).

Emergency Department Management and Disposition

Cerebrovascular accident or spinal cord compression is managed as outlined in the section on cerebral emergencies and the section on back pain and spinal cord compression, respectively. When the evaluation discloses tumor progression with or without associated increase in edema, initial emergency department therapy includes administration of dexamethasone (a bolus of 10–20 mg given intravenously, followed by 4–6 mg given intravenously every four to six hours). When leptomeningeal tumor is suspected, an MRI with gadolinium enhancement can be diagnostic. Cytological examination of CSF is the best study for the diagnosis of leptomeningeal metastases.

Back Pain and Spinal Cord Compression in Patients with Cancer

Back pain is a common complaint and has an annual incidence of 5% and a lifetime prevalence of 60–90% in the general population.[23] The back pain of most patients is benign and self-limited. In patients with systemic or CNS cancer, it is often the first sign of a serious underlying neurological process.

The structural components of the spinal column are common sites for bony metastases. Vertebral metastases are common in patients with prostate cancer, breast cancer, renal cancer, lung cancer, melanoma, and myeloma (see Table 23.2).[8,22,24] Epidural spinal cord compression (ESCC), the most serious sequela of spinal column metastasis, is relatively common, occurring in 5–14% of patients with systemic cancer.[8,22,24] Each year in the United States, approximately 20,000 patients with cancer are at risk for ESCC, caused by metastases in and around the spinal column.[8,9,22,24] Although, ESCC is more common in patients with diagnosis of cancer and widespread disease, it can be the first manifestation of cancer in up to 25% of patients. After the development of back pain, neurological deterioration can occur rapidly in patients with ESCC. Without treatment, ESCC results in paraplegia, loss of lower extremity sensation, and incontinence. Patients with ESCC require rapid and accurate diagnosis, and stabilization in the emergency department in order to minimize morbidity and mortality.

Neuroanatomy and Pathophysiology

Back pain caused by ESCC arises from metastases to the vertebral column (85%), paravertebral spaces (10–12%), and epidural space (1–3%).[8,22] Within the vertebral column, metastases occur most commonly in the vertebral bodies (usually thoracic); the laminae, transverse processes, and spinous processes can also be affected. The concentration of growth factors found in bone marrow stroma and the wide distribution of drainage of the vertebral venous plexus are believed to predispose the thoracic spine to ESCC.[8,10,22] Enlargement of vertebral metastases results in the stretching of the periosteum, causing local or referred pain. Further growth of malignant cells compresses adjacent neural and vascular structures, evoking pain and neurological signs. Compromise of the vertebral venous plexus induces vasogenic edema, hemorrhage, demyelination, and ischemia within the spinal cord.[8,22] Disruption of the arterial supply to the spinal cord can cause ischemia or infarction of the spinal cord, with secondary vasogenic edema. Direct compression of the spinal cord or nerve roots initially causes axonal swelling and white matter edema, followed by reduction of parenchymal blood flow, ischemia, and infarction of the spinal cord.[8,22] The neurological injury of ESCC is not completely understood; however, it appears to be mediated by several biochemical mechanisms, including the release of prostaglandin E_2, 6-ketoprostaglandin $F1\alpha$, and glutamate. The pace of spinal cord compression is an important factor. There is less chance of neurological recovery following treatment when onset of symptoms is rapid (hours to days) than when onset is more protracted (weeks to months).

Prehospital Management

A concise and thorough history of the back pain and related neurological symptoms – including location and severity of pain, presence of weakness or numbness, bladder or bowel incontinence, and gait abnormality – is obtained. A careful evaluation is required to document the baseline severity of back pain, leg strength, and sensory function for monitoring during transport. In patients with severe back pain, partial immobilization of the spine may minimize discomfort. Severe pain may require administration of narcotic analgesics.

Emergency Department Evaluation and Differential Diagnosis

The differential diagnosis of back pain with or without neurological findings is broad. In addition to ESCC, the possible presence of herniated disc, degenerative joint disease, muscle sprain, epidural abscess, spinal osteomyelitis, primary spinal cord tumor, leptomeningeal tumor, facet syndrome, spondylolisthesis, spinal stenosis, and other less common entities is considered.[7,8,22,23] A thorough history includes associated systemic and neurological symptoms and signs, and remote or current diagnoses of cancer. The quality, location, intensity, and evolution of the back pain is noted. In patients with ESCC, pain is the initial symptom and can develop anywhere along the spine, typically in the thoracic region. Initially the pain is mild, but it is always

progressive and is often described as a steady, deep ache that can be axial or radicular (i.e., radiating down a limb or around the rib cage anteriorly). Similar to degenerative conditions of the spine, the back pain from ESCC is commonly exacerbated by movement, Valsalva maneuvers (e.g., straining at stool or sneezing), straight leg raising, and neck flexion. Unlike the back pain from degenerative spine disease, which usually improves with recumbency, the back pain from ESCC is aggravated in the supine position. This may cause the patient to sleep sitting up. Other common symptoms of ESCC include extremity weakness and autonomic dysfunction, occurring in 75% and 55% of patients, respectively. Weakness is typically symmetrical and involves the legs, but occasionally can affect the arms. Autonomic dysfunction manifests as painless urinary retention in most patients, with bladder and bowel incontinence less frequently noted. Other symptoms of autonomic dysfunction include constipation and impotence. Sensory complaints manifest as numbness and paresthesias that start in the feet and extend proximally over time and develop concomitantly with weakness. Certain symptoms can differentiate ESCC from other back conditions. Fever (especially with a history of recent sepsis) indicates an infectious process such as epidural abscess, discitis, or osteomyelitis. Back pain with a rapid onset indicates muscle sprain, acute herniated disc, epidural hemorrhage, or spondylolisthesis, although ESCC evolves rapidly on occasion.

Localized pain to percussion over the involved vertebral bodies is assessed on physical examination of patients with ESCC.[8,10,22] Typically, the tender areas are in the thoracic region. This differs from the pain of degenerative spine disease, which is more common in the cervical or lumbosacral region. The pain may be exacerbated by neck flexion (cervical/upper thoracic lesions) or by straight leg raising (lower thoracic/lumbar lesions) maneuvers. A rectal examination is performed to assess the patient's anal sphincter tone, anal wink, and ability to voluntarily contract the anus, because these functions can be compromised by ESCC affecting the conus medullaris or cauda equina. On neurological examination, leg weakness is the most common finding.[8,10,22] During the early phase of ESCC, neurological findings include weakness of the iliopsoas and hamstring muscle groups, and slightly increased patellar and Achilles reflexes. Progression of ESCC causes myelopathy with an upper motor neuron pattern weakness in the lower extremities (i.e., weak hip flexors, hamstrings, and ankle dorsiflexors), spasticity, bilateral Babinski signs, and further increased reflexes. Rapidly progressive ESCC can cause spinal shock (i.e., flaccidity of limbs and areflexia). When ESCC involves lumbar vertebrae below L_1, the cauda equina is affected, resulting in a lower motor neuron pattern of lower extremity hypotonia, areflexia, atrophy, and muscle fasciculations. Early sensory findings consist of a mild decrease in distal vibratory and proprioceptive sensation. Advanced ESCC disease causes reduction in touch and pinprick sensation below the site of compression, demarcating a "sensory level." Similar findings of myelopathy can be caused by epidural abscess, spinal cord tumor, or hemorrhage.[7,8,10,23]

Emergency Department Management and Disposition

Initial management consists of pain control and diagnostic evaluation such as blood tests and imaging procedures. Typically, the pain of ESCC is severe and requires parenteral narcotic analgesics for adequate control. In patients with a history of fever, the examiner may obtain a white blood cell count, blood cultures, and sedimentation rate, which can help diagnose epidural abscess, discitis, osteomyelitis, and other infectious spinal processes. Plain radiographs of the spine can identify an abnormality in 85–90% of patients with ESCC from solid tumors. The lesions most commonly observed on plain radiographs are vertebral body erosion and collapse, subluxation, and pedicle erosion. Plain radiographs can indicate other diagnoses, such as spondylolisthesis and degenerative spine disease. Epidural abscess is considered when destruction of two adjacent vertebral bodies across the disc space is demonstrated on plain radiograph. Recently, MRI has replaced myelography as the most sensitive and specific imaging technique for evaluation of epidural tumor.[8,10,22] An MRI scan of the complete spine, including T2- and T1-weighted images without and with gadolinium contrast enhancement, can demonstrate epidural or paravertebral masses, ESCC, primary spinal cord tumors, and most in-

stances of leptomeningeal tumor (see Fig. 23.3).[7,8,22] MRI can disclose benign causes of back pain, such as herniated disc and degenerative spine disease. Myelography is not indicated for evaluation of patients with ESCC when MRI is available. CT scans of the spine are more sensitive than plain radiographs for identification of epidural tumor or paravertebral masses and can more accurately demonstrate benign causes of back pain; however, they are inferior to MRI and myelography. Rapid evaluation and treatment of patients with ESCC is important, because the key prognostic factor for posttreatment neurological function is the degree of neurological function at the start of therapy. Among patients who are ambulatory at the start of treatment, 80% remain so after therapy; however, only 45% of paraparetic patients and 5–10% of paraplegic patients are ambulatory following treatment.[8,22,25,26] Intravenous corticosteroids (e.g., dexamethasone) are given promptly to patients with ESCC or when ESCC is suspected clinically. Dexamethasone rapidly reduces spinal cord edema and can improve neurological function, and helps alleviate back pain. An accepted initial dose regimen of dexamethasone is a loading dose of 20–100 mg, followed by 4–24 mg four times a day.[8,22] Definitive therapy such as radiation therapy (RT) or surgical decompression begins as soon as possible and no more than 24 hours after the administration of dexamethasone.

The specific therapy for most patients with ESCC is external beam RT, with or without decompressive surgery.[8,10,22,25,26] The role of decompressive surgery in the treatment of patients with ESCC is poorly defined. Improved clinical outcome with decompressive surgery plus RT as opposed to RT alone is not yet known, although several retrospective and prospective trials support an improved outcome with a combined approach in selected patients.[8,22,27,28] Surgical decompression is accomplished using a posterior (i.e., laminectomy) or anterior (i.e., vertebral body resection) approach to the spine. The anterior technique is preferred because the bulk of the tumor can be removed and the spine typically remains more stable postoperatively. Most patients do not require surgical decompression in addition to RT. However, surgical therapy is considered when a primary tumor is unrecognized, neurological deterioration occurs during or after RT, the involved tumor is known to be radioresistant (e.g.,

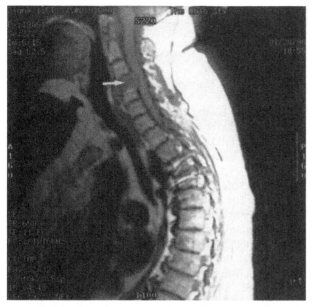

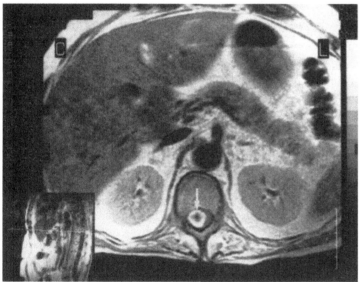

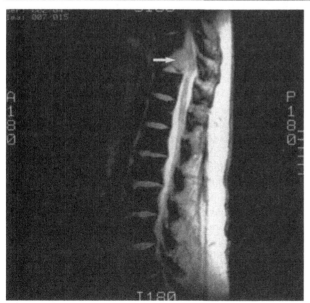

FIGURE 23.3. MRI scans of three patients with different causes of spinal cord compression. (A) 76-year-old woman with breast cancer who developed neck pain and cervical myelopathy. On T1-weighted MRI, the third cervical vertebral body is replaced by tumor, which is compressing the spinal cord, causing it to deviate around the mass (white arrow). (B) 61-year-old man who developed insidious onset of midthoracic spine pain and lower extremity weakness and spasticity. The gadolinium-enhanced T1-weighted MRIs demonstrate an enhancing intradural, extramedullary mass (white arrow) severely compressing the spinal cord. A benign schwannoma was resected. (C) 52-year-old man with multiple myeloma who developed severe lower thoracic spine pain and leg weakness. The gadolinium-enhanced T1-weighted MRIs demonstrate the destruction of the T10 vertebral body by multiple myeloma (white arrow), with compression and kinking of the spinal cord.

renal cell carcinoma), there is spinal instability or bone compression due to ESCC, or there is acute deterioration of neurological function. RT may be necessary after surgical decompression. RT and, in selected cases, surgical decompression is performed in patients with severe deficits that have been present for several days or more, because neurological function can improve.

PEARLS AND PITFALLS

- Toxic encephalopathy from excessive concentrations of various medications is the most common cause of mental status alterations in patients with cancer.
- The best method to lower increased ICP acutely in an obtunded or comatose patient is hyperventilation, which rapidly lowers PCO_2, causing cerebral vasoconstriction and a reduction of cerebral blood flow and volume. The target PCO_2 is approximately 27–33 mm Hg.
- The most common cause of seizures in patients with brain tumor is noncompliance with antiepileptic drug dosing.
- Some patients with cerebrovascular emergencies (e.g., NBTE) present with encephalopathy and not with acute focal deficits, as is more typical in patients with TIA or stroke.
- ESCC can be the first manifestation of cancer in up to 25% of patients and is suspected in any patient with cancer and new back pain.
- The most important prognostic factor for ESCC is the degree of neurological functioning at the time of diagnosis. Following treatment, 80% of patients who can walk at diagnosis remain ambulatory; however, only 5–10% of patients who are paraplegic at diagnosis are ambulatory afterward.

REFERENCES

1. Black PM. Brain tumors. *N Engl J Med.* 1991;324: 1471–6.
2. Newton HB. Primary brain tumors: review of etiology, diagnosis, and treatment. *Am Fam Physician.* 1994;49: 787–97.
3. Pollock IF. Brain tumors in children. *N Engl J Med.* 1994;331:1500–7.
4. Patchell RA. Metastatic brain tumors. *Neurol Clin.* 1995;13:915–25.
5. Sawaya R, Bindal RK. Metastatic brain tumors. In: Kaye AH, Laws ER Jr, ed. *Brain Tumors.* New York, NY: Churchill Livingstone; 1995;48:923–46.
6. Allen JC. Brain metastases. In: Deutsch M, ed. *Management of Childhood Brain Tumors.* Boston, Mass: Kluwer Academic Publishers; 1990;20:457–64.
7. Newton HB, Newton CL, Gatens C, Herbert R, Pack R. Spinal cord tumors. Review of etiology, diagnosis, and multidisciplinary approach to treatment. *Cancer Pract.* 1995;3:207–18.
8. Byrne TN. Spinal cord compression from epidural metastases. *N Engl J Med.* 1992;327:614–19.
9. Klein SL, Sanford RA, Muhlbauer MS. Pediatric spinal epidural metastases. *J Neurosurg.* 1991;74: 70–5.
10. Forman AD. Neurologic emergencies in cancer patients. *Cancer Bull.* 1992;44:197–206.
11. Rogers LR. Cerebrovascular complications in cancer patients. *Oncology.* 1994;8:23–30.
12. Graus F, Rogers LR, Posner JB. Cerebrovascular complications in patients with cancer. *Medicine.* 1985; 64:16–35.
13. Rogers LR, Cho ES, Kempin S, Posner JB. Cerebral infarction from non-bacterial thrombotic endocarditis. Clinical and pathological study including the effects of anticoagulation. *Am J Med.* 1987;83:746–56.
14. Wasserstrom WR, Glass JP, Posner JB. Diagnosis and treatment of leptomeningeal metastases from solid tumors: experience with 90 patients. *Cancer* 1982;49: 759–72.
15. Awad I, Bay JW, Rogers L. Leptomeningeal metastasis from supratentorial malignant gliomas. *Neurosurgery.* 1986;19:247–51.
16. Chitkara N, Sepkowitz K. Central nervous system infections in cancer patients. *Infect Med.* 1994;11: 707–10.
17. Newton HB, Newton C, Pearl D, Davidson T. Swallowing assessment in primary brain tumor patients with dysphagia. *Neurology* 1994;44:1927–32.
18. Kaplan RS, Wiernik PH. Neurotoxicity of antineoplastic drugs. *Semin Oncol.* 1980;9:103–30.
19. Plum F, Posner JB. *The Diagnosis of Stupor and Coma.* 3rd ed. Philadelphia, Pa: FA Davis Co; 1980;1:1–86.
20. Caplan LR, Shuren J, DeWitt LD. Abnormal mental states: decision strategies for imaging referral. *MRI Decisions.* 1990;March/April:14–25.
21. Ropper AH. Treatment of intracranial hypertension. In: Ropper AH, ed. *Neurological and Neurosurgical Intensive Care.* 3rd ed. New York, NY: Raven Press, Ltd; 1993;3:29–52.
22. Posner JB. Spinal metastases. In: Posner JB, ed. *Neurologic Complications of Cancer.* Philadelphia, Pa: FA Davis Co; 1995;6:111–42.

23. Frymoyer JW. Back pain and sciatica. *N Engl J Med.* 1988;318:291–300.

24. Sioutos PJ, Arbit E, Meshulam CF, Galicich JH. Spinal metastases from solid tumors. Analysis of factors affecting survival. *Cancer.* 1995;76:1453–9.

25. Marazano E, Latini P, Checcaglini F, et al. Radiation therapy in metastatic spinal cord compression. A prospective analysis of 105 consecutive patients. *Cancer.* 1991;67:1311–17.

26. Bach F, Agerlin N, Sorensen JB, et al. Metastatic spinal cord compression secondary to lung cancer. *J Clin Oncol.* 1192;10:1781–7.

27. Sorensen PS, Borgesesn SE, Rohde K, et al. Metastatic epidural spinal cord compression. Results of treatment and survival. *Cancer.* 1990;65:1502–8.

28. Sundaresan N, Digiacinto GV, Hughes JEO, et al. Treatment of neoplastic spinal cord compression: results of a prospective study. *Neurosurgery.* 1991;29:645–50.

24 Neuropsychiatry

CRAIG A. TAYLOR AND BARBARA C. GOOD

SUMMARY The neuropsychiatric patient presents unique evaluation and diagnostic challenges in the emergency department. The psychiatric disorder can be one of behavior, mood, or cognition, or a psychosis. It can be caused by or can coexist with an underlying neurological problem. The goals of the emergency evaluation are to: (1) stabilize the agitated or aggressive patient in order to protect him or her and others; (2) establish a presumptive diagnosis or broadly determine whether the cause is medical, neurological, or psychiatric; and (3) determine whether the patient requires inpatient medical, neurological, or psychiatric care, or can be discharged from the emergency department with outpatient follow-up. This chapter reviews neuropsychiatric symptoms associated with a variety of underlying brain disorders.*

Introduction

Neuropsychiatry is a discipline that evaluates and treats a broad array of psychiatric or behavioral symptoms that result from a central nervous system (CNS) dysfunction. Typically, the patient with neuropsychiatric symptoms needs to be assessed and treated quickly in the emergency department. It is critical to determine whether the patient's symptoms are due to an underlying medical, neurological, or psychiatric disorder, or to a combination of causes. Patients with different neuropsychiatric disorders can require very different plans of management. For example, a patient with simple dementia can likely be evaluated as an outpatient, whereas a patient with delirium is likely to require admission to the hospital on an acute medical or neuropsychiatric service. Generating a differential diagnosis in neuropsychiatry is a complex process. The patient's history is obtained and organized to determine underlying organic disease. The evaluation includes an expanded mental status examination that assesses cognitive functions and common organic behavioral signs (Table 24.1).[1]

Neuropsychiatric symptoms can manifest as *disturbances in cognition, behavioral changes, alterations in personality,* or *mood disturbances* (mania, depression, anxiety, poor affective regulation; disturbances in thought processes and content). These symptoms can result from a variety of CNS disorders including infectious disease, vascular disorders, tumors, trauma, epilepsy, hydrocephalus, degenerative disorders, and demyelinating diseases, or from medical diseases such as sepsis, toxin exposure, metabolic disease, immune disorders, and the indirect effects of cancer (see Table 24.2). Despite the number of potential underlying disorders, the neuropsychiatric patient can be placed in one of two major categories: (1) the individual who presents with neuropsychiatric symptoms but no history of a CNS disturbance (this patient requires a thorough evaluation for an underlying disorder);[2] and (2) the individual with known CNS disorder who presents with neuropsychiatric symptoms as evidenced by behavioral change. This patient presents with symptom complex based on an underly-

---

* Adapted with permission from *Principles and Practice of Emergency Medicine,* 4th ed., G. Schwartz, ed. (Baltimore: Williams & Wilkins, in press).

TABLE 24.1. Plan for Evaluation, Treatment, and Disposition of the Patient with Neuropsychiatric Symptoms

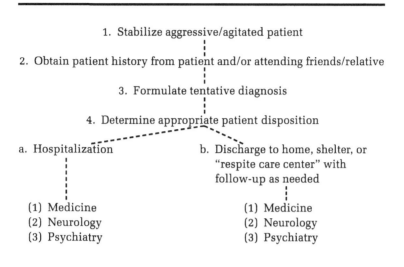

1. Stabilize aggressive/agitated patient

2. Obtain patient history from patient and/or attending friends/relative

3. Formulate tentative diagnosis

4. Determine appropriate patient disposition

a. Hospitalization

(1) Medicine
(2) Neurology
(3) Psychiatry

b. Discharge to home, shelter, or "respite care center" with follow-up as needed

(1) Medicine
(2) Neurology
(3) Psychiatry

---

ing medical or neurological disorder. Conditions associated with primary CNS disturbances are the focus of this chapter.

Emergency Department Evaluation

General Principles

Similar to patients with general psychiatric emergencies, neuropsychiatric patients with underlying CNS disturbance can present to the emergency department because of a change in behavior that requires an urgent evaluation and treatment. Evaluation depends on a thorough history, general physical examination, and neurological examination, with concentration on the mental status examination.[3] It is important to remember that brain dysfunction affects the ability of the patient to give an accurate history and can modify the expression of symptoms and behavior. The psychiatric history and mental status examination can provide specific clues to neurobehavioral symptoms that can help localize the underlying abnormalities of brain function (Table 24.3).[4]

Patient History

A detailed and accurate history is obtained from anyone who presents with a cognitive, behavioral, emotional, or other neuropsychiatric disturbance. Knowledge of a current or past neurological disorder

can help determine whether the symptoms fit a particular pattern. Table 24.4 lists the key factors that are addressed in taking the history of a patient exhibiting neuropsychiatric symptoms. Because many of these patients are unable or unwilling to give complete (or any) descriptions, it is common practice for family members or friends to assist in providing relevant details of the patient's history.[5] Medications the patient has in his or her possession can give the emergency physician clues about the source of the presenting problem and the name of the prescribing physician, who can be contacted for additional information.[6]

General Physical and Neurological Examination

A complete general physical and neurological examination helps differentiate medical and neurological conditions that may be contributing to the neurobehavioral presentation. Particular attention to the patient's appearance and behavior can be revealing and can substitute for part of the formal examination when the patient is uncooperative.[4] Attention to vital signs is important; for example, elevated blood pressure may suggest occult stroke as a cause of neurobehavioral symptoms.[4] The neurological examination is essential in neuropsychiatric evaluation because often it can help localize the site of neurological dysfunction. However, it can have limited

TABLE 24.2. Neurological Disorders that Can Produce Neuropsychiatric Disturbances

Infection
  Encephalitis
  Meningitis
  Brain abscess
  HIV-AIDS
  Syphilis
  Creutzfeldt-Jakob disease
Vascular
  Cerebrovascular accident
  Multi-infarct dementia
  Arteriovenous malformation
Tumors
Trauma
  Subdural hematoma
  Intracerebral hemorrhage
  Frontal and temporal contusions
  Closed-head injury–diffuse axonal injury
Hydrocephalus
Degenerative disease
  Alzheimer's disease
  Pick's disease
  Huntington's disease
  Parkinson's disease
Demyelinating disease
  Multiple sclerosis
Epilepsy
  Leukodystrophies
Medical illness
  Infection/sepsis
  Toxins
    Alcohol and illicit drugs
    Organic compounds
    Metallic poisons
  Metabolic disease
    Thyroid
    Parathyroid
    Pituitary
    Adrenal
  Immune disorders
    Systemic lupus erythematosis
    HIV-AIDS
  Cancer, indirect effects

Source: Adapted from Strub and Wise. Differential diagnosis in neuropsychiatry. In: *Textbook of neuropsychiatry.* Yudofsky SC, Hales RE, eds. Washington, DC: The American Psychiatric Press, 1992.

value in discerning the neurological basis of a specific neurobehavioral disturbance, and results can be normal in a patient with gross brain disease.[4]

Mental status examination is often overlooked in patients evaluated in the emergency department. In an emergency department study of 298 patients whose chief complaint was psychiatric in nature, mental status was not documented in 56% of the patients at triage. Of those patients who had "medical disease," 80% were deemed "medically clear." The most common process deficiencies occurred in the neurological examination.[7] In neuropsychiatric evaluation, the mental status examination is structured and sufficiently detailed so as to enable to: (1) serve as a baseline for future comparisons; (2) give evidence of underlying neurological disturbance (Table 24.5); and (3) detect confusional states. The mental status examination focuses on assessing the patient's level of arousal, attention, concentration, language function, memory, constructions, abstractions, insight, judgment, and praxis. Additionally, observations of appearance, motor behavior, affect, mood, verbal output, thought structure and content, and perceptions of the patient are documented.[8] The patient is evaluated for the presence of depression, anxiety, mania, and thought disorders. These can occur as problems unrelated to a neurological disorder, or they can be due to a stable or progressive neurological disorder. The presence of these symptoms in a "neurologically stable" or "nonacute" patient requires psychiatric intervention. The possibility of alcohol or illicit drug use is investigated thoroughly in any patient who presents with acute mental status or behavioral changes.

The neurological examination also includes the evaluation of cranial nerves, motor and sensory systems, and deep tendon reflexes. Abnormalities of olfaction (CNI) occur in a variety of neurological disorders such as closed-head injury and meningiomas. Anosmia and hyposmia can be associated with changes in sexual behavior, food preference, and appetite. Orbitofrontal injuries can result in disinhibition, impulsivity, and inappropriate social behavior.[9] Right facial weakness can be associated with aphasias. Abnormal findings of the motor and sensory systems and abnormal reflexes can further localize the site of neurological dysfunction associated with specific neuropsychiatric conditions.

TABLE 24.3. Neurobehavioral Symptoms Associated with Specific Areas of Brain Dysfunction

- *Frontal system dysfunction* – apathy, disinhibition, impulsivity, lability, aggressiveness, dysexecutive syndromes (motor perseveration, impersistence, loss of set, stimulus boundness, motor programming deficits, poor word list generation, poor abstraction and categorization, sparse verbal output)
- *Temporal-limbic dysfunction* – general and specific amnestic disorders, personality disturbances associated with temporolimbic epilepsy, Kluever-Bucey syndrome (bilateral amygdala dysfunction: placidity, hyperorality, hypersexuality)
- *Basal ganglia dysfunction* – executive dysfunction, psychomotor slowing, memory impairment, emotional incontinence, personality change, impulsivity, irritability, apathy
- *Thalamic dysfunction* – memory disturbances, apathy, loss of spontaneity and drive, affective flattening (occasional disinhibition and emotional lability with bilateral thalamic lesions)
- *Hypothalamic dysfunction* – obesity, disorders of temperature regulation, diminished drive, emotional reactivity

Source: Adapted from. Lezak MD: *Neuropsychological Assessment*, 3d ed. New York: Oxford University Press, 1995.

Diagnosis and Disposition

Neuropsychiatric symptoms can be difficult to diagnose under any circumstance. When such symptoms occur in patients with a CNS deficit, diagnosis can be particularly problematic. Patients with neurological disorders can present with a wide array of neurobehavioral disturbances (Table 24.6). Aberrant behavior in these patients can be the result of several different processes, each of which may require a separate treatment plan.[10] Symptoms are determined to be acute, subacute, or chronic. This differentiates symptoms that are related to a "state

TABLE 24.4. Medical History of the Neuropsychiatric Patient: Key Questions to Ask

What are the patient's symptoms?
When did the symptoms begin, and have they been continuous?
If not, how long did they last?
What stressors, events, or conditions are related to the symptoms?
What makes the symptoms better or worse?
Is the patient currently taking medication?
Have any changes occurred in medication dosage, or the time or route of their administration?
Have any changes occurred in the baseline medical or neurological condition?
Is there a history of illicit drug or alcohol use?

phenomenon," such as worsening of a neurological or medical condition, which can result in a new onset of neuropsychiatric conditions from symptoms caused by another underlying neuropsychiatric condition. An example of a "state phenomenon" resulting in new neuropsychiatric symptoms is a person with traumatic brain injury or developmental disabilities who has depression that manifests as aggression. Chronic neuropsychiatric symptoms that worsen are commonly associated with psychosocial stressors and a related adjustment disorder rather than with an acute change in a medical, neurological, or psychiatric disorder. Although the cause of a particular neuropsychiatric presentation may not be diagnosed in the emergency department, it is important to determine the nature and extent of the clinical condition so that appropriate disposition can be made.

Certain conditions of a psychiatric nature – including destructiveness, disorganization (as observed in patients with acute intoxication or schizophrenia), depression, disorientation due to severe organic mental disturbances, and conditions requiring detoxification – require psychiatric hospitalization, whether or not the patient has an underlying CNS disturbance. However, not all patients who present with psychiatric symptoms require admission to a psychiatric unit. In patients with known brain injury, it is important to determine whether there is an exacerbation of an underlying medical or neurological condition that presents

TABLE 24.5. Clinical Implications of Selected Cognitive Deficits

Deficit	Clinical Implication
Attentional deficit	Diffuse brain dysfunction (metabolic disturbance, drug intoxication, systemic infection), Alzheimer's disease, bilateral frontal lobe and limbic lesions, depression, anxiety
Language disturbance	Dominant hemisphere lesion (90% left hemisphere)
Memory disturbances	
Immediate recall (digit span)	Disruption of sensory motor areas (inattention, dementia)
Recent memory	Limbic injury (including hippocampus, mammillary bodies, dorsal medial thalamus; head injuries, bitemporal damage, Alzheimer's disease)
Remote memory	Injury to cortical association areas (Alzheimer's disease, Pick's disease, disease involving extensive areas of the cortex)
Constructional impairment	Parietal lobe dysfunction (right parietal lobe produces greater constructional deficits; Alzheimer's disease, multi-infarct dementia)
Higher cognitive function	Widespread brain injury of any pathology (manipulation of well-learned material, abstract thinking, problem solving, arithmetic computations)

Source: Adapted from Strub RI, and Black FW. *The Mental Status Examination in Neurology.* 3d ed. Philadelphia: Davis, 1993.

with neuropsychiatric symptoms. When neuropsychiatric symptoms are due to a change in a medical or an underlying neurological condition, only stabilization of those conditions will result in improvement in the neuropsychiatric symptoms. Neuropsychiatric evaluation is recommended: (1) when the underlying neurological condition is adequately controlled, (2) in absence of active medical illness, and (3) when medications are not considered to be responsible for the symptoms. When major depression, manic episode, or psychosis significantly interferes with the patient's ability to function, inpatient evaluation and treatment are required. This safeguards the patient and those involved in his or her care. Immediate emergency department intervention may be necessary for the acutely agitated or aggressive patient (see Table 24.7).[1]

The acuity of symptoms and their relationship to psychosocial factors determine the need for either hospitalization or discharge to the previous living arrangement with appropriate follow-up. Typically, patients with conditions that appear to be psychosocially mediated (i.e., behavioral or mood distur-

bances that arise as a consequence of environmental stressors) are discharged from the emergency department to the home setting with follow-up by counselors or psychiatrists. A strategic plan with necessary support is arranged in case the patient's symptoms worsen.

Mental Status Change

Patients with brain injury or neurological disorders can present with a variety of acute and chronic cognitive changes. Patients with known neurological conditions who present with an acute change in mental status – including changes in level of arousal, confusion, disorientation, or a disorganized thought process – require evaluation for an acute medical condition or an evaluation of exacerbation of the underlying neurological disturbance. For example, a patient with epilepsy who presents with an acute change in mental status may require an electroencephalogram (EEG). A patient with multi-infarct dementia who presents with an acute change in mental status may be experiencing another cere-

TABLE 24.6. Neuropsychiatric Symptoms Associated with Selected CNS Disorders

Disorder	Symptoms
Alzheimer's disease[13]	Apathy, agitation, anxiety, irritability, depression, disinhibition, delusions
Frontotemporal dementias[13]	Apathy, aberrant motor activity, disinhibition, agitation, anxiety, euphoria, depression, irritability
Parkinson's disease[7,13]	Depression, anxiety, apathy, agitation, mania, irritability, euphoria, executive dysfunction, dementia
Progressive supranuclear palsy[13]	Apathy, disinhibition, irritability, depression
Huntington's disease[14]	Depression, apathy, psychosis, irritability, emotional instability, change in social conduct, executive dysfunction, dementia
Traumatic brain injury[15]	Apathy, impulsivity, distractibility, indifference, poor anger control, rage, poor social skills, irritability, decreased concentration, decreased abstraction, depression, mania
Epilepsy[16]	Mood disorders, irritability, impulsivity, schizophreniform disorder, anxiety, pseudoseizures, personality changes, amnesia-confusion
Cerebrovascular disease[17]	Catastrophic reaction, anxiety, frustration, aggression when presented with cognitive tasks, anosognosia, apathy, depression, poor expression of emotional prosody, poor comprehension of emotion in others, pathological crying/laughing, mania
Brain tumors[18]	
Frontal lobe tumors	Personality changes, impulsivity, disinhibition, emotional instability, poor judgment and insight, distractibility, apathy, indifference, psychomotor retardation, motor perseveration
Temporal lobe tumors	Mood swings; visual, olfactory, tactile, auditory hallucinations, dreamlike or dazed feeling, depression, instability, mania, personality changes, anxiety; verbal and nonverbal memory impairments.
Parietal tumors	Depression, apathy, cognitive changes
Occipital tumors	Personality and behavioral changes, visual hallucinations
Diencephalic tumors	Emotional incontinence, psychosis, depression, hyperphagia, hypersomnia
HIV-AIDS[19]	Cognitive impairment, depression, psychosis
Multiple sclerosis[20]	Dementia, euphoria, depression, emotional dysregulation (pseudobulbar effect)

brovascular event. A CT scan may be helpful in determining a new-onset stroke. A change in mental status in patients with active neurological disease or degenerative disorders is commonly caused by a worsening of the neurological illness. In patients with cognitive disturbance secondary to a neurological condition, it is important to determine whether the current mental status is chronic and stable. This information can be obtained from friends or relatives accompanying the patient. In many instances, patients with brain injuries caused by trauma, stroke, or operative procedures present to the emergency department with chronic cognitive changes. The primary task for the emergency physician is to determine the extent, nature, and course of the cognitive changes. When these changes are acute, it is necessary to determine whether they are caused by an exacerbation of a neurological disorder or of an associated medical disorder. In these cases, evaluation by a neurologist or an internist is indicated. When the mental status changes appear to be related to the evolution of a CNS disorder, or arise in a patient with static CNS dysfunction, psychiatric or neuropsychiatric evaluation and appropriate interventions are indicated. Disposition depends on the acuity of the pa-

TABLE 24.7. Steps to Take in the Control of the Agitated or Aggressive Neuropsychiatric Patient

1. Move the patient to a quiet, secure room and minimize stimuli. The room should not be isolated and should be equipped with an alarm or panic button. It should not be possible to lock the door from the inside.
2. Obtain information about the patient's acute change in behavior or mental status from friends, relatives, or available documentation.
3. Attempt to talk to and/or reason with the patient. Ask relatives or friends to talk to the patient.
4. Obtain a history from the patient, when possible.
5. Administer a sedative or tranquilizer when the patient poses an immediate threat to self or others.
6. Apply physical restraints when the patient is not controlled by medication and poses an immediate threat to self or others.
7. Generate a differential diagnosis.
8. Treat and make appropriate disposition to psychiatry, neurology, or general medicine department. Recommend inpatient or output status evaluation. When the patient responds to treatment in the emergency department and can be discharged, release with appropriate follow up arrangements.

tient's symptoms and their impact on the patient's safety and ability to care for him- or herself.

Behavioral Changes

Behavioral changes in the neuropsychiatric patient commonly causes difficult situations in the emergency department. The agitated or aggressive patient can be difficult to manage, posing a threat to self or others and to those providing care and evaluation. Be-

havioral changes can be acute or chronic. When chronic, they can worsen due to mania, depression, mental status changes including disorganization of thought or psychotic processes, and environmental stressors. In the agitated or aggressive patient, safety is the primary consideration. Typically, the agitated patient cannot provide an adequate history. Input from relatives or friends and from medical records is important. Psychotropic medication may be required to calm the agitated or aggressive patient (Table 24.8).

TABLE 24.8. Psychotropics that Can Be Used to Calm the Agitated or Aggressive Patient

State	Possible Medication
Mildly to moderately agitated/aggressive	Lorazepam, 1–2 mg orally (Rarely, benzodiazepines can paradoxically disinhibit; avoid use in patient with a history of CNS depressant abuse or benzodiazepine-induced disinhibition. Haloperiodol, liquid, 5 mg orally, can be used as an alternative)
Severely agitated/aggressive	Lorazepam, 1–2 mg intramuscularly, or haloperiodol, 5 mg intramuscularly, may be repeated in 20–30 minutes. For extreme agitation, a combination of lorazepam and haloperiodol may be given intramuscularly.

Source: Adapted from Hyman SE: The violent patient. In: *Manual of Psychiatric Emergencies*, 3d ed. Hyman SE, Tesar GE, eds. Boston: Little, Brown, and Company, 1994; 28–37.

PEARLS AND PITFALLS

- A patient with altered behavior and cognition may have an underlying organic illness.
- Iatrogenic factors can be potential causes or contributors to emotional, behavioral, and cognitive disturbances; patients are evaluated for the presence of alcohol or illicit drugs.
- Patients with CNS disturbances can have poor insight and understanding, and can inaccurately describe relevant history and their symptoms; patient information is obtained from family or friends when possible.
- Grossly normal neurological and mental status examinations do not exclude the possibility of a CNS disturbance as the cause of behavioral and psychiatric symptoms.
- Neuropsychiatric patients may require hospitalization on a medical or neurological unit, rather than a psychiatric unit.

REFERENCES

1. Strub RL, Wise MG. Differential diagnosis in neuropsychiatry. In: Yudofsky SC, Hales RE, eds. *Textbook of Neuropsychiatry.* Washington, DC: American Psychiatric Press, 1992.
2. Popkin MK. Syndromes of brain dysfunction presenting with cognitive impairment or behavioral disturbance: delirium, dementia, and mental disorders due to a general medical condition. In: Winokur G, Clayton PJ, eds. *The Medical Basis of Psychiatry.* 2nd ed. Philadelphia, Pa: WB Saunders Co; 1994:17–37.
3. Cain HD. *Flint's Emergency Treatment and Management.* Philadelphia, Pa: WB Saunders Co; 1985:615–27.
4. Mueller J, Fogel BS. Neuropsychiatric examination. In: Fogel BS, Schiffer RB, Rao SM, eds. *Neuropsychiatry.* Baltimore, Md: Williams & Wilkins; 1996.
5. DeKosky ST. Mental status changes in dementia patients. In: Weiner WJ, ed. *Emergent and urgent neurology.* New York, NY: JB Lippincott; 1992:389.
6. Huff S. Altered levels of consciousness. In: Shah SM, Kelly KM, eds. *Emergency Neurology: Principles and Practice.* New York, NY: Cambridge University Press. In press.
7. Tintinalli JE, Peacock FW, Wright MA. Emergency medical evaluation of psychiatric patients. *Ann Emerg Med.* 1994;12:859–62.
8. Folstein MF, Folstein SE, McHugh PR. Minimental state: A practical method for grading the cognitive state of patients for the clinician. *J Psychiatr Res.* 1975;12:189.
9. Sano M, Marder K, Dooneief G. Basal ganglia diseases. In: Fogel BS, Schiffer RB, Rao SM, eds. *Neuropsychiatry.* Baltimore, Md: Williams & Wilkins; 1996:805–25.
10. Sovner R. Behavioral and affective disturbances in persons with mental retardation – a neuropsychiatric perspective: preface. *Semin. Clin Neuropsychiatry.* 1996;1:90–3.
11. Lezak MD. *Neuropsychological Assessment.* 3rd ed. New York, NY: Oxford University Press; 1995.
12. Strub RI, Black FW. *The Mental Status Examination in Neurology.* 3rd ed. Philadelphia, Pa: FA Davis Co; 1993.
13. Cummings JL, Diaz C, Levy M, Binetti G, Litvan I. Neuropsychiatric symptoms in neurodegenerative diseases: frequency and significance. *Semin Clin Neuropsychiatry.* 1996;1:241–7.
14. Roberts GW, Leigh PN, Weinberger DR. *Neuropsychiatric Disorders.* London: M Wolfe; 1993.
15. Taylor C, Price TP. Neuropsychiatric assessment. In: Silver JM, Yudofsky SC, Hales RE, eds. *Neuropsychiatry of Traumatic Brain Injury.* Washington, DC: APA Press; 1994:81–132.
16. Neppe VM, Tucker GJ. Neuropsychiatric aspects of seizure disorders. In: Yudofsky SC, Hales RE, eds. *Textbook of Neuropsychiatry.* Washington, DC: American Psychiatric Press; 1992.
17. Starkstein SE, Robinson RG. Neuropsychiatric aspects of cerebral vascular disorders. In: Yudofsky SC, Hales RE, eds. *APA Textbook of Neuropsychiatry.* Washington, DC: APA Press; 1992.
18. Price TP, Goetz KL, Lovell MR. Neuropsychiatric aspects of brain tumors. In: Yudofsky SC, Hales RE, eds. *APA Textbook of Neuropsychiatry.* Washington, DC: APA Press; 1992.
19. Markowitz JC, Perry SW. Effects of immunodeficiency virus on the central nervous system. In: Yudofsky SC, Hales RE, eds., *APA Textbook of Neuropsychiatry* Washington, DC: APA Press; 1992.
20. Filley CM. Neurobehavioral aspects of cerebral white matter disorders. In: Fogel BS, Schiffer RB, Rao SM, eds. *Neuropsychiatry.* Baltimore, Md: Williams & Wilkins; 1996:913–33.
21. Hyman SE. The violent patient. In: Hyman SE, Tesar GE, eds. *Manual of Psychiatric Emergencies.* 3rd ed. Boston, Mass: Little, Brown, and Co; 1994:28–37.

25 Neuroanesthesiology

KEVIN J. GINGRICH

SUMMARY Patients with acute intracranial pathology and elevated intracranial pressure (ICP) can experience secondary brain injury resulting from factors that include hypoxia and hypercarbia. In the emergency department, patients with an elevated ICP require rapid evaluation of airway and ventilation followed by definitive management. Frequently, endotracheal intubation is used to provide swift control of the airway and mechanical ventilation. Endotracheal intubation is performed while considering the potential for cervical spine injuries and an elevated ICP. Anesthetic agents and muscle relaxants are used not only to facilitate intubation but also to prevent untoward effects on systemic blood pressure and ICP.

Introduction

Acute intracranial pathology with increased intracranial pressure (ICP) has significant potential to cause serious and permanent brain injury. The primary pathological process (e.g., hydrocephalus, intracranial hemorrhage, traumatic brain injury) can induce ischemia, cerebral swelling, abnormalities of cerebral blood flow (CBF), and elevations in ICP, leading to additional brain insult and secondary brain injury.[1] An elevated ICP is the final common pathway of these processes.[2] Pathological elevation of the ICP is called intracranial hypertension (ICH), which can result in brain herniation and cerebral ischemia. ICH may be induced or exacerbated by hypoxia and hypercarbia, which are rapidly and aggressively treated in these patients. Definitive treatment includes endotracheal intubation and mechanical ventilation. In performing the technique for endotracheal intubation, the emergency physician must consider the possibility of cervical spine injuries. Moreover, the technique should prevent pulmonary aspiration, control the ICP, and ensure adequate cerebral perfusion. Specific airway maneuvers, anesthetic agents, and muscle relaxants are used to address these issues.

Prehospital Management

Airway management is the first priority in the patient with an acute intracranial process and possible ICH. When the patient's ability to maintain a patent airway is impaired, endotracheal intubation and bag ventilation are indicated and executed quickly by emergency medical service providers in the field.

Emergency Department Evaluation

Significant intracranial pathology requires rapid evaluation and definitive management of the patient's airway and ventilation to avoid hypoxia and hypercarbia. This is critical in mitigating secondary injury. Indications for endotracheal intubation include the inability to protect the airway, respiratory distress, and a Glasgow Coma Scale score of less than 9 (Table 25.1). Given the relative safety of endotracheal intubation and the gravity of potential

TABLE 25.1. Indications for Endotracheal Intubation

- Respiratory distress
  Respiratory rates >30 or <10 breaths per minute
  Abnormal breathing patterns
- Glasgow Coma Scale <9
- PaO_2 <70 or $PaCO_2$ >50 mm Hg
- Seizures
- Increased intracranial pressure

secondary injury, endotracheal intubation is performed when there are any concerns regarding oxygenation and ventilation.

Neuroanatomy and Physiology

The intracranial compartment is a rigid, bony cranial enclosure coupled with delicate and cushioning support of the cerebrospinal fluid (CSF). The walls of the intracranial compartment are composed of nondistensible cranial bone or dura mater, which results in fixed capacity. The intracranial compartment contains volumes of the brain, CSF, and blood. Elevated ICP results when one of these volumes or that of a fourth pathological volume (e.g., hematoma) expands beyond the capacity of the others to accommodate the increase. Sustained ICP elevation greater than 20 mm Hg is considered intracranial hypertension (ICH). ICH threatens the brain in two ways. First, ICH reduces cerebral perfusion pressure (CPP), the difference between mean arterial pressure (MAP) and ICP. Reduced CPP decreases CBF and can result in cerebral ischemia. Second, ICH can produce pressure gradients within the cranium that cause the brain to herniate through dural or bony passages (see Chap. 26).

CBF, in part, determines the size of the cerebral blood volume (CBV). Increases in CBV exacerbate ICH. Therefore, control of the CBF is equivalent to control of the ICP. Hypoxia and hypercarbia increase CBF through normal physiological mechanisms. Systemic hypertension can also increase CBF. The normal brain exhibits autoregulation, which maintains constant CBF over a wide range of MAP (50–150 mm Hg). However, patients with serious intracranial pathology can have impaired au-

toregulation such that elevations in the MAP result in an increased CBF. Finally, increased brain metabolic activity also increases CBF. Overall hypoxia, hypercarbia, hypertension, and increased brain activity cause ICH to become worse.

Emergency Department Management

Endotracheal intubation of patients with intracranial pathology has a number of accompanying risks. First, patients with full stomachs are at risk for pulmonary aspiration of gastric contents.[3] Second, in patients with traumatic brain injury, cervical spine fractures may threaten the cervical spinal cord. Finally, the stress of endotracheal intubation can induce systemic hypertension, which raises the CBF and CBV, thereby worsening ICH. Endotracheal intubation using direct laryngoscopy, anesthetic agents, and neuromuscular blocking drugs is safe and provides rapid airway control in the emergency department.[2,4]

Intravenous Agents Used in Endotracheal Intubation

Anesthetic agents are used in endotracheal intubation to suppress the hypertensive response and to control ICP. Neuromuscular blocking agents produce skeletal muscle paralysis, facilitating direct laryngoscopy and placement of the endotracheal tube. Overall, neuromuscular blocking agents optimize emergency airway management and are safe and efficacious.[5]

Anesthetic Agents. *Sodium pentothal* is an ultra–fast-acting barbiturate commonly used in rapid-sequence endotracheal intubation for patients with ICH. Sodium pentothal has rapid onset and clearance times, blunts sympathetic responses to laryngoscopy and intubation, and depresses cerebral metabolism, which may ameliorate ICH. However, in clinically unstable patients pentothal can precipitate hypotension, which compromises the CPP. Therefore, the dose is reduced from 3–5 mg/kg to 0.5–1 mg/kg in unstable patients.

Etomidate is a fast-acting hypnotic agent. An advantage of etomidate is that it provides enhanced cardiovascular stability; however, it can still induce hypotension in unstable patients. Therefore, it is prudent to reduce the dose from 0.2–0.3 mg/kg to 0.1–0.2 mg/kg in unstable patients. Etomidate can cause transient myoclonic and tonic-clonic movements as well as adrenal suppression that lasts for hours after a single-bolus injection. With these side effects, etomidate is considered in unstable patients.

Propofol is an ultra–short-acting, nonbarbiturate hypnotic agent. Propofol reduces cerebral metabolism, CBF, and ICH. However, this agent has a propensity to induce hypotension through direct vascular smooth and muscle relaxation. Therefore, propofol is restricted to clinically stable patients without risk for hypovolemia. Dosing is 1–2 mg/kg.

Ketamine is a phencyclidine derivative. This agent is unique among anesthetic agents in that it induces a "dissociative state" in which somatic sensory information is blocked before reaching the supratentorial central nervous system, resulting in unconsciousness and analgesia without cardiovascular depression. However, ketamine dramatically increases CBF and cerebral metabolism, thereby increasing ICP. Therefore, ketamine is *not* used in patients with suspected elevation of the ICP.

Neuromuscular Blocking Agents. *Succinylcholine* is the standard agent of rapid-sequence endotracheal intubation. In dosages for 1.0–1.5 mg/kg, it provides flaccid paralysis within 60 seconds that lasts less than 5 minutes. Succinylcholine is an ideal paralytic agent for patients requiring neurological assessment shortly following intubation. However, succinylcholine has several significant side effects that make its use in patients with ICH and trauma controversial. Succinylcholine increases CBF, CO_2 production, and ICP, and induces potassium release from skeletal muscle due to skeletal muscle fasciculations. CO_2 production is transient and has no implications for weaning from mechanical ventilation. Potassium release can exacerbate hyperkalemia, which can occur following head trauma. Pretreatment with other neuromuscular blocking agents that suppress fasciculations can attenuate, if not eliminate, these effects. Finally, malignant hyperthermia can be triggered by succinylcholine, resulting in a life-threatening hypermetabolic state.

Vecuronium is a neuromuscular blocking agent that lacks some of the negative side effects of succinylcholine. At high doses (0.3 mg/kg), muscle paralysis occurs in approximately 100 seconds,

making it useful in the treatment of patients requiring rapid-sequence endotracheal intubation. Vecuronium has no untoward effects on CBF or the cardiovascular system. This makes vecuronium a popular alternative to succinylcholine. The significant disadvantages of this agent are the slower onset relative to succinylcholine (twice as slow) and paralysis that persists for hours.

Rocuronium is a less potent form of vecuronium and has a more rapid onset of action. Doses of 0.6–1.2 mg/kg induce muscle paralysis in about 60 seconds that lasts about 1 hour. Therefore, rocuronium provides a rapid onset of paralysis comparable to that provided by succinylcholine. Although the duration of action is less than that of vecuronium, it is longer than that of succinylcholine. Given these characteristics, rocuronium is an ideal paralytic when the duration of action is not an issue.

Adjuvant Agents. Agents that suppress the hypertensive response to laryngoscopy and endotracheal intubation are commonly used as adjuvants. *Lidocaine* (1.5–2.0 mg/kg) is used commonly and acts by depressing both central and peripheral nervous systems. *Fentanyl* is a narcotic that has no negative effects on cerebral perfusion and ICP. At a dose of 1–2 mcg/kg in stable patients, it suppresses the hypertensive response to endotracheal intubation. A reduced dose is used or the drug is avoided in unstable patients. Fentanyl is generally safe for the treatment of patients with ICH. However, one study has reported that fentanyl raised the ICP in a patient with head trauma despite hyperventilation.[5]

Modified Rapid Sequence for Endotracheal Intubation

Rapid-sequence intubation refers to the simultaneous administration of an anesthetic agent and a neuromuscular blocking agent in order to induce unconsciousness and muscle paralysis, allowing for rapid endotracheal intubation. This reduces the risk of pulmonary aspiration of gastric contents. This is achieved by minimizing the time between unconsciousness, when the patient can no longer protect the airway, and securing the airway with an endotracheal tube. The technique presented below is called "modified" because gentle bag-mask ventilation is delivered during the 100 seconds required for the onset of muscle paralysis (Table 25.2). Bag-

TABLE 25.2. Rapid-Sequence Endotracheal Intubation

---

1. **Preparation**
   - Stabilize systemic blood pressure when possible
   - Ensure the presence of suction, variety of laryngoscopes, styleted endotracheal tubes, and cricothyroidotomy setup
2. **Preoxygenation**
   - Administer 100% oxygen for 5 minutes or 4 vital capacity breaths
3. **Pretreatment**
   - Administer vecuronium (0.01 mg/kg IV)
   - Administer lidocaine (1.5 mg/kg IV)
   - Administer fentanyl (1–2 mcg/kg IV when patient is not hypotensive)
   - Remove cervical collar and provide manual in-line axial cervical spine stabilization with concern for cervical spine injury (i.e., trauma)
   - Continue preoxygenation and wait 2–3 minutes when possible
4. **Cricoid pressure, unconsciousness, and paralysis**
   - Apply cricoid pressure
   - Administer thiopental (3–5 mg/kg; 0–1 mg/kg when hypotensive)
   - Administer succinylcholine (1.5 mg/kg)
   - Administer gentle bag-mask ventilation with 100% oxygen
5. **Direct laryngoscopy and endotracheal intubation**
6. **Confirm endotracheal intubation**
   - Confirm endotracheal intubation using breath sounds and, when necessary, expired CO_2 indicator
   - Following proper endotracheal intubation, release cricoid pressure, replace cervical collar, and institute mechanical ventilation. Consider surgical airway when unsuccessful (i.e., cricothyroidotomy)

---

mask ventilation was excluded in the original description of rapid-sequence intubation.

The emergency physician initiates modified rapid sequence endotracheal intubation by stabilizing the clinical hemodynamics. The emergency physician first stabilizes the patient's hemodynamic parameters, because hypotension is associated with secondary injury, and hypovolemic patients manifest an exaggerated hypotensive response to anesthetic agents. Proper equipment must be available for endotracheal intubation, including a setup for a surgical airway (cricothyroidotomy). The patient is preoxygenated, thereby postponing arterial oxygen desaturation, which occurs during apnea. Preoxygenation is achieved by delivering 100% oxygen for five minutes of normal tidal volume ventilation, or during four vital capacity breaths. Vecuronium, fentanyl, and lidocaine are administered to prevent ICP elevation during direct laryngoscopy and endotracheal intubation. When the patient has sustained multiple trauma, the hard collar is removed and the cervical spine is immobilized with manual in-line axial stabilization. Stabilization continues until the collar is replaced after successful endotracheal intubation. After two to three minutes the intravenous medications attain their desired effects. Cricoid pressure is applied to inhibit gastric aspiration. Sodium pentothal and succinylcholine are given quickly in succession. The patient is gently ventilated by bag-mask while these medications take effect. This allows continuous delivery of oxygen to the lungs to prevent hypoxia but is done gently to prevent possible inflation of the stomach, which leads to diaphragmatic restriction or vomiting. After the onset of paralysis (approximately 100 seconds, depending on the drug regimen) laryngoscopy is performed, the vocal cords are visualized, and the trachea is intubated. Proper position of the endotracheal tube is confirmed using auscultation of the chest and epigastrium, the presence of mist in the tube, and detection of expired CO_2. Detection of expired CO_2 by simple color-changing devices or other means is the only reliable method of confirming endotracheal intubation. After confirmation of endo-

TABLE 25.3. Settings for Mechanical Ventilation

- Tidal volume of 10–14 ml/kg
- Rate of 8–12 per minute
- FIO_2 of 100%, then reduced to maintain PaO_2 >80 mm Hg or until FIO_2 or 50% is reached
- Initial settings should be modified based on the serial arterial blood gas analysis and the clinical status

tracheal intubation, the cervical collar is replaced and mechanical ventilation is instituted. When intubation fails, bag-mask ventilation is continued and followed quickly by another attempt. Providing bag-mask ventilation remains effective, additional attempts can be made. However, when bag-mask ventilation becomes ineffective or intubation cannot be achieved after several attempts, cricothyroidotomy is performed as a last resort. Cricothyroidotomy is the puncture of the cricothyroid membrane with a large-gauge needle catheter (#14) or scalpel. The puncture is followed by insertion of a formal tracheostomy or endotracheal tube, which provides for traditional controlled ventilation. For needle cricothyroidotomy, the catheter is connected to a controlled high-pressure oxygen supply (50 psi) that allows for jet ventilation. Jet ventilation provides oxygenation and ventilation,[6] but is a temporizing measure until a definitive airway can be achieved. Because cricothyroidotomy provides an important surgical airway in the emergency department,[7] emergency physicians should be skilled in this technique.

Mechanical Ventilation

Controlled ventilation is indicated in patients who are paralyzed or have no spontaneous respirations. Initial settings (Table 25.3) are modified based on serial arterial blood gas analysis and the patient's clinical status. Commonly available modes of mechanical ventilation are intermittent mandatory ventilation (IMV) and spontaneous intermittent mandatory ventilation (SIMV). Both modes provide a fixed number of full tidal volume breaths per minute either at constant intervals (IMV) or triggered by spontaneous ventilatory efforts (SIMV). SIMV allows the patient to breathe between mechanical breaths, permitting the actual ventilatory rate to be greater than the ventilator setpoint. Mechanical ventilation is advantageous because it provides a known inspired oxygen concentration and tidal volumes that overcome dead space and inhibit atelectasis. Positive end-expiratory pressure (PEEP) can also be applied to increase functional residual capacity and enhance ventilation–perfusion matching, thereby improving oxygenation. However, PEEP is used with caution because it can increase ICP.

Hyperventilation. Hyperventilation can reduce CBF and thereby decrease ICP. However, extreme hyperventilation ($PaCO_2$ <30 mm Hg) can also cause cerebral ischemia[8] and worsen neurological outcome following traumatic brain injury.[1,9] Therefore, extreme hyperventilation is no longer recommended as a first-line therapy for the management of patients with ICH, but it may be useful in the management of patients with sudden neurological deterioration.[2,9] The goal of mechanical ventilation in patients with ICH is mild hyperventilation ($PaCO_2$ 30–35 mm Hg).[1,2,9]

Sedatives, Analgesics, and Neuromuscular Blockade. Intubated patients commonly receive analgesics and sedation to limit agitation, discomfort, and pain. Muscle relaxants are used to control patients who actively oppose mechanical ventilation. These factors may cause systemic hypertension, elevated cerebral metabolism, or increased intrathoracic pressure, which can further elevate ICH. Sedation without analgesia can lead to agitation and increased combativeness. Therefore, a sedative/analgesic combination can be more effective. Intermittent intravenous administration of midazolam (0.02–0.05 mg/kg) and morphine sulfate (0.05–0.1 mg/kg) is effective and should not significantly compromise the neurological examination. However, care must be exercised with an unstable patient. These drugs can depress the respiratory drive[10] and are used with extreme caution in patients who are not receiving mechanical ventilation, because they are at particular risk for hypoventilation, hypoxia, and hypotension. Neuromuscular blockade can be easily achieved with intermittent doses of vecuronium (0.1 mg/kg).

PEARLS AND PITFALLS

- Adequacy of airway and ventilation must be assessed rapidly in order to avoid hypoxia, hypercarbia, and secondary brain injury.

- Definitive airway management involves modified rapid-sequence endotracheal intubation and mechanical ventilation.

- Goals of mechanical ventilation are PaO_2 greater than 80 mm Hg and $PaCO_2$ between 30 mm Hg and 35 mm Hg (mild hyperventilation).

- Extreme hyperventilation ($PaCO_2$ <30 mm Hg) is used only for brief periods in patients with acute neurological deterioration and suspected impending herniation.

- Sedation of patients with head injury without a secured airway or with possible elevated ICP is done with caution or not at all.

REFERENCES

1. Wald SL. Advances in the early management of patients with head injury. *Surg Clin North Am*. 1995;75:225–42.
2. Pickard JD, Czosyka M. Management of raised intracranial pressure. *J Neurol Neurosurg Psychiatry*. 1993;56:845–58.
3. Redan JA, Livingston DH, Tortella BJ, et al. The value of intubation and paralyzing patients with suspected head injury in the emergency department. *J Trauma*. 1991;31:371–80.
4. Abrams KJ. General management issues in severe head injury: airway management and mechanical ventilation. *New Horiz*. 1995;3:479–87.
5. Sperry RJ, Bailey PL, Reschman MV, et al. Fentanyl and sufentanil increase intracranial pressure in head trauma patients. *Anesthesiology*. 1992;77:416–20.
6. Zornow MH, Thomas TC, Scheller MS. The efficacy of three different methods of transtracheal jet ventilation. *Can J Anesth*. 1989;36:624–8.
7. Salvino CK, Dries D, Garnelli R, et al. Emergency cricothyroidotomy in trauma victims. *J Trauma*. 1993;34:503–5.
8. Sheinberg GM, Kanter MJ, Robertson CS, et al. Continuous monitoring of jugular venous oxygen saturation in head-injured patients. *J Neurosurg*. 1992;76:212–17.
9. Marion DW, Firlik A, McLaughlin MR. Hyperventilation therapy for severe traumatic brain injury. *New Horiz*. 1995;3:439–47.
10. Ward D, Perkins F. Control of ventilation. *Prog Anesthesiol*. 1993;12:15–35.

26 Increased Intracranial Pressure

AMY BLASEN AND RONALD JAKUBIAK

SUMMARY Many pathological conditions can result in increased intracranial pressure (ICP). Traditional therapies for treatment of increased ICP have changed in several ways. Routine hyperventilation is no longer recommended. Controlled ventilation with adequate oxygenation and a $PaCO_2$ within the normal range is the therapy of choice. Mannitol continues to be the preferred pharmacological treatment of increased ICP. Corticosteroids have no role in the treatment of increased ICP caused by trauma, but are beneficial in the reduction of edema caused by tumors and abscesses. The use of barbiturate coma is limited to those patients with increased ICP who do not respond adequately to other ICP-lowering measures. Advances in the understanding of the pathophysiology of increased ICP and new strategies for its early detection and treatment continue to emerge with ongoing studies.

Introduction

Several distinct pathological processes follow a common pathway that leads to increased ICP.[1,2] These varied disorders include traumatic brain injury (TBI), space-occupying intracranial lesions, and many others. Initial identification and management of patients at risk for developing increased ICP commonly occurs in the emergency department. Many of these patients have TBI. A review of the mechanism of the development of increased ICP and its treatment is presented in this chapter.

Prehospital Care

Definitive diagnosis of increased ICP is generally not possible in out-of-hospital evaluation. As with any other potentially life-threatening condition, management of airway, breathing, and circulation is undertaken immediately. TBI is the most commonly encountered condition by prehospital care providers that can result in increased ICP. When TBI is suspected, adequate cervical spine immmobiliza-

tion is required. Hypoxia, hypercapnea, and systemic hypotension can exacerbate brain injury via cellular hypoxia and cerebral edema, causing further increases ICP.[3] Prehospital care providers can perform endotracheal intubation to protect the airway and to achieve controlled ventilation. Hyperventilation has been used traditionally to lower ICP by decreasing the $PaCO_2$, resulting in vasoconstriction and decreased cerebral blood flow (CBF). However, recent evidence suggests that the *prophylactic* use of hyperventilation to achieve a $PaCO_2$ of less than 35 mm Hg during the first 24 hours after severe brain injury can compromise cerebral perfusion during a time when CBF is reduced; therefore, it is not performed.[3,4]

Hyperventilation may be necessary for brief periods of time to treat patients with acute neurological deterioration, or for longer periods when intracranial hypertension is refractory to other methods of control such as sedation, paralysis, cerebrospinal fluid (CSF) drainage, and osmotic diuresis. In the prehospital care setting, elevating the patient's head to 30 degrees to augment venous drainage is an im-

Sid M. Shah and Kevin M. Kelly, eds., *Emergency Neurology: Principles and Practice.* Copyright © 1999 Cambridge University Press. All rights reserved.

TABLE 26.1. Prehospital Care for Patients with Suspected Increased ICP

1. Aggressive airway management for controlled ventilation with adequate oxygenation and normalization of $Paco_2$
2. Immobilization of the cervical spine when indicated
3. Assessment of the neurological deficits
4. Establishment of an initial Glasgow Coma Scale score
5. Elevation of head to 30 degrees
6. Correction of hypotension due to possible extracranial injuries

portant initial step in controlling increased ICP. Prior to elevation of the head, the neck is immobilized. These procedures are performed quickly and efficiently because the sooner these patients reach an emergency department with available computerized tomography (CT) scanning and definitive intervention, the better the outcome.[3,4] Table 26.1 provides guidelines for prehospital care.

Emergency Department Evaluation

Primary survey of the patient includes a brief neurological examination and establishment of a Glasgow Coma Scale (GCS) score. The secondary survey includes a detailed history from family and the prehospital care providers, and more detailed and specific physical and neurological examinations.[17]

Examination of the eyes is singularly useful in patients with suspected increased ICP. Pupils are examined for size, symmetry, and reactivity. A dilated pupil can give evidence of increased ICP, with a lesion typically ipsilateral to the pupillary dilatation. Bilaterally fixed, dilated pupils can indicate brain death, whereas bilaterally dilated and poorly responsive pupils can be caused by sympathetic overactivity from a variety of catecholamines or from anticholinergic medications such as atropine sulfate. Midposition and fixed pupils reflect sympathetic and parasympathetic failure at the midbrain level. Extremely miotic pupils are characteristic of either a narcotic overdose or a pontine lesion. Visual field defects can occur with postchiasmal hemispheric lesions, including ischemia in the dis-

tribution of the posterior cerebral artery, which can cause cortical blindness when bilateral. Pupillary constriction can occur initially in response to an expanding supratentorial mass, followed by unilateral dilatation. When ICP is markedly increased, the pupils become dilated and fixed. It is important to note that pupillary responses are associated with the immediate clinical condition and have little or no predictive value of subsequent clinical course or outcome.[18]

Papilledema is the only reliable clinical sign of increased ICP. In the acute phase, TBI rarely causes papilledema, which may take several hours or days to develop. Other findings associated with an initial rise in ICP include a sixth nerve palsy. Papilledema, nuchal rigidity, and subhyaloid hemorrhage occur with subarachnoid hemorrhage (SAH).

Emergent CT of the brain is used to evaluate the patient for cerebral edema, hematoma, neoplasm, diffuse brain swelling, or midline shift of structures. CT findings of diffuse cerebral edema include compression of the ventricular system, and effacement of cortical sulci, basal cisterns, and the junction of gray and white matter. When focal areas of edema are present, a mass effect can cause midline shift of structures or deviation of the posterior fossa structures.[19]

Pathophysiology

The three main compartments within the intracranial space are brain, CSF, and blood. Normal brain volume is approximately 1400 cc. CSF volume is 120–140 ml, comprising 40 ml within the ventricles and 30 ml in the spinal subarachnoid space; the remainder is within the intracranial cisterns and the cranial subarachnoid space.[2] Adult cerebral blood volume (CBV) is approximately 150 ml, which represents 10% of the total intracranial volume. Seventy percent of CBV is venous.[1] Because the intracranial sphere is rigid, a change in the volume of the brain causes a reciprocal change in the volume of the other intracranial components. The ability of the brain to adjust to space-occupying masses is limited by the inelasticity of the skull. The cranial intradural space is nearly constant in volume, and its contents are noncompressible. Therefore, addition of any volume inside the cranium has the potential to increase ICP. Slight reciprocal modifica-

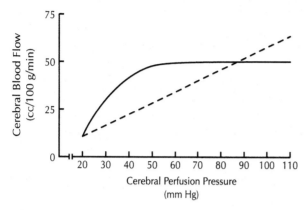

FIGURE 26.1. Autoregulation of cerebral blood flow. Flow is plotted against cerebral perfusion pressure (mean arterial pressure–ICP). The solid line describes the normal relationship: There is little change in flow over a wide range of perfusion pressures. When perfusion pressure decreases below 50–60 mm Hg, cerebral blood flow begins to fall. The dashed line depicts the relation between perfusion pressures and flow when autoregulation has been lost. Cerebral blood flow changes passively, and in linear fashion, with the perfusion pressure (from JE McGillicuddy, Cerebral protection: Pathophysiology and treatment of increased intracranial pressure. *Chest.* 1985; 87:85–93.)

tions in volume can occur; these account for many of the clinically significant aspects of ICP dynamics.

Because the brain lacks the metabolic reserves present in other organ systems, it relies on steady arterial perfusion to meet its metabolic demands. Cerebral ischemia of any cause is directly proportional to decreased CBF to the affected area. Clinical determination of CBF is difficult to make; therefore, measurement of cerebral perfusion pressure (CPP) is used as an indirect measurement of CBF. CPP is calculated by the following equation: CPP = mean arterial pressure (MAP) − ICP.

Cerebral autoregulation refers to the constant maintenance of blood flow to the neural tissue despite pressure changes in the vessels that transport blood. CBF is able to remain constant at 60 ml/100 g of brain tissue per minute over a wide range of MAPs due to autoregulatory factors that control cerebrovascular resistance (Fig. 26.1). These factors include local levels of carbon dioxide, oxygen, and neurogenic influences of the autonomic nervous system. Moderate hypoxemia and hypercapnea can cause cerebrovascular dilatation without subsequent increases in ICP. Because the vasculature is

more sensitive to changes in $PaCO_2$ than to changes in PaO_2, small changes in $PaCO_2$ can cause disproportionate changes in CBF. The brain can usually tolerate modest hypoxia while keeping CBF essentially unchanged.[5]

ICP represents resting pressure, which reflects the equilibrium of CSF production and absorption. CSF is produced in the choroid plexus at a rate of 20–25 ml per hour. This rate does not change unless the CPP changes. Absorption of CSF by the arachnoid granulations is a passive process and generally increases with increasing ICP. Resting ICP in the normal adult and child over 7 years of age is 0–10 mm Hg; 15 mm Hg is the upper limit of normal. In young children, the upper limit of normal ICP is 0–5 mm Hg;[6] in neonates, the normal ICP is 0–2 mm Hg.[7] Current data support the lowering of ICP when it is equal to or higher than 20–25 mm Hg. When the ICP is elevated to 40 mm Hg in the adult, the mortality rate is 65%. At ICPs of 60 mm Hg or higher, the mortality is virtually 100%.[8] Brain herniation can occur at ICPs less than 20–25 mm Hg; therefore, an absolute ICP threshold for instituting treatment is not uniform. The likelihood of brain herniation depends on the location of the intracranial mass lesion.

Normalizing ICP does not assure a good clinical result, due to the presence of cerebral injury caused by the traumatic event or by prior high ICP. ICP due to generalized cerebral edema or hydrocephalus is much better tolerated by the patient than increased ICP due to a focal mass lesion. In addition, an insidious rise in ICP occurring over a prolonged period is much better tolerated than an abrupt increase in ICP.[7]

Brain Herniation

The cranial contents are compartmentalized by a layering of dura mater. The folding of the dura mater forms distinct compartments of brain. The falx cerebri separates the two hemispheres of brain, and the tentorium cerebelli separates the infratentorial structures from the supratentorial structures, forming the third compartment of brain. Expansion of intracranial contents is severely limited due to the presence of compartmentalization and the rigid outer shell of the skull. The presence of generalized cerebral edema or increasing ICP does not directly affect neuronal activity; its main consequence is compromised CBF, leading to ischemia and the de-

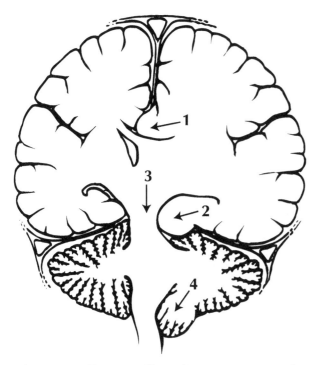

FIGURE 26.2. Patterns of brain herniation: (1) cingulate herniation under the falx; (2) uncal herniation through the tentorial incisura; (3) central transtentorial herniation through the incisural notch; (4) cerebellar tonsillar herniation through the foramen magnum (from RH Wilkins and SS Rengochary, eds. *Neurosurgery.* 2nd ed. New York, NY: McGraw-Hill Book Co, 1996:349. Used with permission.)

velopment of pressure gradients between the intracranial compartments.

Brain herniation, an end-stage manifestation of increased ICP, refers to displacement of brain tissue from one intracranial compartment to another through an opening in the dural sheath (uncal herniation through a tentorial notch; tonsillar herniation through the foramen magnum), or beneath edges (falx cerebri herniation) of the dural sheath. This causes hemorrhagic necrosis, direct vascular injury, and lateral compression of vital structures. Several herniation syndromes are described in Figure 26.2.[7]

Cingulate herniation is also referred to as subfalcine or supracallosal herniation. Cingulate herniation may not produce any significant clinical symptoms in the initial stage and is frequently identified only radiologically. It occurs when an expanding hemispheric mass forces all or part of the cingulate gyrus beneath the free edge of the falx.[9] This can

cause compression of the anterior cerebral artery with resultant ischemia.

Uncal herniation is associated with supratentorial masses and masses in the temporal fossa. An expanding mass can cause the medial portion of the temporal lobe (uncus) to displace over the tentorial notch, causing compression of the ipsilateral oculomotor nerve and displacement of the brainstem. Compression of the ipsilateral posterior cerebral artery can also occur. An early clinical sign is dilatation of the ipsilateral pupil with loss of light reflex and the development of ptosis of the ipsilateral eyelid. Pupillary changes are typically followed by contralateral hemiparesis caused by compression of the contralateral cerebral peduncle against the free edge of the tentorium.[9] Consciousness is depressed with these events and can be accompanied by respiratory changes and bradycardia. However, systemic vital signs may not change until just prior to fatal herniation.[7]

Central transtentorial herniation results from lesions of the frontal, parietal, and occipital lobes. This occurs when there is downward movement of the diencephalon and rostral midbrain through the tentorial notch. Clinically, this displacement results in impairment of cognitive function and can result in loss of upward gaze secondary to midbrain compression.[7] When central herniation is severe, bilateral pupillary dilatation occurs. Vital signs do not change until late in the clinical course, which underscores the importance of serial mental status evaluations in a patient with suspected increased ICP.

Cerebellar tonsillar herniation typically is observed in the setting of posterior fossa mass lesions but can occur with supratentorial lesions. The most severe cases are seen when a sudden pressure gradient develops, as in the sudden release of CSF in the presence of raised ICP. When this herniation syndrome occurs, the cerebellar tonsils are displaced through the foramen magnum. Respiratory arrest occurs because of compression of the respiratory centers in the medulla oblongata. Blood pressure falls, pupils dilate, and coma ensues. These signs can occur precipitously. Once the medulla is severely compressed, death is virtually inevitable.[9]

A herniation syndrome is a neurosurgical emergency. When immediate intervention is not taken, death can ensue rapidly. Initial therapy is aimed at

TABLE 26.2. Differential Diagnosis of Increased Intracranial Pressure

Condition	Pathogenesis
Traumatic Brain Injury	Intracerebral Hematoma
	Brain Contusion and Swelling
Cerebrovascular accidents	Subarachnoid hemorrhage
	Intracerebral hematoma
	Cerebral infarct
	Cerebral venous thrombosis
Hydrocephalus	Obstructive
	Communicating
Brain tumor	
CNS infection	Meningitis
	Abscess
	Encephalitis
Metabolic encephalopathy	Hepatic coma
	Hypoxic encephalopathy
	Reye's syndrome
	Diabetic ketoacidosis
	Hyponatremia
Status epilepticus	

Source: Adapted from Pickard JD and Czosnka M. Management of raised intracranial pressure. *J Neuro Neurosurg and Psychiatry* 1993;56:845–58.

lowering ICP while determining and treating the underlying cause.

Differential Diagnosis

Common conditions resulting in increased ICP include TBI, cerebrovascular events, hydrocephalus, brain tumor, CNS infections, metabolic and hypoxic encephalopathies, and status epilepticus (see Table 26.2). The common factor linking the development of increased ICP in these various conditions appears to be the production of cerebral edema. *Cerebral edema* is categorized into vasogenic, cytotoxic, and interstitial types depending upon the pathogenesis, location of edema, fluid composition, extracellular fluid volume, and effects on the blood–brain barrier (Table 26.3). This specific classification helps to dictate appropriate management.

Vasogenic edema is characterized by an increase in vascular permeability. This allows exudative plasma fluid to be extracted into gray and white matter, accumulating predominantly in white mat-ter. Common causes of vasogenic edema include TBI, neoplasm, abscess, meningitis, infarct, and hemorrhage.[10]

Cytotoxic edema occurs with an intact blood–brain barrier and is likely due to "cell membrane pump failure," causing intracellular swelling of neurons and endothelial cells with an overall reduction in the extracellular fluid volume. Gray and white matter are generally affected. Although hypoxia is classically associated with cytotoxic edema, other conditions such as diabetic ketoacidosis, Reye's syndrome, water intoxication, and many "toxic encephalopathies" are associated with cytotoxic edema.[7]

Interstitial edema occurs with an intact blood–brain barrier and generally involves the periventricular white matter. The edema results from an increased amount of CSF caused by blocked CSF absorption, as occurs in hydrocephalus.

Traumatic Brain Injury

The various mechanisms leading to increased ICP in patients with TBI are intracerebral hemor-

TABLE 26.3. Types of Cerebral Edema

Type of Edema	Pathogenesis	Blood-Brain Barrier	Fluid	Possible Causes
Cytotoxic	Cellular swelling	Intact	Water/sodium chloride	Hypoxia Diabetic ketoacidosis Reye's syndrome Water intoxication
Vasogenic	Increased capillary permeability	Disrupted	Plasma filtrate and proteins	Traumatic brain injury CNS neoplasms CNS abscess Meningitis Stroke Hemorrhage
Interstitial	Increased fluids from blocked CSF absorption	Intact	CSF	Obstructive hydrocephalus

Source: Adapted from Critchley. Raised intercranial pressure. In: *Neurological Emergencies.* Philadelphia, Pa: WB Saunders, 1989.

rhage, extracerebral mass lesions such as subdural or epidural hematomas, SAH, occlusion of venous drainage, generalized cerebral edema, and hydrocephalus.[11] Serious TBI often results in multiple areas of brain contusion. The resultant hyperemic areas in the injured regions of the brain cause an increase in ICP by increasing CBF and CBV. The loss of integrity of the blood–brain barrier leads to the production of vasogenic edema. TBI causes dysfunction at the cellular membrane level, in turn causing intracellular accumulation of water, or cytotoxic edema. (See Chapter 30, "Traumatic Brain Injury.")

Cerebrovascular Events

The various cerebrovascular etiologies for increased ICP include SAH, intracerebral hematoma, cerebral venous thrombosis, and cerebral infarct.[12] SAH, a common event following TBI, is associated with aneurysmal or arteriovenous malformation ruptures. Patients generally present with a sudden onset of an explosive, severe headache typically described as "the worst headache of my life." Accom-

panying nausea, vomiting, photophobia, and nuchal rigidity can be present. Increased ICP associated with aneurysm rupture is at times secondary to obstructive hydrocephalus due to blood within the ventricular system obstructing ventricular flow. Major complications of SAH are rebleeding and vasospasm. Rebleeding can account for sudden and harmful rises in ICP. The risk of vasospasm is greater in the first two weeks after the hemorrhage and can result in areas of ischemic infarct, which can act as mass lesions with adjacent cerebral edema. Because of the severe disabling consequences of vasospasm, early surgical treatment of the aneurysm is recommended for many patients.

Intracerebral hemorrhage is a typical consequence of poorly controlled hypertension and is a common cause of increased ICP. The most common locations of hemorrhage include the internal capsule, thalamus, pons, basal ganglia, subcortical white matter, and cerebellum. In the emergency department, recognition of cerebellar hemorrhage is important because these patients can benefit from early neurosurgical intervention.[12] These patients typically present with headache, vomiting, vertigo, and occasionally, loss of consciousness. Physical findings include sixth nerve palsy and respiratory depression due to brainstem compression.

By decreasing venous return, cerebral venous thrombosis can cause interstitial edema of brain parenchyma. This results in a rise in ICP and can occur with thrombotic events such as sagittal sinus thrombosis, cavernous sinus thrombosis, and superior vena cava syndrome.

Cerebral infarction generally does not cause an acute rise in ICP. The resultant vasogenic edema develops over a period of about three days postinfarction and often causes generalized elevation in ICP which, in turn, can produce a herniation syndrome. Clinical presentation depends on the anatomical location of the infarction.

Hydrocephalus

Hydrocephalus can be regarded clinically as a pathological accumulation of intracranial CSF, usually within the cerebral ventricles. Hydrocephalus is broadly classified as either *obstructive*, that is, associated with an impairment of circulation or absorption of CSF, or *nonobstructive*, which refers to the enlargement of the ventricular system and CSF spaces due to loss of brain tissue (ex vacuo hydrocephalus). Obstructive hydrocephalus is subcategorized into *communicating obstructive hydrocephalus*, which refers to a blockage outside the ventricular system such that the ventricular fluid is in communication with the subarachnoid space. Communicating hydrocephalus occurs from an inflammatory process such as bacterial meningitis or subarachnoid hemorrhage. *Noncommunicating obstructive hydrocephalus* results from blockage within the ventricular system, which prevents communication of CSF with the subarachnoid space.[13] Etiologies of obstructive hydrocephalus include intraventricular mass lesions such as colloid cyst, obstructive intraventricular hemorrhage, and aqueductal stenosis.[7] Interstitial edema results from the obstruction, and patients typically present with headache, vomiting, and other symptoms, depending on the etiology and the site of the obstruction.

Brain Tumor

Brain tumors and associated vasogenic edema can produce a gradual rise in ICP.[14] Slow-growing tumors such as meningiomas can be silent clinically until sudden deterioration from increased ICP is identified. More rapidly growing malignant tumors such as glioblastomas present with a more rapid increase in ICP. Benign tumors and cysts can also have dramatic presentations, depending on the rate of growth and location of the lesion.

Central Nervous System Infection

Eighty-five percent of adults with meningitis have opening pressures greater than 300 mm CSF at lumbar puncture.[15] The elevation of pressure is due to meningeal inflammation. Hydrocephalus can develop, which exacerbates the increase in ICP.

Intracranial abscesses are mass lesions associated with a subacute or chronic rise in ICP, and vasogenic edema. Patients are commonly febrile without or with focal symptoms. Sixty percent of all abscesses arise from contiguous spread of infection from the middle ear or paranasal sinuses. The remainder result from blood-borne infection.

Metabolic and Hypoxic Encephalopathies

Cerebral edema is the most common cause of death in patients with hepatic failure. The exact mechanism is likely due to disruption of the blood–brain barrier. Increased ICP that occurs in hyperglycemic states results from the development of cerebral edema, which can be due to the underlying disease entity or a complication of therapy. Severe hyponatremia, a typical result of water intoxication, can lead to an increase in ICP secondary to cytotoxic edema. Patients at risk include schizophrenics and hospitalized patients receiving hypotonic fluids.

Reye's syndrome is a rare disorder associated with the use of aspirin during a viral infection, particularly varicella zoster. Incessant vomiting, hypoglycemia, and deteriorating mental status are some of the dominant features of this syndrome. Mortality from this syndrome is directly related to the increased ICP from accumulating cytotoxic edema.[10]

Hypoxic encephalopathy is associated with postresuscitation cardiac arrest, TBI, airway obstruction, near-drowning states, or birth.

Status Epilepticus

Status epilepticus can cause significant cerebral neuronal injury resulting in increased ICP. The neuronal injury is likely due to ischemia and hypoxia. The mortality rate ranges from 3% in children to 25% in adults.[16]

Management

As with the management of patients with any other potentially life-threatening event, management of patients with increased ICP requires immediate at-tention to airway, breathing, and circulation (see Fig. 26.3). The goals of airway management are pro-tection of the airway and controlled ventilation. Routine hyperventilation, especially within the first 24 hours after brain injury, is not indicated. Rapid-sequence intubation (RSI) is the preferred method of securing the airway in order to prevent laryngeal spasm, which can raise the ICP (see Chapter 25, "Neuroanesthesiology"). When succinylcholine is

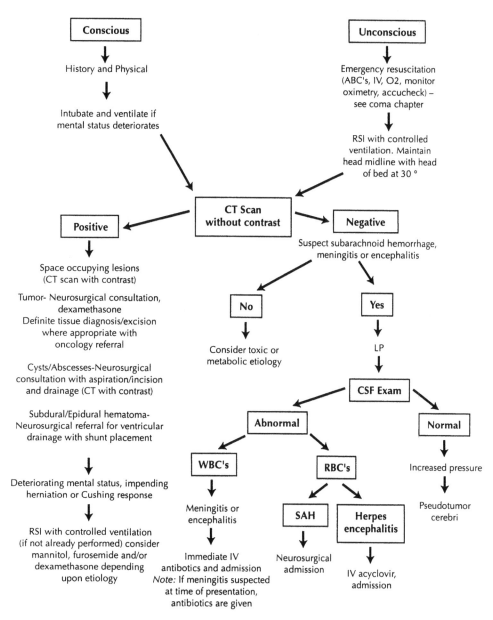

FIGURE 26.3. Management of patient with suspected raised intracranial pressure. ABCs = airway, breathing, and circulation; CSF = cerebrospinal fluid; CT = computerized to-mography; IV = intravenous; LP = lumbar puncture; RBCs = red blood cells; RSI = rapid sequence intubation; SAH = subarachnoid hemorrhage; WBCs = white blood cells.

used for intubation, a priming dose of pancuronium or a minidose of succinylcholine is used to decrease the likelihood of fasciculations, which can increase ICP and lead to emesis and aspiration of gastric contents. Pretreatment with lidocaine (1–1.5 mg/kg, given two minutes before intubation) can blunt the increase in ICP associated with tracheal intubation.[20]

Maintenance of Adequate Systemic Blood Pressure

An increase in ICP associated with TBI (except for concomitant heavy blood loss from scalp injuries) does not cause hypotension and shock. Because systemic hypotension is associated with increased morbidity and mortality, systemic blood pressure is maintained above 90 mm Hg. Adequate fluid resuscitation is carried out using either lactated Ringer's solution or normal saline. Recently, the use of hypertonic saline solution in fluid resuscitation has been shown to result in less cerebral edema and lower ICP values than isotonic saline.[21] More comprehensive clinical trials studying the use of hypertonic saline in patients with TBI and increased ICP are needed. Profound increases in ICP and ensuing brain herniation may be associated with hypertension and bradycardia (Cushing's phenomenon) as a terminal event. Spinal injuries above T1 can cause hypotension and bradycardia, which are treated with inotropic support.

Role of Hyperventilation

Controlled ventilation is an important procedure in the management of patients with increased ICP. The traditional role of hyperventilation has been challenged recently. Routine use of hyperventilation to "prevent" increased ICP is no longer recommended. Controlled hyperventilation with maintenance of $Paco_2$ levels between 25 mm Hg and 40 mm Hg and PaO_2 levels at or above 80 mm Hg for a short duration is recommended when intracranial hypertension is refractory to sedation, paralysis, CSF drainage, or the use of osmotic diuretics. Chronic prophylactic hyperventilation is avoided in the first five days after severe TBI and particularly during the first 24 hours because CBF measurements in patients with severe TBI demonstrate a "low" CBF state.[22] Hyperventilation reduces CBF further, does not consistently lower ICP, and can

contribute to a loss of autoregulation. Cerebrovascular response to hypercapnea is reduced in those patients with the most severe injuries such as diffuse brain contusions. The CBF level at which irreversible ischemia occurs is not clearly known, but ischemic cell injury has been demonstrated in 90% of those who die following TBI.[23,24]

Role of Diuretics

Mannitol, an osmotic diuretic, is currently the diuretic of choice for treating increased ICP. Mannitol acts by two distinct mechanisms. There is an initial rapid fall in ICP after the administration of mannitol due to reflex vasoconstriction that results from its ability to increase flow velocity in cerebral vessels. Following this, mannitol gradually causes dehydration of areas of brain where the blood–brain barrier is intact. An osmotic gradient is established between intra- and extracellular compartments with dehydration of normal and edematous brain.[5,9] Mannitol has the capacity to diffuse across injured areas of the brain and, in some instances, can increase edema in focally injured areas of the brain. When mannitol is given in therapeutic doses, significant diuresis results, which requires close monitoring of the patient's volume status and serum osmolality. Hyperosmotic states (>320 mOsm/dl) are avoided. Plasma osmolality of more than 320 mOsm/dl can result in renal tubular toxicity and renal failure. The dosage of mannitol is 1 g/kg given over a period of 10–20 minutes, followed by smaller doses of approximately 0.25–0.50 g/kg every 4–6 hours.[10]

Furosemide, a loop diuretic, is effective in lowering ICP. It seems to have a synergistic effect when used with mannitol. The adverse effect associated with combined therapy is accelerated electrolyte loss, which requires close monitoring of the patient's volume status and serum electrolyte levels.

Role of Corticosteroids

Recent studies have not shown a beneficial effect of steroid use in the management of patients with increased ICP resulting from trauma.[12,25,26] However, corticosteroids have proven effective in the reduction of vasogenic edema caused by abscesses and by primary or metastatic neoplasms of the brain. Although the edema surrounding brain hemorrhage is known to be vasogenic, corticosteroids typically are not recommended. Dexamethasone, at an initial dose of 10 mg followed by 4 mg every six hours, is used when indicated. When the cause of increased ICP is uncertain, and a neurodiagnostic test is not immediately available, a single dose of corticosteroids does not adversely affect the outcome.

Role of Barbiturate Coma

Barbiturate therapy is effective in lowering ICP in a select subset of patients such as those with persistently high ICP despite aggressive management.[27] Barbiturates lower ICP through vasoconstriction of the cerebral vessels and depression of cerebral metabolism.[28] Therapy is usually begun with pentobarbital in a dose of 3–5 mg/kg given over several minutes. A change in ICP is noted in about 15 minutes. When the response is favorable, treatment is continued at a dose of 1–2 mg/kg per hour. Serum pentobarbital levels are followed and should not exceed 4 mg/dl. However, the complications of pentobarbital coma often preclude its use. Hypotension is the most common and serious complication; typically it occurs when pentobarbital levels exceed 4 mg/dl. This is due to a decrease in the systemic vascular resistance and a direct myocardial depressant effect, which can lead to a reduction in CPP despite a lowered ICP. Additional complications include an increase in incidence of pneumonia and systemic infections. Thus barbiturate therapy can be effective in lowering ICP when uncontrolled ICP is refractory to all conventional medical and surgical ICP-lowering treatments. The use of barbiturates for prophylactic management of patients with increased ICP is not indicated.

Miscellaneous Management Points

Patients with suspected ICP, particularly patients with TBI, should have the head of their bed elevated to 30 degrees. The head is positioned in the midline to augment venous drainage.[29]

Endotracheal suctioning causes a transient but significant rise in ICP that cannot be ameliorated with preoxygenation. Some patients actually show a cumulative increase in ICP based on the number of suction catheter passes. Therefore, it is recommended to pretreat patients with lidocaine, 1 mg/kg given intravenously, and to limit the number of suction catheter passes to two per procedure.[30,31]

Seizures can increase ICP by increasing metabolic and electrical activity within the brain, and are managed aggressively and prevented when possible.[1,2,14] Generalized seizures in a patient with an elevated ICP can be life-threatening.

High fever is treated aggressively in patients with elevated ICP, because it increases cerebral metabolism and CBF. Mild hypothermia of a few degrees has been shown to be beneficial, for unknown reasons.

Monitoring Techniques

There is no reliable clinical sign of increasing ICP. A high index of suspicion of its presence is based on the clinical presentation and guides the evaluation of an underlying cause. Of the several noninvasive methods of measuring ICP on an emergency basis, transcranial Doppler examination and tympanic membrane displacement are commonly advocated but are not practiced routinely.[1,2] The most widely used method to monitor ICP continuously is an invasive procedure of intraventricular catheter placement (see Fig. 26.4). The catheter is inserted through a burr hole over the convexity just anterior to the coronal suture and in relation to the ipsilateral pupil. The method allows for continuous and reliable monitoring of ICP, and it provides a poten-

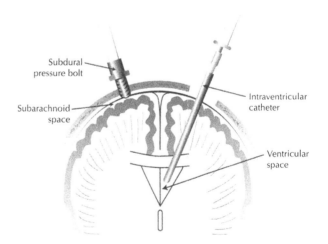

FIGURE 26.4. Schematic representation of a subdural pressure bolt *(left)* and an intraventricular catheter *(right)*. Both systems are connected by nonexpansile tubing to a pressure transducer (from JE McGillicuddy, Cerebral protection: Pathophysiology and treatment of increased intracranial pressure. *Chest.* 1985;87:85–93. Used with permission).

tial route for the drainage of CSF in instances of refractory increases of ICP. Other methods include a fiberoptic system, with placement of the monitor in an intraparenchymal or subdural location.[32] Another method, rarely used, is placement of a subdural bolt in the subdural space through a twist hole at the right frontal convexity. The bolt is connected to a pressure transducer for ICP readings.

PEARLS AND PITFALLS

- Increasing ICP cannot be reliably detected clinically. Increased ICP is considered in patients with TBI, known brain tumor, or CNS infection.
- Adequate oxygenation with controlled ventilation is required in the treatment of patients with increasing ICP either out-of-hospital or in the emergency department.
- Maintenance of a normal arterial blood pressure is critical in a patient with increased ICP. Fluid resuscitation, pressors, or antihypertensives are used as indicated.
- Keep the head of the bed at 30 degrees to augment venous drainage in patients with elevated ICP.
- Seizures are prevented or treated rigorously when present.
- Prophylactic hyperventilation is not indicated in the management of patients with increased ICP.
- The absence of papilledema does not exclude the diagnosis of increased ICP.
- A repeat CT scan of the brain is considered in a patient with declining mental status despite aggressive management.

REFERENCES

1. Pickard JD, Czosnyka M. Management of raised intracranial pressure. *J Neurol Neurosurg Psychiatry.* 1993;56:845–58.
2. Pickard JD, Czosnyka M. Raised intracranial pressure. In: Hughes RAC, ed. *Neurological Emergencies.* 1st ed. London: BMG, 1994:150–86.
3. Pepe PE, Copass MK, Joyce TH. Prehospital endotracheal intubation: rationale for training emergency medical personnel. *Ann Emerg Med.* 1985;14:1085–92.
4. Fink ME. Emergency management of the head-injured patient. *Emerg Med Clin North Am.* 1987;5:783–95.
5. Wilkinson HA. Intracranial pressure. In: Youmans JR, ed. *Neurosurgery.* Philadelphia, Pa: WB Saunders Co; 1990:661–91.
6. Duncan CC, Ment LR. Central nervous system: head injury. In: Toulorian RJ, ed. *Pediatric Trauma,* 2nd ed. Philadelphia, Pa: CV Mosby; 1990.
7. Critchley EM. *Neurological Emergencies.* Philadelphia, Pa: WB Saunders Co; 1989:97–149.
8. McGillicuddy JE. Cerebral protection: pathophysiology and treatment of increased cranial pressure. *Chest.* 1985;87:85–93.
9. Miller ER. Nursing care of the head injured patient. In: Becher DF, Euderman SK, eds. *Textbook of Head Injury.* 1st ed. Philadelphia, Pa: WB Saunders Co; 1989:386–419.
10. Bingaman WV, Frank JI. Malignant cerebral edema and intracranial hypertension. *Neurol Clin.* 1995;13:479–509.
11. Bleck T. Increased intracranial pressure. In: Schwartz E, ed. *Emergency Medicine.* Philadelphia, Pa: WB Saunders, 1992 :1573–80.
12. Critchley EM. *Neurological Emergencies.* 1st ed. Philadelphia, Pa: WB Saunders Co; 1989;233–75.
13. Roth PA, Conen AR. Management of hydrocephalus in infants and children. In: Tindall N, Cooper PR, Barrow DL, eds. *The Practice of Neurosurgery,* Baltimore, Md: Williams and Wilkins; 1995;2707–10.
14. Hareri RJ. Cerebral edema. *Neurosurg Clin N Am.* 1994;5:687–706.
15. Ashwal S. Neurologic evaluation of the patient with acute bacterial meningitis. *Neurol Clin.* 1995;13:529–48.
16. Chang CW, Blech TP. Status epilepticus. *Neurol Clin.* 1995;13:529–48.
17. American College of Surgeons Committee on Trauma Staff. *Advanced Trauma Life Support.* 3rd ed. Chicago, Ill: American College of Surgeons; 1991.
18. Kreiger D, Adams WR, Schwartz S, et al. Prognostic and clinical relevance of pupillary responses, intracranial pressure monitoring, and brainstem auditory evokes potentials in comatose patients with acute supratentorial mass lesions. *Crit Care Med.* 1993;21:1944–50.
19. Purdy PO, Eckard DA. Traumatic brain injury. In: Redman HC, Purdy PD, Miller GL, et al., eds. *Emergency Radiology.* 1st ed. Philadelphia, Pa: WB Saunders Co; 1993:1–38.
20. Gabriel EM, Boul CO. Emergency treatment of patients with severe head injury. *J Crit Illn.* 1996;11:75–83.
21. Gunnar W, Jonasson I, Merlotti G, et al. Head injury and hemorrhagic shock: studies of the blood brain barrier and intracranial pressure after resuscitation with normal saline solution, 3% saline solution and dextran 40. *Surgery.* 1988;103:398–407.
22. Obrist WD, Langfitt TW, Jaggl JL, et al. Cerebral blood flow and metabolism in comatose patients with acute head injury. *J Neurosurg.* 1984;61:241–53.

23. Muizlaar JP, Marmaron A, Ward JD, et al. Adverse effects of prolonged hyperventilation in patients with severe head injury. A randomized clinical trial. *J Neurosurg.* 1991;75:731–9.

24. Brain Trauma Foundation. Guidelines for the management of severe head injury. 1995; Section IX:2–7.

25. Dearden NM, Gibson JS, McDowall DG, et al. Effect of high dose dexamethason on outcome from severe head injury. *J Neurosurg.* 1986;61:81.

26. Braakman R, Schoulten HI, Braau-Van Diskoech, et al. Megadose steroids in severe head injury. Results of prospective double blind clinical trial. *Neurosurg Clin North Am.* 1994;5:573–605.

27. Eisenberg HM, Frankowski RF, Contant CF, et al. High dose barbiturate control of elevated intracranial pressure in patients with severe head injury. *J Neurosurg.* 1988;69:15–23.

28. Cassell NF, Hitchon PW, Gerk MK, et al. Alterations in cerebral blood flow, oxygen metabolism, and electrical activity produced by high dose thiopental. *Neurosurgery.* 1980;7:598–603.

29. Ropper AH, O'Rourke D, Kennedy SK. Head position, intracranial pressure and compliance. *Neurology.* 1982;32:1288–91.

30. Rudy EB, Baun M, Stone K, Turner B. The relationship between endotracheal suctioning and changes in intracranial pressure: a review of the literature. *Heart Lung.* 1986;16:488–94.

31. Rudy EB, Turner BS, Baun M, Stone KS, Brucia J. Endotracheal suctioning in adults with head injury. *Heart Lung.* 1991;20:667–74.

32. Chambers IR, Mendelow AD, Simar EJ, Modha P. A clinical evaluation of the camino subdural screw and vent monitoring kits. *Neurosurgy.* 1990;26:421–3.

33. Wilkins RH, Rengochary SS, eds. *Neurosurgery.* 2nd ed. New York, NY: McGraw-Hill Book Co; 1996:349.

27 Idiopathic Intracranial Hypertension

ERIC EGGENBERGER, SID M. SHAH, MARSHA D. RAPPLEY

SUMMARY Idiopathic intracranial hypertension (IIH) should be considered in the younger patient who presents to the emergency department with headaches or papilledema. IIH can cause severe and permanent visual sequlae. Diagnosis is focused on excluding other conditions that can cause disc edema and symptoms suggestive of increased intracranial pressure most notably space occupying lesions. The pace of visual loss in IIH is typically slow, and similar to glaucoma in affecting peripheral vision before central visual acuity. Therapy is initiated with a weight loss program and oral diuretics such as acetazolamide; however, surgery with either optic nerve sheath fenestration or lumboperitoneal shunting is required in a minority of patients.

Introduction

Idiopathic intracranial hypertension (IIH) and pseudotumor cerebri (PTC) (previously known as otitic hydrocephalus, hypertensive meningeal hydrops, intracranial pressure without brain tumor, and benign intracranial hypertension) are the most common terms applied to a clinical syndrome resulting from increased intracranial pressure (ICP) without a known pathophysiology. The only major permanent sequela of IIH is visual loss.

Epidemiology and Pathophysiology

IIH typically is a disease of obese young females: over 90% of IIH patients are overweight and over 90% are women, with a mean age of 30 years at diagnosis. IIH is rare, with an annual incidence of approximately 1 per 100,000 persons; however, among obese women between the ages of 20 and 44, the incidence increases to approximately 19 per 100,000 persons.[1] Pediatric cases of IIH are uncommon.

The pathophysiology of IIH remains enigmatic. The epidemiology of IIH suggests a relationship to hormonal alterations; however, the exact association remains unknown. Recent hypotheses suggest that cerebral venous outflow obstructions are related to the final common pathway, leading to increased ICP.[2]

Numerous case reports linking IIH and various conditions include medication use [nitrofurantoin, vitamin A, isoretinoin, nalidixic acid, indomethacin or ketoprofen (with Bartter's syndrome), lithium, anabolic and corticosteroids, chlordecone (Kepone), amiodarone, tetracyclines, cyclosporin, levonorgestrel implants (Norplant), psychotropics, and corticosteroid withdrawal], endocrinopathies, paraproteinemia, systemic lupus erythematosus (SLE), pregnancy, menstrual irregularities, iron deficiency anemia, renal failure, and Guillain-Barré syndrome. Among the medication use that is associated with IIH, vitamin A derivatives and the tetracycline family of antibiotics are the most common. However, no causal link between these conditions has been established, and controlled studies have demonstrated significant associations only with obesity and recent weight gain.[3] Many of the reported associations with IIH are common conditions among females of childbearing years and may represent chance occurrences.

TABLE 27.1. Various Conditions Associated with IIH

Endocrine/ Metabolic	Drugs/Toxins	Hematological disorder	Connective tissue disorders	Conditions of high CSF protein	Infections	Empty Sella Syndrome	Miscellaneous
Obesity	Vitamin A	Iron deficiency anemia	Lupus erythematosus	Spinal cord tumors	Bacterial meningitis		Sydenham's chorea
Menstrual disorders	Retinoic acid	Cryofibrino-genemia		Polyneuritis	Viral meningitis		After head trauma
Menarche	Tetracycline				Inf. Mono-nucleosis		Primary or idiopathic sinus thrombosis
Addison's disease	Nalidixic acid						Intracranial venous-sinus thrombosis
Hypopara-thyroidism	Amiodarone						Idiopathic
Hyperadrenalism	Lithium						
Rapid growth in infancy	Nitrofurantoin						
	Progesterone preparations						

Clinical Features

Recognition of IIH is important because it is not necessarily a benign condition and often requires specialized treatment. Typically, the patient with IIH is a young, obese, white female with a headache. In a prospective, controlled study of 50 patients with IIH, headache was the most common initial symptom (94%), followed by transient visual obscurations (68%), pulsatile intracranial noises (58%), photopsia (54%), retrobulbar pain (44%), diplopia (38%), and visual loss (30%).[4] Other investigators have reported similar findings.[5–7] The headache typically is worse on awakening or in the mornings and may be aggravated by straining or coughing. Transient visual obscurations occur in association with optic disc edema, and are characterized by brief episodes (seconds to minutes) of marked diminution, blackout, graying, or complete visual loss often precipitated by postural changes or straining. Although these episodes are benign, they suggest possible optic disc edema, which in the early stages is associated with normal vision. Commonly, patients do not report pulsatile tinnitus unless asked specifically. Diplopia reflects either unilateral or bilateral abducens nerve palsies, a nonlocalizing, potential consequence of increased ICP from any cause. Other disturbances of ocular motility suggest diagnoses other than IIH.

The clinical signs of IIH are generally limited to the visual and ocular motor systems, and examination of patients with suspected IIH focuses on visual acuity, visual fields, eye movements, and fundoscopy (see Fig. 27.1 A–D). Papilledema is present in the vast majority of patients with IIH, and it is indistinguishable from that resulting from any other cause of elevated ICP. Papilledema is usually bilateral but can be asymmetrical or unilateral in some cases. When ICP is elevated at the time of ophthalmoscopy, spontaneous venous pulsations typically are absent; however, approximately 20% of healthy individuals lack spontaneous venous pulsations, thereby diminishing the diagnostic value of their absence. Occasionally, papilledema may be accompanied by a macular exudate or other retinal pathology that may affect vision. Rare cases of IIH without papilledema have been reported.[8]

Visual loss is typically absent in the early stages of papilledema, and it may be minimal on routine examination despite severe chronic papilledema including retinal hemorrhages. Only 13% of patients

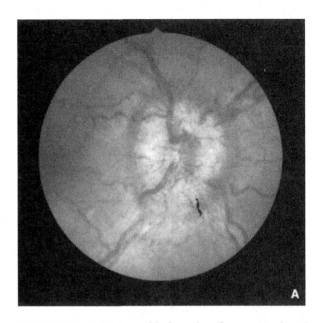

FIGURE 27.1. A 25-year-old obese female presented with increasing headache and diplopia. (A) Initial examination revealed 20/20 vision in each eye with normal color vision and pupils; chronic-appearing fully developed disc edema was present in each eye. [Right eye shown] (B) Even with this degree of papilledema, the afferent visual examination revealed only an enlarged blind spot in each eye. Neuroimaging was unremarkable, and lumbar puncture revealed OP 458 mm H_2O. With the addition of acetazolamide, headaches and diplopia resolved. Follow-up examination 3 months after presentation revealed resolution of (C) disc edema and (D) enlarged blind spots.

with IIH demonstrate Snellen visual acuity (VA) less than 20/20 upon initial evaluation.[4] However, visual fields are often abnormal. Whether patients with IIH are tested by kinetic or static perimetry, approximately 50–75% demonstrate significant visual field defects.[5,9] Enlargement of the blind spot, resulting from swelling-induced peripapillary refractive error, is the most common defect (see Fig. 27.1B). Other defects include paracentral scotomas and arcuate or altitudinal field loss. Constriction of the peripheral field may be present in chronic cases. The rate of vision loss in patients with IIH is variable, but typically it is slow and characterized by peripheral visual field defects that develop long before central vision is affected, as measured by Snellen VA. Like glaucoma, visual loss can go unreported until it is profound, and formal visual field testing (Goldmann or Humphrey perimetry) is crucial in managing these patients.[10] Patients with IIH

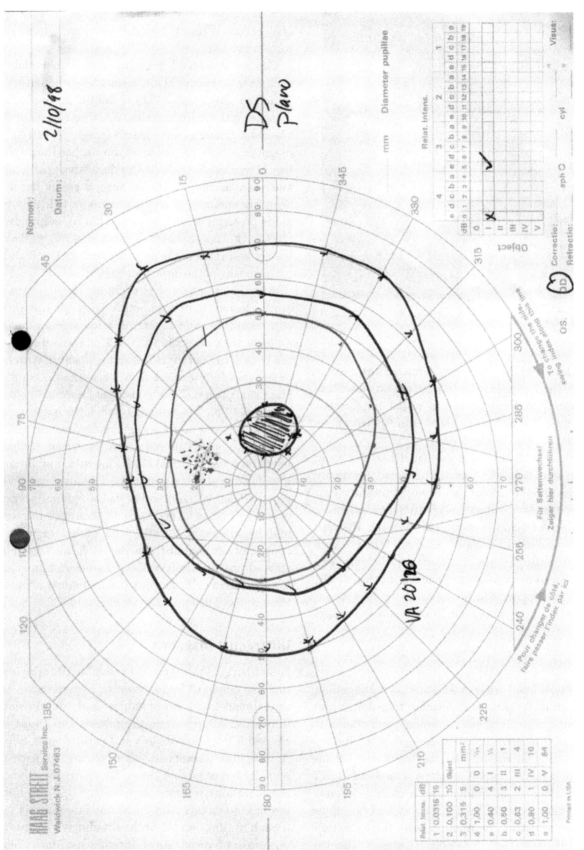

FIGURE 27.1. *(Continued)*

B

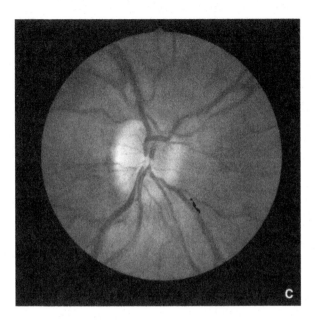

FIGURE 27.1. (*Continued*)

rarely lose vision acutely; systemic or intraocular hypertension appear to be risk factors for acute loss of vision. Blindness or severe visual impairment occurs in up to 25% of patients with IIH who have extended follow-up evaluations.[5]

Clinical evidence suggests that IIH is a chronic disease and that ICP remains elevated for many years despite the resolution of symptoms and signs. Approximately 8% of patients with IIH experience a recurrence of symptoms and papilledema after apparent resolution of the syndrome.[5] When severe optic disc atrophy has occurred, papilledema may not be present with recurrence of increased ICP. Therefore, long-term follow-up of patients is essential even in those whose condition seems to resolve.

Diagnosis

IIH is considered when evaluating a young patient with symptoms such as headache, transient visual obscurations, or diplopia, or when papilledema is detected; however, IIH is a diagnosis of exclusion. IIH is characterized by four major criteria: (1) increased ICP; (2) normal cerebrospinal fluid (CSF) composition; (3) no evidence of a central nervous system mass lesion or hydrocephalus; and (4) a nonfocal neurological examination, with the exception of papilledema with its potential visual sequelae

and occasional abducens nerve palsies. Rarely, IIH can occur without papilledema and does not threaten vision.

Contrast-enhanced neuroimaging is essential to exclude other causes of increased ICP. Although computerized tomography (CT) is helpful in excluding mass lesions, hydrocephalus, or other causes of increased ICP, magnetic resonance imaging (MRI) is the diagnostic study of choice because it has the advantage of increased sensitivity for dural sinus pathology and vascular malformations. Several subtle imaging signs are common accompaniments of IIH; they include posterior scleral flattening (80%), empty sella (70%), optic nerve sheath distension (45%), prelaminar enhancement of the optic nerve (50%), and vertical tortuosity of the optic nerve (40%).[11]

After neuroimaging has excluded the presence of a mass lesion, lumbar puncture with opening pressure recording and CSF examination are required in patients with suspected IIH. ICP is measured with the patient in the lateral decubitus position with his or her legs fully extended. An opening pressure of less than 250 mm CSF is considered normal in obese patients.[12] Patients with IIH can have large variations in ICP, and rarely, a single measurement of ICP may be normal.[13] Patients who are suspected of having IIH but have normal ICP as measured by lumbar puncture need to be evaluated for other causes of papilledema. When no other cause is found, repeat or serial LPs may be necessary to document intracranial hypertension. A diagnosis of IIH requires a completely normal CSF analysis. CSF findings of increased protein levels or the presence of more than 5 white blood cells suggests inflammatory, neoplastic, or infectious etiologies for elevated ICP.

Differential Diagnosis

Pathological conditions that resemble IIH clinically include cerebral mass lesions, hypertensive encephalopathy, hydrocephalus, and dural sinus thrombosis. Dural sinus thrombosis can cause increased ICP with cephalgia and papilledema. Superior sagittal thrombosis often occurs in patients with hypercoagulable disorders. Seizures, hemorrhagic venous infarcts, and bloody CSF are often present in patients with dural sinus thrombosis. Although findings on CT of the brain may suggest the diagnosis of dural sinus thrombosis (the "delta"

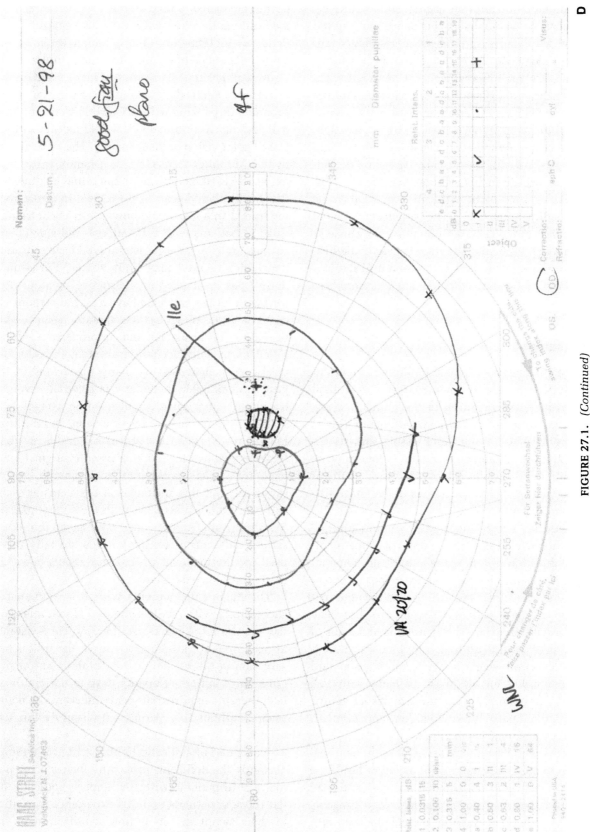

FIGURE 27.1. *(Continued)*

D

sign of blood clot within the sagittal sinus), MRI is a more sensitive test to detect this condition (sagittal T1-weighted images and magnetic resonance angiography sequences are very useful). Chronic forms of meningitis such as cryptococcal meningitis can resemble IIH initially because of headache and papilledema. CSF results are diagnostic with a positive cryptococcal antigen and cellular reaction. Rarely, certain tumors can cause symptoms and signs suggestive of IIH, especially early in the clinical course. These include gliomatosis cerebri (diffuse neoplasia involving astrocytes) and soft tissue tumor seeding of the CSF.[14] The patient is evaluated for associated medical conditions that can cause or aggravate IIH. Particular attention is paid to medication use, especially in those who do not fit the profile typical of patients with IIH, such as nonobese males.

Management

IIH is best managed by a team including a neurologist, ophthalmologist, and neurosurgeon. Treatment is individualized according to the clinical setting and the condition of the patient. Goldmann kinetic or Humphrey 24–2 visual field testing, and stereoscopic fundus photographs guide follow-up care and treatment decisions. Changes in visual acuity or visual evoked potentials are signs of end-stage IIH-related optic nerve injury.

The initial management of asymptomatic patients who have no evidence of optic neuropathy includes education regarding the nature and potential complications of the condition, treatment of potential secondary causes, and a supervised weight loss program in obese patients. Weight loss has been documented to improve the symptoms and signs of IIH, but is often difficult to accomplish.[15–17] A medically supervised weight loss program is a standard recommendation for all obese patients with IIH. Regular follow-up with attention to visual acuity, visual fields, ocular motor function, and ophthalmoscopic appearance is required.

Patients who have no evidence of optic neuropathy and whose only complaint is mild headache can be treated with nonnarcotic analgesics. Severe headaches may respond to pharmacological agents such as beta blockers, calcium channel blockers, antidepressants, or ergot derivatives. Headaches that ap-

pear to be related to increased ICP can improve with medications that lower ICP such as acetazolamide. Patients with refractory, incapacitating headache, despite the absence of abnormal visual symptoms and signs, require surgical lowering of increased ICP.

A trial of medical therapy to lower ICP may be appropriate in patients with IIH who have mild visual deficits, such as minimal visual field defects without loss of color vision or visual acuity. The carbonic anhydrase inhibitor acetazolamide (Diamox) is the most frequently used medication in the initial treatment of IIH. Acetazolamide can be prescribed in doses ranging from 1 to 4 g per day; however, it is contraindicated in patients with sulfa allergy, and side effects such as limb paresthesias and altered taste sensation ("metallic" quality) may limit dosage. Furosemide (Lasix) has been used as alternative or adjunctive treatment for patients who have a partial response to acetazolamide. When medical therapy is successful, resolution of headache and improvement of papilledema usually occurs within about two to four weeks. Although used by many physicians in the past, systemic steroid therapy is generally avoided because of concomitant fluid retention, weight gain, systemic and intraocular hypertension, and multiple long-term adverse effects; however, steroids may be a final medical treatment option prior to surgical intervention.[18] Serial lumbar punctures may be used to lower ICP, but this treatment is often unsuccessful and over time is associated with the suboptimal patient followup. Other medical options are limited by serious side effects. Corticosteroids are only rarely used in the treatment of IIH, and should never be used for prolonged periods.

The majority of patients with IIH are managed successfully with medical therapy alone; relatively few require more aggressive therapy. The existence of a significant optic neuropathy at the initial presentation of the patient or the development or progression of optic neuropathy despite optimal medical therapy requires surgical intervention before severe, and possibly, permanent visual dysfunction occurs.

Placement of a silastic lumboperitoneal shunt is currently the definitive procedure for restoring normal ICP in patients with IIH. Reports indicate that 65–100% of patients with IIH experience resolution of their symptoms, including stabilization or improvement of visual function, following this procedure.[19–22] Although shunt function can be difficult to assess, and shunt complications such as obstruction, infection, and symptoms of low ICP (e.g., postural headache and dizziness) occur in some patients and may require shunt revision, lumboperitoneal shunting remains one of the preferred treatments for IIH.

Optic nerve sheath fenestration (ONSF) has been performed for the treatment of papilledema. ONSF creates one or more openings in the dural sheath of the orbital portion of the optic nerve just posterior to the globe. The exact mechanism of the success of ONSF in the treatment of papilledema is controversial. Mechanisms that have been postulated include a filtering function of the fenestration, and postfenestration nerve sheath scarring, which prevents the transmission of ICP to the optic nerves. Numerous reports have documented improved visual function and a relatively low rate of complication.[23–29] Following unilateral optic nerve sheath decompression, approximately 50% of patients experience relief of headache, and 50% of patients show improvement in the contralateral visual field, papilledema, or both.[26,27] The success and relative ease of this procedure have led many to recommend ONSF as the initial surgical procedure in the treatment of IIH. Nonetheless, the failure of ONSF to lower ICP consistently,[25,30–39] the potential for postoperative complications such as diplopia, pupillary dysfunction, and visual loss, and a failure rate of ONSF as high as 20%[40] are weighed against its potential benefits and underscore the clinical perception that there is no ideal treatment for IIH. Regardless of the treatment modality, posttreatment failures occur in many patients and highlight the need for diligent care of the patient subsequently.

Because swollen optic nerves require increased perfusion pressures, prophylactic surgical intervention is considered in certain circumstances such as in anticipation of potential hypotensive episodes (e.g., dialysis or the administration of medications with antihypertensive effects). Similarly, protective surgical intervention is considered when accurate monitoring of the patient's visual function is not possible.

IIH associated with evidence of severe or rapidly progressive optic neuropathy is a neuro-ophthalmological emergency. When untreated, these patients can become blind in a matter of days, and lost visual function can be regained rarely. Treatment in these situations is the immediate reduction of ICP, especially surrounding the optic nerves, and can include the use of mannitol and furosemide given intravenously, lumbar puncture, or lumbar drain. Attention is directed at minimizing coexistent risk factors for visual loss in IIH and avoiding extremes of blood pressure and intravascular volume. Although these measures may be appropriate for the short-term treatment of patients with acute loss of visual function, lumboperitoneal shunting or ONSF is performed within 24–48 hours after it has been determined that urgent treatment of IIH is required.

Disposition

Hospitalization is required when rapid visual loss or serious complications of IIH are suspected. Consultation with a neurologist, ophthalmologist, and neurosurgeon is indicated according to the severity of symptoms and the current treatment. When mild, recurrent symptoms of IIH – particularly headache – result in numerous evaluations in the emergency department, referral is given to the appropriate outpatient setting.

PEARLS AND PITFALLS

- IIH is suspected in an obese female patient of childbearing age who presents with headache, visual obscuration, or papilledema.
- Over 90% of patients with IIH are overweight; over 90% are females.
- In a patient with IIH, headaches frequently are worse on awakening or in the morning. Headaches can be aggravated by straining or coughing.
- Transient visual disturbances occur in association with optic disc edema and are characterized by brief episodes of diminished vision, blackout, or complete vision loss precipitated by postural changes or straining.
- Because 20% of the normal population lack spontaneous venous pulsations on funduscopy, absence of venous pulsations cannot reliably confirm the presence of increased ICP.
- Because only 13% of patients with IIH demonstrate Snellen visual acuity less than 20/20 upon initial evaluation, visual acuity cannot be relied on to document visual loss associated with IIH.

- The examination of visual fields (not commonly performed in the emergency department) is often abnormal in patients with IIH.
- Severe, episodic headache associated with known IIH refractory to diuretic use may respond to beta blockers, calcium channel blockers, antidepressants, or ergot derivatives.
- Hospitalization of a patient with IIH associated with rapid vision loss is prudent.

REFERENCES

1. Durcan FJ, Corbett JJ, Wall M. The incidence of pseudotumor cerebri. Population studies in Iowa and Louisiana. *Arch Neurol.* 1998;45:875–7.
2. Karahalios DG, Rekate HL, Khayata MH, et al. Elevated intracranial venous pressure as a universal mechanism in pseudotumor cerebri of varying etiologies. *Neurology.* 1996;46:198–202.
3. Giuseffi V, Wall M, Siegel PZ, Rojas PB. Symptoms and disease associations in idiopathic intracranial hypertension: a case-control study. *Neurology.* 1991; 41:239–44.
4. Wall M, George D. Idiopathic intracranial hypertension (pseudotumor cerebri): a prospective study of 50 patients. *Brain.* 1991;114:155–80.
5. Corbett JJ, Savino PJ, Thompson HS, et al. Visual loss in pseudotumor cerebri: follow-up of 57 patients from five to 41 years and a profile of 14 patients with permanent visual loss. *Arch Neurol.* 1982;39:461–74.
6. Round R, Keane JR. The minor symptoms of increased intracranial pressure: 101 patients with benign intracranial hypertension. *Neurology.* 1988;30:1461–4.
7. Rush JA. Pseudotumor cerebri: clinical profile and visual outcome in 63 patients. *Mayo Clin Proc.* 1980;55:541–6.
8. Marcelis J, Silberstein SD. Idiopathic intracranial hypertension without papilledema. *Arch Neurol.* 1991; 48:392–9.
9. Wall M, George D. Visual loss in pseudotumor cerebri. Incidence and defects related to visual field strategy. *Arch Neurol.* 1987;44:170–5.
10. Radhakrishnan K, Ahlskog JE, Garrity JA, Kurland LT. Idiopathic intracranial hypertension. *Mayo Clin Proc.* 1994;69:169–80.
11. Vaphiades MS, Brodsky MC. Neuroimaging signs of elevated intracranial pressure. Presented at North American Neuro-ophthalmologic Society, Orlando, Fla., March 1998.
12. Corbett JJ, Mehta MP. Cerebrospinal fluid pressure in normal obese subjects and patients with pseudotumor cerebri. *Neurology.* 1983;33: 1386–8.
13. Gucer G, Viernstein L. Long-term intracranial pressure recording in the management of pseudotumor cerebri. *J Neurosurg.* 1978;49:256–63.
14. Aroichane M, Miller NR, Eggenberger ER. Glioblastoma multiforme masquerading as pseudotumor cerebri. *J Neuroophthalmol.* 1993;13:105–12.
15. Newborg B. Pseudotumor cerebri treated by rice/reduction diet. *Arch Intern Med.* 1974;133:802–7.
16. Sugerman HJ, DeMaria EJ, Felton WL, et al. Increased intra-abdominal pressure and cardiac filling pressures in obesity-associated pseudotumor cerebri. *Neurology.* 1997;49:507–11.
17. Kupersmith ML, Gamell L, Turbin R, et al. Effects of weight loss on the course of idiopathic intracranial hypertension in women. *Neurology.* 1998;50:1094–8.
18. Liu GT, Glaser JS, Schatz NJ. High-dose methylprednisolone and acetazolamide for visual loss in pseudotumor cerebri. *Am J Ophthalmol.* 1994;118: 88–96.
19. Eggenberger ER, Miller NR, Vitale S. Lumboperitoneal shunt for the treatment of pseudotumor cerebri. *Neurology.* 1996;46:1524–30.
20. Burgett RA, Purvin VA, Kawasaki A. Lumboperitoneal shunting for pseudotumor cerebri. *Neurology.* 1997; 49:734–9.
21. Rosenberg M, Smith C, Beck R, et al. The efficacy of shunting procedures in pseudotumor cerebri. *Neurology.* 1989;39(suppl 1):209.
22. Johnston I, Besser M, Morgan MK. Cerebrospinal fluid diversion in the treatment of benign intracranial hypertension. *J Neurosurg.* 1988;69:195–202.
23. Goh KY, Schatz NJ, Glaser JS. Optic nerve sheath fenestration for pseudotumor cerebri. *J Neuroophthalmol.* 1997;17:86–91.
24. Acheson JF, Green WT, Sanders MD. Optic nerve sheath decompression for the treatment of visual failure in chronic raised intracranial pressure. *J Neurol Neurosurg Psychiatry.* 1994;57:1426–9.
25. Brourman ND, Spoor TC, Ramocki JM. Optic nerve sheath decompression for pseudotumor cerebri. *Arch Ophthalmol.* 1988;106:1378–83.
26. Sergott RC, Savino PJ, Bosley TM. Modified optic nerve sheath decompression provides long-term visual improvement for pseudotumor cerebri. *Arch Ophthalmol.* 1988;106:1384–90.
27. Corbett JJ, Nerad JA, Tse DT, Anderson RL. Results of optic nerve sheath fenestration for pseudotumor cerebri. The lateral orbitotomy approach. *Arch Ophthalmol.* 1988;106:1391–7.
28. Kelman SE, Sergott RC, Cioffi GA, Savino PJ, Bosley TM, Elman MJ. Modified optic nerve decompression in patients with functioning lumboperitoneal shunts and progressive visual loss. *Ophthalmology.* 1991; 98:1449–53.

29. Pearson PA, Baker RS, Khorram D, Smith TJ. Evaluation of optic nerve sheath fenestration in pseudotumor cerebri using automated perimetry. *Ophthalmology.* 1991;98:99–105.

30. Herzau V. Behandlung des pseudotumor cerebri. In: Berneaud-Kotz G, ed. *Versammlung des vereins Rheinisch-Westfalischer augenarzte.* Balve, West Germany: Zimmerman-Druck & Verlag; 91–6.

31. Davies G, Zilkha KJ. Decompression of the optic nerve in benign intracranial hypertension. *Trans Ophthalmol Soc UK.* 1976;96:427–9.

32. Kilpatrick CJ, Kaufman DV, Galbraith JEK, et al. Optic nerve decompression in benign intracranial hypertension. *Clin Exp Neurol.* 1981;18:161–8.

33. Kellen RI, Burde RM. Optic nerve decompression. *Arch Ophthalmol.* 1987;105:889.

34. Kaye AH, Galbraith JEK, King J. Intracranial pressure following optic nerve decompression for benign intracranial hypertension. Case report. *J Neurosurg.* 1981;55:453–7.

35. Billson FA, Hudson RL. Surgical treatment of chronic papilledema in children. *Br J Ophthalmol.* 1975; 59:92–5.

36. Burde RM, Karp JS, Miller RN. Reversal of visual deficit with optic nerve decompression in long-standing pseudotumor cerebri. *Am J Ophthalmol.* 1974; 77:770–2.

37. Knight RSG, Fielder AR, Feith JL. Benign intracranial hypertension: visual loss and optic nerve sheath fenestration. *J Neurol Neurosurg Psychiatry.* 1986;49:243–50.

38. Tomkins CM, Spalton DJ. Benign intracranial hypertension treated by optic nerve sheath decompression. *J R Soc Med.* 1984;77:141–4.

39. Gutgold-Glen H, Kattah JC, Chavis RM. Reversible visual loss in pseudotumor cerebri. *Arch Ophthalmol.* 1984;102:403–6.

40. Spoor TC, Ramocki JM, Madion MP, Wilkinson MJ. Treatment of pseudotumor cerebri by primary and secondary optic nerve sheath decompression. *Am J Ophthalmol.* 1991;112:177–85.

28 Normal Pressure Hydrocephalus

HENRY R. LANDSGAARD AND OLIVER W. HAYES

SUMMARY Normal pressure hydrocephalus is a syndrome of progressive dementia, gait disturbance, and urinary incontinence that is associated with ventriculomegaly and normal cerebrospinal fluid pressure. The symptoms associated with this adult form of chronic hydrocephalus may improve after ventriculoperitoneal shunting.

Introduction

Normal pressure hydrocephalus (NPH) is a clinical syndrome of progressive dementia, gait disturbance (gait apraxia), and urinary incontinence. NPH typically occurs in the elderly and progresses over weeks to years.[1] It is associated with enlarged ventricles and normal cerebrospinal fluid (CSF) pressures. NPH is a form of communicating hydrocephalus in which intracranial hypertension is absent or unrecognized. In some patients, NPH is a correctable cause of dementia and gait disturbance. Although NPH typically is not diagnosed or treated in the emergency department, recognition of the clinical syndrome and its associated clinical findings directs referral for further evaluation and possible treatment.

Pathophysiology

CSF is formed by the choroid plexus in the lateral ventricles, flows through the foramen of Monro into the third ventricle, through the aqueduct of Sylvius into the fourth ventricle, and exits the fourth ventricle through the foramina of Luschka and Magendie. Once outside the brainstem, the CSF enters the subarachnoid space and flows into the superior sagittal sinus via the arachnoid villi.[2]

The mechanisms that cause NPH are not clear because the relationship between ventriculomegaly, normal CSF pressures, and the resulting symptoms of NPH is not fully established. Isotope cisterno-graphic studies of patients with NPH demonstrate a communicating hydrocephalus that is likely due to partial obliteration of the subarachnoid space with defective reabsorption through the arachnoid villi.[3]

Most patients with NPH have normal or slightly increased CSF pressure at the time of examination, suggesting that the hydrocephalus was initiated by increased CSF pressure in the past. Continuous monitoring of CSF pressure in patients with NPH have shown intermittent elevation of CSF pressures above normal.[3] Delayed hydrocephalus can occur after head injury, subarachnoid hemorrhage, or meningoencephalitis. However, most patients with NPH have no history of these conditions, and in many cases the etiology is not known.

Clinical Manifestations

NPH is a clinical syndrome described as a triad of progressive dementia, gait disturbance (apraxia), and urinary incontinence that progresses over a period of weeks to years.[1] Examination of the patient shows varying signs of dementia, abnormal gait, increased tone in the lower limbs, hyperactive tendon jerk reflexes of the legs, and extensor plantar reflexes.

Gait disturbance is commonly the first symptom of NPH. It is an important clinical feature that helps to distinguish NPH from other dementias and is likely the best predictor of clinical improvement

Sid M. Shah and Kevin M. Kelly, eds., *Emergency Neurology: Principles and Practice.* Copyright © 1999 Cambridge University Press. All rights reserved.

378

following ventriculoperitoneal shunting.[4] No specific gait disorder occurs. The abnormal gait includes a broad-based stance, hesitant initiation of walking (apraxia), and frequent falling.

The dementia presents with lack of judgment and insight followed by impairment of immediate and recent recall. Initiative and spontaneity are decreased, and the patient typically is described by the family as disinterested, apathetic, or lethargic.[5,6] The dementia of NPH is commonly less severe and less rapidly progressive than that of Alzheimer's disease. Generally, patients do not have seizures, aphasia, agnosia, or other focal neurological deficits.

Urinary incontinence occurs in less than 50% of patients and is usually a late symptom of NPH. It is typically accompanied by a lack of awareness or concern by the patient. When untreated, NPH can progress resulting in the inability to stand and the eventual development of akinetic rigidity and withdrawn behavior.

Differential Diagnosis

The differential diagnosis includes syndromes that can cause dementia. The most common neurological conditions include Parkinson's disease, bifrontal brain disease due to tumor, metastases, or cerebral infarction, aqueductal stenosis, metabolic encephalopathy, and Alzheimer's disease. The characteristic gait disorder of NPH is its most reliable clinical feature.

Diagnostic Testing

The diagnosis of NPH is typically not made in the emergency department because of the common association of ventricular enlargement in patients with degenerative brain conditions, particularly Alzheimer's disease (see Table 28.1). When NPH is suspected clinically, computerized tomography (CT) with contrast enhancement is performed. Findings consistent with NPH include ventriculomegaly, minimal or absence of cortical atrophy, periventricular lucencies, and nearly normal-sized subarachnoid space. Magnetic resonance imaging (MRI) is the study of choice to evaluate ventriculomegaly and for functional imaging of CSF motion.[7] CSF velocity MRI is useful in the selection of patients with NPH to undergo ventriculoperitoneal shunting.[8]

Lumbar puncture with measurement of CSF pressure is necessary in the evaluation of patients with suspected NPH; however, lumbar puncture is rarely indicated in the emergency department unless other disease processes are suspected. CSF pressure readings in patients with NPH are usually in the range of 80–150 mm of water (H_2O). Serological and chemical studies of CSF are normal in NPH. Some patients with NPH experience temporary improvement in gait disturbance and cognitive functioning

TABLE 28.1. A Comparison of Findings of Normal Pressure Hydrocephalus and Alzheimer's Disease

Sign or Symptom	NPH	Alzheimer's Disease
Imbalance in gait or stance	Early symptom	Late symptom
Dementia	Subacute progression	Slow progression
Memory loss	Late occurrence	Early clinical finding
Gait type	Imbalance in turns	Shuffling, scuffing gait
	Broad-based, ataxic with hesitation	
Incontinence	Urinary, rarely fecal	Uncommon symptom

Source: Adapted from Gleason, Black, and Matsumae;[11] George, Holodny, and Deleon.[12]

following removal of 20–50 ml of CSF (i.e., with the CSF tap test).[5,9]

Treatment

When subacute progressive dementia and gait disturbance are accompanied by ventriculomegaly and normal CSF pressure, surgical correction with ventriculoperitoneal shunting is considered. Between 40% and 70% of patients improve after surgery, although recent literature suggests that surgical shunting may be less effective than originally believed.[5,10] The most important role of the emergency physician is to consider the diagnosis of NPH in patients with subacute progressive dementia and gait disturbance, and to initiate appropriate referral.

PEARLS AND PITFALLS

- NPH is a clinical syndrome of progressive dementia, gait disturbance, and urinary incontinence.
- NPH is associated with enlarged ventricles and normal CSF pressure.
- NPH is typically not diagnosed or treated in the emergency department. Recognizing the possibility of NPH in the emergency department directs appropriate referral.
- It is important to differentiate the dementia of NPH from that of other neurodegenerative processes.
- Ventriculoperitoneal shunting in selected patients with NPH can improve dementia and/or gait disturbance.

REFERENCES

1. Adams RD, Fisher CM, Hakim S, Ojemann RG, Sweet WH. Symptomatic occult hydrocephalus with "normal" cerebrospinal fluid pressure: a treatable syndrome. *N Engl J Med.* 1965;273:117–26.
2. Davson H, Welch K, Segal MB. The physiology and pathophysiology of cerebral spinal fluid. New York, NY: Churchill Livingstone; 1987.
3. Sahuqullo J, Rubio E, Codina A, et al. Reappraisal of the intracranial pressure and cerebrospinal fluid dynamics in patients with so-called "normal pressure hydrocephalus" syndrome. *Acta Neurochir.* 1991;112:50–61.
4. Sorenson PS, Jansen EC, Gjerris F. Motor disturbances in normal pressure hydrocephalus, special reference to stance and gait. *Arch Neurol.* 1986;43:34–8.
5. Ojemann RG, Black PM. Evaluation of the patient with dementia and treatment of normal pressure hydrocephalus. *Neurosurgery.* 1985;1:312–21.
6. Larsson A, Wikkelso C, Bilting M, Stephensen J. Clinical parameters in 74 consecutive patients shunt operated for normal pressure hydrocephalus. *Acta Neurol Scand.* 1991;84:475–82.
7. Feinberg DA. Neuroimaging. *Clin North Am.* 1995; 5:125–34.
8. Bradley WG, Scalzo D, Queralt J, Nitz WN, Atkinson DJ, Wong P. Normal pressure hydrocephalus: evaluation with cerebrospinal fluid measurements at MR imaging. *Radiology.* 1996;98:523–9.
9. Malm J, Kristensen B, Karlson T, Fagerlund M, Elfvevson J, Ekstedt J. The predictive value of cerebrospinal fluid dynamic tests in patients with idiopathic adult hydrocephalus syndrome. *Arch Neurol.* 1995;52:783–9.
10. Vanneste J, Augustijn P, Tan WF, Dirven C. Shunting normal pressure hydrocephalus: the predictive value of combined clinical and CT data. *J Neurol Neurosurg Psychiatry.* 1993;56:251–6.
11. Gleason PL, Black PM, Matsumae M. The neurobiology of normal pressure hydrocephalus. *Neurosurg Clin North Am.* 1993;4:667–75.
12. George AE, Holodny A, Golomb J, Deleon MJ. The differential diagnosis of Alzheimer's disease. Cerebral atrophy versus normal pressure hydrocephalus. *Neuroimaging Clin North Am.* 1995;5:19–31.

29 Sleep Disorders

A. SINAN BARAN

SUMMARY   Although uncommon, patients do present to the emergency department with problems related to a sleep disorder. Excessive daytime sleepiness is a symptom of many sleep disorders and can predispose patients to accidental trauma. Behaviors while asleep (parasomnias) can lead directly to injury. Obstructive sleep apnea can cause or contribute to cardiovascular disorders observed in the emergency department. Cataplexy, an auxiliary symptom of narcolepsy characterized by sudden muscle weakness, can be mistaken for other acute medical problems. Sleep-related panic attacks can occur in patients without daytime panic attacks and may mimic acute cardiovascular symptoms. Insomnia (difficulty falling asleep or staying asleep) due to various causes, including primary sleep disorders or primary medical/psychiatric disorders, can compromise daytime functioning and predispose to trauma.

Introduction

Although sleep disorders are not generally regarded as medical emergencies, the emergency physician may encounter patients whose presenting complaints may be a direct consequence of, or relate to, a primary sleep disorder. Patients with sleep disorders may present to an emergency department for evaluation of injury or with other medical problems related to a primary sleep disorder. Injury can be a result of excessive daytime sleepiness (EDS) or behaviors during sleep. In addition to the patient with acute injury, the emergency physician may encounter patients who present with more chronic medical manifestations of their sleep disorder (obstructive sleep apnea). Furthermore, the presence of an underlying sleep-related breathing disturbance may predispose a patient to complications due to medications with sedating effects that may be administered in the emergency department.

Because sleep medicine is an interdisciplinary field, this chapter addresses sleep disorders that are most likely to have emergency medicine implications, rather than only those thought to have a neu-

rological etiology. The definitive diagnosis of sleep disorders almost always requires an evaluation and testing at a sleep disorders center. Therefore, the emphasis of this chapter is on the recognition of relevant sleep disorders, rather than treatment and management issues.

Normal Sleep

The function of sleep is not fully known, but this physiological state has been extensively characterized. The duration of nightly sleep required by the average adult is thought to be approximately eight hours. Sleep is composed to two distinctly different states: rapid eye movement (REM) sleep and non-REM sleep. REM sleep normally accounts for 25% of sleep time, and non-REM sleep occupies the remaining 75%. Non-REM sleep is further divided into four stages (stages 1, 2, 3, and 4) that are progressively deeper, as defined by electroencephalographic (EEG) criteria. Stage 1 is a short-lived transitional stage that normally occupies less than 10% of the total sleep time, and is followed by stage 2,

Sid M. Shah and Kevin M. Kelly, eds., *Emergency Neurology: Principles and Practice.* Copyright © 1999 Cambridge University Press. All rights reserved.

which is characterized by discrete EEG phenomena known as K-complexes and sleep spindles. Stages 3 and 4 are defined by the predominance of delta waves on the EEG (hence the synonymous terms *delta sleep* and *slow-wave sleep*), and it is thought that these stages play an important role in the restorative function of sleep. The majority of slow-wave sleep occurs during the first third of the night; this may sometimes help to identify sleep disorders that occur exclusively during these stages of sleep (stage 3 and 4 non-REM sleep parasomnias such as sleepwalking and sleep terrors).[1,2]

The majority of dreaming occurs during REM sleep, which is characterized by a mixed-frequency fast EEG, conjugate rapid eye movements, and relative atonia of the skeletal musculature. The peri–locus coeruleus area of the dorsal pontine tegmentum appears to be responsible for REM sleep–related skeletal muscle atonia, which is interrupted by brief, intermittent, excitatory inputs responsible for the characteristic rapid eye movements and muscle twitches of REM sleep. Variations in respiratory rate, heart rate, and blood pressure reflect the autonomic instability that occurs during REM sleep.

REM sleep first occurs approximately 90 minutes after sleep onset, and approximately every 90 minutes thereafter throughout the night. REM sleep periods lengthen progressively during the course of the night, so that the last third of the night is predominantly composed of REM sleep. The timing of the onset of the first REM sleep period is of great importance in the diagnosis of narcolepsy.

Diagnostic Procedures in Sleep Medicine

The nocturnal polysomnogram (PSG) remains the standard procedure to evaluate patients for sleep disorders. The PSG includes: the electroencephalogram (EEG); electrooculogram (EOG); electromyogram (EMG) of the intercostal, chin, and anterior tibialis muscles; electrocardiogram (EKG); and oximetry – along with measurement of respiratory airflow (by a thermistor that detects the temperature of inspired and expired air) and effort (typically by piezoelectric belts that quantify chest and abdominal movement). The study is best performed in the controlled setting of a sleep laboratory; although portable home study units are available, they do not conform to the standards of a laboratory study.[1,2]

The Multiple Sleep Latency Test (MSLT) is a daytime test to assess objectively for EDS and the occurrence of REM sleep at sleep onset. This test is performed in selected cases to clarify the diagnosis, and is generally preceded by a nocturnal PSG. The patient is given four or five opportunities to nap, starting at 2 hours following awakening from the PSG, and every 2 hours afterward. No sleep is allowed between naps. When sleep occurs during a nap period, it is terminated 15 minutes after the first 30-second epoch of sleep. The nap period is otherwise terminated when sleep onset has not occurred within 20 minutes. From the results, the mean sleep latency is calculated, and values of less than 10 minutes are considered abnormal. As mentioned previously, special attention is given to any presence of REM sleep, because this stage of sleep is an abnormal occurrence during any short nap and should not occur until a person has slept for approximately 90 minutes. Conditions that can cause an abnormally short REM sleep latency include narcolepsy, other sleep disorders that severely fragment sleep, withdrawal from REM sleep–suppressing agents, or a sleep–wake schedule abnormality.

Disorders that Predispose to Trauma

Disorders Associated with Excessive Daytime Sleepiness

Many automobile and occupational accidents are thought to be at least in part due to sleepiness and associated impairment of vigilance. Although insufficient sleep is the leading cause of EDS, sleep disorders can also cause sleepiness either by disrupting nocturnal sleep or, in the case of narcolepsy, by as yet uncharacterized neurological mechanisms. Hence, patients with sleep disorders seem to be at increased risk for automobile accidents.[3] Table 29.1 lists features of sleep disorders pertinent to evaluation in the emergency department. Table 29.2 lists general treatment approaches to sleep disorders.

Obstructive Sleep Apnea and Upper Airway Resistance Syndrome. Loud snoring is the hallmark of obstructive sleep apnea (OSA), which is caused by the instability of the upper airway during sleep. OSA can occur at any age, but most patients come to medical attention between the ages of 40 and 60

TABLE 29.1. Features of Sleep Disorders Pertinent to Emergency Medicine

	EDS*	Behaviors During Sleep*	Associated Medical Conditions	Mimic Other Medical Problems
Obstructive sleep apnea/upper airway resistance syndrome	X		X	
Periodic limb movement disorder	X			
Narcolepsy	X			X
Recurrent hypersomnia	X			
Sleep terrors		X		
Sleepwalking		X		
REM sleep behavior disorder		X	X	
Sleep panic attacks				X

*Potential for trauma.

years. In the United States, an estimated 1–2% of the population have OSA, with a male to female ratio of 8:1 in adults.[1,2,4]

Reduction in upper airway muscle tone with sleep onset is a normal occurrence. However, when this occurs in a compromised upper airway, partial or complete occlusion can result, associated with an interruption of normal air exchange. Factors that can contribute to upper airway collapse include: adipose infiltration of the parapharyngeal structures (due to obesity); mass effect of an enlarged neck; nasal obstruction; and oropharyngeal obstruction as a result of redundant parapharyngeal tissues; a long, soft palate; macroglossia; or tonsillar hypertrophy. Craniofacial features of retrognathia and micrognathia can cause or predispose to upper airway obstruction by affecting the posterior extension of the tongue. OSA can also occur in association with neurological disorders that cause abnormal control of pharyngeal muscles.

Weight gain and obesity are common in patients with OSA, and even relatively minor weight gain

TABLE 29.2. Typical Treatment Approaches to Sleep Disorders

Disorder	Treatment
Obstructive sleep apnea/upper airway resistance syndrome	CPAP/ENT surgery/oral appliances
Periodic limb movement disorder/RLS	Benzodiazepines/dopamine agonists/opiates
Narcolepsy	Stimulants (for EDS) and tricyclic antidepressants (for cataplexy)
Sleep terrors/sleepwalking	Benzodiazepines/tricyclic antidepressants
REM sleep behavior disorder	Benzodiazepines (clonazepam)

may be sufficient to cause upper airway obstruction during sleep in an anatomically predisposed patient. Furthermore, slender individuals may have sleep-disordered breathing by virtue of their facial and oropharyngeal anatomy.

Upper airway obstruction leads to a progressive increase in respiratory effort, culminating in an arousal – a brief awakening that may last only several seconds or minutes – with associated activation of the pharyngeal musculature and resolution of the obstruction. Because of their brief duration, these arousals are neither consciously acknowledged by the patient nor remembered the following morning. However, in some cases the patient may complain of unexplained awakenings or awakenings accompanied by shortness of breath, gasping, or choking. Rarely, difficulty falling asleep (due to awakenings associated with respiratory disturbance) can be a prominent feature of the disorder. Repeated episodes of respiratory compromise with associated arousals result in sleep fragmentation and consequent EDS due to the nonrestorative sleep. The associated impairment of daytime vigilance places the patient at increased risk for injury due to automobile or occupational accidents.

Upper airway resistance syndrome (UARS) is a variant of OSA. Mild to moderately increased upper airway resistance as a result of narrowing of the upper airway during sleep may be overcome by increased respiratory effort, without a significant reduction in airflow. The increased resistance requiring increased effort can nevertheless result in an EEG arousal that fragments sleep. Thus, the patient with UARS may have EDS without evidence of obvious respiratory disturbance (other than snoring, in most cases) on the standard PSG. Monitoring of intraesophageal pressure with a thin, water-filled catheter during the PSG is the definitive method of detecting UARS.

In addition to the short-term consequences of sleep fragmentation and EDS, untreated OSA has been associated with an increased risk of cardiovascular and cerebrovascular morbidity and mortality. Disorders including systemic hypertension, pulmonary hypertension, cor pulmonale, cardiac arrhythmias, myocardial infarction, and stroke have been associated with untreated OSA.[5]

Patients with OSA or UARS may experience worsening of their respiration during sleep after ingesting any sedatives, including alcohol. Sedatives may not only worsen preexisting sleep-disordered breathing, but may cause increased upper airway resistance and obstruction in some otherwise normal patients. There are two primary mechanisms for this phenomenon: (1) pharyngeal muscle tone is reduced, promoting upper airway obstruction, and (2) the arousal threshold is raised, so that respiratory events may last longer before the patient arouses to terminate an episode. This effect of sedative medications is of relevance in the emergency department, because patients with sleep-disordered breathing may require sedation or analgesia for other reasons, and may develop respiratory compromise as a result.

Periodic Limb Movement Disorder. Previously known as nocturnal myoclonus, this disorder of periodic and highly stereotyped involuntary movements of the limbs during sleep can cause sleep fragmentation and resultant EDS. Onset is usually during middle adulthood, with a tendency to progress with advancing age. Rare cases occur during childhood. The prevalence is unknown.[1,2,4]

Periodic limb movements typically occur in the legs, but may also involve the arms. The leg movements involve extension of the great toe, along with partial flexion of the ankle, knee, and occasionally the hip. Both legs are usually affected, and movements can occur in intervals lasting minutes to hours, or throughout the sleep period. Sleep disruption associated with periodic limb movements may result in a complaint of insomnia (awareness of awakenings) or EDS, which can compromise daytime functioning, placing the patient at increased risk for accidents.

Narcolepsy. Narcolepsy is characterized by the so-called narcoleptic tetrad: excessive daytime sleepiness, cataplexy, sleep paralysis, and hypnagogic hallucinations. EDS is the hallmark of narcolepsy, and the other three symptoms (the "auxiliary symptoms") are not necessary for the diagnosis of this disorder. All three auxiliary symptoms are thought to be REM sleep–related phenomena.[1,2,4]

Narcolepsy occurs in 0.03–0.16% of the population in the United States and typically begins during the second decade of life. EDS is the first symptom in most cases, and cataplexy may appear simultaneously, as late as 30 years later, or not at all.

Rarely, cataplexy precedes EDS. Cataplexy without narcolepsy is extremely rare.

Cataplexy is a sudden loss of voluntary muscle tone typically precipitated by emotional excitement, particularly laughter. The duration is usually several seconds or minutes but may be longer. Severity can range from a subtle, barely noticeable sagging of facial muscles or slurring of speech to a generalized and profound weakness resulting in a collapse to the floor. Inhibition of the monosynaptic H and muscle stretch reflexes occurs, as in REM sleep. Particularly strong emotion may cause *status cataplecticus,* which is more than one episode of cataplexy in succession, lasting as long as an hour. Although not life-threatening in itself, cataplexy may lead to injury. However, it is usually EDS, not cataplexy, that increases the risk of injury for the narcoleptic patient.

Cataplexy can be mistaken for, and should be distinguished from syncope, transient ischemic attacks, and partial seizures. Consciousness is fully intact during cataplexy, although patients may sleep following an episode. A history of emotional excitement as a precipitant of the events, EDS, and other auxiliary symptoms of narcolepsy help to clarify the diagnosis.

Sleep paralysis and hypnagogic hallucinations are other REM sleep–related phenomena that the narcoleptic patient may experience. Sleep paralysis is the occurrence of atonia during the transition from wakefulness to REM sleep (during a sleep-onset REM episode) or from REM sleep to wakefulness. Typically, the patient reports a transient inability to move (lasting no longer than several minutes) as he or she is falling asleep or awakening, and this may be particularly frightening the first time it occurs. Hypnagogic hallucinations are dreamlike images or sounds that may occur at sleep onset, as the patient is entering REM sleep. Hypnapompic hallucinations are their counterpart experienced while awakening from REM sleep. Hypnagogic or hypnapompic hallucinations may accompany sleep paralysis, adding to the frightening nature of the occurrence. In some cultures, these phenomena are given supernatural interpretations such as a demon or witch casting a spell on the patient. Hypnagogic and hypnapompic hallucinations can be misinterpreted as psychotic symptoms, but they are not indicative of psychosis.

Sleep paralysis and hypnagogic/hypnapompic hallucinations can occur in normal individuals, especially during an irregular sleep schedule or REM sleep rebound caused by sleep deprivation or withdrawal from a REM sleep–suppressing agent. However, frequent episodes of these REM sleep–related phenomena and EDS suggest narcolepsy. A history of EDS in conjunction with a clear history of cataplexy is essentially pathognomonic for narcolepsy.

Patients with narcolepsy may experience worsening of their auxiliary symptoms (cataplexy, hypnagogic hallucinations, and sleep paralysis) when a REM sleep–suppressant medication (typically an antidepressant) is discontinued or reduced in dose. The cause for this is the REM sleep rebound that follows REM sleep suppression. Since all three auxiliary symptoms are REM sleep–related phenomena, an increased propensity for REM sleep may transiently increase the severity or frequency of episodes. Exacerbation of cataplexy has also been reported with administration of the $alpha_1$ antagonist prazosin, and is supportive of altered $alpha_1$ adrenoreceptor function in narcoleptic patients.[6]

Disorders Associated with Behaviors While Asleep (Parasomnias)

Injury can result from behaviors that occur during sleep. The patient's ability to recall the episode depends partly on the type of the parasomnia (occurrence during non-REM versus REM sleep).

Sleep Terrors and Sleepwalking. Sleep terrors and sleepwalking are both non–REM sleep phenomena that specifically occur during stage 3 or 4 sleep (slow-wave sleep). Because the majority of slow-wave sleep occurs in the first third of the night, sleep terrors and sleepwalking are most likely to occur at that time. Patients may demonstrate dangerous behaviors, including jumping through a closed window in an attempt to escape a perceived threat or danger, leading to significant injury.[1,2,4]

Both sleep terrors and sleepwalking are common during childhood, and usually resolve during adolescence. However, the episodes can persist into adulthood, and can be exacerbated by stress, sleep deprivation, alcohol consumption, or other sleep disrupters, including primary sleep disorders such as obstructive sleep apnea or periodic limb movement disorder. Rarely, onset may occur during adulthood. Sleep terrors occur in approximately 3% of children and less than 1% of adults. The incidence of sleepwalking is 1–15% of the population in the United States, with a peak onset between 4 and 8 years of age.

Sleep terrors are characterized by a sudden arousal from slow-wave sleep, accompanied by a scream and manifestations of autonomic arousal including tachypnea and tachycardia. The patient is disoriented, difficult to console, and unlikely to remember the event the following day, but may have vague recall. In some cases there may be an associated visual component, and the patient may refer to the episode as a nightmare. Upon further questioning, it becomes apparent that the memory is of a frightening static image rather than a sequence of dream events.

Sleepwalking involves behaviors initiated during slow-wave sleep, and shares many of the features of sleep terrors, with the exception of intense fear. Behaviors may involve movements without leaving the bed. In extreme cases, complex activities including driving have been reported during apparent sleepwalking episodes.[7] During an episode, the patient may violently attack anyone who attempts to awaken him or her.

Since the patient with either of these disorders is at risk for injury, specific safety precautions should be taken even after a patient has been adequately treated. All sharp and breakable objects should be removed from the bedroom, and windows and doors should be locked. Bedroom windows should additionally be barricaded or covered with heavy drapery, and a bell or alarm should be placed on the door to alert family members to the patient's nocturnal wandering.

REM Sleep Behavior Disorder. The atonia of skeletal muscles during REM sleep may be conceptualized as a protective mechanism that prevents the physical enactment of dreams. When atonia is abolished, movements become possible, and are dictated by the content of dreams. Patients with REM sleep behavior disorder (RBD) have intermittent loss of REM atonia, and as a result may engage in various behaviors, with a potential for injury to themselves or their bed partners.[1,2,4]

RBD typically occurs in men over the age of 50, but it may occur in both sexes and begin at any age.

Sixty percent of cases are idiopathic. Animal research has localized the peri–locus coeruleus area of the pontine tegmentum as the site that causes atonia during REM sleep. Tumors, infarctions, or hemorrhages in this area, or other more generalized types of intracranial pathology (including dementia), are associated with RBD in the remaining 40% of cases. For this reason, brain imaging is strongly indicated in patients confirmed to have RBD.

RBD is confirmed polysomnographically by the presence of abnormally high muscle tone during REM sleep, as measured by chin, lower extremity, and upper extremity EMG recordings, even in the absence of behaviors or significant movements. As in cases of non-REM parasomnias, patients are advised to exercise the safety precautions described previously.

Other Sleep Disorders

Recurrent Hypersomnia

Kleine-Levin syndrome, a disorder thought to be due to hypothalamic dysfunction, is characterized by recurrent hypersomnia and disinhibited behaviors. Cases involve recurrent episodes of hypersomnia and hyperphagia that typically begin in adolescent males and resolve by adulthood. The syndrome occurs less commonly at a later age, and in women. A monosymptomatic form of the syndrome with only hypersomnia has been described. Episodes occur 2–12 times per year and may last several days to weeks. During an episode, patients may sleep up to 20 hours per day, with awakenings to eat and void. With concurrent hyperphagia, weight gain is common, but weight loss may occur in the monosymptomatic type. There may be associated hypersexuality, confusion, memory impairment, and hallucinations. In the intervals between episodes, patients do not have any waking or sleep-related abnormalities.[1,2,4]

The patient with recurrent hypersomnia is more likely to spend excessive time in bed than to become drowsy while driving or engaging in other activities. Hence, patients with this disorder may be brought to medical attention by family members because they are difficult to arouse and may behave inappropriately.

Insomnia

Insomnia is characterized by difficulty falling asleep or staying asleep. Although patients with insomnia typically do not complain of EDS, they can nevertheless have impaired daytime functioning that can increase their risk for accidents and injury. Insomnia can result from multiple causes including psychiatric or general medical disorders, medication effects, substance abuse, other sleep disorders, or conditioned cognitive mechanisms. Idiopathic insomnia is extremely rare; insomnia should generally be regarded as a symptom of an underlying primary disorder. Patients with sleep disorders previously mentioned under the category of excessive daytime sleepiness (OSA and periodic limb movement disorder) may present with insomnia as the primary complaint in some cases.[1,2,4]

Restless legs syndrome (RLS) is another important cause of insomnia. RLS is thought to be related to periodic limb movement disorder, and is characterized by lower extremity dysesthesias that occur at rest and are particularly bothersome as patients lie in bed at bedtime. The discomfort is relieved transiently by movement, and patients are compelled to keep their legs active, sometimes requiring them to get up and walk. As a result, sleep onset is delayed until the symptoms subside, sometimes taking hours in severe cases. Most cases are idiopathic, but a minority have been associated with deficiencies of iron, vitamin B_{12}, and folic acid. Renal failure has also been associated with RLS.

Panic Attacks During Sleep

Panic attacks during sleep constitute not a primary sleep disorder, but a sleep manifestation of various psychiatric disorders. Panic attacks may occur in association with panic disorder or other anxiety disorders, as well as with major depression. An episode is characterized by a sudden onset of intense anxiety accompanied by somatic symptoms and signs that can include tachypnea, tachycardia, palpitations, chest pain, diaphoresis, lightheadedness, paresthesias, trembling, nausea, or abdominal distress. During sleep, panic attacks begin during late stage 2 or early stage 3 non-REM sleep, when the patient suddenly awakens with typical panic symptoms.[1,2,4,8]

Most patients with panic disorder have attacks during sleep at some point in the course of the ill-ness; 30–45% have repeated episodes during sleep, but only a minority have attacks exclusively during sleep. It is not uncommon for a patient to present to the emergency department for evaluation of the somatic manifestations of a panic attack, particularly in the early phase of the illness before formal diagnosis and treatment. After cardiovascular or other relevant etiologies have been investigated, these patients should be referred for psychiatric evaluation and treatment whether the attacks occur during wakefulness or sleep.

Sleep panic attacks should be distinguished from sleep terrors and nightmares. With an awakening due to a panic attack, mentation is clear, and the patient will recall the episode the next day, as compared to sleep terrors, which are associated with confusion and partial or total amnesia for the event. Nightmares are distinguished by the associated dream content.

Conclusion

Sleep disorders are typically chronic and insidious conditions that may evade diagnosis even by the most astute primary care physician. The potential acute complications of sleep disorders give the emergency physician the opportunity to raise the question of an otherwise unsuspected chronic disorder and contribute to its ultimate diagnosis and treatment. In particular, patients presenting with accidental trauma – during waking hours or associated with nighttime sleep – and acute cardiovascular or cerebrovascular events may have an underlying sleep disorder. Furthermore, vague neurological complaints may be explained by sleep-related phenomena such as cataplexy. Obtaining a brief sleep history from such patients can readily identify those who warrant a formal sleep evaluation.

PEARLS AND PITFALLS

- Excessive daytime sleepiness, regardless of its etiology, can lead to trauma.
- Excessive daytime sleepiness can be masked by physical activity and is most apparent when the patient is sedentary; this should be taken into account when inquiring about this symptom.

- Patients may underestimate and minimize the severity of their daytime sleepiness.
- Patients with obstructive sleep apnea may experience respiratory compromise when given sedating medications.
- Not all patients with sleep-disordered breathing (upper airway resistance syndrome and obstructive sleep apnea) are obese.
- Cataplexy, an auxiliary symptom of narcolepsy, may be mistaken for syncope, transient ischemic attacks, and partial seizures.
- Panic attacks can occur during sleep and may include symptoms suggestive of cardiac ischemia.

REFERENCES

1. Kryger M, Roth T, Dement W. *Principles and Practice of Sleep Medicine*. 2nd ed. Philadelphia, Pa: WB Saunders Co; 1994.
2. Chokroverty S. *Sleep Disorders Medicine: Basic Science, Technical Considerations, and Clinical Aspects*. Boston, Mass: Butterworth-Heinemann; 1994.
3. Aldrich MS. Automobile accidents in patients with sleep disorders. *Sleep*. 1989;12:487–94.
4. American Sleep Disorders Association. *The International Classification of Sleep Disorders. Diagnostic and Coding Manual*. Rochester, Minn: American Sleep Disorders Association; 1990.
5. Bassetti C, Aldrich MS, Chervin RD, Quint D. Sleep apnea in patients with transient ischemic attack and stroke: a prospective study of 59 patients. *Neurology*. 1996;47:1167–73.
6. Aldrich MS, Rogers AE. Exacerbation of human cataplexy by prazosin. *Sleep*. 1989;12:254–6.
7. Schenck CH, Mahowald MW. A polysomnographically documented case of adult somnambulism with long distance automobile driving and frequent nocturnal violence: parasomnia with continuing danger as a noninsane automatism? *Sleep*. 1995;18:765–72.
8. American Psychiatric Association. *Diagnostic and Statistical Manual of Mental Disorders*. 4th ed. Washington, DC: American Psychiatric Association; 1994.

FOUR Neurological Trauma and Environmental Emergencies

30 Traumatic Brain Injury

PATRICIA LANTER AND BRIAN ZINK

SUMMARY Traumatic brain injury (TBI) is one of the leading causes of preventable death and disability. The management of patients with TBI includes appropriate oxygenation, ventilation, and fluid resuscitation to maintain adequate cerebral perfusion. Rapid and accurate diagnosis and treatment of patients with TBI includes computerized tomography of the brain with neurosurgical evaluation that can decrease the morbidity and mortality of this form of brain injury.

Introduction

Traumatic brain injury (TBI) is one of the leading preventable causes of death and disability worldwide. It is the leading cause of death in Americans younger than 45 years of age and is the most common cause of traumatic death in children. It accounts for 100,000 deaths in the United States each year, of which 25,000 are pediatric. Of all traumatic deaths in the United States, 25–30% result from TBI. Reported death rates from TBI range from a low of 9 per 100,000 people in the United Kingdom to 32 per 100,000 people in inner-city Chicago.[1,2] Hospital admission rates for patients with TBI vary with practice standards and the availability of neuroimaging. In the United States and the United Kingdom, the incidence of admission for patients with TBI is between 160 and 400 per 100,000 people. Approximately 500,000 patients with TBI per year require hospital admission in the United States; 30–40% of these admissions are for moderate to severe injury.[1-3] Many of these patients experience permanent neurological disability. Many young and healthy individuals experience TBI. The resultant cost to society in terms of disruption of families, lost productivity, and health care expenditures over a lifetime is enormous.[4,5]

The incidence of TBI is biphasic, peaking in adolescence and early adulthood, and in the elderly.

TBI occurs more commonly in males than in females, by a ratio of nearly 2 : 1 in many studies.[5] The mechanism of injury varies with age. Bicycle accidents are common in children; the elderly are typically injured by falling.[2,6] Most serious head injuries are caused by motor vehicle crashes, followed by falls, assaults, and recreational injuries.[2] The incidence of TBI due to assault is inversely related to socioeconomic status; in many economically depressed areas, assault is the leading cause of TBI. Although the majority of TBIs occur from blunt impact, penetrating injury from gunshot wounds is responsible for about 40% of fatal TBI cases in some large cities in the United States.[2] Alcohol use and abuse is clearly associated with TBI. In most series, alcohol intoxication is present in 25–50% of patients with TBI.[5,7,8] TBI is usually not an isolated injury, at least 75% of patients with TBI have serious injuries to other organ systems.[9]

Despite these statistics, mortality from TBI has decreased over the past 10 years.[10] Clinical research has focused on the early management of TBI. The biomolecular mechanisms responsible for brain cell dysfunction and death following TBI are under active investigation. One of the most important concepts to emerge from this research is that early recognition and treatment of hypoperfusion, hypoxia, and high intracranial pressure (ICP) in the in-

Sid M. Shah and Kevin M. Kelly, eds., *Emergency Neurology: Principles and Practice.* Copyright © 1999 Cambridge University Press. All rights reserved.

jured brain are crucial to a good neurological outcome.[11] This information has directly improved the care of patients with TBI. Computerized tomography (CT) scanners are more readily available, faster, and show finer detail, contributing to more expeditious patient transfer and aggressive management of severe TBI, resulting in decreased mortality and morbidity.

Pathophysiology

Many changes occur in the brain following a traumatic injury. Historically, the pathophysiology of TBI has been divided into primary and secondary injury. With primary injury, the mechanical forces applied to or occurring within the cranium result in functional and physical disruption of brain tissue. Secondary brain injury occurs when postinjury factors such as hypoxemia or hypotension adversely affect the already injured brain. Most patients with TBI have both primary and secondary injuries.

Primary brain injury can result from a blow to the cranium, or from rapid acceleration, deceleration, or rotation of the brain within the skull. The initial force is counteracted by reactive forces inside the brain, called *stresses.* Forces within the cranium, such as acceleration, deceleration, or rotation, create *shear-strain* stresses and ICP gradients.[11,12] Primary injury can be further subdivided into focal and diffuse injury. Postmortem microscopic inspection of the injured brain reveals that most brain injuries have both diffuse brain injury and foci of increased cellular or vascular damage. Examples of focal injury include subdural and epidural hematomas, intraparenchymal hemorrhages, and contusions. The most recognized type of diffuse injury is diffuse axonal injury.

Subdural Hematoma

Acute subdural hematoma (SDH) results from tearing of the veins or cortical arterioles in acceleration/deceleration injuries such as motor vehicle crashes and falls. After impact, the brain continues to move within the calvarium, and the parasagittal and bridging veins are stretched and torn. SDHs can occur without trauma to the head. An acute SDH appears as a crescent-shaped, heterogeneous density that fills in the space between the dura and the brain on CT of the head. They are usually found on the surface of the cerebral hemispheres and account for approximately 5% of traumatic brain lesions.[13] Patients with SDH have relatively high morbidity and mortality compared to patients with other types of TBI. Mortality rates range from 35–80%.[13–15] In one study, 67% of the patients who underwent operative removal of the SDH had coexistent injuries such as contusions and other parenchymal injuries.[14] The morbidity and mortality of SDHs may be related to the extent of these coexisting injuries.[13,15]

A typical history for a patient with an SDH is loss of consciousness with the event, initial improvement, and deterioration. Patients with an SDH can present with a severe headache and personality changes, or can be unresponsive with unilateral pupillary dilatation and contralateral hemiparesis. Management of patients with SDH depends upon the size of the hematoma, the associated injuries, the amount of edema, and the condition of the patient. Patients with small SDHs (<3 mm thick) without other brain injuries can often be observed on a hospital trauma or neurosurgical service. Larger SDHs, and smaller SDHs associated with parenchymal injury are evacuated operatively. Removal of small SDHs can markedly decrease elevated ICP and improve outcome.[13]

Epidural Hematoma

Epidural hematoma (EDH) results from direct trauma to the skull. EDHs occur with or without associated skull fracture. The incidence of EDHs peaks in the second and third decades of life and is rare during infancy and in the elderly. EDHs account for 0.5–1% of all TBIs and are less common than SDHs.[16] They usually result from falls or the impact of motor vehicle crashes and are caused by blood vessel disruption and detachment of the dura mater from the inner table of the skull. The middle meningeal artery is the blood vessel most commonly associated with an EDH; middle meningeal vein and dural sinus injuries also occur. When an EDH is caused by venous bleeding, its size is limited by the space between the dura and the skull.[17] The pressure from an arterial hemorrhage can cause further separation of the dura from the skull, resulting in a larger and increasing mass. On CT of the head, EDHs form a lenticulate homogeneous hyperdense image on the surface of the brain, usually in the temporal area.

Patients with an EDH can present with a history of an initial loss of consciousness, or concussion, followed by a "lucid interval" with a subsequent rapid deterioration resulting from the increasing mass of the EDH. As is the case with SDHs, the patient's symptoms depend upon the size and rapidity of growth of the hematoma, the time from the event, and the associated brain and systemic injuries. Treatment of an acute EDH is prompt surgical evacuation. It is imperative to make the diagnosis of EDH as soon as possible in the postinjury period, because many patients have excellent recovery following timely surgical evacuation.[13]

Diffuse Axonal Injury

Diffuse axonal injury (DAI) can occur in virtually all patients with TBI, and is not limited to the obtunded or comatose patient with a "normal" CT of the head. Magnetic resonance imaging (MRI) is the imaging modality most likely to show the areas of severe DAI. However, MRI is typically not available during emergency evaluation and takes much longer to perform. DAI is likely the primary reason for persistent coma following TBI. DAI can be found scattered throughout the brain and brainstem but is more common in the deeper cerebral white matter, corpus callosum, and cerebral peduncles. Historically, DAI was thought to be a disruption or tearing of the axon, however, recent studies have shown that it is a result of a mechanical insult to the axonal cytoskeleton.[18] This change in the cytoskeleton impedes anterograde transport. In severe DAI, the axon disconnects from the neuronal soma within 6–12 hours. The distal (i.e., disconnected) segment of the axon degenerates, "withdraws," and subsequently is phagocytized. There is deafferentation and subsequent degeneration of the target field. In mild to moderate injury, axons may regenerate. DAI can occur without adjacent microvascular or neuronal damage, or ischemia. DAI causes much of the long-term neurological impairment in patients with TBI. The morbidity associated with TBI correlates with the extent and severity of DAI.[18]

Cerebral Contusion

Cerebral contusions and intraparenchymal hemorrhages (IPH) are areas of hemorrhage within the brain parenchyma. They vary from very small punctate lesions of brain structures and brain on the crests of the gyri to large hemorrhages in the deep white matter and are associated with edema, shift, and herniation. Parenchymal injuries typically occur where the brain is injured by bone, including the frontal and temporal lobes over the spicules, at the base of the skull, or from bony fragments. They also can occur from shear strain and rotational stresses.[13]

Concussive Syndromes

Concussive syndromes are transient alterations in neural functioning. Patients can present with or without a history of loss of consciousness. Consciousness is regained within six hours following concussive injury. The mildest forms are characterized by a brief period of confusion, commonly experienced by athletes who are struck in the head. A more severe concussive syndrome entails a loss of consciousness of up to six hours with retrograde and postinjury (anterograde) amnesia, and subtle changes in cognitive functioning. Of note is that patients with EDHs can present with an initial loss of consciousness followed by subtle neurological findings. Patients with more severe concussions can exhibit a brief period of focal neurological signs immediately after the event, including posturing or apnea. Persistent focal neurological findings imply more severe injury than a concussion.[19]

Brain Regulatory Mechanisms and Secondary Brain Injury

Secondary brain injury occurs in the postinjury period and is due to associated physiological impairments resulting from the primary injury.[20] Decreased cerebral perfusion, elevated ICP, hypoxemia, and circulatory shock can increase brain injury and worsen outcome in patients with TBI.

Cerebral perfusion pressure (CPP) is the difference between the mean arterial pressure (MAP) and the ICP. Decreased CPP can occur with a decrease in MAP, as in circulatory shock, or from an increase in the ICP from edema or an expanding intracranial mass. A CPP of 60–70 mm Hg is adequate for normal perfusion. When the CPP is less than 50 mm Hg, cerebral autoregulation is compromised and perfusion becomes inadequate, resulting in focal or global ischemia.

Cerebral autoregulation is the protective mechanism that maintains cerebral blood flow (CBF) in a narrow physiological range despite changes in MAP and ICP. Normal autoregulation of cerebral vascular resistance is maintained by local chemical and endothelial factors, and neurotransmitters released from adjacent neurons.[21,22] An intact blood–brain barrier (BBB) is necessary for normal autoregulation. The BBB prevents passive diffusion of electrolytes (primarily sodium, chloride, and potassium), plasma proteins, and other large molecules into the brain extracellular space.[23] The BBB is composed of specialized cerebral vascular endothelial cells and continuous tight junctions between them. When CPP is inadequate, CBF is dependent on systemic arterial pressure, and autoregulation begins to fail. Abnormally low CBF leads to an acute or focal global ischemic brain injury and can lead to breakdown of the BBB, which further impairs autoregulation. The BBB becomes incompetent when the autoregulatory control of the upper limit of CBF is exceeded, resulting in brain edema, intracranial hypertension, and possible hemorrhage.[10,21,23]

CBF is influenced by arterial P_{CO_2} and P_{O_2}, brain temperature, and various pharmacological agents.[22] Typically, in the first hour postinjury, a decrease in CBF occurs. In experimental models, reduced CBF occurs more commonly as the injury force is increased.[24] Studies of regional CBF differences following TBI indicate variation of the CBF response in different brain regions. Focal areas of hypoperfusion can exist despite normal global CBF. It is likely that mediators of injury such as oxygen radicals, excitatory amino acids, and nitric oxide play important roles in the global and focal loss of cerebral autoregulation and disruption of the BBB.[10,21,24,25]

Increased Intracranial Pressure

ICP in the intact cranium is determined by brain parenchyma tissue pressure, cerebral blood volume (CBV), intracranial cerebrospinal fluid (CSF) volume, and, in trauma, mass lesions. Normal ICP is 0–10 mm Hg. At an ICP of 15–20 mm Hg, capillary beds are compressed and the microcirculation is compromised. Venous drainage is compromised at an ICP of 30–40 mm Hg, resulting in increased edema. A sustained ICP of >60 mm Hg is usually fatal.[26] Elevated ICP is likely caused by increased brain edema. However, a patient with TBI can have an elevated ICP with minimal edema. Conversely, a patient with TBI can have edema and no elevation of ICP. Following TBI, a compensatory decrease in CBV or CSF can lessen increased ICP due to hemor-

rhage and brain edema. However, cerebral autoregulation can increase CBF with associated increased CBV, thereby increasing ICP. Compression of CSF out of the cranial space and into the spinal canal occurs passively and has a transient benefit in cases of increased ICP. When ICP elevation is not decreased by these compensatory mechanisms, brain tissue can be compressed and brain herniation can occur. Brain herniation can be unilateral uncal transtentorial herniation, central herniation, or transfalcine cingulate herniation, depending on the presence of mass lesions, hemorrhage, or elevated ICP.[27] Brain herniation due to severely elevated ICP is usually a premorbid event. Elevated ICP causes global and focal reductions in CBF with subsequent brain ischemia. The brain can withstand increased compressive forces but cannot recover from prolonged ischemia.[10,23,28,29]

Brain Edema

Brain edema is defined as an increase in brain water content with resultant increased brain tissue volume.[28] Brain edema can be interstitial (vasogenic) or intracellular (cytotoxic). When injury causes a disruption of the BBB, electrolytes, water, and proteins diffuse into the main interstitium. Initially, brain compliance can offset the increased tissue pressure. With time, this compensatory mechanism fails and the patient develops increased ICP. The elevated ICP causes focal and global ischemia secondary to decreased CBF. When autoregulation is normal, CBF increases, resulting in higher ICP. The CBF response with BBB disruption and cerebral autoregulation dysfunction is not well characterized. In this situation, regional CBF changes may be more important than global CBF.

Cytotoxic edema is a secondary form of edema that results from alterations in cell membrane function and ion transport. Cytotoxic edema occurs after the initial injury and is caused by ischemia, or induced by toxic mediators. The sodium/potassium pump does not function, and sodium and water diffuse into the cell. Glial cells and neurons are susceptible to cytotoxic edema. An early finding of ischemic injury is astrocyte swelling.[5] Vasogenic edema likely starts almost immediately after injury; cytotoxic edema occurs later. Brain edema is maximal at about 24–48 hours postinjury.[10,23,28]

Hemorrhage can cause elevated ICP by increasing CBV and by causing the release of injury mediators. When an intraparenchymal hemorrhage occurs, the vascular endothelial cells and thus the BBB are disrupted, and autoregulation is no longer functional. Blood collections in EDHs or SDHs increase CBV and ICP. In the surrounding brain parenchyma, increased pressure causes tissue ischemia and brain edema. This zone of ischemia expands as tissue is shifted by an enlarging hemorrhage. Subarachnoid hemorrhage (SAH) commonly occurs with closed-head injury. Blood in the subarachnoid space can initiate many of the same neurochemical reactions as IPH. A delayed sequela of SAH is cerebral arterial vasospasm. This can worsen ischemia in the injured brain.[20,30] Mediators of injury such as excitatory amino acids, oxygen radical molecules, nitric oxide, and endogenous opioids may be released from the injured endothelium.[23,31] Extravasated blood contains large amounts of iron, which promotes oxidant reactions.[29,32] Blood in the interstitial space triggers an inflammatory immune response that is partly regulated by local cytokine release.

In the above discussion, the recurrent themes of altered CBF and ischemia relate directly to the concept of secondary brain injury. In some instances, secondary injury results from the physiological changes induced by primary injury; in other cases, it is caused by extraneous or iatrogenic events. Hypoxia and systemic arterial hypotension are the two most important secondary abnormalities in the early postinjury period. Hypoxemia causes increased mortality from TBI.[9,33] Apnea typically occurs immediately after TBI, and respiratory depression can follow this initial apneic period. Failure to maintain adequate oxygenation and ventilation in these situations increases injury due to hypoxia. Alcohol and other drugs can worsen initial respiratory depression.[20,34] Similarly, systemic hypotension is associated with poor outcome and increased mortality following TBI.[9,20] Factors such as hemorrhagic shock from internal or orthopedic injury, decreased cardiac output due to tension pneumothorax, cardiac contusion, infarction, or tamponade, or neurogenic shock due to spinal cord injury may decrease CPP to critically low levels. In ischemic brain areas due to elevated ICP or local factors, a decrease in CPP, failure of cerebral autoregulation,

and hypoxia can result in severe ischemia and brain cell necrosis.[10]

Prehospital Management

Prehospital care providers are faced with the challenge of correctly assessing and identifying patients with TBI in suboptimal conditions. They must maintain adequate oxygenation and recognize and treat circulatory hypotension in patients who may be belligerent and combative, while providing rapid transport to the nearest appropriate hospital. Patients with TBI may be intoxicated, confounding the presentation of TBI. Because intoxicated patients have an increased incidence of TBI, an altered mental status is not attributed solely to intoxication. Thirty percent of patients with TBI are hypoxemic upon presentation to the emergency department. Hypoxia causes confusion and combativeness, and increases the morbidity of TBI. Patients with suspected TBI are given high-flow oxygen en route the hospital.[9,20] More than 50% of patients with serious TBI have multiple injuries and are at risk for hemorrhage and hypotension. Fifteen percent of patients with TBI present to the emergency department with hypotension.[9,20,35,36] Administration of intravenous fluids to restore and maintain adequate CPP is an important aspect of prehospital trauma resuscitation, provided it does not delay transport to the hospital.

The Glasgow Coma Scale (GCS) (see Table 30.1) is widely used by emergency medical service and emergency department personnel and has greatly improved the ability to assess and communicate information about patients with TBI, whether at the scene, during transport, or in the emergency department. The initial GCS score and any subsequent change in the mental status or neurological examination at the scene or en route is documented. Essential information provided by emergency medical services for early hospital management includes: (1) the mechanism of the trauma (e.g., speed, ejection, rollover, caliber of the gun); (2) findings at the scene (e.g., position of the patient, blood loss, shattered windshield); and (3) the early neurological findings (e.g., pupils, mental status, GCS score).[37]

A patient who has a GCS score of less than 9 undergoes tracheal intubation at the scene, when pos-

TABLE 30.1. Glasgow Coma Scale

Eye opening	
Opens eyes spontaneously	4
Opens eyes to verbal command	3
Opens eyes to pain	2
Does not open eyes	1
Verbal response	
Alert and oriented	5
Converses but disoriented	4
Speaking but nonsensical	3
Moans or makes unintelligible sounds	2
No response	1
Motor response	
Follows commands	6
Localizes pain	5
Movement or withdrawal from pain	4
Abnormal flexion (decorticate)	3
Abnormal extension (decerebrate)	2
No response	1
Total	3–15

sible (see Fig. 30.1). The comatose or apneic patient can undergo tracheal intubation through the oral route. Head-injured patients commonly have irregular respirations and can be intermittently combative. Prehospital care providers typically are not trained in rapid-sequence intubation techniques, and therefore use forced oral intubation, nasotracheal intubation, or assisted ventilation with a bag-valve mask apparatus. The risk of increasing ICP during endotracheal intubation in a nonsedated, nonparalyzed patient is weighed against the risk of ongoing hypoxia to the injured brain. Other considerations include proximity to the emergency department, skill of the technician, the likelihood of vomiting and aspiration, and the risk of cervical spine injury. Cervical spine precautions are maintained during extrication, intubation, and transport of a patient with TBI.

Emergency Department Evaluation

Primary Survey

This includes early use of the GCS, which gives a standardized measure of neurological function that can be recorded and repeated as the patient under-

goes diagnostic and therapeutic maneuvers. A rapid evaluation of the airway and oxygenation status of the patient is important because the mortality and morbidity of TBI is related to cerebral oxygenation. Adequate intravenous access is maintained, and vital signs are observed closely. Tachypnea and hyperventilation can be an initial response to rising ICP. Hypotension can result from acute hemorrhage or hypothermia. Hypertension with bradycardia (Cushing response), suggests severe intracranial hypertension and impending brain herniation. Abnormal breathing patterns can be due to brainstem injury. Irregular breathing and apnea occur when ICP is very high, with impending herniation.[10]

Secondary Survey

The head is inspected for depressed skull fractures, facial fractures, deformities, abrasions, lacerations, bony stepoffs, and entrance or exit wounds. The ears and nose are inspected for CSF or blood. A more detailed neurological examination is done during the secondary survey, including mental status, pupillary function, eye movements, and motor symmetry. The neurological examination of patients with TBI can change rapidly, requiring serial examinations to detect improvement or deterioration. A decrease in the GCS score by two points or more, a deterioration in mental status, or the development of a new focal finding warrants aggressive management, including rapid CT of the head. An awake, talking patient diagnosed with concussion can become comatose within minutes due to an expanding intracranial hematoma such as an SDH or an EDH. Conversely, a comatose trauma patient can become alert when the coma is due to alcohol intoxication, not severe TBI.

Glasgow Coma Scale

A "normal" Glasgow Coma Scale does not exclude TBI. Patients with a GCS score of 14 or 15 can have significantly altered mental status and TBI. Altered mental status includes disorientation, retrograde and anterograde amnesia, and confusion. These findings can be associated with hypotension, hemorrhage, hypoxia, drug or alcohol intoxication, a concussion, or ICH. Correctable causes of altered

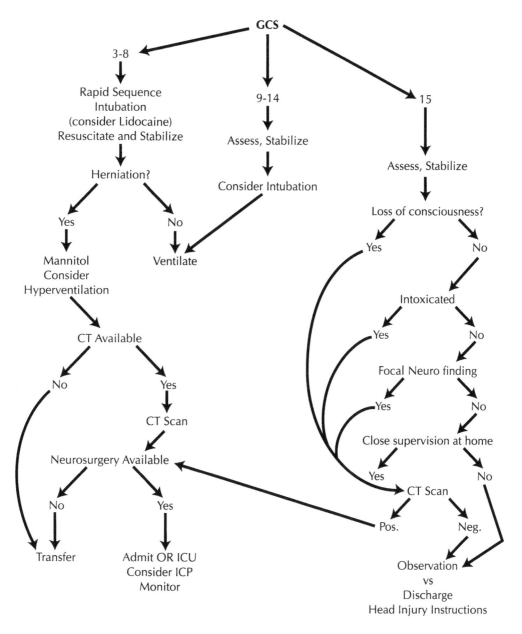

FIGURE 30.1. Algorithm for the treatment of head injury. CT = computerized tomography; GCS = Glasgow Coma Scale; ICP = intracranial pressure; ICU = intensive care unit; OR = operating room.

mental status are treated, and any improvement or lack of improvement is noted.

Pupillary Function

Pupillary function provides important information in the secondary survey. The size of each pupil and the reaction to light is evaluated. Pupillary size and reactivity are not altered by neuromuscular blockers that are given during patient transport or management. Anisocoria can be associated with an expanding intracranial mass. The ipsilateral pupil dilates in response to increasing ICP and impending transtentorial herniation.[38] Bilateral dilated and fixed pupils are commonly associated with severe TBI and a very poor prognosis. Extraocular eye movements are observed and tested. No movements may be observed in the unconscious patient. Forced conjugate deviation of the eyes toward the side of an intracranial lesion can occur. Patients with TBI can have disconjugate gaze or roving eye movements. Rhythmic eye movements and persistent nystagmus suggest seizure activity. Testing of the oculocephalic reflex, or the "doll's eyes" maneuver, is done in a comatose patient after the cervical spine is cleared radiographically. In a normal awake patient, the eyes turn as the head does, with the patient continuing to look in the face-pointing direction. In the patient with an intact brainstem and an injured cortex, the eyes move in the opposite direction of the head. This is referred to as an intact doll's eyes, or oculocephalic, reflex. In the patient with severe brainstem injury, the eyes remain fixed within the orbits and the reflex is absent. Cold caloric testing to assess the oculovestibular reflex can be used in patients with brainstem dysfunction or when the cervical spine may be injured. The ear canal is inspected for obstruction, and the tympanic membrane is observed for patency. Ice water (10 ml) is instilled into the ear canal. Awake patients have slow movement to the side of stimulation and rapid movement back to the midline. The direction of the rapid movement defines the nystagmus. When the cortex is not functioning, both eyes deviate toward the stimulated side. There is no eye movement with absent brainstem function. Loss of corneal and oculocephalic reflexes occurs in patients with severe TBI and suggests minimal brainstem function.

Focal motor findings in the unconscious patient with TBI suggest hematoma or significant injury to the contralateral cerebral hemisphere. Lateralizing weakness can be difficult to determine in the patient with multiple trauma. Asymmetry in extremity posturing or in localizing pain is noted. Hemiplegia and contralateral pupillary dilation are findings that typically occur shortly before transtentorial herniation.[36,38,39] Flaccid quadriplegia occurs in patients with cervical spine injury with or without TBI.

Laboratory Testing

Laboratory tests have a limited but important role in the initial evaluation of the patient with TBI. Arterial blood gases can give evidence of hypoxemia and hypoperfusion, and can direct appropriate hyperventilation. Metabolic acidosis with adequate oxygenation suggests poor tissue perfusion, despite vital signs that are mildly abnormal. Poor tissue perfusion results from hemorrhage or decreased car-

diac output. Similarly, a low or decreasing hematocrit suggests persistent blood loss and the potential for shock. A normal hematocrit does not exclude significant hemorrhage. Electrolytes are typically normal shortly after TBI, but the hyperadrenergic state that accompanies trauma and TBI can induce temporary hypokalemia and hyperglycemia. Hyperglycemia can adversely affect cerebral metabolism following TBI, and is monitored and treated when necessary. A blood ethanol level and a serum or urine drug screen are essential in adults with suspected TBI. These studies aid in determining whether toxins are likely contributing to an altered mental status. Many patients with TBI are intoxicated; consequently, an altered mental status due solely to alcohol or drugs is a diagnosis of exclusion.

Neuroimaging

After the initial stabilization and evaluation, patients with suspected TBI are imaged by CT scanning of the brain. CT scanning is a rapid and noninvasive imaging modality that has reduced not only the morbidity and mortality of TBI, but also the need for surgical exploration.[40] A typical CT of the brain for a trauma evaluation consists of 10–15 10-mm axial images parallel to the skull base. Typically, images through the posterior fossa and images in pediatric CTs of the head are 5 mm apart. Newer CT scanners provide high-resolution images with total imaging times of two minutes and have improved detection of smaller hemorrhagic areas and edema formation. This technology can provide an anatomical diagnosis of TBI within minutes of patient arrival. Intravenous contrast is not administered in patients with TBI because it can obscure the presence of blood in the brain on CT. CT scanning of the brain is done before any other study that involves a contrast agent.[41]

CT of the brain is done as soon as possible in patients with a GCS score of 13 or less, or in patients with a GCS score of 14 or 15 with a focal neurological finding or persistent altered mental status.[35] When CT scanning is not obtainable, the patient is transferred immediately to the closest medical center with emergency CT scanning and neurosurgical availability. CT scanning may not be needed in patients with a GCS score of 15, a normal physical and neurological examination, and no vomiting or severe headache upon presentation to the emergency department.[43]

CT scanning provides anatomical and pathological information that is useful in determining intracranial lesions such as ICHs, SDHs, EDHs, cerebral edema, mass effect and shift of brain structures, cerebral contusions, skull fractures, pneumocephali, and cerebral infarctions. The need for lesion evacuation is determined more accurately with CT than with clinical examination alone. However, CT scanning is limited in defining nonhemorrhagic injured areas such as the gray–white matter interface disruption that occurs with DAI.[12] This limitation can result in a relatively normal-appearing CT of the head in a patient with TBI and a low GCS score. CT scanning cannot provide information on the blood flow, metabolism function, or of the brain. Xenon-enhanced CT scanning or positron emission tomography (PET) scanning can provide this information.

There are few indications for skull radiographs in the emergency department evaluation of patients with TBI. Some centers obtain plain radiographs of the skull to evaluate for fractures. However, a linear nondepressed skull fracture does not affect patient management, and patients with depressed skull fractures require CT scanning and neurosurgical evaluation.[41,42]

Management

The initial management of the patient with TBI is the same as that for all patients in the emergency department. Airway, breathing, and circulation are assessed and stabilized. Cervical spine precautions are taken while stabilization is ongoing. The incidence of cervical spine injury in patients with severe TBI (GCS score of 8 or less) is approximately 8%, compared with approximately 1–2% in all patients with multiple trauma.[44]

Airway

Initial management of the airway is of primary importance. Patients with severe TBI are intubated and hyperventilated. Endotracheal intubation is indicated in any patient with a GCS score of less than 9 who cannot follow commands.[35] Patients with TBI who have a GCS score of more than 9 are managed

without endotracheal intubation when proper oxygenation and ventilation are maintained. Patients with moderate TBI can be agitated and combative, putting themselves and staff at risk for further injury. Agitation can cause hypoventilation and inadequate oxygenation, and interfere with management. Intubation and mechanical ventilation may be indicated in these situations. Trauma patients who have spine precautions are at risk for aspiration of vomitus, blood, or debris. Endotracheal intubation is the best method to maintain oxygenation and protect the patient from aspiration.

Rapid-sequence intubation (RSI) is the most effective and safest method for providing immediate airway control in patients with severe TBI and has a straightforward technique.[22,45–47] The neurological examination is documented prior to the administration of sedating and paralyzing agents. Two large-bore intravenous lines are inserted. The selection of paralytic and induction agents for RSI is intended to provide good conditions for intubation rapidly, without adversely affecting ICP or CPP. Thiopental, etomidate, and fentanyl are dissimilar pharmacological agents that provide rapid onset of unconsciousness or deep sedation while maintaining cerebral perfusion and preventing increased ICP (see Chapter 25, "Neuroanesthesiology"). Of these agents, etomidate is least likely to induce systemic hypotension.[48] Most protocols for RSI use succinylcholine for induction of paralysis. A dose of 1.5–2.0 mg/kg of lidocaine by intravenous infusion can be given three minutes before succinylcholine to prevent a possible succinylcholine-induced transient rise of ICP. Alternatively, a small dose of a nondepolarizing agent can be given before succinylcholine to prevent fasciculations and an elevation of ICP. Nondepolarizing agents can be used for emergency intubation but are not as rapidly acting as succinylcholine. The use of longer-acting nondepolarizing agents precludes assessment of possible changes in the neurological condition until their effects have ended.[10]

Cervical spine precautions are maintained during endotracheal intubation. Neck movement is minimized by a rigid cervical collar, and by in-line stabilization of the neck procedure. Traction on the neck is avoided.[49] No detrimental effect was reported when RSI was used for airway control in patients with cervical spine injuries in several studies.[10,50]

Fluid Resuscitation

In patients with hemorrhagic shock, decreased CBF to critically low levels is a greater threat to brain cells than is concurrent anemia. The decision to transfuse blood in the patient with TBI is based on issues related to other body injuries. In a stable patient with TBI and no evidence of shock, standard intravenous crystalloid solutions (0.9 normal saline, or lactated Ringer's solution) are used to provide maintenance fluid requirements. Monitoring of the CPP helps guide the rate of fluid administration. Guidelines for the optimal administration of fluids in the setting of brain edema are not established. Fluid restriction may limit brain edema in the patient with severe TBI, but animal studies have not demonstrated the effectiveness of this method of treatment.[51] Because hypotension and decreased CPP are detrimental to patients with TBI, appropriate fluid resuscitation is administered to trauma patients with hemorrhagic complications.

Hypotensive patients are fluid-resuscitated with crystalloid and blood products when indicated. Seventy-five percent of patients with TBI have serious injuries to other organ systems including the abdomen, chest, and skeleton. Splenic or liver injury, hemothorax, scalp or multiple skin lacerations, and pelvic and long bone fractures can induce hemorrhagic shock. Hypotension (systolic blood pressure less than 90 mm Hg) on presentation to the emergency department is associated with worse outcome in patients with TBI, requiring rapid evaluation and treatment of acute hemorrhagic shock.[9,36] Persistent tachycardia can be the first indication of hemorrhage. Hypotension can be a late sign of shock, especially in young patients. Treatment of circulatory shock in trauma patients includes the rapid intravenous infusion of 2–3 liter of crystalloid solution, followed by administration of blood in patients with persistent shock.[37] Assessment of shock includes examination of skin perfusion, urine output, arterial blood gases, serum bicarbonate, and ongoing fluid requirements. The initial hematocrit in patients with circulatory shock can be normal. Patients with moderate to severe TBI require cardiac monitoring with frequent assessment of blood pressure. Intra-arterial catheters provide continuous blood pressure readings and are used to obtain blood for frequent assessment of arterial blood

gases. When intra-arterial monitoring is not performed, oxygen saturation monitors assist in assessing oxygenation status. Patients who are hypotensive or cold and clammy may not have accurate readings. An arterial blood gas is checked initially to determine the correlation between measured oxygen saturation and the monitored reading.

The choice of resuscitation fluid in patients with TBI is not established. Concerns of elevated ICP and brain edema have prompted an interest in other resuscitation fluids such as hypertonic saline. Hypertonic saline is typically administered as a small bolus of dextran in 7.5% saline. In patients with hemorrhagic shock, hypertonic saline improves hemodynamics and increases CPP and oxygen delivery.[52] It can cause osmotic shifts in the brain, resulting in movement of water out of brain tissue and into the systemic intravascular compartment. This can decrease edema and, consequently, ICP. The effects of hypertonic saline are transient, because intravascular sodium chloride diffuses into the interstitial space.[51] The effects of hypertonic saline in the brain are dependent on BBB integrity. When the BBB is intact, osmotic shifts can occur, and hypertonic saline may be helpful. However, when the BBB is injured and normal ionic gradients are lost, hypertonic saline does not produce osmotic effects. In this setting, hypertonic saline can exacerbate brain edema by increasing systemic arterial pressure and CBF. Although hypertonic saline administration may produce acute changes that are desirable in the injured brain, hypertonic saline may injure the BBB and is not recommended as the initial resuscitation fluid in patients with severe TBI.[53]

Ventilation

Following initial stabilization, oxygenation and ventilation are titrated to provide the best possible conditions for the injured brain. Ventilatory management of patients with severe TBI no longer includes hyperventilation, except when there is evidence of acute herniation or deterioration.[54] Hyperventilation and hypocapnia lower blood pH. Cerebral blood vessels constrict and CBF falls in response to the lower pH. CBF in the injured brain is likely lower than normal and, at times, low enough to cause ischemia.[55] By further decreasing CBF with hyperventilation, cerebral perfusion can be compromised and can increase the extent of TBI.[54,56]

Mannitol

Patients with acute brain herniation, or those with neurological deterioration or focal neurological signs and anisocoria may benefit from *brief* periods of hyperventilation and from osmotic diuretics such as mannitol. Because mannitol can potentially worsen hemodynamic instability by causing a large diuresis, its use in patients without brain edema is controversial. When given as a rapid intravenous infusion or bolus, mannitol decreases the extracellular fluid volume by increasing the osmolarity of the blood and by forming an osmotic gradient across the BBB. This reversal of the osmotic gradient occurs in the injured and the uninjured brain.[57] The optimal dose of mannitol is not established. Low doses of 0.25–0.5 g/kg are short-acting but are as effective as higher doses. The usual dosing regimen is 0.25–0.50 g/kg every four to six hours to maintain ICP in a normal range.[58] Repeated doses of mannitol can cause a hyperosmolar state and adversely affect other organ systems. Therefore, the effects of mannitol are evaluated frequently by serum osmolarity and electrolytes, beginning in the emergency department.[58] Mannitol can also be given to hemodynamically stable patients with severe TBI, brain edema, and suspected elevated ICP.

Antiepileptic Drugs

Drugs are commonly given early in the management of patients with moderate to severe TBI. Patients with focal brain injury and hemorrhage can develop an epileptogenic focus that results in seizures. Seizures are detrimental to patients with TBI because of increased metabolic demands and possible hypoxemia and elevations in ICP. It is difficult to detect seizures in a sedated and paralyzed patient.[59] Phenytoin is used to treat patients with convulsive seizures and is used as prophylaxis for patients with severe TBI who have focal lesion.[10,59] Intravenous loading of phenytoin (15–18 mg/kg) is administered at a rate of no more than 50 mg per minute. Recently made available, phosphenytoin can be administered rapidly (see Chap. 12). Treatment of seizures in the patient with TBI is the same as in the nontraumatized patient. Lorazepam (2–4 mg by intravenous infusion) or diazepam (5–10 mg by intravenous infusion) can be used every 5 minutes until the seizure stops, or to a maximum dose of 8–10 mg for lorazepam or 20 mg for diazepam. Because these agents can cause respiratory depression, the airway is protected when higher doses are used. Phenobarbital is the next drug of choice for patients with persistent convulsive seizures.

Opiate Analgesics

Patients with moderate to severe TBI can be agitated and combative. Resisting the ventilator can elevate and exacerbate ICP. Comatose patients with TBI perceive pain demonstrated by hemodynamic and ICP changes that occur when stimulated. Medication for pain is provided, especially to those patients with concurrent painful injuries. Opiate agents, such as morphine and fentanyl, can be administered by bolus or infusion. However, following the use of sedating agents, it is more difficult to assess the neurological state of the patient. Management of patients is assessed individually.[10] Early paralysis is not beneficial to patients with TBI unless it facilitates evaluation and management. Patients who receive neuromuscular blockade spend more time in the intensive care unit and have a higher incidence of pneumonia without improvement in outcome.[60] Corticosteroids are not beneficial in the management of patients with TBI.[10,54]

Pediatric Traumatic Brain Injury

TBI in children results from motor vehicle crashes, falls, bicycle accidents, pedestrian accidents, and nonaccidental injury. The cause of TBI in children varies with age and geographic location. In the inner city, homicide, including that resulting from child abuse, is the leading cause of TBI in infants and adolescents. In infants, TBI results primarily from nonaccidental injury, motor vehicle collisions, and falls. The incidence of pediatric TBI in the United States is 185–200 per 100,000 children per year, and TBI is the cause of death in approximately 40% of childhood injuries. It occurs in males more commonly than in females, and in infants and adolescents more commonly than in children.[61,62] Children with TBI recover more quickly and with less residual impairment than do adults with similar injuries. However, children under 3 years of age have a poorer prognosis than those over age 3 years. Infants have a thinner and more pliable skull that is less protective of the underlying brain. The head is also disproportionately larger in infants, compared with older children and adults.

Many pediatric TBIs result from situations that are unique to childhood. Infants and young toddlers are placed in walker devices, which can result in serious falls, especially down the stairs. TBI can result from car restraint systems that are not intended for children and do not provide sufficient protection for them. Appropriate car seats are required for adequate protection. The inappropriate use, or lack of use, of car seats can result in more severe TBI due to motor vehicle collisions. Although bicycle accidents are not unique to childhood, the majority of cyclists are children, who are less likely to wear a helmet.[63] The severity of TBI due to bicycle accidents is related to the use (or nonuse) of helmets.[62]

PEARLS AND PITFALLS

- TBI is one of the leading preventable causes of death and disability worldwide.
- Primary brain injury is caused by functional and physical disruption of brain tissue; secondary brain injury occurs when postinjury factors such as hypoxemia and hypotension further adversely affect the injured brain.
- DAI is likely the primary reason for persistent coma following TBI.
- Patients with TBI can be intoxicated, confounding the presentation of TBI.
- A "normal" Glasgow Coma Scale does not exclude TBI.
- CT scanning is the neuroimaging study of choice in the emergency department when evaluating patients with TBI.
- Hyperventilation is not performed in the patient with TBI, except when there is evidence of acute brain herniation or neurological deterioration.

REFERENCES

1. Bennett BR, Jacobs LM, Schwarz JR. Incidence, cost and DRG-based reimbursement for traumatic brain injured patients: A 3 year experience. *J Trauma.* 1989;29:556–65.
2. Jennett B, Frankowski RF. The epidemiology of head injury. In: Braakman R, ed. *Handbook of Clinical Neurology.* New York, NY: Elsevier Science Publishers; 1990;13:1–16.
3. Shackford SR, Mackersie RC, Davis JW, et al. Epidemiology and pathology of traumatic deaths occurring at a level I trauma center in a regionalized system: the importance of secondary brain injury. *J Trauma.* 1989;29:1392–97.
4. Van Zomeren AH, Saan RJ. Psychological and social sequelae of severe head injury. In: Braakman R, ed. *Handbook of Clinical Neurology.* New York, NY: Elsevier Science Publishers; 1990;13:397–420.
5. Kraus J. Epidemiology of head injury. In: Cooper PC, ed. *Head Injury.* Baltimore, Md: Williams & Wilkins; 1993:1–25.
6. Kraus JF, Black MA, Hessol N, et al. The incidence of acute brain injury and serious impairment in a defined population. *Am J Epidemiol.*1984;119: 186–201.
7. Brismar B, Engstrom A, Rydberg U. Head injury and intoxication: a diagnostic and therapeutic dilemma. *Acta Chir Scand.* 1983;149:11–14.
8. Gurney JG, Rivara FP, Mueller BA, et al. The effects of alcohol intoxication on the initial treatment and hospital course of patients with acute brain injury. *J Trauma.* 1992;33:709–13.
9. Miller JD. Changing patterns in acute management of head injury. *J Neurol Sci.* 1991;103:S33–7.
10. Zink BJ. Traumatic brain injury. *Emerg Med Clin North Am.* 1996;14:115–50.
11. Stalhammar DA. The mechanism of brain injuries. In: Braakman R, ed. *Handbook of Clinical Neurology.* New York, NY: Elsevier Science Publishers; 1990;13: 17–41.
12. Gentry LR. Imaging of closed head injury. *Radiology.* 1994;191:1–17.
13. Cooper PR. Post-traumatic intracranial mass lesions. In: Cooper PR, ed. *Head Injury.* Baltimore, Md: Williams & Wilkins, 1993:275–329.
14. Sprick C, Bettag M, Bock WJ. Delayed traumatic intracranial hematomas – clinical study of seven years. *Neurosurg Rev.* 1989;12(suppl 1):228–30.
15. Klun B, Fettich M. Factors influencing the outcome in acute subdural hematoma. A review of 330 cases. *Acta Neurochir.* 1984;71:171–8.
16. Cook RJ, Dorsch NWC, Rearnside MR, et al. Outcome prediction in extradural hematomas. *Acta Neurochir.* 1988;95:90–4.
17. Ganz JC, Zwetnow NN. Analysis of the dynamics of experimental bleeding in swine. *Acta Neurochir.* 1988;95:72–81.
18. Povlishok JT. Traumatically induced axonal injury: pathogenesis and pathobiological implications. *Brain Pathol.* 1992;2:1–12.

19. Dacey RG, Dikman SS. Mild head injury. In: Cooper PR, ed. *Head Injury.* Baltimore, Md: Williams & Wilkins; 1993:159–83.

20. Doberstein CE, Hovda DA, Becker DP. Clinical considerations in the reduction of secondary brain injury. *Ann Emerg Med.* 1993;22:993–7.

21. Cold GE. Cerebral blood flow in acute head injury: the regulation of cerebral blood flow and metabolism during the acute phase of head injury, and its significance for therapy. *Acta Neurochir.* 1990;49(suppl):1–64.

22. Wahl M, Schilling L. Regulation of cerebral blood flow – a brief review. *Acta Neurochir.* 1993;59(suppl):3–10.

23. Betz AL, Crockard A. Brain edema and the blood brain barrier. In: Crockard A, Hayward R, Hoff JT, eds. *Neurosurgery: The Scientific Basis of Clinical Practice,* 2nd ed. Oxford: Blackwell Scientific Publications; 1992:353–72.

24. Pitts LH, McIntosh TK. Dynamic changes after brain trauma. In: Braakman R, ed. *Handbook of Clinical Neurology.* New York, NY: Elsevier Science Publishers; 1990;13:65–100.

25. Fessler RD, Diaz FG. The management of cerebral perfusion pressure and intracranial pressure after severe head injury. *Ann Emerg Med.* 1993;22:998–1003.

26. Marmarou A, Tabaddor K. Intracranial pressure: physiology and pathophysiology. In Cooper PC, ed. *Head Injury.* Baltimore, Md: Williams & Wilkins, 1993:203–224.

27. Olshaker JS, Whye DW. Head trauma. *Emerg Med Clin North Am.* 1993;11:165–86.

28. Murr R, Berger S, Schürer L, et al. Relationship of cerebral blood flow disturbances with brain edema formation. *Acta Neurochir.* 1993;59:11–17.

29. White BC, Krause GS. Brain injury and repair mechanisms: the potential for pharmacologic therapy in closed-head trauma. *Ann Emerg Med.* 1993;22:970–9.

30. Krasznai L, Grote EH. Acute vasoparalysis after subarachnoid hemorrhage and cerebral trauma: general reflex phenomenon? *Neurol Res.* 1994;16:40–3.

31. Siesjo BK. Basic mechanisms of traumatic brain damage. *Ann Emerg Med.* 1993;22:959–69.

32. Gutteridge JMC, Rowley DA, Holliwell B. Superoxide-dependent formation of hydroxyl radicals in the presence of iron salts. Detection of free iron in biological systems by using bleomycin-dependent degradation of DNA. *Biochem J.* 1981;199:263–5.

33. Becker DP. Common themes in head injury. In: Becker DP, Gudeman SK, eds. *Textbook of Head Injury.* Philadelphia, Pa: WB Saunders, 1989:1–22.

34. Zink BJ, Feustel PJ. Effects of ethanol on respiratory function in traumatic brain injury. *J Neurosurg.* 1995; 82:112–8.

35. Gentleman D, Dearden M, Midgley S, et al. Guidelines for resuscitation and transfer of patients with serious head injury. *Br Med J.* 1993;307:547–52.

36. Miller JD. Assessing patients with head injury. *Br J Surg.* 1990;77:242.

37. Alexander RH, Proctor HJ, eds. *Advanced Trauma Life Support Course for Physicians.* 5th ed. Chicago, Ill: American College of Surgeons; 1993.

38. Andrews BT, Pitts LH. *Traumatic Transtentorial Herniation and Its Management.* Mt. Kisco, NY: Futura Publishing Co; 1991:59–72.

39. Mendelow AD. Clinical examination in traumatic brain damage. In: Braakman R, ed. *Handbook of Clinical Neurology.* New York, NY: Elsevier Science Publishers; 1990;13:123–42.

40. Johnson MH, Lee SH. Computed tomography of acute cerebral trauma. *Radiol Clin North Am.* 1992;30: 325–50.

41. Hughes M, Cohen WA. Radiographic evaluation. In: Cooper PR, ed. *Head Injury.* Baltimore, Md: Williams & Wilkins, 1993:65–90.

42. Masters SJ, McClean PM, Arcarese JS, et al. Skull x-ray examinations after head trauma: recommendations by a multidisciplinary panel and validation study. *N Engl J Med.* 1987;316:84–91.

43. Miller EC, Derlet RW, Kinser D. Minor head trauma: is computed tomography always necessary? *Ann Emerg Med.* 1996;27:290–4.

44. Hills MW, Deane SA. Head injury and facial injury: is there an increased risk of cervical spine injury? *J Trauma.* 1993;34:549.

45. Rotondo MF, McGonigal MD, Schwab CW, et al. Urgent paralysis and intubation of trauma patients: is it safe? *J Trauma.* 1993;34:242–6.

46. Walls RM. Rapid-sequence intubation in head trauma. *Ann Emer Med.* 1992;22:1008–13.

47. Morris IR. Pharmacologic aids to intubation and the rapid sequence induction. *Emerg Med Clin North Am.* 1988;6:753–68.

48. Harris CE, Murray AM, Anderson JM, et al. Effects of thiopentone, etomidate and propofol on the hemodynamic response of tracheal intubation. *Anaesthesia.* 1988;43:32–6.

49. Bivins HG, Ford S, Bezmalinovic Z, et al. The effect of axial traction during orotracheal intubation of the trauma victim with an unstable cervical spine. *Ann Emerg Med.* 1988;17:25–9.

50. Wright SW, Robinson GG II, Wright MB. Cervical spine injuries in blunt trauma patients requiring emergent endotracheal intubation. *Am Emerg Med.* 1992;10:104–9.

51. Sutin K, Ruskin K, Kaufman B. Intravenous fluid therapy in neurologic injury. *Crit Care Clin.* 1992;8:367–408.

52. Schmoker J, Zhuang J, Shackford S. Hypertonic fluid resuscitation improves cerebral oxygen delivery and reduces intracranial pressure after hemorrhagic shock. *J Trauma.* 1991;31:1607–13.

53. Gunnar WP, Jonasson O, Merloti G, et al. Head injury and hemorrhagic shock: studies of the blood-brain barrier and intracranial pressure after resuscitation with normal saline solution, 3% saline solution and dextran-40. *Surgery.* 1988;103:398.

54. Bullock R, Chesnur RM, Clifton G, et al. *Guidelines for the Management of Severe Head Injury.* Washington, DC: Brain Trauma Foundation; 1995.

55. Bouma GJ, Muizelaar JP, Stringer WA, et al. Ultra-early evaluation of regional cerebral blood flow in severely head injured patients using xenon-enhanced computerized tomography. *J Neurosurg.* 1992;77:360–8.

56. Muizelaar JP, Marmarou A, Ward JD, et al. Adverse effects of prolonged hyperventilation in patients with severe head injury: a randomized clinical trial. *J Neurosurg.* 1991;75:731–9.

57. McGraw CP, Howard G. Effect of mannitol on increased intracranial pressure. *Neurosurgery.* 1983;13:269–71.

58. Smith H, Kelly D, McWhorter J, et al. Comparison of mannitol regimens in patients with severe head injury undergoing intracranial monitoring. *J Neurosurg.* 1986;65:820–4.

59. Biros MH. Anticonvulsants. In: Barsan WG, Jastremski MS, Syverud SA, eds. *Emergency Drug Therapy.* Philadelphia, Pa: WB Saunders Co; 1991:120–46.

60. Hsiang JK, Chesnut RM, Crisp CB, et al. Early routine paralysis for intracranial pressure control in severe head injury: is it necessary? *Crit Care Med.* 1994,22:1471–6.

61. Shapiro K, Smith LP. Special considerations for the pediatric age group. In: Cooper PC, ed. *Head Injury.* Baltimore, Md: Williams & Wilkins; 1993:427–59.

62. Ghajar J, Haririi RJ. Management of pediatric head injury. *Pediatr Clin North Am.* 1992;39:1093–123.

63. Noakes TD. Fatal cycling injuries. *Sports Med.* 1992; 20:348–62.

31 Spinal Cord Injuries

CHARLES H. BILL II

SUMMARY The proper care of patients with spinal injury requires adherence to the basic rules of trauma management. Prevention of further injury by spinal immobilization and maintenance of adequate tissue perfusion and oxygenation is emphasized. The neurological examination includes a focused evaluation of motor and sensory function. Injury of paraspinal soft tissue, vertebrae, and the nervous system is described. Proper documentation and communication between the emergency physician and prehospital care providers and family members is stressed.

Introduction

Injury of the spine and spinal cord is one of the most common causes of disability and death following trauma. In the United States, there are an estimated 200,000 new spinal column injuries and approximately 8000–10,000 spinal cord injuries each year,[1–4] and an estimated 300,000–500,000 individuals with chronic paralysis due to spinal cord injury.[5] The incidence of spinal cord injury is highest in young people between 15 and 30 years of age, with a male-to-female ratio of 4:1. The most common causes of spinal cord injury are motor vehicle accidents (approximately 50%); falls (21%), and violence (15%); diving, recreational, and athletic injuries (14%) account for the rest. Regional factors modify the contribution of each of these modes of injuries. For example, gunshot wounds (GSW) cause 34% of the spinal cord injuries in south Florida.[3] Currently, 5–10% of patients with spinal cord injuries die acutely due to concomitant injury, age, or preexisting medical conditions, and not due to the spinal cord injury itself. Successful treatment of patients with spinal cord injury depends on a multidisciplinary team approach that begins at the accident scene and continues through the triage, operating room, intensive care, rehabilitation, and outpatient home care stages.[3]

Prehospital Management

After the initial injury, care is taken to prevent secondary injury. Secondary injuries result from injury to an unstable spine, biochemical abnormality such as hypoxia (from inadequate airway or respiratory drive), or hypoperfusion of an injured spinal cord due to hypotension. Emergency medical services providers are aided by modern extrication equipment and special patient-handling devices that provide for immediate spinal stability. The use of oximeters, early intubation, and fluid resuscitation can reduce the incidence of hypoxia and hypoperfusion. In most situations, it is relatively easy to immobilize the patient on a back board in a neutral position with the head blocked and taped. Occasionally, the patient's head appears to be "fixed" in a position other than neutral due to some aspect of the trauma. In this situation, the patient is blocked without movement and not forced into a neutral position. When hypotension exists, transportation in the Trendelenburg position can be helpful. Care is taken to prevent hypothermia.

Resuscitation at the scene follows the basic requirements of trauma management. It is important to evaluate thoroughly the accident scene for any unusual features that may explain the status of the patient or alter the treatment plan. A focused history is obtained from the patient and others at the scene regarding the nature of the accident, coexisting medical conditions, tobacco, alcohol, and drug use, medications and allergies, and when and how much the patient last ate. The patient is asked about neck pain, back pain, and extremity numbness or tingling. The patient is examined for evidence of head trauma, and Glasgow Coma Scale score is determined. A patient with impaired consciousness or intoxication is treated as if there is an unstable spinal injury and head injury. The neurological examination focuses on motor function and muscle tone. Alert patients are asked to raise their hands over their heads, click their fingers, or open and close their hands rapidly, and individually raise each knee and extend the leg off the board. Strength testing is performed for ankle dorsiflexion, toe dorsiflexion, and plantar flexion. Bowel or bladder incontinence, or priapism is noted. Spinal cord injury and resultant sympathectomy causes reduction in blood pressure, pulse, cardiac contractility, and output. Hypotension can result from ongoing blood loss. Vigorous fluid resuscitation can be dangerous in patients with spinal shock due to a compromised cardiac output. Use of a sympathetic agonist such as dopamine may be required to correct hypotension in patients with spinal shock.

A stable patient is transported to the facility that is best equipped to handle patients with spinal cord injury. An unstable patient is transported to the nearest emergency department for immediate care and stabilization. Subsequent arrangements can be made to transport the patient to a tertiary care center for definitive care. Effective communication between the prehospital care providers and the emergency physician is important to ensure that appropriate preparations are made to receive the patient. The nature of the injury (history), brief general physical examination including vital signs, oxygen saturation (when available), neurological examination (to include Glasgow Coma Scale score and motor examination), condition (whether stable or deteriorating), and treatment rendered is reported in a clear, concise fashion.

Documentation of the patient's pretreatment condition at the time the emergency medical services providers arrive, vital signs, and the initial neurological assessment are critical to patient care. The assessment and documentation of any change in the clinical condition of the patient when treatment is begun at the scene is also important. Acute deterioration of the patient's condition is communicated immediately to the emergency physician. Paralysis can ascend secondary to intraspinal hemorrhage and requires urgent radiographic evaluation and possible immediate surgical intervention. Permanent neurological disability is very expensive in terms of lost wages and long-term care. The medical-legal risk in these circumstances is second only to that seen in neonatology.

Emergency Department Evaluation

Patients with acute spinal cord injuries are evaluated as trauma patients in accordance with the guidelines established by the American College of Surgeons.[8] The primary survey consists of assessment of airway, breathing, circulation, disability (assessment of neurological status), and exposure (patient is fully undressed for examination). Most of the primary survey is conducted prior to the patient's arrival to the emergency department. Multisystem involvement is observed in approximately 50% of patients with spinal cord injury. Spinal cord injury may not be the most life-threatening injury. Resuscitation begins with an evaluation of the adequacy of the patient's airway. Quadriplegic patients lose neural control of intercostal muscles and are largely dependent on the diaphragm (which may be compromised) for respiration. Signs of respiratory fatigue require immediate tracheal intubation and ventilatory support. Patients at high risk for respiratory fatigue are those with preexisting pulmonary problems, obesity, acute aspiration or upper airway compromise, or advanced age. Tracheal intubation is achieved by the oral route with in-line support of the head and neck, or by the nasotracheal route, preferably using fiberoptic visualization. The patient's head, neck, and shoulders are kept in axial alignment during this procedure. Cervical traction is not performed, because ligamentous stability is not fully known at this point in the delivery of care. Cervical traction could result in inadvertent spinal cord injury, especially in the very young patient.

Fluid resuscitation requires two large-bore intravenous lines and bladder catheterization to monitor urine output. The influence of perfusion pressure on spinal cord recovery has been studied in models of dog and monkey spinal cord trauma. In these studies inadequate spinal cord perfusion was observed when the diastolic blood pressure was 69 mm Hg or lower. When patients have sustained incomplete spinal cord injuries where further recovery is possible, adequate blood pressure and volume support are crucial. Older patients with advanced atherosclerosis may require a higher-than-average baseline blood pressure, and hypotension is poorly tolerated. In the presence of spinal cord injury with resultant sympathectomy, a continuous infusion and titration of vasopressors such as dopamine in the emergency department to keep the diastolic blood pressure over 70 mm Hg is indicated. In older individuals, high blood pressures may be maintained. When the spinal cord injury is at the T8 level or higher, the patient is at a higher risk for hypothermia, and appropriate precautions are taken.

The neurological examination begins with assessment of the level of consciousness, and a Glasgow Coma Scale score is assigned. Function of the pupils and the extraocular muscles is tested, and the obvious smell of alcohol or other evidence of drug use is noted.

Spinal evaluation begins with the examination of the patient's motor system. The phrenic nerves originate primarily from the fourth cervical nerves and some from the third and fifth cranial nerves. Spinal cord injuries at or above the C4 level result in respiratory arrest. When the level of injury is just below the origins of the phrenic nerves, the intercostal muscles cannot contract and the patient can be completely dependent on diaphragmatic contraction for respiration. The upper extremities are assessed by asking patients to hold their arms straight up in the air, and then over the head. These movements are possible for patients with lower cervical cord injury, provided there are no other limiting injuries. Lower cervical spine injury can be assessed by having the patients open and close their hands tightly, and snap their fingers. These actions are impaired or impossible for patients with lower cervical spine injury. Lifting the head off the examining table causes the patient's abdominal muscles to contract. When the lower abdominal muscles are paralyzed during this maneuver, the umbilicus moves in a cephalad direction (Beevor's sign), indicating

spinal cord damage below the T10 level. The patient is asked to lift the knees (hip flexors, L2) and to extend the legs (knee extensors, L3) to evaluate upper lumbar function. Ankle dorsiflexion (L4), long toe extensors (L5), and plantar flexors (S1) are tested to assess lower lumbar and upper sacral level functions. When all the above segments are intact and rectal tone is normal, serious spinal cord injury is unlikely.

Intoxication complicates the clinical evaluation. Great care is taken in the handling and evaluation of intoxicated patients until the entire spine is "cleared" radiographically and the intoxication resolves. Patients with suspected hysterical paralysis or weakness require a focused neurological and radiographic evaluation. Generally, the hysterical patient presents with a profound motor deficit, typically in the lower extremities, and normal reflexes and rectal tone. These patients are hospitalized until the paralysis resolves.

The sensory examination begins with pinprick testing from insensate areas in a cephalad direction to determine the level of spinal cord injury. There may be a zone of abnormal sensation below the intact level. It may be helpful to draw a line on both sides of the patient's body for future comparison and to help localize the area of injured spine for radiographics. A standardized scoring sheet, such as that prepared by the American Spinal Injury Association: International Standards for Neurological Classification of Spinal Cord Injury,[16] is used for each patient (Fig. 31.1). Posterior column function is assessed by applying deep pressure to the extremities, by testing with a tuning fork over bony prominences, and by testing position sense in a distal to proximal fashion.

"Spinal shock" results from physiological transection of the spinal cord, which commonly lasts for 24–48 hours. During this time, flaccid paralysis occurs below the level of the spinal cord injury, and all reflexes are typically absent below this level. Following recovery from spinal shock, there is return of reflex arcs below the level of injury. Patients who experience continued paralysis after the return of reflex arcs following spinal shock have a poor prognosis. One of the first reflexes assessed is the bulbocavernosus reflex, involving the S3 and S4 nerve roots. This reflex is tested by squeezing or pulling the glans penis or the clitoris and noting

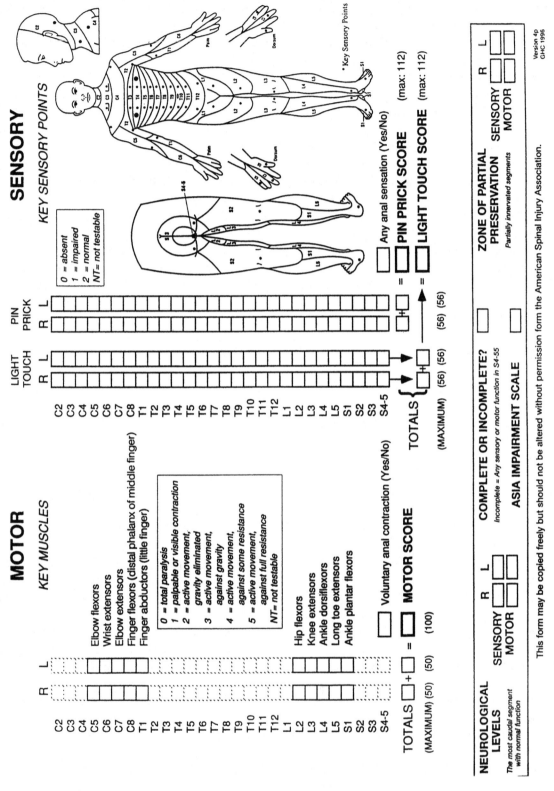

FIGURE 31.1. Standard score sheet for classification of spinal cord injury (from *International Standards for Neurological and Functional Classification of Spinal Cord Injury*. Revised 1996. American Spinal Injury Association/International Medical Society of Paraplegia, Chicago, Illinois. Reprinted by permission).

TABLE 31.1. Soft Tissue Injuries

Acute cervical sprain
Disc herniation
  Pain syndrome
  Nerve root syndrome
  Spinal cord compression
  Cauda equina syndrome
Vascular injury
  Arterial (stroke)
  Venous (epidural hematoma)

contraction of the anal sphincter. This test can be accomplished by pulling on an inserted Foley catheter. A similar contraction of the anal sphincter, the "anal wink," is elicited by stroking the skin of the perianal area. This reflex tests the S2–4 nerve roots. A transition from early spinal shock with flaccid extremities to spastic extremities, hyperactive deep tendon reflexes, and extensor plantar responses occurs 6–16 weeks following complete spinal cord injuries.

Anal tone is evaluated in each patient. Voluntary contraction of the anus is tested in an alert and cooperative patient by having him or her squeeze down on the examiner's finger. Sensation in the perianal area is also noted. Voluntary anal contraction or perianal sensation indicates "sacral sparing," an incomplete injury to the spinal cord, and a more favorable prognosis.

Breakdown of Injury

Soft Tissue Injury

Acute cervical sprain is the most common injury following a vehicular accident (see Table 31.1 for a list of soft tissue injuries). The typical mechanism of injury is hyperflexion-hyperextension of the cervical spine, without or with concomitant head injury. There is partial tearing of ligaments, muscle, connective tissue (fascia), discs, and joint capsules, but most of the fibers remain intact. Typically, radiographs are normal and there is no significant instability. The term *whiplash* was introduced in 1928 to describe "the manner in which a head was moved

suddenly to produce a sprain in the neck."[11] The term is not a medical diagnosis and does not describe a pathological condition; its use should be avoided. Most patients improve with time and require reassurance. Treatment includes nonsteroidal anti-inflammatory drugs (NSAIDs), heat/cold, a soft cervical collar, and physical therapy.

Disc herniation can result from trauma. A nerve root syndrome (radiculopathy) resulting from mechanical pressure on a single nerve root is the typical presentation. Posterior herniation of the disk in the cervical, thoracic, or upper lumbar spine can cause spinal cord compression (Fig. 31.2). Occasionally, the spinal cord and the nerve root are compressed, resulting in myeloradiculopathy. An isolated disc herniation due to trauma is rare but can accompany more serious ligamentous disruptions (dislocations) or fracture dislocations. Older patients who have significant degenerative changes of the spine (spondylosis) can develop new nerve root syndromes or spinal cord syndromes (e.g., central cord syndrome) from preexisting stenosis without associated soft tissue injury or fracture.

Over 90% of carotid artery injuries in the United States result from penetrating injuries. Injuries to the carotid arteries, the vertebral arteries, and jugular veins are commonly associated with spinal cord injuries caused by GSW.[12] A series of 15,935 victims of blunt trauma in San Diego, California, included only 14 patients with carotid artery dissections. Two of these patients had concomitant cervical spine fractures.[13]

The vertebral arteries enter the foramina transversaria of C6, continue through the same in all the cephalad vertebrae, and penetrate the dura mater to join the opposite vessel in the formation of the basilar artery. The vertebral arteries can be compressed where they enter the C6 foramina, and degenerative osteophytes can compromise the vessels at the C2–5 foramina. Subluxations of the cervical vertebrae can cause vertebral artery occlusions, resulting in stroke. Over 80% of vertebral artery injuries are the result of the "sudden thrust" of chiropractic manipulation.[12] Most chiropractic injuries occur in relatively young individuals who have no risk factors for stroke.[14] The vertebral artery is surrounded by a venous plexus. Spinal cord ischemia can result from a traumatic arteriovenous fistulae. Vascular oc-

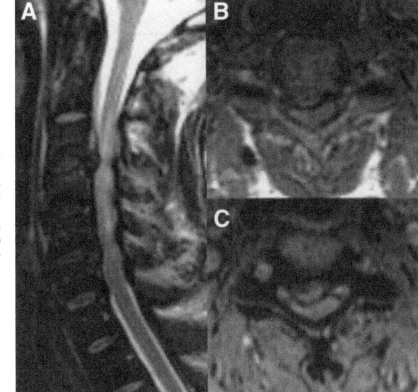

FIGURE 31.2. Traumatic cervical disc herniation in a 38-year-old unrestrained man who lost control of his car and struck a tree. (A) T2 sagittal MRI showing the C3–4 disc herniation stripping the posterior longitudinal ligament from the vertebral bodies. Compression of the spinal cord and increased signal in the spinal cord are observed. (B, C) T1 and gradient refocused images.

clusion is suspected when stroke follows initial trauma. Diagnostic evaluation begins with duplex ultrasound and magnetic resonance angiography, but is best performed by selective angiography. Treatment can be as simple as establishing normal vertebral alignment with prompt skeletal traction. Treatment may require heparinization or ligation of one of the vertebral arteries. Patients at increased risk for epidural hemorrhage following spinal fracture are those with ankylosing spondylitis ("bamboo spine"), in which there is complete circumferential bony fusion of the spine, or those with diffuse idiopathic skeletal hyperostosis (Forestier's disease), in which there is thickening and ossification of the anterior longitudinal ligament.[15] Progression of neurological deficit in these patients following injury suggests the possibility of epidural hemorrhage. Plain radiographs demonstrate ankylosing spondylitis and Forestier's disease and fractures when present. Patients with bleeding disorders or those treated with anticoagulant agents are also at increased risk for epidural hemorrhage following spinal trauma. When acute neurological deteriora-

tion occurs, magnetic resonance imaging (MRI) is performed as soon as possible to evaluate for hemorrhage (Fig. 31.3). When MRI is not available or there is a contraindication to this imaging modality, myelography and postmyelogram computerized tomography (CT) are performed. Coagulation abnormalities are corrected promptly. When compression of the spinal cord or cauda equina is demonstrated, prompt surgical exploration and evacuation are necessary to preserve neurological function.

Patients who have severe rheumatoid arthritis can have severe degenerative spondylosis of the spine and a preexisting C1–2 ligamentous instability, which predisposes them to spinal cord injury.

Nervous System Injuries

Nerve Root Injury

Compression of a nerve root by a disc or bone can result in loss of sensory innervation of a dermatome, motor innervation of a myotome, or both. Pain is nonspecific in the location shortly following

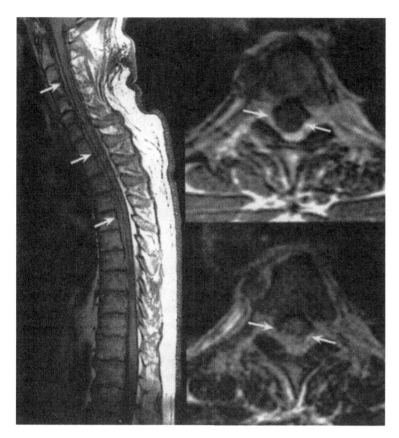

FIGURE 31.3. Spinal epidural hematoma in a 57-year-old man who had a minor fall and presented with progressive quadriplegia, neck, and back pain. He was taking coumadin for a prosthetic mitral valve. (A) T1 sagittal MRI. Arrows outline the epidural hematoma, which is anterior to the spinal cord with which it is isointense. (B, C) T1 and T2 axial images. Arrows demarcate the cleft between the hematoma and the posteriorly displaced spinal cord. The increased signal in the spinal cord is observed on T2 imaging (C).

nerve root compression but eventually can localize in a dermatomal distribution. Isolated nerve root irritation without spinal cord damage can be observed in patients with cervical sprains who have significant spondylosis, traumatic disc herniations, and subluxations, in which disc disruption is a part of the overall injury (e.g., a unilateral facet dislocation). More commonly, these accompany spinal cord injury at the level of disruption. Nerve root irritation results in radicular or nonspecific pain without or with motor deficit. Pain and weakness can improve following surgical decompression or closed reduction of cervical subluxations. Recovery of function of one spinal cord level in a quadriplegic patient can result in partial, as opposed to complete disability. Assessment of severity of neurological impairment is listed in Figure 31.4.

Complete Spinal Cord Injury

The 1996 revised standard of the American Spinal Injury Association (Fig. 31.1) defines complete injury as one in which no motor or sensory function is preserved in the sacral segments S4–5.[16]

The "zone of partial preservation" is defined as the number of segments below the neurological level that remain partially innervated. The "neurological level" is defined as the most caudal level with normal function. Sensory function (pinprick and light touch) are tested bilaterally in a dermatomal fashion (the presence or absence of any perianal sensation represents S4–5), and is graded in each dermatome as follows: 0 indicates absent; 1, impaired; 2, normal. Motor testing of elbow flexors (C5), wrist extensors (C6), elbow extensors (C7), finger flexors (C8), finger abductors (T1), hip flexors (L2), knee extensors (L3), ankle dorsiflexors (L4), long toe extensors (L5), and ankle plantar flexors (S1) is performed. The presence of voluntary anal contraction represents integrity of the S4–5 spinal cord level. Grading of motor function is done by international convention as follows: 0 indicates total paralysis; 1, palpable or visible contraction; 2, active movement, gravity eliminated; 3, active movement against gravity; 4, active movement against some resistance; 5, active movement against full resistance. In the acute setting, definitive testing as described above is of-

ASIA IMPAIRMENT SCALE

☐ **A = Complete:** No motor or sensory function is preserved in the sacral segments S4-S5.

☐ **B = Incomplete:** Sensory but not motor function is preserved below the neurological level and includes the sacral segments S4-S5.

☐ **C = Incomplete:** Motor function is preserved below the neurological level, and more than half of key muscles below the neurological level have a muscle grade less than 3.

☐ **D = Incomplete:** Motor function is preserved below the neurological level, and at least half of key muscles below the neurological level have a muscle grade of 3 or more.

☐ **E = Normal:** motor and sensory function is normal.

CLINICAL SYNDROMES

☐ Central Cord
☐ Brown-Sequard
☐ Anterior Cord
☐ Conus Medullaris
☐ Cauda Equina

FIGURE 31.4. ASIA impairment scale for grading the degree of neurological impairment (from International Standards for Neurological and Functional Classification of Spinal Cord Injury. Revised 1996. American Spinal Injury Association/International Medical Society of Paraplegia, Chicago, Illinois. Reprinted by permission).

tennot possible or practical and is not always meaningful for long-term prognosis. The presence of alcohol or other intoxicating substances, coexistence of head or multisystem trauma, and the evolution of injury with intervention make a definitive examination difficult until approximately three to seven days after the initial injury. Frequent reevaluation

and a comprehensive record of neurological findings are crucial.

Patients with spinal shock due to physiological transsection of the spinal cord are flaccid, areflexive, and without sensation below the zone of injury. Rarely does complete spinal shock last longer than 24 hours. When no recovery is noted within 24 hours, permanent paralysis and sensory loss is likely to occur. In 6–16 weeks following the injury, a spastic hyperreflexive state evolves, indicating loss of function of upper motor neurons. There is a 3–5% probability of significant spontaneous recovery following spinal shock.[3]

Incomplete Spinal Cord Injuries

As defined by the American Spinal Injury Association,[16] these injuries are divided into three categories. In the first category, sensory, but not motor, function is preserved below the neurological level and extends through the sacral S4–5 segments. In the second category, motor function is preserved below the neurological level; most of the key muscles below the neurological level have a muscle strength grade lower than 3. In the third category, motor function is preserved below the neurological level; most of the key muscles below the neurological level have a muscle strength grade of 3 or higher.

Spinal Cord Syndromes

Spinal cord syndromes were first described in the 1950s and 1960s.[17] The most frequent spinal cord syndrome, the *central cord syndrome,* was thought to be due to hemorrhage of the central gray matter with subsequent swelling of the surrounding white matter. Recent information suggests that "buckling of hypertrophied ligamentum flavum, associated with hyperextension, creates a shearing injury to the underlying cord tissue."[18] This hyperextension injury occurs most commonly in middle-aged and elderly males with preexisting spinal stenosis (Fig. 31.5). Plain radiographs and CT imaging usually demonstrate spondylosis. MRI typically demonstrates spinal cord contusion. Pathology is observed predominantly in the central gray and adjacent white matter. In the corticospinal tracts, medial placement of fibers to the upper extremity likely results in disproportionately greater weakness of the upper extremities compared to the lower extremities. Sensory abnormalities include hypesthesia, dysesthesia, and hyperesthesia of the upper extremities. Bladder, bowel, and sexual dysfunction can occur initially. A gradual but limited improvement typically occurs. These patients have a 75% probability of functional recovery. Surgical decompression of the stenosis is controversial. In the acute phase, the patient's neck is kept immobilized with a hard cervical collar.

The second most common syndrome, the *anterior cord syndrome,* usually results from an axial loading or flexion mechanism where either bone, disk, or both become dislodged into the anterior canal and the spinal cord. In addition to the complete motor deficit that begins at the level of injury, pain and temperature sensation is lost, usually starting a few levels below that of the motor loss. The dorsal columns are spared. The prognosis for recovery with anterior cord syndrome is poor, with a 10–20% probability of recovering functional motor control. Surgery usually is indicated to stabilize the spine.

The *Brown-Sequard syndrome* (spinal cord hemisection), as the result of penetrating injury (e.g., stab wound), was first described in 1850.[19] This classic description includes an ipsilateral motor paralysis, ipsilateral dorsal column injury (loss of two-point discrimination, proprioception, vibration, and deep pressure), and contralateral loss of pain and temperature beginning two levels below the level of injury. This syndrome is rarely observed as described initially, but can occur with nonpenetrating injury or with spinal cord injury in patients with severe spondylosis. The probability of functional recovery is greater than 90%.

The *posterior cord syndrome* is rare. It occurs with selective injury to the posterior columns and results in the loss of deep pressure and pain, vibration sense, and proprioception.

The *conus medullaris syndrome* has components of both spinal cord and nerve root (i.e., cauda equina) injury. These occur commonly with thoracolumbar spine injury, where anterior elements of bone and disc are thrust posteriorly into the caudal end of the spinal cord. A complete or incomplete spinal cord injury and nerve root injury follow. Incomplete spinal cord lesions have a more favorable prognosis than complete spinal cord lesions. Nerve

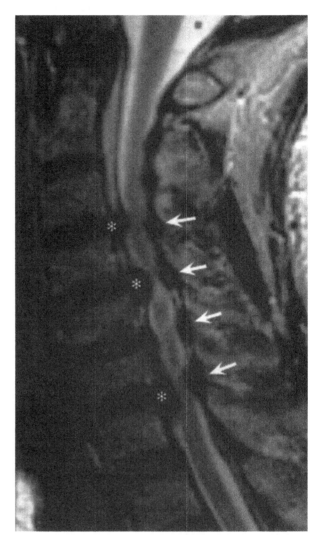

FIGURE 31.5. Cervical stenosis in a 78-year-old man who fell forward, striking his forehead on the sidewalk. He presented with a central cord syndrome. T2 sagittal MRI. Asterisks indicate disc herniations that are chronic (degenerative spondylosis). Arrows indicate buckling of ligamenta flava resulting from the loss of disc height.

root injury has a potentially favorable prognosis when these nerve roots are decompressed surgically. Surgery is required for spinal stabilization and decompression of the contents of the spinal canal. The spinal level involved in the conus medullaris syndrome is T11–L1. Typically, early urinary dysfunction and symmetrical saddle-type anesthesia are common and early pain uncommon in conus medullaris syndrome.

The *cauda equina syndrome* occurs with injury below the termination of the spinal cord (L1/L2).

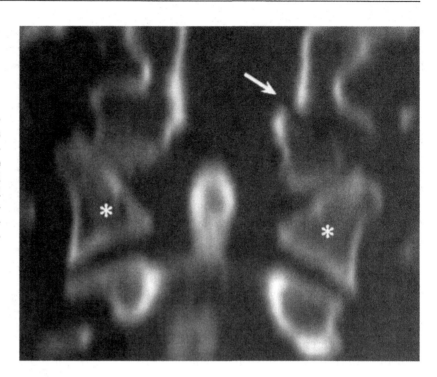

FIGURE 31.6. Occipital condyle fracture in a 26-year-old man who was involved in a high-speed motor vehicle accident and sustained multiple injuries, including diffuse axonal injury of the brain, broken ribs, and a femur fracture. CT axial reconstruction showing unilateral fracture (arrow). Asterisks indicate lateral masses of C1.

Injury to these nerve roots results in a lower motor neuron type of deficit (i.e., flaccid paralysis). Typically, early pain is common in cauda equina syndrome. However, assymetrical sensory loss and urinary dysfunction are relatively late findings. The deficits are typically asymmetrical. Nerve root destruction results in atrophy of muscles and plegic lower extremities. This syndrome contrasts with that of the patient with complete spinal cord paralysis where leg muscles do not atrophy and can have sufficient tone to facilitate movement.

Spinal Injury

Occipital condyle fractures are rare and involve the articulation of the head with the spinal column. In patients with cervico-occipital (suboccipital) pain, the fracture may be demonstrated by CT (Fig. 31.6). Alternatively, these fractures may be observed by conventional tomography. Of the three types of occipital condyle fracture described, only the type III fracture involves avulsion of the occipital condyle by the alar ligament, in which the contralateral alar ligament and tectorial membrane can be disrupted. This can result in instability and require craniocervical fusion.[20] These injuries are commonly associated with "brain concussion" or closed-head injury. Cranial nerve palsies can occur. Immobilization is required. These fractures are not commonly associated with spinal cord injury.

Cervical Spine Injury. A list of cervical spine injuries is provided in Table 31.2. *Atlanto-occipital dislocation* typically is a terminal injury in which distraction forces are great. A typical setting in which this injury occurs is that of a pedestrian hit by a motor vehicle. For most individuals, this causes immediate death. However, rarely a few patients survive to the emergency department due to improved prehospital care. Neurological integrity is rare. The injury is commonly apparent on lateral cervical spine films as an increased distance between the tip of the odontoid process and the end of the clivus (basion). The Powers ratio is defined as the distance between the basion (tip of the clivus) and the posterior arch of the atlas, divided by the distance from the posterior margin of the foramen magnum (opisthion) to the anterior arch of the atlas.[21] Dislocation is suggested by a ratio greater than 1.0. The normal ratio is 0.7 ± 0.09. This ratio may be unaffected by posterior dislocation. The Powers ratio is not valid if the atlas

TABLE 31.2. Cervical Spine Injuries

Atlanto-occipital dislocation
Atlas fractures
Axis fractures
Traumatic spondylolisthesis
Atlantoaxial combination fractures
Compression fractures
Burst fracture
Unilateral facet dislocation
Bilateral facet dislocation
Teardrop fracture
Clay shoveler's fracture
Laminar fracture
Hyperextension-dislocation injury
Hyperextension-fracture-dislocation injury

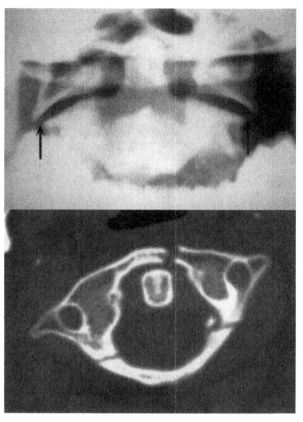

FIGURE 31.7. Jefferson fracture in an 18-year-old unrestrained backseat passenger who struck the top of his head on the dashboard. (A) Open-mouth odontoid view reveals overhanging of the lateral masses of C1 with respect to the articular facets of C2 bilaterally. (B) Expanded ring of C1 is observed on axial CT image. The three breaks in the ring are observed.

is fractured or in cases of congenital anomalies of the skull base. Placement of a halo and subsequent occipitocervical fusion is generally required. Care is exercised so that the head is not manipulated or any traction placed on it. This injury is usually observed in young children.

Fractures of the atlas account for approximately 5–10% of cervical spine injuries.[20] Four basic patterns are observed. The posterior arch fracture likely results from hyperextension-compression of the arch between the occiput and spinous process of C2. The fracture causes pain, but neurological deficit is rare. Immobilization in a collar is required. Axial loading can produce *lateral mass fractures.* These fractures can be demonstrated on radiographs with an open-mouth view, but CT is best for visualization. Atlas fractures can be associated with lateral mass fractures of C2 or with occipital condyle fractures. When lateral displacement is minimal, a cervical collar can be adequate for immobilization. Otherwise, a halo is used.

Jefferson fracture occurs when there is a sufficient axial loading force to break the ring of C1. When an open-mouth odontoid view radiograph shows lateral displacement of the lateral masses totaling 7 mm or more from their original location, the transverse ligament is likely disrupted. CT scan can be diagnostic (Fig. 31.7). MRI may show disruption of the transverse ligament. The disrupted ring moves away from the spinal cord, resulting in rare injury to the nervous system. Halo vest placement

is the treatment of choice. A transverse fracture of the anterior arch can be caused by the attachment of the longus colli muscle. In isolation, this fracture usually heals in a cervical collar.

In *axis fractures,* the unique anatomy of the axis allows for several types of fracture patterns, including three types of odontoid fractures; fractures of the pars interarticularis or pedicles; and miscellaneous fractures. *Odontoid fractures* are characterized into three categories.[22] Type I, a fracture at the tip of the odontoid process, is due to an avulsion by an alar ligament. This extremely rare fracture is of minimal clinical significance and is typically managed conservatively by immobilization in a cervical collar. Type II, a fracture at the base of the odontoid process, is the most common type but can go unrecognized, especially when there is no displacement

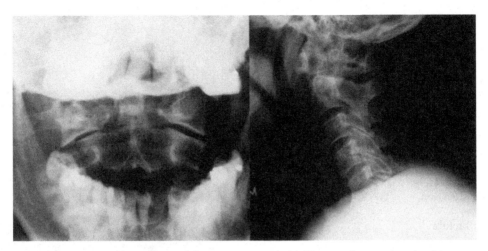

FIGURE 31.8. Type II odontoid fracture in a 48-year-old man who was involved in a roll-over accident and presented to the emergency department with high cervical neck pain. (A) Open-mouth odontoid radiograph. (B) Lateral radiograph. The fracture is seen only on the open-mouth view.

of the fractured tip. When the fracture is not observed on lateral radiograph, it may be identified on the open-mouth odontoid view. A good-quality film is important. This fracture can be inapparent on CT scan because the scan's plane of section is the same as that of the fracture. The best imaging method is anteroposterior and lateral tomography. CT utilizing thin-slice (1 mm, contiguous) scans with reconstruction demonstrates these fractures well (Fig. 31.8) and eliminates the need for conventional tomography. Type III, a fracture of the body of C2, results in a separation of the odontoid (and part of the body of C2) from the rest of the body of C2. This is the second most common fracture type and, like type II, is unstable and requires immobilization in a halo. Additionally, the type II fracture may require fusion or screw placement due to the greater potential for nonunion. Traction may be required to realign the fractured segments. These injuries are potentially fatal when subluxation causes compression of the spinal cord by bone. Lateral mass fractures can be treated with a cervical collar or halo immobilization.

Traumatic spondylolisthesis (also known as "hangman's fracture,") is a fracture through the pedicles or pars interarticularis bilaterally, and is fairly common. It involves ligamentous disruption between C2 and C3 and is divided into four types, depending upon the translation and angulation between C2 and C3. Although neurological injury is rare, this injury is unstable and may require traction, surgery, halo placement, or all three.

Atlantoaxial combination fractures occur and, unlike either atlantal or axial fractures alone, there is a greater incidence of spinal cord injury when both vertebrae are fractured. Dislocation of these two vertebrae is rare and usually fatal (Fig. 31.9).

Subaxial Fractures. *Compression fractures* are caused by flexion and axial loading, and they result in structural failure of the anterior portion of the vertebral bodies (Fig. 31.10). These fractures are typically stable. Radiographs with flexion and extension views are obtained to confirm ligamentous stability. Treatment is usually supportive with immobilization in a cervical collar.

Burst fractures are caused by axial loading and structural failure of the anterior and posterior portions of the vertebral body. Commonly, there is retropulsion of bone into the spinal cord. These fractures usually are associated with quadriplegia or an anterior spinal cord syndrome.

Unilateral facet dislocation (or "jumped" facet) typically is caused by a flexion-rotation mechanism. The lateral radiograph shows an anterolisthesis less than 50% of the anteroposterior diameter of the cervical vertebral body (Fig. 31.11). Patients can be "neurologically intact," or present with incomplete quadriparesis or nerve root compression. Patients require closed (tong traction) or open reduction

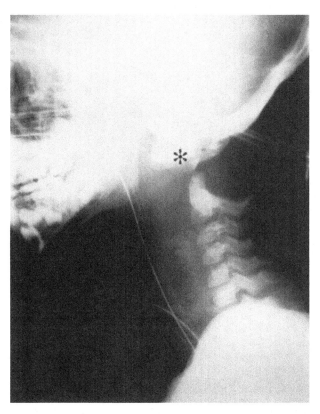

FIGURE 31.9. Atlantoaxial dislocation in a 4-year-old boy who was hit in the head by a car when he ran into the street. There was no evidence of neurological function on arrival. The asterisk is on the atlas, which is still attached to the occiput.

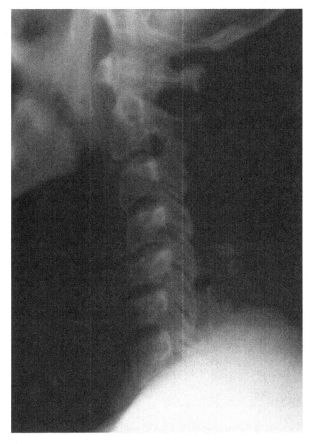

FIGURE 31.10. C5 compression fracture in a 26-year-old woman who dived into a pool head first, striking her head. A Brown-Sequard syndrome resulted.

(tong traction plus surgical reduction), and stabilization.

Bilateral facet dislocation is caused by hyperflexion injury in which there is disruption of all the posterior ligaments, the facet joints, the posterior longitudinal ligament, the disk at the involved interspace, and occasionally the anterior longitudinal ligament. On a lateral radiograph, bilateral facet dislocation is demonstrated as an anterior translation of the upper vertebral body of 50% or more with respect to the vertebral body below (Fig. 31.12). Angular (kyphotic) deformity can be large. This injury is highly unstable and is commonly associated with complete spinal cord injury. Unlike the unilateral facet dislocation, which can clinically resemble a "locked facet" (in that closed reduction may not be easy to perform), there is nothing "locked" about a bilateral dislocation. It is potentially easy to overdistract these injuries. Treatment is realignment via tong traction and sur-

gical stabilization of the spine. *Perched facets* refers to an incomplete ligamentous injury that allows the facet of the vertebra above to ride up, but not over, the superior facet of the vertebra below. Less severe forms of disruption and subsequent translation occur, depending on the amount of ligamentous disruption and fracture of the facets. Cervical spine translation caused by ligamentous injury can be identified on a lateral radiograph. When the spine is reduced, but significant undiagnosed ligamentous injury persists, further radiographic investigation is indicated by the presence of neurological deficit, neurological symptom, or significant neck pain. Failure to recognize this type of injury can occur with a comatose or intoxicated patient. Further investigations include CT to evaluate facet fracture, MRI to evaluate for soft tissue injury, or, under special circumstances, plain radiographs with lateral flexion and extension films, or fluoroscopy.

417

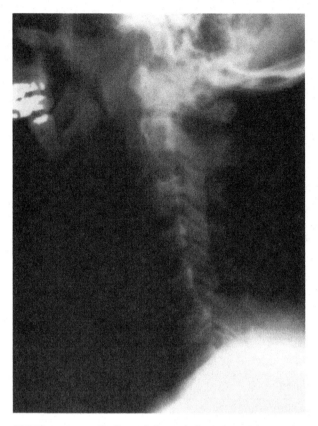

FIGURE 31.11. Unilateral facet dislocation in a 58-year-old man who was rear-ended while driving his pickup truck. He presented with arm and neck pain. The subluxation at C5–6 is less than 50% of the vertebral body anteroposterior diameter.

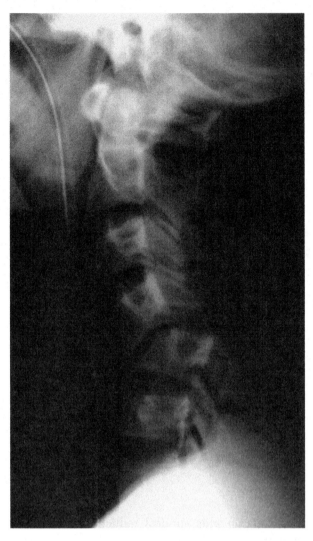

FIGURE 31.12. Bilateral facet dislocation in a young man who was in a high-speed motor vehicle accident. He presented with a complete quadriplegia. Near-complete subluxation of C4 anterior to C5 is observed.

Teardrop fracture is another type of hyperflexion injury. On a lateral radiograph, a large triangular fragment displaced from the anterior inferior aspect of the involved vertebral body is the first indication of this severe injury. Associated with the vertebral body fracture, there is complete ligamentous, intervertebral disc, and bilateral facet disruption (Fig. 31.13). The radiograph typically shows the spine in a flexed position with evidence of anterior soft tissue swelling. Usually, the patient has an anterior spinal cord syndrome. Reduction and stabilization with spinal fusion are indicated.

Clay (or coal) shoveler's fracture is the description of a spinous process fracture of C7, C6, or T1, occurring in that order of frequency.[23] It occurs when the head and upper cervical segments are forced into flexion against the opposing action of the interspinous and supraspinous ligaments, an action common when shoveling overhead. It can be caused by a direct blow to the spinous process itself. The lateral radiograph is diagnostic. When neck pain limits the evaluation of the patient by flexion and extension view radiographs, the study can be obtained later. Generally, these injuries do not cause neurological deficits and can be managed conservatively with immobilization in a soft collar, NSAIDs, and local application of ice (or heat).

Laminar fracture is a hyperextension injury that is nondisplaced or displaced into the spinal cord with associated neurological injury.

Hyperextension dislocation and *hyperextension fracture-dislocation injuries* are uncommon hyper-

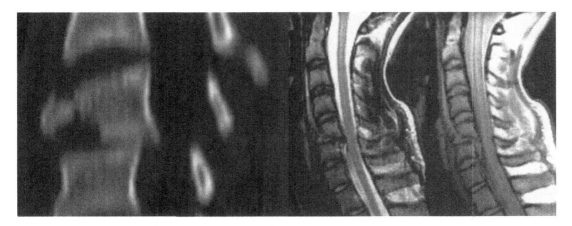

FIGURE 31.13. Teardrop fracture. (A) Two-dimensional sagittally reformatted image (B, C) T2 and proton density images showing blood, and disruption of the posterior longitudinal ligament and disc.

extension injuries. Dislocation without fracture involves ligamentous disruption that begins with the anterior longitudinal ligament and disc, and continues with the joint capsules and posterior ligamentous complex. Dislocation with fracture can involve simple avulsion fractures of the anterior inferior aspect of the upper vertebral body, fractures through the vertebral body endplates, or of the facets. The latter results in the horizontal or "absent" facet signs observed on a lateral radiograph.[23] Disruption of the anterior longitudinal ligament without or with fracture results in diffuse anterior soft tissue swelling observed on a lateral radiograph. The normal prevertebral soft tissue width observed on a lateral radiograph is approximately 5 mm at C1 and C2, 2–7 mm at C3 and C4, and approximately 10–20 mm at C6 and C7.[24] The alignment of the cervical spine observed on a radiograph usually is normal in this injury. The disc space can be widened as a result of disruption, and there may be air in the disc space (vacuum defect). The most common spinal cord injury caused by hyperextension is the *central cord syndrome*. This syndrome is caused by the spinal cord coming in contact with the base of the spinous process of the lower vertebra or by the inbuckling of the ligamentum flavum. This injury is commonly observed in elderly patients where the ligamentum flavum buckles due to the loss of disc height and hypertrophies (Fig. 31.5). Spinal alignment typically returns to normal after posterior dislocation and radiographics are normal, making this diagnosis difficult. This injury is suggested by a

triad of signs: (1) A soft tissue injury to the face or forehead, (2) typical neurological findings, and (3) diffuse prevertebral soft tissue swelling on the lateral radiograph where the alignment appears normal.[20] CT scan can define the facet fractures, and MRI can identify the ligamentous and disc disruption, and spinal cord contusion. These patients require stabilization and possible decompression of neural elements.

Thoracic Spine Injury. A list of thoracic spine injuries is provided in Table 31.3. In contrast to cervical spine injuries, where there is a 39% incidence of associated spinal cord injury, only 10% of thoracic spine injuries are associated with spinal cord injury.[25] Upper thoracic fractures (T2–10) are stabilized by the rib cage, and costotransverse and costovertebral ligamentous attachments.[31] Rotational injuries are rare. Severe fracture dislocations of the thoracic spine require great force and are less com-

TABLE 31.3. Thoracic Spine Injuries

Compression fractures
Burst fractures
Fracture dislocation
Seat belt–type injuries
Sagittal slice fractures

mon than those of the cervical spine, thoracolumbar junction, and lumbar spine. The thoracic canal is narrow and this increases the likelihood of spinal cord injury with spinal trauma. Because of the stabilizing effect of the rib cage, herniated discs are less common in the thoracic spine. However, when disc herniation occurs, spinal cord compression commonly results. As in the lumbar spine, there is a rich epidural venous plexus that can bleed profusely with trauma, increasing spinal compression.

"Clinical instability" of the spine refers to the inability of the spine to maintain its normal pattern of displacement under physiological loads so that there is no neurological injury, major deformity, or incapacitating pain.[28] The three-column injury model of thoracic and lumbar fractures includes anterior, middle and posterior columns.[26] The anterior column consists of the anterior longitudinal ligament, the anterior annulus fibrosis, and vertebral body. The middle column consists of the posterior annulus fibrosis, vertebral body, and posterior longitudinal ligament. The posterior column consists of the facet joints, the posterior laminar arch, and the ligamentous attachments between laminae and spinous processes. Clinical instability and surgical treatment have been reviewed comprehensively.[26,27]

Compression fractures are common and are caused by axial loading. Injury is predominantly restricted to the anterior column (wedge compression fracture). Neurological injury is rare. Injuries are described as a percentage of loss of the anterior height of the vertebral body involved. When the vertebral fracture reduces the anterior vertebral height by 50% or more, there is an increased probability that the anterior and middle columns are injured and spinal stability is compromised. Kyphotic deformity greater than 30 degrees or a prior laminectomy at the site of fracture increases the incidence of long-term progression of the deformity. Posterior stabilization is recommended.

Burst fractures occur under axial load, and anterior and middle columns (Fig. 31.14). Radiographic signs of a burst fracture are: (1) comminution of the vertebral body; (2) increase of the interpedicular distance (a spreading of the pedicles typically is observed on the anteroposterior view of the spine); (3) vertical fracture of the lamina; (4) retropulsion of the fractured posterior vertebral body into the canal; and (5) loss of posterior vertebral body height.

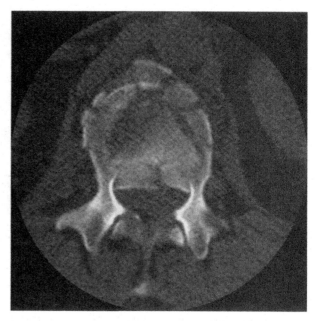

FIGURE 31.14. Burst fracture in a 40-year-old man who fell out of a deer stand. He sustained a complete spinal cord injury at the T11 level. Comminution of the vertebral body and the retropulsed bony fragments are observed. The latter compromise the spinal canal by about 50% of the anteroposterior diameter.

These fractures are commonly associated with spinal cord injury, are typically unstable, and require decompression and internal fixation.

Fracture-dislocation injuries involve failure of all of the three columns. The forces responsible include compression, tension, rotation, shear, and extension. Most patients have complete spinal cord injuries.

Seat belt–type injuries were first described in 1948.[29] They can be purely ligamentous, osseous involving the spinous processes, transverse processes, pedicles, and the vertebral body ("a perfect slice"; Fig. 31.15), or involve a combination of ligamentous dislocation and fracture. They are caused by flexion and distraction forces that are peculiar to sudden deceleration in which the patient is wrapped around the lap belt. The entire spine is subjected to tensile loading, similar to a rubber band being stretched. These injuries are most common in the thoracolumbar junction and lumbar spine. Intra-abdominal injuries are common with this type of injury and require evaluation.

Sagittal slice fracture typically occurs in the upper thoracic spine (above the thoracolumbar junc-

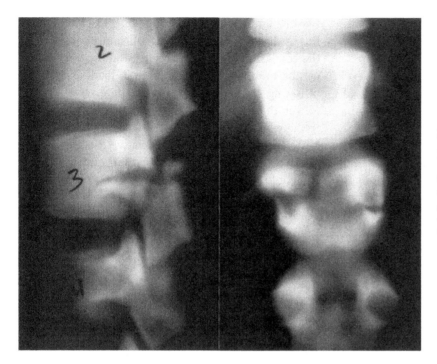

FIGURE 31.15. Chance fracture in a 35-year-old man who was a restrained backseat passenger in a head-on collision. He was neurologically intact with severe back pain. (A) Sagittal and (B) coronal CT reconstructions show the transverse fracture through the vertebral body and pedicles.

tion). This is an osseous injury in which the vertebra from above "slices" down in a sagittal plane through the vertebra below, displacing half of the vertebra laterally.[1] An anteroposterior radiograph shows the upper vertebra telescoped over the one below. The more cephalad portion of the vertebral column is displaced laterally to the side of the shear fracture. A lateral radiograph shows a near complete overlapping of the two involved vertebrae. These injuries typically present with complete spinal cord injury.

Thoracolumbar Junction (T11–L1) and Lumbar Spine Fractures. A list of thoracolumbar junction and lumbar spine fractures is provided in Table 13.4.

The thoracolumbar region is located between the rigid thoracic complex and the mobile lumbar spine and is predisposed to forces of axial compression, flexion, and rotation.[28,30] During axial loading, the thoracic spine deforms in kyphosis while the lumbar spine deforms in lordosis. Thus, the thoracolumbar region is exposed to pure compression. Rotational forces are particularly effective in causing spine dislocations. The upper thoracic spine is protected from rotational forces (as described above), and the lower lumbar spine is protected by the direction of the inwardly directed facet joints. Thus, the thora-

columbar junction is more susceptible to rotational injury and consequent dislocations.[32]

Wedge compression fractures, burst fractures, seat belt injuries, and fracture-dislocations occur at the thoracolumbar junction. When a patient with a dislocation injury is placed in the supine position, a spontaneous reduction can occur. There are two caveats associated with spontaneous reduction. First, plain radiographs may appear normal. Severe back pain or neurological deficit suggest spinal injury and possible spinal instability. Second, the mechanism and extent of ligamentous injury may not be determined on initial radiographic studies. Lumbar fractures below the L1–2 junction spare the conus medullaris but can result in cauda equina injuries, where there is good potential for neurological

TABLE 31.4. Thoracolumbar Junction and Lumbar Spine Fractures

Wedge compression fractures
Burst fractures
Seat belt–type injuries
Fracture dislocations

recovery. In the "neurologically intact" patient, many of these fractures heal with rigid bracing.

Sacral Fractures

Sacral fractures account for less than 1% of spinal fractures and occur with pelvic fractures in 30% of reported cases.[33] These fractures are commonly not identified, especially in patients with multiple trauma. Sacral fractures are divided into three anatomical zones.[34] *Zone I fractures* occur through the ala of the sacrum without causing injury to the foramina or the central canal. The typical mechanism of injury is a vehicular-pedestrian accident. These fractures usually are stable, and neurological injury usually does not occur. However, when injury is severe, the L5 nerve root can be involved between the fracture fragment and the transverse process of L5. *Zone II fractures* involve one or more sacral foramina, but not the central canal. The mechanism of injury can be the same as in zone I fractures, but zone II fractures are commonly vertical shear fractures that occur in passengers involved in high-speed motor vehicle accidents. A zone II fracture can involve zone I but may not involve zone III. Neurological injuries occur in 28–54% of zone II fractures and commonly involve the S1 nerve root. *Zone III fractures* involve the sacral canal medial to the foramina and can involve zones I and II. Zone III fractures include vertical shear injuries, high and low transverse fractures, and traumatic lumbosacral fracture-dislocations. Zone III fractures can produce a cauda equina syndrome.[35] The following findings on standard anteroposterior pelvic radiographs suggest sacral fracture: (1) fracture of lower lumbar transverse process; (2) significant anterior pelvic ring fracture without an identifiable posterior pelvic lesion; (3) asymmetry of the sacral notch; (4) clouding of the radiating trabecular pattern in the lateral sacral mass; or (5) irregularity of the arcuate lines of the upper three sacral foramina.[36] When sacral fracture is suspected, an anteroposterior sacral radiograph performed with the radiation beam directed 30 degrees cephalad (Ferguson's view) and a lateral sacral radiograph including the coccyx are obtained. Further investigation can include thin-slice CT scan with reconstruction and, possibly, MRI.

The coccyx is formed from rudimentary segments. Ossification of the first segment begins between 1 and 4 years of age. The fourth segment ossifies by 20 years of age. Although usually segmented, the coccyx can fuse occasionally. Rarely, the coccyx can be traumatized, and fractured, leading to a debilitating pain that does not radiate. It can take longer than 1 year for the pain to resolve. In extremely rare cases, the fractured segment may require surgical removal. Conservative treatment consists of sitz baths, pain medication, and use of an inflatable "life preserver."

Emergency Department Management and Disposition

Emergency department evaluation and resuscitation of a critically injured patient proceed simultaneously. The patient's airway, breathing, and circulation are managed as detailed previously. Adequate spinal immobilization is required. Adequate tissue perfusion and oxygenation are maintained to prevent secondary spinal cord ischemia.

The Third National Acute Spinal Cord Injury Randomized Controlled Trial concluded that high-dose methylprednisolone administration is associated with improved neurological outcome in spinal cord–injured patients, compared with placebo or tirilazad mesylate.[37] Patients with acute spinal cord injury who receive methylprednisolone within 3 hours of injury are maintained on the treatment regimen for 24 hours. When methylprednisolone is initiated 3–8 hours after injury, patients are managed on steroid therapy for 48 hours. Beyond 8 hours, the use of corticosteroids is contraindicated because the second trial showed a poorer outcome in this delayed drug treatment group. Methylprednisolone is administered as a loading dose of 30 mg/kg given intravenously over 1 hour, followed by a constant infusion of 5.4 mg/kg per hour for the next 23 hours when started within the first 3 hours of the injury or for the next 47 hours when the injury occurred 3–8 hours from the time of onset of therapy. An H_2 blocker is included in the medical regimen for patients for gastrointestinal prophylaxis.

The most important factors of spinal injury are alignment, displacement, and extent of canal compromise.[38] Anteroposterior and lateral radiographs of the entire spine are essential for patients with multitrauma, or comatose or intoxicated patients.

Approximately 10–15% of patients with a spinal fracture have a second noncontiguous spinal fracture. The lateral cervical spine radiograph should expose the top of T1 vertebra, possibly requiring a "swimmer's view." Full evaluation of the cervical spine requires oblique and open-mouth odontoid views, and flexion and extension views to assess possible ligamentous injury. Typically, it is necessary to continue to immobilize the cervical spine using a hard cervical collar for one to two weeks after the initial injury before patients are sufficiently comfortable to undergo a dynamic study (e.g., flexion and extension radiographs). A dynamic study can demonstrate soft tissue swelling and reversal of normal cervical, thoracic, or lumbar curves, which suggest possible ligamentous disruption or fracture that may not be apparent on standard radiographs. It is important that radiographic quality is not compromised by artifacts, jewelry, or other objects.

In a patient with a fixed neurological deficit, the neurological examination is directed at determining the anatomical level of involvement. Plain radiographs are obtained at the level of spinal injury prior to evaluation with CT. Because 5-mm image slices are inadequate to assess clinically significant spinal fractures, 3-mm CT contiguous image slices are obtained through the involved area. MRI has largely replaced the need for myelography. MRI is ideal for demonstrating herniated discs, neuroforaminal encroachment, hematoma, and spinal cord edema. Many MRI facilities are equipped to scan patients on a ventilator. MRI-compatible tongs and halo rings are available, so that patients requiring reduction or traction can be treated before imaging is obtained.

The concept of "clearing the spine" must be kept in perspective. Life-threatening problems are managed first. Transfer to surgery or the intensive care unit without complete spinal clearance is necessary at times. In these cases, "spinal clearance" is the responsibility of the trauma surgeon or the admitting physician. A good-quality lateral cervical spine radiograph is obtained as one of the initial studies on presentation to the emergency department.

Back boards are critical to the initial stability of the acutely spine-injured patient. Patients with no neurological deficits and normal spine radiographs are taken off the back board as soon as possible. Back boards are responsible for serious skin breakdown when the spinal cord–injured patient is allowed to lie on it for too long. Because there is little or no movement or sensation in parts of the body in contact with the back board (sacrum, heels, shoulders, back of the head), these areas are under constant pressure once the patient is on the back board. Assessment, diagnostic testing, and emergency procedures are done without delay in these patients, who are transferred to an appropriate hospital bed as soon as possible.

The decision to remove a hard cervical collar is easy when the patient is awake and has no neurological deficit or neck pain. Following significant head trauma, cervical spine radiographs are obtained; when these radiographs are normal, the collar is removed. In the patient with "cervical sprain," flexion and extension views are obtained to assess for significant ligamentous injury. Commonly, these studies are delayed because of significant neck pain, and the neck is immobilized with a hard cervical collar until the studies can be performed. These guidelines include patients who are intoxicated and unconscious, patients who are being ventilated, and patients requiring sedation. In a patient with a neurological deficit related to the cervical spinal cord (without or with evidence of fracture or dislocation), the decision to remove a cervical collar is made by the treating physician.

When a patient presents to the emergency department with spine or spinal cord injury, the emergency physician contacts a neurosurgeon or an orthopedic spine surgeon. When they are not available, following the initial resuscitation and primary and secondary surveys of the patient, the patient is transferred to a tertiary care center for comprehensive care. In a stable patient, evaluation of the relevant spinal areas by CT scan can be helpful to the receiving hospital. Original radiographs are sent with the patient because copies of radiographs are typically of inadequate quality.

Evaluation and Management of Pediatric Spinal Injuries

Epidemiology

Injuries of the spine and spinal cord are rare in individuals under 17 years of age. The incidence of pediatric spinal injury is 1–10% of all spinal injuries.[38] The majority of injuries occur during the summer months. In the 0–9 years of age group, pedestrian–motor vehicle accidents and falls account for more than 75% of the injuries. As children grow older, accidents due to motor vehicles (including motorcycles) and sports-related activities become more common The incidence of spinal injuries is approximately the same for boys and girls under 10 years of age. After this age, the incidence of spinal injuries is much greater among boys than among girls.

The Pediatric Spine

Interpretation of plain radiographs of the developing spine requires knowledge of the timing of the ossification process. For example, ossification of the atlas proceeds from three centers through the cartilaginous arches over a period of six to nine years. Prior to the ossification of the anterior arch C1, a plain radiograph of the pediatric cervical spine can be misinterpreted as showing a fracture of the C1 ring. The pediatric cervical spine has the following radiographic features: (1) The atlanto–dens interval, measured as a distance between the posterior border of the anterior arch of the atlas and the anterior margin of the dens, can be greater than 3 mm in flexion in 20% of patients. The upper limit of normal in children is 5 mm. (2) The anterior arch of the atlas can override the unossified tip of the dens in extension, giving the appearance of odontoid hypoplasia. (3) Among children under 8 years of age, 40% have evidence of "physiological" anterior displacement of C2 on C3 that is equal to or greater than 3 mm. (4) Among children under 8 years of age, 14% can have a "physiological" anterior displacement of C3 on C4 that exceeds 3 mm.[39] Other normal findings include marked angulation at a single intervertebral space, absent cervical lordosis in the neutral position, and absence of a flexion curve between the second and the seventh cervical vertebrae, suggesting muscle splinting.[38] The newborn spine is elastic, and the supporting ligaments allow longitudinal distraction up to two inches. However, the spinal cord, which is held in place by the brachial plexus, the lumbar plexus, and dentate ligaments, stretches only a quarter of an inch before failing.[40] The combination of a large head on a small body contributes to the torque applied to the neck with acceleration and deceleration. The cervical musculature becomes supportive at puberty.

Spinal cord injury tends to be more severe in children under 9 years of age than in older children, who experience more fractures and ligamentous disruptions resembling those that occur in adults. Spinal cord injury without radiographic abnormality (SCIWORA) is the most common severe injury to the pediatric spine (see p. 425).

Age and Injury Site

The combination of large head and ligamentous laxity contributes to the high incidence of upper cervical spine and craniovertebral junction injuries in children up to 3 years of age. The leading cause of neonatal spinal cord injury is delivery of the fetus with a hyperextended head from either a transverse lie or a breech presentation.[41] Injury to the lower cervical and thoracic spine occur with approximately equal frequency in the age groups of 0–9 years and 10–17 years, because maturation of these joints occurs much more gradually with age than upper cervical articulations. Thoracolumbar and lumbar injuries occur primarily in children between 10 and 17 years of age.

Management

The spine is immobilized immediately when a spinal injury is suspected. Up to 8 years of age, the difference between head and chest circumference results in cervical kyphosis when these patients are placed on a back board. It is necessary to prop up the body on folded blankets from the shoulders down. When there is possible or recognized spinal trauma, a complete spinal radiographic survey is obtained. The methylprednisolone protocol is initiated if indicated. This is started no later than eight hours after the onset of neurological change. The complete spinal evaluation includes complete anteroposterior and lateral spinal radiographs. When these do not show any fracture despite apparent neurological deficit, MRI is obtained through the suspected anatomical area(s) of injury. When spinal fracture is seen on plain radiographs, or when bony abnormality or fracture is suspected, thin-slice CT with reconstruction in sagittal and axial plane or conventional tomography is considered. When fracture and neurological impairment coexist, MRI is performed.

TABLE 31.5. Pediatric Spinal Injuries

Avulsions
Growth plate fractures
Upper cervical spine injuries
Craniovertebral junction injuries
Epiphyseal separation
Spinal cord injury without radiographic abnormality

Pediatric Spinal Injuries. Because the immature spine is progressively ossifying, injuries in children under 8 years of age tend to be avulsions, epiphyseal separations, and fractures of the growth plate – not true fractures.[42] Common injuries of the upper cervical spine in the pediatric age group include occipitoatlantal dislocation, atlantoaxial rotary subluxation, and fixation and fracture of the odontoid process (Table 31.5).

Occipitoatlantal dislocation is seen twice as often in the pediatric population as in the adult population and is usually fatal. It is typically the result of a child being hit by a car.

Atlantoaxial rotary subluxation occurs in children as a result of trauma or with infections of the upper respiratory system (Grisel's syndrome). It has occurred following surgical procedures such as cleft lip and palate repair, and removal of orthodontic devices. The clinical presentation is the "cock-robin" appearance of the head. The patient's head is turned in the opposite direction to the subluxation of the articular process of C1 with that of C2. This is referred to as a "jumped facet" (Fig. 31.16). CT is obtained with the patient's head rotated in the extremes of both directions. The two scans are compared and the diagnosis is confirmed when the position of C1 vertebra remains fixed with respect to C2 vertebra. Neurological deficit is uncommon. These patients require cervical traction for reduction, and immobilization.[38]

Odontoid fractures in patients under 8–10 years of age occur as an epiphyseal separation of the growth plate at the base of the dens. Reduction and immobilization for six to eight weeks is required for healing.

The acronym *SCIWORA* (*spinal cord injury without radiographic abnormality*) was first used in

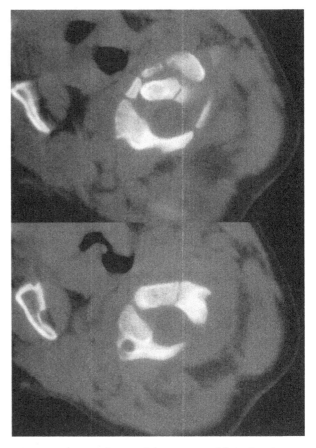

FIGURE 31.16. Atlantoaxial rotatory subluxation in a 2-year-old girl who was injured by her older brother. Allegedly, he twisted her head. She was taken to the emergency department on a back board with her head fixed in rotatory subluxation. The subluxation was reduced with in-line traction under sedation and direct fluoroscopy, and neck was immobilized in a cervical collar. (A, B) Axial views by CT, adjacent 3-mm cuts showing the counterclockwise rotation of C1 with respect to C2.

1982.[43] By definition, children with this syndrome have traumatic myelopathy without identifiable fractures or subluxation on plain spine radiography, plain tomography, or CT. The mechanisms of injury include hyperextension, flexion, distraction, and spinal cord ischemia. Buckling of ligaments and discs, and shifting of vertebrae can result in trauma to the spinal cord. Disruption of blood flow in the vertebral or radicular arteries can cause spinal cord ischemia. This injury typically involves the upper cervical spine in infants and young children. The lower cervical spine is at risk in children up to age 16 years of age.[38] This injury can occur in the upper thoracic and thoracolumbar regions. Some children with SCIWORA do not have detectable neurological deficits immediately following trauma but develop deficits within 30 minutes to 4 days after injury. Recurrent SCIWORA can occur up to 10 weeks following the initial injury. Delayed onset and recurrence of the syndrome suggest the possibility of ligamentous laxity and vulnerability of the spinal cord to further damage. Cervical immobilized in a hard cervical collar for 3 months in order to prevent subsequent injury is recommended. The spinal cord injury can be complete or a spinal cord syndrome can be present. Five patterns of spinal cord injury in SCIWORA, as defined by MRI, are: (1) complete anatomical disruption of the spinal cord; (2) major hemorrhage observed in over 50% of the cross-sectional area of the spinal cord; (3) minor spinal cord hemorrhage; (4) edema only, without hemorrhage; and, (5) a normal study.

Vertebral endplate fractures or separations from the vertebral body can occur through the epiphysis, similar to physical injuries of long bones. Many of these abnormalities remain unidentified but can be associated with an increase in the disc height. They can be observed on MRI and can be accompanied by adjacent bony fracture in older children.

The best predictor of long-term outcome in children with SCIWORA is the neurological status at presentation. Children with complete spinal cord lesions rarely improve. Those with severe but incomplete lesions typically have limited improvement with time, but rarely regain normal function. When the deficits seen in the emergency department are mild-to-moderate, the likelihood for complete recovery is good.

Congenital hemivertebrae can be mistaken for acute fractures (Fig. 31.17). Lack of pain over these vertebrae and no neurological deficit are consistent with the diagnosis of congenital hemivertebrae, but MRI or bone scan may be necessary to confirm the absence of acute fractures.

Infection or neoplasm can mimic traumatic fracture, especially when symptoms occur following real or imagined trauma. A careful history and the use of laboratory studies, such as the erythrocyte sedimentation rate, can assist in determining the etiology. The imaging study of choice is MRI.

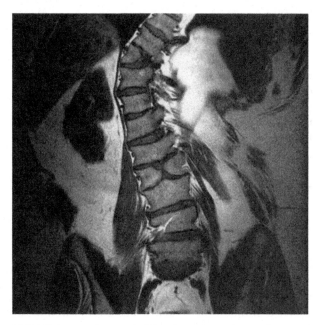

FIGURE 31.17. Congenital hemivertebrae. Coronal MRI of a young boy with a hemivertebra at T9 and a "butterfly" hemivertebra at L2.

Metabolic disease can lead to osteopenia with resultant fracture. Children with osteogenesis imperfecta typically present with spine fractures at different levels. Morquio's syndrome is characterized by involvement of all the vertebrae. Careful history, physical examination, and laboratory studies assist in determining metabolic bone disease.

Scheuermann's disease is characterized by wedging of multiple consecutive thoracic vertebrae. These patients have a characteristic round back deformity and a rigid kyphosis with chronic thoracic spine pain.

Child Abuse

The incidence of spinal injuries caused by child abuse is 0–3%.[44] It is important to obtain a skeletal survey in all cases of suspected child abuse that includes anteroposterior and lateral radiographs of the entire spine. The average age of abuse in a series of 45 children with 85 spinal fractures was 22 months.[45] Most of the injuries involve the vertebral bodies. Most fractures occur in the thoracolumbar junction and lumbar spine as a result of the child being held above a counter or table and slammed down, with the buttocks impacting the surface. The outstretched arms usually are fractured as the child tries to break the impact. Vertebral body fractures and subluxations suggest child abuse.

PEARLS AND PITFALLS

- Adequate stabilization of the spine is of paramount importance in patients with suspected spine injuries.
- Maintenance of adequate tissue oxygenation and perfusion to minimize subsequent injury to the nervous system is the next most important step in caring for the spine-injured patient.
- The emergency department evaluation focuses on motor function. In the presence of spinal cord injury, "sacral sparing" is associated with a better prognosis.
- A thorough radiographic evaluation is essential in identifying spinal abnormalities. It is important to evaluate the entire spine radiographically in patients with multiple trauma and in unconscious or intoxicated patients.
- In patients with neurological injury at a specific spinal cord level, it is important that the imaging studies are focused on the corresponding spinal level. The remainder of the spine is evaluated with plain radiographs.
- In the traumatized patient without neurological deficit, areas of spinal tenderness can indicate fracture without or with ligamentous disruption. These are evaluated radiographically. When indicated, CT or MRI are obtained.
- Neurological or spine orthopedic surgeons are involved early in the care of the spine-injured patient.

REFERENCES

1. Bohlman HH, Ducker TD. Spine and spinal cord injuries. In: Rothman RH, Simeone FA, eds. *The Spine.* 3rd ed. Philadelphia, Pa: WB Saunders Co; 1992:973–1104.
2. Stover SL, Fine PR. *Spinal Cord Injury: The Facts and Figures.* Birmingham, Ala: University of Alabama at Birmingham; 1986.
3. Green BA, David C, Falcone S, Razack N, Klose KJ. Spinal cord I injuries in adults. In: Youmans JR, ed. *Neurological Surgery: A Comprehensive Reference Guide to the Diagnosis and Management of Neurosurgical Problems.* 4th ed. Philadelphia, Pa: WB Saunders Co; 1996;3:1968–90.
4. Sonntag VKH, Hadley MN. Management of upper cervical spinal instability. In: Wilkins RH, Rengachary SS, eds. *Neurosurgery.* 2nd ed. New York: NY: McGraw-Hill Book Co; 1996;2:2915–26.
5. Gerhart KA. Spinal cord injury outcomes in a population-based sample. *J Trauma.* 1991;31:1529–35.
6. Elsberg CA. The Edwin Smith surgical papyrus – and the diagnosis and treatment of injuries to the skull. *Ann Med Hist.* 1931;3:271–9.
7. Hippocrates. On the articulations. In: Adams F, ed. *The Genuine Works of Hippocrates, Translated from the Greek with a Preliminary Discourse and Annotations.* New York, NY: William Wood; 1886;2:114–24.
8. American College of Surgeons Committee on Trauma. *Advanced Trauma Life Support Course Student Manual.* Chicago, Ill: American College of Surgeons; 1989.
9. Ducker TB, Salcman M, Perot PL, et al. Experimental spinal cord trauma, I: correlations of blood flow, tissue oxygen and neurologic status in the dog. *Surg Neurol.* 1978;10:60–3.
10. Ducker TB, Salcman M, Lucas JT, et al. Experimental spinal cord trauma, II: blood flow, tissue oxygen, evoked potentials in both paretic and plegic monkeys. *Surg Neurol.* 1978;10:64–70.
11. Newman PK. Whiplash injury. *Br Med J.* 1990;301:395–6.
12. Kaufman HH. Trauma to the carotid artery and other cervical vessels. In: Youmans JR, ed. *Neurological Surgery: A Comprehensive Reference Guide to the Diagnosis and Management of Neurosurgical Problems.* 4th ed. Philadelphia, Pa: WB Saunders Co; 1996;3:1926–38.
13. Davis JM, Zimmermann RA. Injury of the carotid and vertebral arteries. *Neuroradiology.* 1983;25:55–69.
14. Frisoni GB, Anzola BP. Vertebrobasilar ischemia after neck motion. *Stroke.* 1991;22:1452–60.
15. Graham B, Van Peteghem K. Fractures of the spine in ankylosing spondylitis: diagnosis, treatment, and complications. *Spine.* 1989;14:803–7.
16. American Spinal Injury Association. Standards for neurological classification of spinal cord patients. Chicago, Ill: American Spinal Injury Association; 1992.
17. Schneider RC, Crosby EC, Russo RH, Gosh HH. Traumatic spinal cord syndromes and their management. *Clin Neurosurg.* 1973;30:367–81.
18. Quencer RM, Bunge RP, Egnor M, et al. Acute traumatic central cord syndrome: MRI-pathological correlations. *Neuroradiology.* 1992;34:85–94.
19. Brown-Sequard C. Transmission croisee des impressions sensitives par la moelle epiniere. *CR Seances Soc Biol Fil.* 1850;2:70.
20. Eichler ME, Vollmer DG. Cervical spine trauma. In: Youmans JR, ed. *Neurological Surgery: A Comprehensive Reference Guide to the Diagnosis and Manage-*

ment of Neurosurgical Problems. 4th ed. Philadelphia; Pa: WB Saunders Co; 1996;3:1939–68.

21. Powers B, Miller JD, Kramer RS, et al. Traumatic anterior atlanto-occipital dislocation. *Neurosurgery.* 1979; 4:12–17.

22. Anderson LD, D'Alonzo RT. Fractures of the odontoid process of the axis. *J Bone Joint Surg.* 1974;56:1663–774.

23. Harris JH, Edeiken-Monroe B. *The Radiology of Acute Cervical Spine Trauma,* 2nd ed. Baltimore, Md: Williams & Wilkins; 1987.

24. Penning L. Prevertebral hematoma in cervical spine injury: incidence and etiological significance. *Neuroradiology.* 1980;1:557–65.

25. Riggins RS, Kraus JF. The risk of neurologic damage with fractures of the vertebrae. *J Trauma.* 1977;17:126–33.

26. Denis F. The three-column spine and its significance in the classification of acute thoracolumbar spinal injuries. *Spine.* 1983;8:817–31.

27. Madsen PW, Lee TT, Eismont FJ, Green BA. Diagnosis and management of thoracic spine fractures. In: Youmans JR, ed. *Neurological Surgery: A Comprehensive Reference Guide to the Diagnosis and Management of Neurosurgical Problems.* 4th ed. Philadelphia, Pa: WB Saunders Co; 1996;3:2043–78.

28. White AA, Panjabi MM. *Clinical Biomechanics of the Spine.* 2nd ed. Philadelphia, Pa: JB Lippincott Co;1990.

29. Chance GQ. Note on a type of flexion fracture of the spine. *Br J Radiol.* 1948;21:452–3.

30. Oxland TR, Lin RM, Panjabi MM. Three dimensional mechanical properties of the thoracolumbar junction. *J Orthop Res.* 1992;10:573–80.

31. Andriacchi T, Schultz A, Belytschko T, et al. A model for studies of mechanical interactions between the human spine and the rib cage. *J Biomech.* 1974;7:497–506.

32. Nockels RP, McCormack B. Diagnosis and management of thoracolumbar and lumbar spine injuries. In: Youmans JR, ed. *Neurological surgery: a comprehensive reference guide to the diagnosis and management of neurosurgical problems.* 4th ed. Philadelphia, Pa: WB Saunders Co; 1996;3:2079–96.

33. Bonnin J. Sacral fractures and injuries to the cauda equina. *J Bone Joint Surg.* 1945;27:113–27.

34. Denis F, Davis S, Comfort T. Sacral fractures: an important problem: Retrospective analysis of 236 cases. *Clin Orthoped.* 1988;227:67–81.

35. Gibbons KJ, Soloniuk DS, Razack N. Neurological injury and patterns of sacral fractures. *J Neurosurg.* 1990;72:889–93.

36. Perin NI, Stanley MI. Sacral fractures. In: Youmans JR, ed. *Neurological Surgery: A Comprehensive Reference Guide to the Diagnosis and Management of Neurosurgical Problems.* 4th ed. Philadelphia, Pa: WB Saunders Co; 1996;3:2097–102.

37. Bracken MB, Shepard MJ, Holford TR, et al. Administration of methylprednisolone for 24 or 48 hours or tirilazad mesylate for 48 hours in the treatment of acute spinal cord injury. Results of the third national acute spinal cord injury randomized controlled trial. *JAMA.* 1997;277:1597–1604.

38. Crawford AH. Operative treatment of spine fractures in children. *Orthop Clin North Am.* 1990;21:325–39.

39. Pang D, Sahrakar K, Sun PP. Pediatric spinal cord and vertebral column injuries. In: Youmans JB, ed. *Neurological Surgery: A Comprehensive Reference Guide to the Diagnosis and Management of Neurosurgical Problems.* 4th ed. Philadelphia, Pa: WB Saunders Co; 1996;3:1991–2036.

40. Cattell HS, Filtzer DL. Pseudosubluxation and other normal variations in the cervical spine in children. A study of 160 children. *J Bone Joint Surg.* 1965;47A:1295–1309.

41. Leventhal HR. Birth injuries of the spinal cord. *J Pediatr.* 1960;56:447–53.

42. Menezes AH, Osenbach RK. Spinal cord injury. In: Cheek WR, ed. *Pediatric Surgery: Surgery of the Developing Nervous System.* 3rd ed. Philadelphia, Pa: WB Saunders Co; 1994:320–43.

43. Pang D, Wilberger JE. Spinal cord injury without radiographic abnormalities in children. *J Neurosurg.* 1982;57:114–29.

44. Chambers HG, Akbarnia BA. Thoracic, lumbar and sacral spine fractures and dislocations. In: Weinstein SL, ed. *The Pediatric Spine: Principles and Practice.* New York, NY: Raven Press, Ltd; 1994;1:743–66.

45. Kleinman PK. *Diagnostic Imaging of Child Abuse.* Baltimore, Md: Williams & Wilkins; 1987.

32 Peripheral Nerve Injuries

ARIO KEYARASH AND MARK BARATZ

SUMMARY This chapter reviews the diagnosis and management of acute and chronic peripheral nerve injuries. Included are the most commonly occurring nerve injuries and compressive neuropathies.

Introduction

The management of peripheral nerve injuries is facilitated by a systematic approach. This chapter is organized to enable the emergency physician to orchestrate appropriate care of patients with peripheral nerve injuries from the field to the time of discharge.

Relevant Neuroanatomy and Physiology

An understanding of peripheral neuroanatomy allows the emergency physician to anticipate the type and location of a nerve lesion for a given injury; an understanding of nerve physiology is the basis for estimating the prognosis for recovery. Nerve injuries are one of three types: neuropraxia, axontemesis, or neurotemesis. *Neuropraxia* is defined as a nerve injury in which there is a temporary ischemic insult to the nerve. Examples include numbness in a sciatic nerve distribution from sitting on the edge of a hard chair, or median nerve compromise from the soft tissue swelling associated with a fracture of the distal radius. Symptoms associated with a neuropraxia resolve within a short time after the source of compression is relieved. *Axontemesis* involves injury to the axons, such as a traction injury, in which separation of part or all of the axons occurs. The nerve sheath remains intact. Recovery from an axontemesis requires regeneration of the injured axons, a process that can take up to three months. *Neurotemesis* is defined as complete disruption of all neural elements of the peripheral nerve. Recovery cannot occur without nerve repair.

Prehospital Management and Evaluation

The patient who reports loss of sensation in an extremity is evaluated in the field for possible injury to the spine or limbs, with careful attention to the limb's vascular supply. The patient with pain in the neck or back is placed on a back board. Pulses are palpated and documented. The injured limb is splinted in a position of comfort with minimal manipulation. Open wounds are covered with a sterile dressing. Active bleeding from a wound can be controlled in virtually all instances with a bulky compressive dressing. A tourniquet is rarely necessary.

Emergency Department Evaluation and Differential Diagnosis

The neurological status of a patient with an injured extremity is assessed quickly by testing the sensation and motor function subserved by the injured nerve (see Figs. 32.1 and 32.2). In the upper extremity, the axillary, radial, median, and ulnar nerves are the most commonly injured (Fig. 32.3). In the lower extremity, most injuries involve the sciatic, femoral, tibial, or peroneal nerves. The "short form" neurological examination (Table 32.1) is completed in a few minutes. When the muscle to be tested is near the site of a fracture or

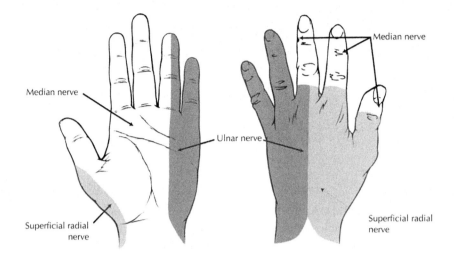

FIGURE 32.1. Sensory distribution in the hand.

dislocation, the examination of motor function is completed by asking the patient to contract the muscle to be tested without actually moving the injured extremity.

A more complete evaluation of sensory function includes two-point discrimination. Patients with normal nerve function can identify a separation of two points by 3–5 mm applied lightly to their fingertips. The "wrinkle test" can be used in young children to diagnose an injured peripheral nerve. The hand is immersed in water until the skin on the fingertips wrinkles. Lack of wrinkling in the injured hand indicates a nerve lesion.

Certain musculoskeletal injuries suggest the possibility of concurrent peripheral nerve injury. Frac-

tures and dislocations with associated nerve lesions are listed in Table 32.2.

Compression of peripheral nerves occurs in locations where the passageway of the nerve is narrow and the nerve excursion is great. This typically occurs around joints where the nerve passes through a "tunnel" and slides back and forth with joint flexion and extension. In a patient with limb numbness, it is useful to identify the nerve supply of that portion of the extremity and to consider all the possible points of compression. A nerve that has had chronic irritation is typically sensitive when examined, a finding that can facilitate diagnosis of a compressive neuropathy. Percussion directly over an irritated nerve produces local pain

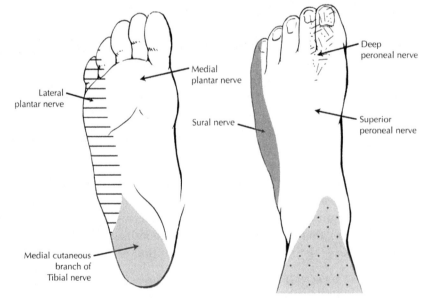

FIGURE 32.2. Sensory distribution in the foot.

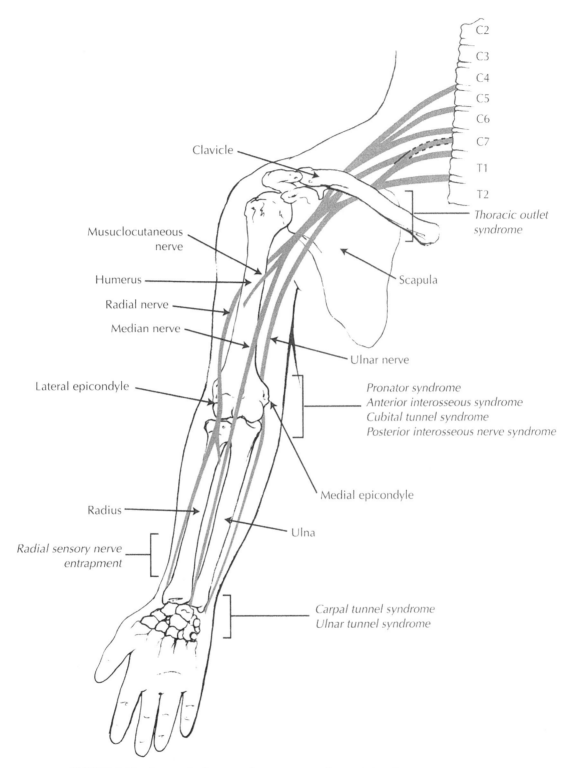

FIGURE 32.3. Anatomical areas of upper extremity peripheral nerve compression and resulting conditions.

TABLE 32.1. "Short Form" Neurological Examination

Nerve	Sensation*	Motor Function*
Axillary	Lateral aspect of shoulder, several centimeters below acromium	Deltoid: shoulder flexion (palpate deltoid and feel contraction
Radial	First web space	Wrist, finger, and thumb extension
Median	Tip of index finger	Thumb apposition: place tip of thumb on tip of small finger, feel contraction of thenar muscles
Ulnar	Tip of small finger	Finger abduction: spread fingers apart; feel contraction of first dorsal interosseous muscle
Femoral	Anteromedial thigh and leg	Quadriceps
Sciatic	Posterior thigh, posterolateral leg	Hamstrings
Tibial	Sole of foot	Gastrocnemius and toe flexors
Common peroneal		
Superficial branch	Dorsum of foot	Foot eversion
Deep branch	First web space	Foot dorsiflexion

*This list of sensory regions and motor functions for each nerve is, in some cases, incomplete. However, testing these functions provides an adequate initial assessment of peripheral nerve function.

and dysesthesias in the sensory distribution of that nerve. This is referred to as *Tinel's sign*.[1] Other provocative maneuvers are designed to increase nerve compression or to stretch the nerve. for example, when sustained wrist flexion causes pain in the wrist and numbness in the thumb, index, or middle fingers, the patient is described as having a positive *Phalen's test*.[2]

Median nerve compression occurs in the forearm or wrist. Compression in the forearm occurs as the median nerve passes between the two heads of the pronator teres muscle, creating *pronator syndrome*.[3] The anterior interosseous portion of the median nerve can develop what is likely a transient neuritis, the *anterior interosseous syndrome*.[4] The most common form of median nerve compression is *carpal tunnel syndrome*.[5] A guide to diagnosing median nerve compression is outlined in Table 32.3.

Compression of nerve fibers that make up the *ulnar nerve* occurs at the shoulder, elbow, or wrist. The medial cord of the brachial plexus can be compressed as it passes from the neck (between the an-

terior and middle scalenes) to the axilla (between the clavicle and first rib). Compromise of the nerve along this course is referred to as *thoracic outlet syndrome*.[6] Compression of the ulnar nerve as it passes from the medial aspect of the upper arm through a narrow passage behind the medial epicondyle of the distal humerus and into the forearm is described as *cubital tunnel syndrome*.[7] This is the most common compressive neuropathy involving the ulnar nerve. *Ulnar tunnel syndrome* occurs when the ulnar nerve is compressed as it passes from the wrist to the hand through Guyon's canal.[8]* The specifics of each syndrome are summarized in Table 32.4.

Radial nerve compression occurs most commonly in the forearm.[9] Extrinsic compression from elbow synovitis or a mass in the proximal forearm on the posterior interosseous portion of the radial nerve results in the *posterior interosseous nerve syndrome*. Patients present with loss of thumb and finger extension. Wrist extension is weak and places the hand in ulnar deviation, because the extensor carpi ulnaris is paralyzed while the extensor

TABLE 32.2. Nerves at Risk with Various Fractures and Dislocations

Fracture or Dislocation	Nerve at Risk
Shoulder dislocation	Axillary
Proximal humerus fracture	Axillary
Humeral shaft (distal third)	Radial
Supracondylar humerus fracture in child	Median* or radial
Intra-articular distal humerus fracture in adult	Ulnar
Elbow dislocation	Ulnar
Proximal ulna fracture with radial head dislocation (Monteggia's fracture)	Radial
Distal radius fracture	Median
Carpal dislocation (especially lunate)	Median
Hip dislocation	Sciatic
Supracondylar femur fracture in child	Peroneal
Knee tibio-femoral dislocation	Peroneal

*Particularly the anterior interosseous portion of the median nerve, which controls "precision pinch" through the action of the flexor pollicis longus tendon in the thumb and the flexor digitorum profundus tendon to the index finger.

carpi radialis longus and brevis continue to be innervated by the main trunk of the radial nerve. *Radial tunnel syndrome* is likely the result of radial nerve compression as it passes beneath the arcarde of Frohse and through the supinator muscle. Compression of the radial sensory nerve in the distal forearm has been called *cheiralgia paresthetica* or *radial sensory nerve entrapment.* This is the result of radial sensory compression as the nerve passes between the brachioradialis (BR) and extensor carpi radialis longus (ECRB) tendons at the junction of the middle and distal third of the forearm. Diagnostic features of each syndrome are listed in Table 32.5.

Tarsal tunnel syndrome is due to entrapment of the *tibial nerve* or its branches at the ankle. Nerve irritation can occur as it passes beneath the flexor retinaculum, a ligament that stretches between the medial malleolus of the distal tibia and the medial tubercle of the calcaneus. This can be a result of posttraumatic inflammation, soft tissues masses, or foot deformities. (See Fig. 32.4 for the anatomical relationship of the tibial nerve at the ankle.) Chronic compressions of the tibial nerve are described in Table 32.6.

The differential diagnosis of a chronic peripheral nerve dysfunction includes central nervous system lesions, metabolic disorders producing peripheral neuropathy, and limb ischemia.

TABLE 32.3. Chronic Compression of the Median Nerve

Site of Compression	Incidence	Symptoms	Findings	Provocative Maneuvers
Pronator teres	Rare	Forearm pain; numbness absent or of secondary importance	Forearm tenderness	Pain with resisted forearm pronation
Neuritis of anterior interosseous nerve	Uncommon	Weak pinch	Weak flexor pollicis longus and/or flexor digitorum profundus to the index finger	Tinel's sign on anterior aspect of the proximal forearm
Carpal canal	Common	Finger numbness; wrist weakness and ocassional arm pain	Dry fingers; ± thenar atrophy; increased 2-point discrimination	Phalen's and/or Tinel's sign at wrist flexion crease

433

TABLE 32.4. Chronic Compression of the Ulnar Nerve

Site of Compression	Incidence	Symptoms	Findings	Provocative Maneuvers
Thoracic outlet (neck and shoulder)	Uncommon	Diffuse anterior shoulder pain; paresthesias in 4th and 5th fingers	Usually normal	Pressure over anterior scalene;* Roo's test;† military brace position;‡ overhead stress test§
Cubital tunnel (elbow)	Common	Medial elbow pain; paresthesias in 4th and 5th fingers	May have increased 2-point discrimination in 4th and 5th fingers; intrinsic atrophy; weak grip; weak pinch	Tinel's sign behind medial epicondyle of distal humerus; paresthesias in 4th and 5th fingers with sustained elbow flexion
Guyon's canal (wrist)	Uncommon	Wrist pain; paresthesias in 4th and 5th fingers	May have increased 2-point in 4th and 5th fingers; intrinsic atrophy; weak grip; weak pinch	Tinel's sign at wrist over hypothenar emminence; paresthesias in 4th and 5th fingers with sustained wrist flexion

Compression over scalene: Hold pressure over posterior edge of anterior scalene. Positive if produces paresthesias in an ulnar nerve distribution within one minute.
†*Roo's test:* Hyperabduction of arm with elbow bent 90 degrees. Positive if produces paresthesias in an ulnar nerve distribution.
‡*Military brace position:* Arms held at side. Shoulders pulled back as if trying to pinch a quarter between the shoulder blades. Test is positive if patient develops numbness in the ring and small fingers.
§*Overhead stress test:* Hold arms overhead. Make fist in repetitive fashion. Causes fatigue and numbness in ulnar nerve distribution.

Emergency Department Management and Disposition

Penetrating Wounds

Firearms with muzzle velocities of 2000 feet per second or more are considered high-velocity. Wounds inflicted by high-velocity missiles create a concussive effect that damages a wide swath of tissue. Immediate surgical treatment is advisable in cases of nerve injury with vascular compromise or open fracture. Nerve deficits in the absence of fracture or vascular injury can be followed, because many represent neuropraxias or axontemeses.

Lacerations or stab wounds in the upper extremity that result in an abnormal two-point discrimination typically represent a nerve transection. Surgical exploration may be delayed up to two weeks following the injury when the wound is clean. Wounds with gross contamination are debrided and

irrigated. Bleeding is controlled only with a pressure dressing. Coagulation and clamps can cause further nerve injury. An arteriogram is considered for any patient with a nerve injury observed in conjunction with diminished peripheral pulses; it is strongly considered when the patient is not being taken to the operating room for exploration of the wound.

Blunt Trauma and Traction Injuries

Blunt trauma and traction injuries are most likely to cause nerve transection when associated with an open fracture. The majority of other nerve deficits represent neuropraxia and axontemesis.

Traction injury to the *brachial plexus* can lead to avulsion of the nerve off of the spinal cord (preganglionic lesion) or along the length of the axon (postganglionic lesion). Most traction injuries are followed with serial examinations, nerve conduction

TABLE 32.5. Chronic Compression of the Radial Nerve

Site of Compression	Incidence	Symptoms	Findings	Provocative Manuevers
Extrinsic compression proximal forearm (posterior interosseous nerve syndrome)	Uncommon	Weak fingers and wrist	Weak wrist extension, hand radially deviates; weak or absent finger and thumb extension	None
Supinator muscle in proximal forearm (radial tunnel syndrome)	Uncommon	Proximal forearm pain	Tender proximal forearm	Pain with resisted forearm supination and/or middle finger extension
Between BR and ECRL tendons in distal forearm (cheiralgia paresthetica)	Uncommon	Hand and distal forearm pain; sensation dorsum of hand	Tender distal forearm, decreased sensation in first web space	Tinel's sign over burning BR/ECRB interval; increased pain with a clenched fist and wrist ulnar deviation

ECRL = Extensor calpi radialis longus
BR = Brachioradialsis

studies, and, occasionally, a myelogram to document location of injury and prospects for recovery. Once it has been determined that the arm is viable and there are no associated injuries, the patient can be referred for follow-up care.

Fractures and dislocations can be reduced with intravenous sedation and analgesics. Careful documentation of neurological and vascular deficits precedes

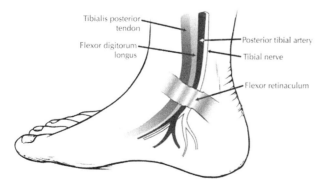

FIGURE 32.4. Anatomical relationship of the tibial nerve at the ankle.

and follows any form of intervention performed in the emergency department including closed manipulation of fractures and joint dislocations.

Compartment Syndrome

Compartment syndromes occur in association with high-energy trauma to an extremity with or without fracture. The first sign is pain with passive motion of the joints adjacent to the compartment. Later the patient develops dysesthesias followed by paralysis and vascular compromise. Measuring compartment pressures assists in the diagnosis. Early surgical decompression is strongly considered in a patient with neurological compromise and tense muscle compartments.

Electrical Injuries

Current from an electrical source courses along the nerve of a limb and dissipates energy throughout the soft tissues. The extent of tissue damage is related to the type of current, and its amperage and

TABLE 32.6. Chronic Compression of the Tibial Nerve

Site of Compression	Incidence	Symptoms	Findings	Provocative Manuevers
Flexor retinaculum of ankle (tarsal tunnel syndrome)	Uncommon	Burning, numbness, plantar aspect of foot	Check for foot deformity or masses	Tinel's sign over tibial nerve behind medial malleolus

voltage. Nerve injury results more commonly from surrounding soft tissue swelling than from direct injury due to the electrical source. The cornerstone of management is detection and early decompression of a compartment syndrome.

PEARLS AND PITFALLS

- Nerve status is documented prior to and after any manipulation of a wound or fracture.
- Attempts to coagulate or tie-off bleeding vessels are not made in the emergency department, particularly when the bleeding is associated with nerve injuries.
- Clavicle fracture with a brachial plexus injury portends a poor prognosis for recovery.
- Nerve compromise occurs in established compartment syndromes and requires prompt surgical decompression.

*Guyon's canal: starts at a hiatus formed by the distal edge of the volar carpal ligament superficially and the proximal edge of the transverse carpal ligament deeply. Through this canal,

REFERENCES

1. Tinel J, "The tingling sign in peripheral nerve lesions." In Spinner M, ed; Kaplan EB, trans. *Injuries to the Major Branches of Peripheral Nerves of the Forearm.* 2nd ed. Philadelphia, Pa: WB Saunders Co; 1978:8–13.
2. Phalen GS. The carpal tunnel syndrome: clinical evaluation of 598 hands. *Clin Orthop.* 1972;83:29–40.
3. Hartz CR, Linscheid RL, Gramser RR, et al. The pronator teres syndrome. Compressive neuropathy of the median nerve. *J Bone Joint Surg.* 1981;63A:885–90.
4. Kihol LG, Nevin S. Isolated neuritis of the anterior interosseous nerve. *Br Med J.* 1952;1:850–1.
5. Pfeffer GB, Gelberman RH, Boyes JH, Rydevik B. The history of carpal tunnel syndrome. *J Hand Surg.* 1988;13:28–34.
6. Leffert RD. Thoracic outlet syndrome. *Hand Clin.* 1992;2:285–97.
7. Adelaar RS, Foster WC, McDowell C. The treatment of the cubital tunnel syndrome. *J Hand Surg.* 1984;9:90–5.
8. Moneim MS. Ulnar nerve compression at the wrist-ulnar tunnel syndrome. *Hand Clin.* 1992;2:337–44.
9. Eaton CJ, Lister GD. Radial nerve compression. *Hand Clin.* 1992;2:345–57.

the superficial branch of the ulnar artery and the arterial branches of the palmaris brevis and overlying skin pass, together with the superficial branches of the ulnar nerve.

33 Neurological Complications of Environmental Emergencies

DAVID ROSSI AND DAVID OVERTON

SUMMARY The evaluation and management of environmental emergencies present unique challenges to the emergency physician. The neurological manifestations of environmental injuries range from benign to life-threatening, and vary in onset from immediate to delayed. Although environmental emergencies commonly involve multiple organ systems, this chapter describes the neurological manifestations of these injuries. Emergency management focuses not only on immediate stabilization, but also on anticipation of future neurological complications and the need for diagnostic testing and specialty referral.

This chapter reviews the neurological manifestations of electrical, thermal, decompression injuries, and hypothermia.

Electrical, Lightning, and Thermal Injuries

Electrical injuries can result in numerous immediate and delayed neurological complications. Electrical injuries kill approximately 1200 individuals annually in the United States.[1] Of these, 25 deaths occur from bathtub electrocution. More than 100 individuals in the United States die each year as a direct result of lightning strikes, and thousands more are injured.[2] In the United States, over 2 million persons sustain burn injuries annually; of these, 70,000–108,000 require hospitalization.[3] The most common cause of death by alternating current or lightning strike is cardiorespiratory arrest,[4] and the most common cause of death in persons with significant thermal injury is multiple organ failure and its complications.[1] Most individuals who experience thermal injury are children and young adult men, and estimates of death from burn injury range between 6000 and 20,000 yearly.[5] Although the majority of these individuals do not die, morbidity from pain and organ system failure is substantial.

Alternating current typically induces ventricular fibrillation; lightning strike commonly causes asys-

tole.[6] Significant burn injury can cause cardiac dysrhythmias. The overall mortality rate from electrical injuries has improved considerably over the last few decades as understanding of the neuropathological processes involved has improved. Permanent neurological sequelae can now be anticipated or possibly prevented in the patient who appears healthy but has underlying serious pathophysiology caused by electrical injury. Therefore, it is important to understand the mechanisms by which electrical injuries cause harm, their immediate stabilization in the prehospital setting, and their appropriate management in the emergency department.

According to Ohm's law of physics, amperage (A), voltage (V), and resistance (R) are related according to the following formula:

$$A = V/R$$

Tissue factors interact to produce electrical injury of varying severity and distribution. Although voltage can be determined from the patient's history, other factors such as amperage, resistance, and susceptibility of tissues may be unknown. Nonetheless, the mechanism of tissue injury is felt to be related to the translation of electrical energy into heat energy, with resultant thermal injury and direct mechanical tissue damage.[7–9] The neurological effects of electrical injury can be classified as immediate (often transient) and delayed (often permanent). Immediate and permanent neurological complications of electrical injuries in many different combinations have been reported.[10]

In the United States, 1 out of 70 individuals is hospitalized for a burn at some point in life.[11] Most burns are minor and can be treated on an outpatient basis. Patients present to the emergency department with a wide range of thermal injuries and potential complications requiring rapid assessment and appropriate management. For example, thermal injury increases the risk of spontaneous abortion and premature labor.[12] A recent study using postmortem examinations of 139 burn patients over a 21-year period demonstrated a 50% incidence of central nervous system (CNS) complications.[11] Peripheral nerve abnormalities following major burn injuries are estimated to occur in 15–29% of patients.[13] Approximately 10–50% of post–burn injury patients have long-term psychological morbidity.[14] Given the young age of most burn patients, this can have a profound impact on their lives.

Prehospital Management

The prehospital management of electrical and burn injuries is unique in several ways. Electrocutions occur rapidly and are often unwitnessed. In cases of bathtub electrocution, oral commissure injuries in children, and lightning strike, there are usually sufficient data available to identify the source of injury. However, for individuals found with unwitnessed injury, there may be no obvious mechanism of injury, and thermal injury can go undetected. Prehospital care providers may be exposed to electrical hazards when caring for these patients and must carefully assess the environment before approaching these individuals. When an individual appears to have been involved in a blast-type injury, the area is scrutinized for additional explosive materials. Smoke may be inhaled from nearby burning material. The rescue of patients injured by lightning can be dangerous because lightning has a propensity to strike again in the vicinity of the first strike, and the restrike can harm rescue personnel.

An unusual prehospital aspect of lightning injury is the often distorted appearance of the injured individuals. The blast effect can hurl the individual several yards, resulting in unconsciousness. Superheated water on skin or clothing results in clothing and shoes being "blown off" as a result of lightning flashover.[15] An immediate vasoconstriction follows, which likely occurs as a result of both vascular thermal injury and direct effects upon the CNS and the peripheral nervous system (PNS).[16] Sudden depolarization of the myocardium causes asystole and centrally mediated apnea, consequently, cardiopulmonary arrest is the primary cause of death in lightning-related injuries.[9] Cardiopulmonary arrest is the leading cause of immediate death among patients with other electrical injuries as well.[4] These processes can result in an on-scene appearance of an unclothed individual with twisted, cyanotic, pulseless extremities, in cardiorespiratory arrest.

In contrast, with severe, full-thickness thermal injuries, the patient may have little associated pain, bleeding, or blistering. This apparent lack of severity can be misinterpretted. The term *keraunoparalysis* is used to describe the transiently insensate, pulseless, and cyanotic extremities that result from high-voltage electrocution. Because of the appearance of the injured individual, there is a tendency to pronounce death at the scene with little intervention by emergency care providers. However, individuals who have sustained an electrical injury have better outcomes even with prolonged arrest than do individuals who have experienced cardiorespiratory arrest from other causes.[17]

Disaster triage protocols for care of multiple patients are altered in cases of electrical and lightning injury. Because cardiorespiratory arrest is the leading cause of death in individuals who have sustained electrical injuries, immediate attention is focused on individuals who appear pulseless and unconscious.[4] When standard triage protocols are used in this setting, victims with a moderate chance of survival can be inappropriately considered expired at the scene. Basic and advanced life support protocols are initiated and do not need to be altered in patients with electrical injuries. Cervical spine immobilization is recommended, because blunt trauma may be undetected early in the course of resuscitation. When the patient appears to have an injury from a high-voltage source, significant surface burns, or the suspicion of significant deep tissue injury, prehospital care providers consider transferring the patient directly to a trauma and burn center. Fluid resuscitation is begun early, because fluid requirements for electrical burn patients exceed those of standard burn protocols.[4] This is most likely due to undetected deep tissue burn injuries. Supplemental oxygen, with or without endotracheal intubation, is administered. It is not uncommon for patients with facial burns to incur oropharyngeal and pulmonary thermal injuries, which can quickly become life-threatening. Continuous cardiac monitoring is indicated in the prehospital setting.

Emergency Department Evaluation

Emergency department evaluation includes rapid assessment using advanced trauma life support (ATLS) guidelines. Patients with evidence of upper airway injury or constricting areas of thermal burns are observed carefully, because they may require early endotracheal intubation or escharotomy to facilitate oxygenation and ventilation. Renal failure secondary to rhabdomyolysis, hypoperfusion, or direct electrical injury is possible.[7] Hypovolemia and shock may occur rapidly. Patients who exhibit dysrhythmias are managed with standard advanced cardiac life support (ACLS) guidelines.

A careful physical examination and frequent repeat examinations follow. Vertebral body injury and articular dislocations, which commonly accompany electrical injuries, are considered. Physical examination of the patient can help differentiate alternating from direct current: Alternating current tends to produce entrance and exit wounds of approximately the same size; direct current produces a small entrance wound and a much larger exit wound. A feather or "ferning" pattern has been described in association with skin surface burns caused by lightning strike.[13] The CNS is the most commonly affected organ system in electrical injuries, with 33–100% of patients developing neurological deficits. Approximately 50% of thermally injured patients exhibit CNS complications.[11] Because neurological deficits initially may be subtle, a detailed neurological examination with frequent reexamination is indicated.[7] Typically, this is difficult because many patients remain unconscious for a period of time. Electrical injury affects the CNS and PNS in numerous ways and the clinical manifesta-

tions can resemble those of other diseases. The CNS and PNS are commonly involved in thermal injuries. Table 33.1 summarizes the most commonly reported neurological abnormalities in patients with electrical injuries.

Differential Diagnosis

Although electrical and thermal injuries can be obvious, the possibility of occult trauma should be considered. Commonly associated injuries include brain, spinal, thoracic, and abdominal injuries, fractures, dislocations, compartment syndromes, and occult deep muscle injury. The differential diagnosis includes assault, sepsis, chemical exposure, and intoxication.

Multiple neuropathies can be observed in patients with burn injuries, caused by nerve compression syndromes secondary to edema formation, complications of escharotomies, prolonged tourniquet applications for wound debridement, prolonged sepsis, multiple organ failure, and prolonged uremia.[13]

Neuropathophysiology

The two mechanisms of neuropathological change resulting from electrical injury are (1) direct injury caused by the effect of the blast (in lightning injury) or mechanical trauma, and (2) thermal injury caused by tissue exposure to current. This type of thermal injury can injure brain tissue and vascular endothelium, resulting in thrombotic or hemorrhagic infarction.[11,18] Thermal injury of peripheral nerves can result in irreversible loss of function.[8]

Histological and electrophysiological changes in peripheral nervous tissue have been implicated in transient peripheral nerve injury. The pathological findings are summarized as cavitation, chromatolysis of anterior horn cells, fragmentations of axons, myelin degeneration, petechial hemorrhages, reactive gliosis, and swelling and softening of the spinal cord.[20] In patients with large burns (over 35% of body surface area) there is evidence that a neurotoxic high-molecular-weight lipoprotein is released, causing both encephalopathy and peripheral neuropathies.[13]

Emergency Department Management

Following initial stabilization, the electrically injured patient is assessed for spinal injury. A complete physical examination, including a detailed

TABLE 33.1. Common Neurological Manifestations of Electrical Injury

Neurologic Region	Early Manifestations	Late Manifestations
Central	Confusion	Progressive cerebellar syndrome
	Unconciousness	Parkinsonism
	Retrograde amnesia	Reflex sympathetic dystrophy
	Hemorrhage	Hemionopia
	Apnea	Cerebral venous thrombosis
	Anxiety	Necrosis of brain tissue
	Intracerebral hematoma	Retinopathy
		Neuropsychological complications
		Decreased cognition
		Post traumatic syndrome
		Amytrophic lateral sclerosis-like syndrome
		Hyperreflexia
		Ascending paralysis
		Seizure disorders
		CN VII nerve deficits
		CN VIII nerve deficits
		Visual disturbances
		Cerebral edema
		Transverse myelitis
		Chronic headache
Spinal	Babinski reflex	Progressive spinal atrophy
	Unsustained clonus	Quadriplegia
	Snout reflex	Hemiplegia
	Karaunoparalysis	Paraplegia
		Monoplegia
Peripheral	Hypothesia	Demyelination of peripheral nerve tissue
	Hyperalgesia	Polyneuropathy
	Median nerve deficits	Raynaud's syndrome
	Ulnar nerve deficits	Progressive muscular atrophy
	Entrapment syndrome	
	Brachial plexus deficits	

Source: Reproduced with permission from Danzl DF, Pozos RS. Accidental hypothermia. *New Eng J Med.* 1994;331(26):1756–60.

neurological examination, follows. Continuous cardiac monitoring is established. Urine output is monitored and maintained at 1.5–2.0 cc/kg per hour.[7] Fluid management becomes more difficult in the setting of traumatic brain injury, increased intracranial pressure (ICD), or cerebral edema. Hyperventilation, steroid therapy, and diuresis may be necessary to prevent further CNS injury. Other early complications of thermal injury include fluctua-

tions in serum electrolytes, especially sodium, magnesium, and calcium.[21] Tetanus immunization status is assessed.

A variety of diagnostic tests are used to evaluate the patient with electrical or thermal injury. Some have a higher sensitivity, and some offer a method of evaluating specific neurological pathways. Although some diagnostic tests may not be useful in acute management, they can provide valuable information for subsequent care. Cranial computerized tomography (CT) is performed in patients with altered mental status, when there is evidence of traumatic brain injury or when focal neurological deficits exist.

The electroencephalogram (EEG) (see Chapter 3, "Electroencephalography") may demonstrate the absence of alpha rhythms and a predominance of low-amplitude slow waves.[21] Technetium 99m scanning outlines deep muscle injury of the extremities.[22] ICP monitoring devices have been used successfully in managing patients injured by lightning strike.[23] The early use of electromyography helps document PNS injuries.[8] Baseline hearing and visual acuity measurements are performed. Early referral to a neurologist, neurosurgeon, or burn specialist is considered.

Disposition

Most patients injured by a high-voltage electrical source require hospital admission with cardiac monitoring. It is not unusual for such patients to remain in the intensive care unit or burn unit for several weeks. These patients typically undergo long-term therapy with neurological rehabilitation and psychological counseling. In patients with very mild electrocution, the prognosis is good, and a period of monitoring in the emergency department may be adequate to allow discharge from the emergency department. Many burn patients experience subsequent psychological difficulties; estimates of long-term psychological morbidity are as high as 50%.[14] Patients with mild burns can be taught to care for the burns at home. Silver sulfadiazine ointment is commonly used on deep burns and is a good choice for wounds likely to become infected. These patients can be reevaluated daily or every two to three days as indicated.

Neurological Decompression Sickness

Each year in the United States, 500–600 diving-related injuries occur, with 75–100 fatalities occurring.[25] In the 1980s there were over 3 million recreational self-contained underwater breathing apparatus (SCUBA) divers in the United States,

with many thousands more in the commercial, scientific, and military sectors.[26] Approximately 500,000 individuals are newly certified each year.[27] In a 13-year study of U.S. Navy diving injuries, 426 (41% of diving accidents) involved decompression sickness.[28] Although these divers received hyperbaric oxygen therapy, they were found to have increased rates of hospitalization, headache, and vascular abnormalities.[28]

Dysbarism is a term used to describe three main clinical syndromes resulting from SCUBA diving. These syndromes are barotrauma, dysbaric air embolism, and decompression sickness. Synonyms for these entities exist; dysbaric air embolism is commonly referred to as arterial gas embolism (AGE).

Decompression sickness is divided into two specific categories based on severity of injury. Type I decompression sickness is a mild form, from which the term *the bends* originated. Shoulder and elbow periarticular joint pain are the most common symptoms of type I decompression sickness. However, descriptions have included more unusual presentations such as temporomandibular joint pain.[29] All joint spaces can develop periarticular pain secondary to the effects of decompression sickness. Type I decompression sickness syndrome is characterized by skin, lymphatic, and musculoskeletal system involvement and typically results in very low morbidity when treated appropriately.

Type II decompression illness is more severe than type I, and can involve the CNS, PNS, and inner ears. Hence, the term *neurological decompression sickness* is often used interchangeably with *type II decompression sickness*. Treatment of patients with type II (neurological) decompression sickness involves prolonged and repeated hyperbaric oxygen therapy. Despite treatment, long-term neurological deficits or death can occur.

For an understanding of the pathophysiology of decompression sickness, specific properties of gases are reviewed. Divers are able to compress gases into portable, confined tanks for use while submerged according to Boyle's law. This law states that at any given temperature (k), the volume of a gas (V) is inversely proportional to the pressure exerted on that gas (P). This may be represented as:

$k = VP$

Thus, a doubling of pressure at a constant temperature causes the volume of the gas to decrease by one half. Conversely, halving the pressure causes the volume of gas to double.

Dalton's law states that the total pressure exerted by a gas in a mixture of gases is equal to the sum of the partial pressures of each component gas. Using the example of a SCUBA tank with a mixture of gases, this can be expressed as:

P(total) = P(oxygen) + P(nitrogen) + P(others)

Thus, the partial pressures of oxygen, nitrogen, and the other gases in the tank are additive and equal the total pressure of gases within the tank.

Henry's law states that in a given volume of fluid, the amount of gas dissolved in that fluid at any given time is proportional to the pressure of the gas with which it is in equilibrium. This law is sometimes referred to as the "carbonated beverage law," and explains how gas can be dissolved in a carbonated beverage while under pressure only to bubble out quickly when the bottle is opened and the gas pressure above the beverage is reduced. Analogously, divers have increasing amounts of external (or ambient) pressure exerted upon them with increasing depth of dive. This causes inert nitrogen to dissolve into tissues, in accordance with Henry's law. Once the nitrogen has dissolved into tissues and the divers surface too quickly, the effect is likened to uncapping a bottle of soda with rapid formation of nitrogen bubbles in tissues and vascular spaces in response to the decreased pressure exerted upon the divers as they rise in the water. Given the previous example, this may be mathematically written as:

%N = [P(N)/P(T)] × 100

where %N is the percentage of nitrogen gas dissolved in liquid, P(N) is the partial pressure of nitrogen gas, and P(T) is the total external (atmospheric) pressure exerted.

Prehospital Management

Management of patients with neurological decompression sickness in the prehospital environment usually does not involve advanced life-saving measures. Although it is possible that a diver may become unresponsive shortly after a dive, immediate loss of consciousness is more commonly associated with AGE. Most decompression sickness presents as delayed joint pain. Among symptomatic divers, 90% exhibit joint pains, and 20–50% exhibit neurological symptoms as a delayed consequence of diving.[30]

Approximately 50% of patients with decompression sickness demonstrate symptoms within 30 minutes postdive, 95% within 3 hours, and nearly 100% within 6 hours. When dysbaric air embolism is suspected, the Trendelenburg and left lateral decubitus positions are maneuvers that may prevent further gas embolism.[26] Additionally, these maneuvers increase venous distension and pressure and facilitate the elimination of air emboli through the venous pulmonary system. Wet clothing is removed, and the diver is protected from the wind in order to minimize loss of body heat. When available, 100% oxygen is administered immediately to increase tissue oxygenation. Supplemental oxygen helps to remove excess nitrogen gas dissolved in tissues, a process called "nitrogen washout," and aids in preventing further bubble formation. Patients with immediate loss of consciousness and suspected air embolism are transferred to a recompression chamber as soon as possible. A fixed-wing aircraft capable of low-altitude flying and cabin pressures of 1 atm is optimal. However, other modes of transportation are considered when they provide faster transport time. Patients are not left unattended, because loss of consciousness can occur without warning and compromise airway patency. Because most divers exhibit some degree of dehydration, isotonic fluid resuscitation, either intravenously or orally, is begun. Both dehydration and hemoconcentration compound ischemia, which develops as a consequence of bubble formation.[31]

Emergency Department Evaluation

Immediate assessment includes evaluation of the airway patency, breathing, and circulation. The history is most important in diagnosing decompression sickness, and witnesses are consulted. The following questions can elicit useful information: How long and how deep was the dive? What type of equipment was used? Were there repeat dives? What was the water temperature? Where did the dive take place? Was this dive particularly fatiguing? Advanced age, obesity, dehydration, recent alcohol intoxication, and local physical injury have all been anecdotally related to increased risk of developing decompression sickness.[26]

The patient is kept in a Trendelenburg or left lateral decubitus position, and intravenous access is established. Although administration of high-dose intravenous steroids is controversial, their use may reduce edema associated with ischemia or trauma. Aspirin has been advocated to decrease platelet adhesiveness and provide prophylaxis against thrombosis secondary to nitrogen bubble accumulation.[32]

Physical examination precedes recompression therapy, because patients can have associated medical problems. A Foley catheter is inserted to facilitate the monitoring of urine output and obviates the need of the male patient to stand in order to urinate. Several studies have confirmed that neuropsychological testing is at least as sensitive as clinical examination.[33] In patients with pulmonary barotrauma, chest pain, cough, dyspnea, or tachypnea is usually present. The oropharynx may be deeply red. Skin lesions may also be present. These lesions are typically tender, warm to touch, and pruritic. Typically, they occur over the chest and may represent nitrogen bubble emboli in the smaller vessels of the skin.[30]

Numerous neurological manifestations of decompression sickness include headache, confusion, delirium, coma, visual loss, blurred vision, vestibular deficits, nausea, equilibrium disorder, paraplegia, quadriplegia, paresis, lower extremity paresthesias, tremor, bladder dysfunction, and death.[1,27,30, 34,35] Case reports of patients with barotraumatic injuries and loss of consciousness due to AGE without demonstrated neurological dysfunction have been reported.[36] These reports reinforce the fact that history is usually the best way to differentiate between AGE and decompression sickness. Consultation with a neurologist and pulmonologist for recompression therapy is recommended in order to facilitate definitive treatment. "Definitive care" includes the earliest possible hyperbaric oxygen treatment, whether the patient exhibits symptoms of dysbaric arterial embolism or neurological decompression sickness.

Laboratory evaluation of decompression sickness should not delay recompression therapy. Tests include a complete blood count and blood glucose levels. An electrocardiogram and chest radiograph are performed prior to recompression therapy, when possible. Serum creatine kinase levels can reflect the size and severity of AGE.[37] Evidence suggests that serum creatine kinease levels help to differentiate AGE from decompression sickness with manifestations resembling embolism. When carbon monoxide poisoning is suspected, a carboxyhemoglobin level is obtained. Arterial blood gas analysis is beneficial when complications of pulmonary barotrauma are present. Blood alcohol levels, drug screens, and electrolyte levels are required in selected patients.

Neuroimaging and neurophysiological studies are helpful in evaluating a patient with decompression sickness. Magnetic resonance imaging (MRI) provides a more sensitive technique than conventional CT scanning in localizing spinal cord lesions related to decompression sickness.[27] Intravenous injection with gadolinium-diethylene-triamine-pentacetic acid (Gd-DTPA) increases the sensitivity of MRI scans in patients with decompression sickness and AGE.[25] Additionally, electronystagmography (ENG) is useful in evaluation of inner ear decompression sickness.[25] Brainstem auditory evoked responses (BAERs), somatonsensory evoked potentials (SSEPs), and visual evoked potentials (VEPs) are less sensitive than neurological examination in detecting abnormalities of spinal cord decompression sickness.[38] One diagnostic test that can be used quickly in the emergency department involves inflating a blood pressure cuff over an affected limb joint, such as the elbow, and inflating the pressure above 200 mm Hg. This may result in relief of symptoms of pain at the joint. Doppler studies can be used when AGE is suspected; in rare instances, it can detect small amounts of air within the ventricles of the heart.

Additional factors can predispose to decompression illness. Neurological symptoms can develop due to AGE after decompression in a diver who has an atrial septal defect. Similarly, a patent foramen ovale is a risk factor for the development of decompression sickness. Echocardiography is performed when cardiac abnormalities are suspected. Recompression therapy is not withheld when there has been a long delay in presentation, because virtually complete recovery from decompression sickness can occur with recompression therapy initiated more than a week after the inciting event.[39]

Differential Diagnosis

Although the patient history provides an obvious diagnosis in the case of diving injuries, other conditions are considered in the differential diagnosis. Conditions that resemble decompression sickness include motion sickness, near drowning, envenomations, carbon monoxide poisoning, nitrogen toxicity, psychological disorders, hypothermia, and cardiac dysfunction. Patients with decompression sickness can present in delayed fashion with headache, nausea, and fatigue, and can be misdiagnosed as with a viral illness.[29] Diagnoses that can coexist with diving injuries include pulmonary barotrauma, aural barotrauma, squeeze syndromes, hypoxia, alternobaric vertigo, physical trauma, and exhaustion.

Pathophysiological Process

Decompression sickness occurs when there is a sufficient volume of gas (usually nitrogen) dissolved in tissue, which under decreased pressure comes out of solution and forms bubbles within vascular and tissue spaces. The mechanisms of injury include direct tissue injury, obstruction of blood flow, and foreign body reaction.[35]

Clinical manifestations reflect the amount and location of bubble formation. Bubbles that obstruct the paravertebral venous system result in spinal cord symptoms. Bubbles that embolize to the CNS cause cerebral, cerebellar, or other CNS symptoms. Preferential involvement of the lower thoracic, upper lumbar, and lower cervical spinal cord have been described in postmortem studies of divers with decompression sickness who had significant residual impairments following recompression.[41] The vascular anatomy of the spinal cord allows bubbles in the paravertebral veins to form a stagnant collection, creating stasis and infarction.[37] Cerebral and cerebellar lacunes, hyalinization of vessel walls, perivascular white matter vacuolization, and foci of necrotic gray matter have also been identified in patients with fatal diving accidents. Other pathological findings include neuronal (medulla) changes, diffuse increase of astrocytes and microglia, and thickening of the adventitial wall by the expansion of collagen fibers.[40] These findings suggest an inflammatory (foreign body) reaction

secondary to vascular damage induced by bubble formation.

Disposition

In cases of very mild (type I) decompression sickness, patients commonly have resolution of symptoms with recompression therapy and can be discharged from the emergency department shortly thereafter. Alternatively, patients with mild cases of decompression sickness may be hospitalized overnight for monitoring, because recompression therapy is time-intensive. When neurological symptoms or signs are present, patients are hospitalized, because manifestations of neurological decompression sickness can recur after the first recompression treatment. Some patients never recover full function, and experience lifelong sequelae.

Accidental Hypothermia

Accidental hypothermia is sometimes referred to as *thermal disequilibrium*. With more individuals participating in outdoor recreational activities than in the past in the United States, increased accidental cold-related injuries are anticipated. Many cases of hypothermia are avoidable with appropriate education and preparation. The overall mortality rate for patients treated for hypothermia is estimated to be nearly 40%.[42] Very young and very old individuals are particularly susceptible to the effects of hypothermia. Alcohol ingestion is commonly associated with hypothermia, although there is no clear correlation between alcohol intoxication and the initial body temperature recorded and patient survival.[43,44] Therefore, although alcohol ingestion can precipitate events that lead to hypothermia, this factor does not appear to affect patient outcome adversely. In contrast, underlying cardiovascular status plays an important role in patient outcome.

Although full resuscitation with intact neurological function is possible, persistent neurological deficits are common.[45–48] The rapid detection and correction of core body temperature is the ultimate goal of prehospital care providers and emergency physicians. Long-term neurological abnormalities may not be immediately apparent, and may be detected only after complete neurological evaluation. Global ischemia, as a consequence of prolonged alterations of cardiac functioning, is perhaps the most significant pathological process of hypothermia.

Hypothermia is defined by a range of core temperature abnormalities. Mild hypothermia is defined as a core temperature of 34–35.9°C, moderate hypothermia as 30–33.9°C, and severe hypothermia as less than 30°C. The lowest recorded temperature for revival after hypothermia was a 23-month-old boy with an initial temperature of 15°C.[49] Although full neurological recovery has occurred after severe accidental hypothermia in patients who have undergone active core rewarming, neurological outcome remains difficult to predict in the acute setting. A hypothermia outcome score has been developed that uses the presenting neurological and cardiac status as well as laboratory abnormalities to define prognostic factors for patient outcome.[50]

Prehospital Management

The management of hypothermic patients in the prehospital setting focuses on recognition of hypothermia (using a low-reading thermometer), establishment of intravenous catheter(s), administration of supplemental oxygen, cardiac monitoring, and the initiation of rewarming (see Table 33.2).

Hypothermic patients are handled extremely gently, because cardiac irritability is related to the degree of core temperature depression below 28°C.[52] Performance of cardiopulmonary resuscitation (CPR), endotracheal intubation, or nasogastric intubation or merely moving the patient can induce ventricular fibrillation.[52,53,54] The patient's clothing is removed, and warmed blankets are provided. Once initiated, rewarming is continued in order to prevent "afterdrop" and its consequences. *Afterdrop* is defined as a drop in core temperature once rewarming has been initiated. It has been demonstrated to affect the cardiovascular system adversely by lowering mean arterial pressure (MAD) and peripheral vascular resistance, and by promoting the development of ventricular fibrillation.[51,52]

Emergency Department Evaluation

Patients are assessed quickly for adequacy of airway, breathing, and circulatory function. Intra-venous access, when not obtained in the prehospital setting, is established. Although central venous catheterization has been reported to precipitate cardiac arrhythmias, it is a potential alternative to peripheral venous catheterization in the emergency department. Supplemental oxygen is humidified and warmed to 46°C. Severely hypothermic patients can have adequate oxygenation with a respiratory rate as low as four to six breaths per minute.[52] The presence of occult trauma, especially of the cervical spine, is considered.

Differential Diagnosis

Table 33.3 lists factors that are considered in the differential diagnosis of primary causes of hypothermia. These conditions can occur concomitantly (but as separate disease entities) in patients with hypothermia. In addition, disorders of the CNS may induce hypothermic states. These disorders include Wernicke's encephalopathy, cerebrovascular accidents, head trauma, brain tumors, spinal cord transection above T1, anorexia nervosa, Shapiro's syndrome, spontaneous periodic hypothermia, sarcoidosis, and hypothalamic infarction.[51,55,56] (See Fig. 33.1.)

Pathophysiology of Hypothermia

Nuclei within the preoptic anterior hypothalamus regulate physiological heat conservation in humans.[51] Within the skin lie end organs that are very sensitive to alterations in ambient temperature. As ambient temperature declines and blood begins to cool, cells within the posterior hypothalamus respond by triggering cutaneous vasoconstriction and shivering.[57,58] When these compensatory mechanisms are inadequate and temperature continues to decline, the patient becomes hypothermic. Heart rate and cardiac output can decrease by over 50%, culminating in asystole or ventricular fibrillation. There can be a 75% reduction in oxygen consumption, and renal blood flow may decrease by 50%. There is a 7% decrease in cerebral metabolism for every 1°C fall in temperature.[59] Up to an 80% decrease in basal metabolic rate is noted. Inactivation of insulin has been reported.[58] At 36°C, the PNS responds with an increase in sympathetic neuronal discharge, leading to increased deep tendon reflexes. At lower tem-

TABLE 33.2. Physiologic Changes Associated with Hypothermia

Severity of Hypothermia	Body Temperature	Central Nervous System	Cardiovascular	Respiratory	Renal and Endocrine	Neuromuscular
Mild	35°C (95°F) to 32.2°C (90°F)	Linear depression of cerebral metabolism; amnesia; apathy; dysarthria; impaired judgment; maladaptive behavior	Tachycardia, then progressive brady-cardia; cardiac-cycle prolongation; vaso-constriction; increase in cardiac output and blood pressure	Tachypnea, then progressive decrease in respiratory minute volume; declining oxygen consumption; bronchorrhea; bronchospasm	Cold diuresis; increase in catecholamine, adrenal steroids, triodothyronine, and thyroxine; in-crease in metabolism with shivering	Increased preshivering muscle tone, then fatiguing shivering-induced thermogenesis; ataxia
Moderate	<32.2°C (90°F) to 28°C (82.4°F)	Electroencephalographic abnormalities; progressive depression of level of consciousness; pupillary dilatation; paradoxical undressing; hallucinations	Progressive decrease in pulse and cardiac output; increased atrial and ventricular arrhythmias; non-specific and suggestive (J-wave) electrocardio-graphic changes; prolonged systole	Hypoventilation; 50% decrease in carbon dioxide production per 8°C drop in temperature; absence of protective airway reflexes; 50% decrease in oxygen consumption	50% increase in renal blood flow; renal autoregulation intact; no insulin activity	Hyporeflexia; diminishing shivering-induced thermo-genesis; rigidity
Severe	<28°C (82.4°F)	Loss of cerebrovascular autoregulation; decline in cerebral blood flow; coma; loss of ocular reflexes; progressive decrease in electroen-cephalographic activity	Progressive decreases in blood pressure, heart rate, and cardiac output; reentrant dys-rhythmias; decreased ventricular arrhythmia threshold; asystole	Pulmonic congestion and edema; 75% decrease in oxygen consumption; apnea	Decrease in renal blood flow parallels decrease in cardiac output; extreme oliguria; poikilo-thermia; 80% decrease in basal metabolism	No motion; decreased nerve-conduction velocity; peripheral areflexia

Source: Reproduced with permission from Danzl DF, Pozos RS. Accidental hypothermia. *New Eng J Med.* 1994;331(26):1756–60.

TABLE 33.3. Risk Factors for Decreased Thermostability

Decreased Heat Production	Increased Heat Loss
Endocrinologic failure	Induced vasodilation
Hypothyroidism	Pharmacologic
Hypopituitarism	Toxin-induced
Hypoadrenalism	Dermatologic causes
Insufficient fuel	Burns
Hypoglycemia	Dermatitis
Malnutrition	Iatrogenic causes
Extreme physical exertion	Exposure
Neuromuscular physical exertion	Cold infusions
Age extremes	Emergency deliveries
Impaired shivering	Environmental causes
Inactivity	Immersion
Lack of adaptation	Nonimmersion

Impaired Thermoregulation	Miscellaneous Associated Clinical States
Peripheral failure	Multisystem trauma
Neuropathies	Shock
Acute spinal cord transection	Cardiopulmonary disease
Diabetes	Systemic acidoses
Central nervous system failure or	Infections-bacterial,
neurologic abnormalities	viral, parasitic
Pharmacologic causes	Carcinomatosis
Metabolic causes	Vascular insufficiency
Toxins	Pancreatitis
Cerebrovascular accident	Uremia
Central nervous system trauma	Recurrent or episodic
Neoplasm	hypothermia
Degenerative disease	

Source: Reproduced with permission from Danzl DF, Pozos RS. Accidental hypothermia. *New Eng J Med.* 1994;331(26):1756–60.

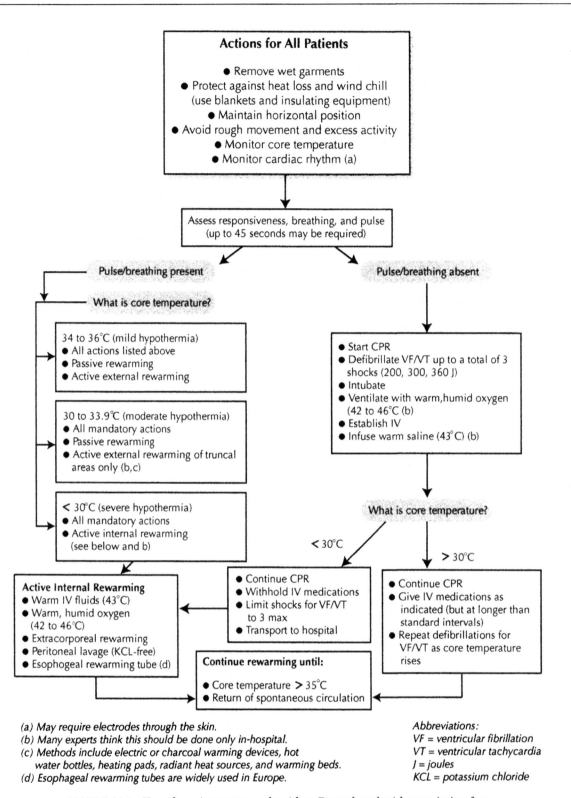

Actions for All Patients

- Remove wet garments
- Protect against heat loss and wind chill (use blankets and insulating equipment)
- Maintain horizontal position
- Avoid rough movement and excess activity
- Monitor core temperature
- Monitor cardiac rhythm (a)

Assess responsiveness, breathing, and pulse (up to 45 seconds may be required)

Pulse/breathing present

What is core temperature?

34 to 36°C (mild hypothermia)
- All actions listed above
- Passive rewarming
- Active external rewarming

30 to 33.9°C (moderate hypothermia)
- All mandatory actions
- Passive rewarming
- Active external rewarming of truncal areas only (b,c)

< 30°C (severe hypothermia)
- All mandatory actions
- Active internal rewarming (see below and b)

Pulse/breathing absent

- Start CPR
- Defibrillate VF/VT up to a total of 3 shocks (200, 300, 360 J)
- Intubate
- Ventilate with warm, humid oxygen (42 to 46°C (b)
- Establish IV
- Infuse warm saline (43°C) (b)

What is core temperature?

< 30°C

> 30°C

Active Internal Rewarming
- Warm IV fluids (43°C)
- Warm, humid oxygen (42 to 46°C)
- Extracorporeal rewarming
- Peritoneal lavage (KCL-free)
- Esophogeal rewarming tube (d)

- Continue CPR
- Withhold IV medications
- Limit shocks for VF/VT to 3 max
- Transport to hospital

- Continue CPR
- Give IV medications as indicated (but at longer than standard intervals)
- Repeat defibrillations for VF/VT as core temperature rises

Continue rewarming until:

- Core temperature > 35°C
- Return of spontaneous circulation

(a) May require electrodes through the skin.
(b) Many experts think this should be done only in-hospital.
(c) Methods include electric or charcoal warming devices, hot water bottles, heating pads, radiant heat sources, and warming beds.
(d) Esophageal rewarming tubes are widely used in Europe.

Abbreviations:
VF = ventricular fibrillation
VT = ventricular tachycardia
J = joules
KCL = potassium chloride

FIGURE 33.1. Hypothermia treatment algorithm. Reproduced with permission from Weinberg, A.D., Hypothermia. *Annals of Emergency Medicine* 1993;22(2):370–377.

perature, ataxia and muscular rigidity may develop. At approximately 32°C, hyporeflexia develops.[51] At 28°C, nerve conduction is delayed by 25% and physical activity becomes difficult due to muscular rigidity. Patients typically exhibit ataxia, confusion, or obtundation and dysarthria. Below 8°C, nerve conduction ceases entirely.[60]

Effects of hypothermia on the CNS are similar, with apathy being an early finding. As the patient's temperature continues to fall, judgment becomes impaired and hallucinations may develop. By 30°C, patients typically have dilated, sluggish pupils, and cardiovascular irritability can lead to dysrhythmias. Patients exhibit loss of muscular reflexes, loss of pain responses, and fixed, dilated pupils by the time core temperature has reached 28°C. The corneal reflex, mediated by CNS pathways, disappears at approximately 25°C.[58] EEC recordings are isoelectric at a core temperature of 19°C but reappear at approximately the same temperature when the patient is rewarmed.[47]

Emergency Department Management

Hypothermic patients in the emergency department are evaluated by ATLS (Advanced Trauma Life Support) guidelines developed by the American College of Surgeons. Assessment of airway, breathing, and circulation is performed in a gentle manner. Patients are handled very carefully. Hypoventilation or inability to protect the airway requires tracheal intubation. Intravenous access is established and warmed isotonic solutions are infused, because most severely hypothermic patients demonstrate some degree of volume depletion.[56] Humidified oxygen (warmed to 46°C) is administered and cardiac and continuous rectal temperature monitoring is established.

A variety of active, external, and core warming modalities exist, including warmed blankets, heated ceiling tiles, radiant heat lamps, aerosol masks, gastric lavage, bladder lavage, peritoneal lavage, thoracic lavage, dialysis, and cardiopulmonary bypass. The method(s) used depend on the extent of hypothermia and the cardiovascular status of the patient. Cardiopulmonary bypass is rapid, with little afterdrop phenomenon, but is typically not readily available. Unconscious patients receive naloxone, thiamine, and glucose. Patients in whom hypothermia

develops gradually are prone to hypoglycemia, because prolonged shivering utilizes glycogen stores.[58] However, the inactivation of insulin that occurs with hypothermia can lead to hyperglycemia.[52,56,58] Severely hypothermic patients who have not sustained cardiac arrest may benefit from prophylactic treatment with bretylium, 10 mg/kg.[52]

Laboratory evaluation includes: arterial blood gases; complete blood count; liver function tests; coagulation studies; blood glucose, electrolyte, blood urea nitrogen, serum creatinine, and amylase levels; electrocardiogram; urinalysis; and chest radiograph. Aggressive correction of acidosis is not recommended in hypothermic patients, because the acidosis corrects itself with rewarming and alkalosis may precipitate dysrhythmias.[44] Studies have reported a wide range of significant clinical and laboratory factors in hypothermic patients.[62] Poor prognostic signs include prehospital cardiac arrest, low or absent presenting blood pressure, elevated blood urea nitrogen levels, and the need for endotracheal or nasogastric tube placement in the emergency department.[50]

Disposition

Many patients with mild hypothermia can be rewarmed in the emergency department and discharged once evaluation for accompanying injuries and illness is complete. Patients with more severe hypothermia are hospitalized for thorough assessment, rewarming, and stabilization. Neurological abnormalities are evaluated and documented. Occasionally, slowing of mentation or other subtle neurological complications may persist with slow resolution. Complications such as these are followed closely after discharge.

Conclusion

Numerous environmental emergencies and their potential neurological complications are evaluated and treated in the emergency department. In the United States, approximately 1200 individuals die from electrical injuries annually. Over 2 million individuals sustain burn injuries. Recreational activities are responsible for many of the neurological complications resulting from dysbarism and hypothermia. Education plays a significant role in reducing morbidity and mortality. The most challenging task for the treating physician, however, is to develop an appropriate differential diagnosis and remain vigilant for occult injuries. Neurological complications from environmental emergencies requires a team approach, from first responders to subspecialists. Treatment delays result in more pronounced neurological deficits, which may be permanent.

PEARLS AND PITFALLS

Electrical, Lightning, and Thermal Injuries

- Cardiopulmonary arrest is the leading cause of death in individuals with electrical injuries.
- The presence of occult deep tissue thermal injuries is considered.
- Decisions to transfer individuals with severe electrical injury to burn and trauma centers are made out of hospital or early in the emergency department evaluation.
- Significant head, chest, and abdominal injuries are considered present until proven otherwise in the electrically injured patient.
- Fractures and dislocations are commonly associated with electrocution.
- Tetanus immunization status is assessed in all patients.
- Alternating current commonly causes ventricular fibrillation and exhibits entry and exit wounds of nearly equal size.
- Direct current commonly causes ventricular asystole and exhibits a larger exit wound.
- Oral commissure injuries in children are monitored for labial artery rupture in the days following injury.
- Baseline hearing and visual acuity tests are performed and the results documented.
- Electromyography may aid in diagnosing patients with PNS injuries.

Decompression Sickness

- The most common form of decompression sickness is type I, "the bends," and nearly 90% of patients exhibit musculoskeletal symptoms only.
- Associated injuries, envenomations, or intoxications are reviewed with suspected decompression sickness.

- The patient history is of greatest importance in diagnosing decompression sickness.
- The left lateral decubitus or Trendelenburg position is used for patient transport.
- Use of a Foley catheter may restrict body position changes and thereby prevent AGE from the heart's ventricles.
- Immediate supplemental oxygen can help to remove excess nitrogen dissolved in tissues.
- The history and physical examination may be normal initially in patients eventually requiring recompression therapy.
- Diagnostic evaluations should not delay definitive recompression treatment.
- The use of positive airway pressure devices is avoided, because associated pulmonary barotrauma may be present.

Accidental Hypothermia

- Movement of patients with hypothermia can precipitate cardiac dysrhythmias and is done as gently as possible.
- Nearly all hypothermic patients exhibit some degree of volume depletion.
- Once rewarming has been initiated, it is not discontinued until core temperature has reached a minimum of 30°C.
- Target organs become progressively more unresponsive to pharmacological agents as core temperature drops. This may lead to toxic levels when pharmacological therapy is aggressively pursued prior to rewarming.
- Correction of metabolic acidosis occurs with rewarming and usually is not be treated.
- Associated illnesses or injuries often exist in patients with apparently uncomplicated hypothermia.

REFERENCES

1. Beckner E, Hooshmand H, Radfar F. The neurophysiological aspects of electrical injuries. *Clin Electroencephalog.* 1989;20:111–20.
2. Harviel DJ, Jarffin JH, Jordan MH. Lightning strike to the head: case report. *J Trauma.* 1994;36:113–15.
3. Demling RH. Medical progress. *N Engl J Med.* 1985; 313:1389–98.
4. Fontanarosa PB. Electrical shock and lightning strike. *Ann Emerg Med.* 1993;22(pt 2):112–21.

5. Griglak MJ. Thermal injury. *Emerg Med Clin North Am.* 1992;10:369–83.
6. Parkin G, Petty PG. Electrical injury to the central nervous system. *Neurosurgery.* 1986;19:282–4.
7. Billowitz EB. Lightning and electrical injuries. In: Cayten CG, Hanke BK, Mangelsen MA, et al., eds. *Principles and Practice of Emergency Medicine.* 3rd ed. Philadelphia, Pa: Lea & Febiger; 1992:2833–8.
8. Bruynincks F, Dendooven AM, Lissens M, Vanhecke J. Electrical injuries to peripheral nerves. *Medica Physica.* 1990;13:161–5.
9. Stanley LD, Suss RA. Intracerebral hematoma secondary to lightning stroke. Case report and review of literature. *Neurosurgery.* 1985;16:686–8.
10. Cherington M, Lammereste D, Yarnell P. Lightning strikes: nature of neurological damage in patients evaluated in hospital emergency departments. *Ann Emerg Med.* 1992;21:133–6.
11. Galloway PG, Winkleman MD. Central nervous system complications of thermal burns: a postmortem study of 139 patients. *Medicine.* 1992;71:271–82.
12. Block CE, Boes EG, Cywes S, et al. Thermal injury in pregnancy – the neglected tragedy. *South African Med J.* 1990;77:346–8.
13. Dagum AB, Douglas LG, Neligan PC, Peters WJ. Severe multiple mononeuropathy in patients with major thermal burns. *J Burn Care Rehabil.* 1993; 14:440–3.
14. Blalock SJ, Bunker BJ, Devolliss RF. Psychological distress among survivors of burn injury: the role of outcome expectations and perceptions of importance. *J Burn Care Rehabil.* 1994;15:421–7.
15. Edlich RF, Kenney JG, Morgan RF, Persing JA, Tribble CG. Lightning injuries. *Trauma Emerg Med.* 1985; 11:32–40.
16. Craig SR. When lightning strikes: pathophysiology and treatment of lightning injuries. *Postgrad Med.* 1986;79:109–24.
17. Masui M, Wakasugi C. Secondary brain hemorrhages associated with lightning stroke: report of a case. *Japanese Journal of Legal Medicine.* 1986;40:42–6.
18. Patel A., Lo R. Electric injury with cerebral venous thrombosis. *Stroke.* 1993;24:903–5.
19. Mani MM, Redford JB, Varghese G. Spinal cord injuries following electrical accidents. *Paraplegia.* 1986;24:159–66.
20. Pruitt BA. The burn patient, I: Initial care. *Curr Probl Surg.* 1979;16:1–55.
21. Das A, Khanna R, Nizamie SH. Electrical trauma, non-ictal EEG changes, and mania: a case report. *J Clin Psychiatry.* 1991;52:280.
22. Pattern BM. Lightning and electrical injuries. *Neurol Clin.* 1992;10:1047–57.
23. Lehman LB. Successful management of an adult lightning victim using intracranial pressure monitoring. *Neurosurgery.* 1991;28:907–10.
24. Frayne JH, Gilligan BS. Neurological sequelae of lightning strike. *Clin Exper Neurol.* 1987;24:195–200.
25. Greer HD, Massey EW. Neurologic injury from undersea diving. *Neurol Clin.* 1992;10:1032–43.
26. Kizer KW. Management of dysbaric diving casualties. *Emerg Med Clin North Am.* 1983;1:659–70.
27. Anthony DC, Burger PC, Camporesi EM, et al. Neuroimaging of scuba diving injuries to the CNS. *Am J Radiol.* 1988;151:1003–8.
28. Hoiberg A. Consequence of U.S. Navy diving mishaps: decompression sickness. *Undersea Biomed Res.* 1986; 13:383–94.
29. Rudge FW. Decompression sickness presenting as a viral syndrome. *Aviat Space Environ Med.* 1991;62: 60–1.
30. Hanke BK, Schwartz GR. Diving and altitude emergencies. Cayten CG, Hanke BK, Mangelsen MA, et al., eds. *Principles and Practice of Emergency Medicine.* 3rd ed. Philadelphia, Pa: Lea & Febiger; 1992:2934–48.
31. Gallagher TJ. Initial evaluations of the diving accident victim. *J Florida Med Assoc* 1992;79:614–15.
32. Bove AA. Basis for drug therapy in decompression sickness. *Undersea Biomed Res.* 1982;9:91.
33. Kelly PJ, Levin HS, Peters BH. Neurologic and psychologic manifestations of decompression illness in divers. *Neurology.* 1977;27:125–7.
34. Aarli JA, Hjelle JO, Kambestad BK, et al. Analysis of neurological symptoms in deep diving: implications for selection of divers. *Undersea Biomed Res.* 1990; 17:95–107.
35. FitzPatrick DT. Visual manifestations of neurological decompression sickness. *Aviat Space Environ Med.* 1994;65:736–8.
36. Hallenbeck JM, Neuman TS. Barotraumatic cerebral air embolism and the mental status examination: a report of four cases. *Ann Emerg Med.* 1987;16:125–7.
37. Neuman TS, Smith RM. Elevation of serum creatin kinase in divers with arterial gas embolization. *N Engl J Med.* 1994;330:19–24.
38. Dutka A, Farm F Jr, Overlock R, et al. Somatosensory evoked potentials measured in divers with a history of spinal cord decompression sickness. *Undersea Biomed Res.* 1989;16:89.
39. Kizer KW. Delayed treatment of dysbarism; a retrospective review of 50 cases. *JAMA.* 1982;247:2555–8.
40. Calder IM, Palmer AC, Yates PO, Cerebral Vasculopathy in divers. *Neuropathol Appl Neurobiol.* 1992;18: 113–24.
41. Francis TR, Glasspool E, Murrison AW, Pethybridge RJ, Sedgwick EM. Neurophysiological assessment of divers with medical histories of neurological decompression illness. *Occup Environ Med.* 1994;51:730–734.
42. Epstein F, Ferguson J, Van de Leuv J. Accidental hypothermia. *Emerg Med Clin.* 1983;1:619–37.
43. Anardi D, Copass MK, Luna GK, Maier RV, Pavlin EG, Oreskovisch MR. Incidence and effect of hypothermia in seriously injured patients. *J Trauma.* 1987;27:1014–18.

44. White JD. Hypothermia: The Bellevue experience. *Ann Emerg Med.* 1982;11:49–56.

45. Auerback PS, Garmel GM, Tom PA. Environment-dependent sports emergencies. *Sports Med.* 1994;78: 305–25.

46. Barnes PD, Bellinger DC, Castaneda AR, et al. Developmental and neurologic status of children after heart surgery with hypothermic circulatory arrest or low-flow cardiopulmonary bypass. *N Engl J Med.* 1995; 332:549–55.

47. Bjaertnes L, Jolin A, Rekand T, Sulg L. Neuromonitoring in hypothermia and in hypothermic hypoxia. *Arctic Med Res.* 1991;50:22–6.

48. Exton-Smith AN, Fox RH, Woodward PM. Body temperature in the elderly: a national study of physiological, social and environment conditions. *Br Med J.* 1973;1:200–6.

49. Kelly KJ, Glaeser P, Rice TB. Profound accidental hypothermia and freeze injury of the extremities in a child. *Crit Care Med.* 1990;18:670–80.

50. Danzel DF, Hedges JR, Pozos RS. Hypothermia outcome score: development and implications. *Crit Care Med.* 1989;17:227–31.

51. Danzl DF, Pozos RS. Accident hypothermia. *N Engl J Med.* 1994;331:1756–60.

52. Kurtz KJ, Zell SC. Severe exposure hypothermia: a resuscitation protocol. *Ann Emerg Med.* 1985;14:339–45.

53. Dalglish PH Jr, Southwick FS. Recovery after prolonged asystolic cardiac arrest in profound hypothermia. A case report and literature review. *JAMA.* 1980;243:1250–3.

54. Gunby P. Cold facts concerning hypothermia. *JAMA.* 1980;243:1403–9.

55. Carton H, Lammens M, Lissoir F. Hypothermia in three patients with multiple sclerosis. *Clin Neurol Neurosurg.* 1989;91:117–21.

56. Weinberg AD. Hypothermia. *Ann Emerg Med.* 1993; 22:104–11.

57. Barr ML, Kiernan JA. *The Human Nervous System: An Anatomical Viewpoint.* 5th ed. Philadelphia, Pa: JB Lippincott Co; 1988:196–204.

58. Granberg P. Human physiology under cold exposure. *Arctic Med Res.* 1991;50:23–7.

59. Ehrmantraut RR, Fazekras JF, Ticklin HE. Cerebral haemodynamics and metabolism in accidental hypothermia. *Arch Intern Med.* 1957;99:57–61.

60. Enander A. Performance and sensory aspects of work in cold environments – a review. *Ergonomics.* 1984; 27: 365–78.

61. Barish RA, Browne B, Solomon A, Tso E. The electrocardiographic features of hypothermia. *J Emerg Med.* 1989;7:169–73.

62. Shields CP, Sixsmith DM. Treatment of moderate-to-severe hypothermia in an urban setting. *Ann Emerg Med.* 1990;19:1093–7.

FIVE Pediatric Neurology

34 Hydrocephalus and Shunts in Children

STEPHEN GUERTIN

SUMMARY This chapter reviews emergency department recognition and management of cerebrospinal fluid (CSF) shunt dysfunction. Due to the rapid and potentially lethal result of complete shunt failure, systematic identification of the shunt components, evaluation of shunt patency, recognition of peripheral shunt–related complications, and effective therapeutic measures should proceed in tandem.[1-5] The symptoms and signs of shunt failure are discussed, followed by interpretation of specific findings. A stepwise approach to assessing shunt function is provided. Appropriate therapeutic regimens are recommended. A brief review of the non–central nervous system complications of CSF shunts is presented.

Introduction

Almost all cerebrospinal fluid (CSF) shunt systems fail over time. On average, within 1 year of placement, 30–40% of shunts fail; 80–90% fail over a 10-year period.[6-8] More than 50% of children who receive a CSF shunt for neural tube defects require shunt revisions within 3 years and, of that number, 20% require multiple revisions.[9] Approximately 5% of children with birth weights under 1500 g require CSF shunting due to hydrocephalus secondary to intraventricular hemorrhage.[10-12] Up to 80% of these children require revision within months of placement.[12] The greatest single risk of shunt failure is the age of the patient.[13] Children under 2 years of age are at the highest risk for shunt obstruction. Approximately 10% of shunts become infected within the first year, and children under 6 months of age carry the highest risk of infection.[13] The most common cause of shunt failure is occlusion of the ventricular tubing by cellular debris, fibrous tissue, choroid plexus, the ventricular walls, and, in the case of catheter migration, the brain itself.[3] Distal catheter blockage or migration of the catheter is the second most common cause. Valve survival directly relates to the presence or absence of cells and debris in the CSF.[14] The presence of cells (CSF pleocytosis) contributes significantly to the high rate of shunt failure when the system is infected.

With rare exception, shunt systems consist of several distinct components,[15] and disconnections in the systems account for 15% of all shunt malfunctions.[16] Complex systems that incorporate more than one valve have a median survival rate of only 11 months.[13] The siliconized rubber tubing used within the system is subject to degradation, leakage, and fracture.[17]

Once the shunt system is compromised, the pace of clinical deterioration and the severity of presentation depends on the size of the ventricles and the age of the child. Children with large dilated ventricles have tremendous volume-buffering capacity. These children tolerate large increases in volume with relatively small increases in intracranial pressure (ICP) over longer periods of time than do children with small ventricles.[18] Once a CSF shunt is in place, this volume-buffering capacity is lost. Intracranial compliance reverts to that of healthy children. In response to accumulating CSF, a child with normal-sized ventricles experiences greater increases in ICP more rapidly than would be experienced by an adult.[19] The rise in ICP is exacerbated once chronic shunting results in small "slit ventricles" where drained ventricular volume is compensated by growing brain that fills the intracranial space.[20]

When evaluating shunt dysfunction, usually the chief concern is the presence of "shunt blockage." However, life-threatening effects of sudden "overdrainage" of CSF are also of major importance. This overdrainage occurs in children with neural tube defects and Chiari malformations. When there is a rapid drop in the ICP, brainstem traction and shift can lead to immediate compromise of the hindbrain.[21-23] The symptoms and signs of mechanical dysfunction of a CSF shunt system thus can be associated with intracranial hypertension or intracranial hypotension.

Prehospital Care

The prehospital evaluation and management of a child with a CSF shunt is similar to that of any other ill child who does not have a CSF shunt. Airway, breathing, and circulation are assessed and managed first. Intravenous access is important in a child who appears ill. Increased ICP due to shunt dysfunction is a major concern in ill children with CSF shunts. Prehospital clinical determination of increasing ICP is difficult, and, when it is suspected, clinically controlled ventilation with endotracheal intubation is appropriate (see also Chapter 25, "Neuroanesthesiology"). When long transport time is anticipated, the control of airway is of prime importance. The ill child is transported to the nearest emergency department, appropriately stabilized, and transferred to a tertiary care hospital for definitive treatment.

Emergency Department Evaluation and Diagnosis

Symptoms and Signs of Shunt Dysfunction

Most children with CSF shunts who present with irritability, headache, vomiting, and fever are more likely to have a "viral illness" than a shunt malfunction.[7] Fever makes the diagnosis of shunt dysfunction less likely; drowsiness or lethargy makes the diagnosis of shunt dysfunction more likely. Typically, the parent indicates that the child is, in some way, "disturbingly changed." These vague general complaints and parental concerns are considered seriously. Unless a convincing finding exists to support a diagnosis of "viral" infection, CSF shunt dysfunction is assumed, particularly with changes in sensorium, autonomic instability, or cranial nerve findings.[2,7,24]

Symptoms and signs of elevated ICP due to shunt dysfunction include headache, changes in sensorium (lethargy, irritability, disorientation, coma), nausea, and vomiting.[25] Especially ominous are a precipitous change in sensorium, decerebrate posturing, pupillary changes, and components of Cushing's triad (systemic vascular hypertension, bradycardia, and respiratory ataxia), which can occur when blood supply to the medulla is compromised. These changes suggest impending brain herniation. An enlarging or bulging fontanelle, fluid extravasation along the shunt tract, upward gaze palsy, diplopia, dilated scalp veins, and increased muscle tone are the other findings of increasing ICP.

Neuro-ophthalmological signs of shunt dysfunction can precede findings on computerized tomography (CT) scanning. These include palsies of cranial nerves III, IV, and VI, anisocoria, dilated and slowly reactive pupils, upward gaze paresis, tonic downward eye deviation, and eyelid retraction.[24] Sudden blindness secondary to compromise of posterior cerebral artery circulation is reversible with correction of the shunt malfunction; however, permanent blindness can occur when not treated promptly.[26] Any preexisting abnormality of movement or muscle tone is accentuated when ICP is increased. Asymmetrical dilatation of the ventricles can cause focal weakness and the signs of uncal herniation.

Symptoms and signs of gradual ventricular enlargement caused by partial CSF shunt system dysfunction include gait disturbance, urinary incontinence, worsening of cerebral palsy, deteriorating school performance, visual deterioration, and hypothalamic signs.[25,27] Hypothalamic signs include a markedly increased or absent appetite, growth abnormalities, and pituitary insufficiency.[28] Chronic cortical visual impairment can occur and be improved following shunt correction.[29]

Brainstem signs such as stridor, laryngospasm, syncope, disturbed consciousness, pallor, respiratory ataxia or arrest, opisthotonus, and a vacillating heart rate can result from high ICP.[25] These findings also occurs with sudden "overdrainage" of CSF, which results in low ICP and consequent upward traction on the brainstem.[21,22] Brainstem signs can occur in congenital neural tube defects including Chiari malformation.[23] Low ICP is suspected clinically by marked indentation of a cranial defect or collapse of the fontanel. This life-threatening condition can be ameliorated by placing the child into a Trendelenburg position at 15–30 degrees and providing supportive ventilation.

The relationship between seizures and CSF shunts is complex. The electroencephalogram is abnormal in up to 98% of children prior to shunting.[31] Spike and sharp wave activity (see Chapter 3, "Electroencephalography") is present preoperatively in more than 40% of children who require CSF shunting. At least 25% of children who require a CSF shunt have preexisting seizures.[32] The incidence of new-onset seizures after shunt insertion is 5–10%, with 80% of these occurring within the first postoperative year. Onset of new seizures after shunt insertion, or an acute seizure in a child with a known seizure disorder and a CSF shunt, may or may not indicate shunt dysfunction. However, seizures can be temporally related to shunt malfunction. A seizure in a child with a CSF shunt prompts evaluation of the shunt system, particularly when antiepileptic drug levels are therapeutic.[30]

Evaluation of Shunt Function

Almost all CSF shunt systems have intraventricular tubing, a valve apparatus, and distal tubing (see Fig. 34.1). When a separate reservoir is included in the system, it is located proximal to the valve. The most common reservoir used is a Rickham-type reservoir, seated in the skull with proximal connection to the ventricular tubing and distal connection to the valve apparatus.[1–5,15] The components are identified and tracked. For diagnostic and therapeutic reasons, close examination of connections and knowledge of the number and locations of reservoirs are essential (see Figure 34.2). Tracking of the distal tubing allows inspection for possible disconnection.

Intraventricular tubing is located anteriorly or posteriorly within the lateral ventricles, or within the fourth ventricle. CSF enters the tubing through multiple small holes or though larger perforations protected by longitudinal slots. The unique flanged intraventricular tube is designed to prevent envel-

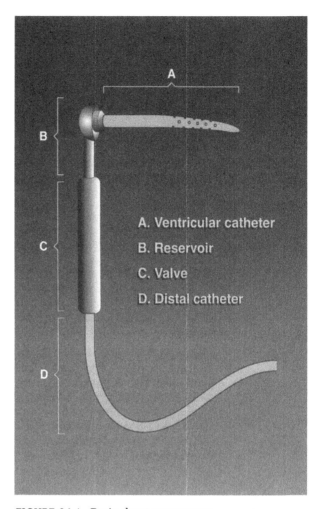

FIGURE 34.1. Basic shunt components.

opment by choroid plexus and reduce the incidence of proximal obstruction (see Fig. 34.2). The presence of flanges allows for firmer investiture of the tubing by choroid plexus, making its removal especially hazardous.[15]

Valves are identified by inspection, palpation, and plain radiography as "tubular" or "domed" (see Figs. 34.3 and 34.4). Tubular valves consist of two one-way valves with an intervening pumping chamber. The two most commonly used types of tubular valves are slit valves and ball-and-cone valves. CSF pressure opens the slit flap, and back pressure closes the flap, resulting in one-way flow. Ball-and-cone valves open when CSF pressure pushes a ball out of a cone into which it is ordinarily wedged by a spring. Back pressure immediately wedges the ball back into the cone, resulting in one-way flow. Domed system valves can be miter valves or dia-

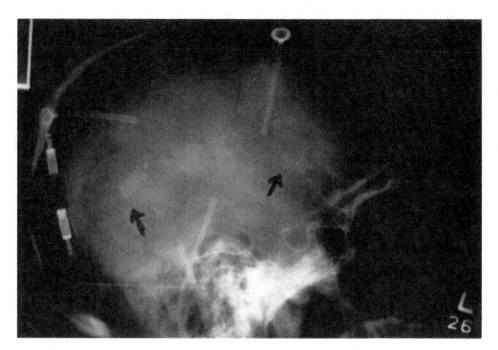

FIGURE 34.2. Superior: Domed shunt system consisting of intraventricular catheter, Rickham reservoir, "dome" valve, and distal tubing. The distal tubing is disconnected and separated from the valve by a long gap. Midfield: Two abandoned "flanged" ventricular catheters (arrows), left in place because they could not be extracted. The abandoned distal tubing has been left in place. Far left: Tubular shunt system consisting of intraventricular catheter, Rickham reservoir, "tubular" valve, and distal tubing. All connections are intact. This is the only functional system in this child's head.

phragm valves. Miter valves are made of folded, siliconized rubber leaflets. CSF pressure opens the leaflets, allowing outflow; however, any back pressure immediately apposes the leaflets, resulting in one-way flow. Diaphragm valves are hinged over or under an aperture like a trapdoor. CSF pressure pushes the diaphragm off the aperture, allowing CSF outflow; back pressure closes the trap door, resulting in one-way flow. When palpation and plain radiographs do not reveal a valve apparatus, close examination of the end of the distal tubing should reveal a rounded convex catheter tip indicating a distal terminal slit valve.[15]

Detailed history obtained from the patient, the family, and medical records focuses on occurrence of a fall, the number of shunt systems, the pressure gradient and types of each of the shunt systems, which (if any) of the shunts are known not to be working, where the shunt systems terminate, and which system (with more than one) was the last shunt system to be revised, and when.

Low-pressure valves maintain ICP at 2–5 cm CSF; medium pressure valves at 5–12 cm CSF; and high-pressure valves at 10–18 cm CSF. When more than one shunt system is in place, each is tapped when infection is suspected. A shunt system that is known not to work is not assessed for function, but when more than one system is working, each one is assessed. Tubing that ends in the heart, the pleural space, or the peritoneal cavity can cause symptoms and signs referable to each location.

Inspection of the shunt system is the next step in evaluation. Craniotomy scars and skull defects suggest shunt locations or previous cranial expansion and shunt revision. Distended scalp veins or bulging of the fontanelle or a craniotomy site indicates high ICP. A sunken fontanelle and sunken craniotomy site indicate low ICP. Swollen sites on the scalp or cranial vault associated with Rickham reservoirs, "domed" systems, "tubular" systems, and distal tubing require closer examination. Unusual or recent swelling over the shunt site is con-

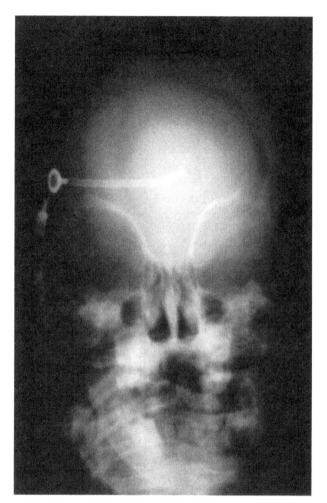

FIGURE 34.3. "Tubular" CSF shunt system consisting of intraventricular catheter, Rickham reservoir, "tubular" valve, and distal tubing. All connections are intact. The ventricular catheter is bent against the septum pellucidum.

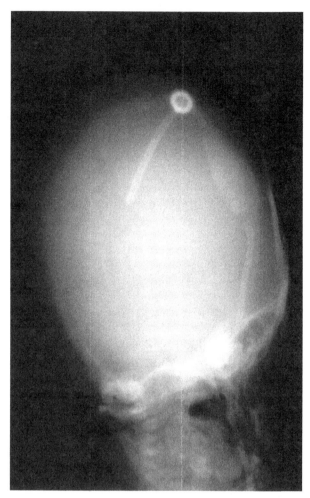

FIGURE 34.4. "Domed" CSF shunt system consisting of intraventricular catheter, Richkam reservoir, "domed" valve, and distal tubing. All connections are intact.

sidered diagnostic of shunt failure.[33] Recent swelling over any portion of the system can indicate an underlying disconnection or perforation. Cellulitis, frank pus, or erosion of the scalp, especially among infants, is associated with a high incidence of ventriculitis leading to mechanical dysfunction.[25] The distal tubing usually can be tracked visually across the neck, chest, and abdomen on its way to the peritoneal space, pleural space, or heart. Swelling at the distal insertion site indicates fluid tracking up the catheter because of distal loculation (Fig. 34.5).

Palpation of the system allows the examiner to check for gaps between components and establishes

the presence and location of reservoirs and pumping chambers. Palpation of a "floating reservoir" confirms the following events: (1) misplacement of Rickham reservoir from its position within the skull and (2) CSF leak around the reservoir and the ventricular tubing. Local warmth indicates underlying infection. Palpation of the abdominal wall can identify an extraperitoneal loculation of fluid, and deep abdominal palpation can reveal an underlying pseudocyst (Fig. 34.5).

Manual Evaluation to Test Cerebrospinal Fluid Shunt Patency. The pumping chambers of both tubular and domed systems are designed to allow the examiner to assess shunt patency by manually testing the system. In domed systems, an attempt is

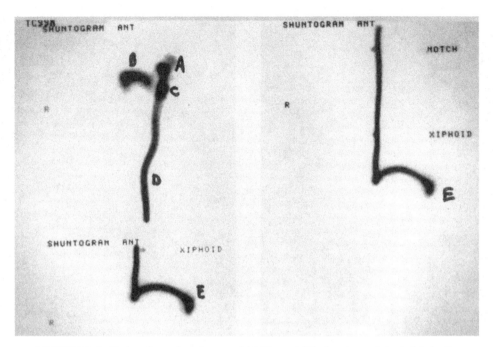

FIGURE 34.5. Technetium shuntogram. (A) The nuclide has been injected into the reservoir. (B) There is reflux into the lateral ventricle. (C) The technetium passes into a valve and (D) is carried through the distal tubing. (E) The technetium does not freely diffuse throughout the peritoneum, but terminates in a distal loculation. This pseudocyst is the cause of the shunt obstruction.

made to occlude the system proximal to the pumping chamber. When the pumping chamber is depressed, CSF is ejected distally. When the chamber is released, it refills with CSF from the ventricle. Easy compression implies that the distal components are patent. Difficult compression or high resistance indicates that distal tubing is blocked, or that CSF is loculated distally and is under pressure. The pumping chamber should refill within seconds. When the chamber remains depressed or fills slowly, the proximal (ventricular catheter) may be partially occluded.[34] An audible "click" that occurs during valve compression or refill indicates incompetence of the valve.[35] Normal pumping and refill correctly predict a normally functioning shunt system about 80% of the time.[36] In contrast, a delay in refill of the chamber confirms an obstructed system in 20% of cases.

The *plain radiograph shunt survey* includes anterior–posterior (A-P) and lateral views of the skull and neck, and an A-P view of the chest. Lateral as well as right and left lateral decubitus views of the abdomen and pelvis are also obtained. Disconnection of the shunt components can occur after minimal trauma (see Fig. 34.6), yet the fibrous sleeve around the shunt tubing often is able to conduct CSF. In these cases, ICP is invariably elevated and death can occur rapidly if not treated promptly.[37,38] Radionuclide flow studies of shunt patency result in up to one-third of the studies being interpreted as normal because of the conduction of CSF through the fibrous sheath. Therefore, radiographs of the skull are always included in the complete radiographic shunt survey.

Plain radiographs demonstrate the origin, connections, and destinations of the various components of a shunt system. The A-P and lateral views of the skull and neck are necessary to evaluate the number and type of ventricular catheters, and to confirm the integrity of the connections. Reservoirs are localized from radiographs for subsequent tapping. Valve configurations (tubular or domed) and the locations of the pumping chambers can be established, and connections to the distal tubing can be confirmed on plain radiograph. The A-P chest radiograph demonstrates any valves located on the chest, confirms atrial or pleural destinations for the distal tubing, and verifies intact connections. Right

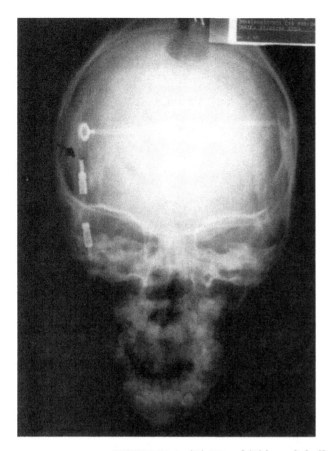 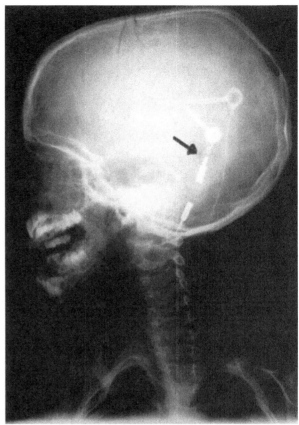

FIGURE 34.6. (A) AP and (B) lateral skull radiographs. A close look plainly reveals a gap and a misalignment between the reservoir and the valve of the "tubular" valve system (arrows). The valve is disconnected from the reservoir.

and left lateral decubitus films of the abdomen demonstrate the final destination of the ventricle-to-peritoneum tubing. The peritoneal catheter changes position with changes in body position, indicating that the peritoneal catheter is free-floating. Tube migration outside of the peritoneal cavity, fixed or stuck distal tubing, curling of the catheter within the abdominal wall or within pseudocysts, and kinking and defects of the tube itself are observed on plain radiograph. Fusiform swelling of the distal tubing, observed on plain radiograph indicates distal shunt obstruction.[39] The lateral view of the abdomen can demonstrate the distal tubing in preperitoneal space, another cause of distal shunt obstruction and failure.[3]

When shunt dysfunction is suspected, a CT scan of the brain is compared with previous studies.[35,40] Comparison with previous studies can demonstrate relative changes in the ventricular volume. Ventricular enlargement compared with previously small ventricles indicates an obstructed system under high pressure. Markedly enlarged ventricles commonly indicate shunt malfunction. However, in some cases, enlarged ventricles can be a normal finding, particularly in the presence of well-defined gyri and sulci. Large ventricles occur in a child with minimum cortical mantle, cerebral atrophy, or porencephaly. Comparison with previous CT scans is helpful in making such a distinction (see Figure 34.7A and B). Normal or small ventricular size does not consistently indicate normal shunt function.[36] CT of the brain can demonstrate asymmetrical dilation of the ventricles and polycystic areas in the brain.[41,42] The CT scan is especially helpful in locating a proximal obstructed catheter that has migrated outside the ventricle. The appearance of well-defined sulci and gyri, especially when surrounded by expansive subarachnoid fluid, is in sharp contrast to that of brain parenchyma flattened against the cranial vault due to high ICP (see Fig. 34.7A and

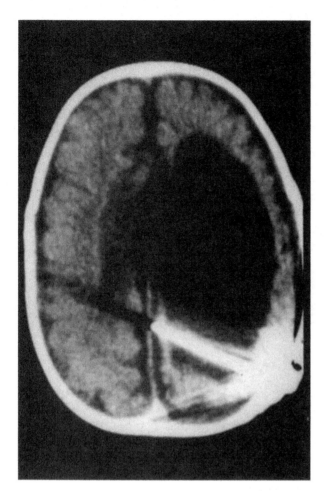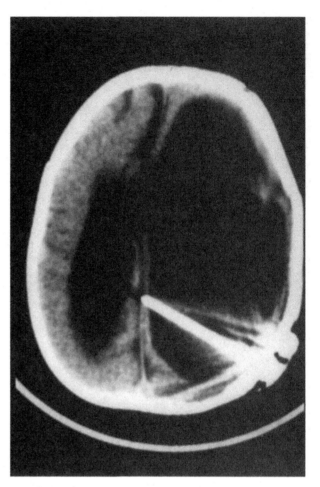

FIGURE 34.7. Comparison CT scans of a child with cerebral atrophy and ventriculomegaly. On the left, well-defined sulci and gyri and generous subarachnoid space are observed. Despite the marked ventriculomegaly, the child has normal ICP and a functioning shunt. On the right, the sulci and gyri are flattened against the cranial vault and ventricular expansion has occurred. The shunt does not work, and the child is symptomatic.

B). Obliteration of the perimesencephalic cistern on the CT scan with other signs of high ICP indicates life-threatening shunt malfunction.[43] Periventricular hypodensity, especially of the anterior horns of the lateral ventricles, indicates transependymal flow of CSF from the ventricles into the parenchyma (see Fig. 34.8).[44] This extravasation of CSF can be confirmed by MRI demonstrating a clearly demarcated periventricular area of hyperintensity around the anterior horns of the lateral ventricles. If radionuclide studies are not available, magnetic resonance imaging can assist in diagnosing an obstructed shunt system.[45]

The combination of shunt tap and radionuclide clearance shuntogram is the most reliable test for investigating shunt obstruction.[35,37,46] The technetium phase of this combination allows visualization of the entire tract, and reveals sites of degradation and separation of the components of the shunt system.[17] It also allows evaluation of the dissemination of nuclide after it has traversed the system (see Fig. 34.5).[37]

A shunt tap is performed through the reservoir whenever possible. When no separate reservoir is present, the pumping chamber of the valve apparatus is accessed. The access scalp site is cleaned with an iodine preparation. A 23-gauge butterfly needle is inserted percutaneously into the reservoir or the pumping chamber. An accurate pressure measurement can be obtained only in a calm

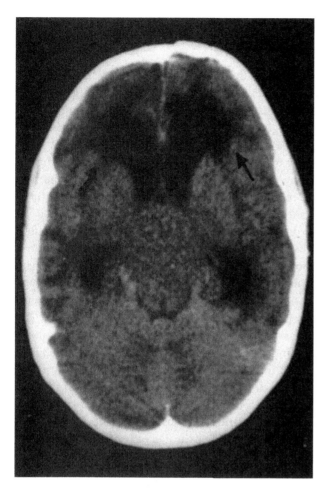

FIGURE 34.8. CT signs of shunt obstruction with elevated ICP. The periventricular transependymal migration of CSF outside of the lateral ventricular anterior horns (arrows) is observed. The sulci and gyri are flattened against the skull. The perimesencephalic cistern remains visible between the enlarged lateral ventricular temporal horns.

patient. Opening pressure is recorded, and CSF drip frequency or free flow is assessed. CSF is collected, closing pressure is measured, and technetium is injected.

In a normally functioning shunt system, the opening pressure is within the normal range for the valve in place and is always lower than 20 cm CSF.[37,46,47] Minor pressure variation with respiration is normal. The CSF pulse pressure amplitude with each heartbeat is minimal, indicating good intracranial compliance. Closing pressure is lower than 20 cm CSF. A spontaneous drip rate of at least one drop per 20 seconds is an excellent predictor of proximal patency.[47] The drip test is performed with the but-

terfly tubing held 5 cm below the ventricles, and is accurate 95% of the time. Technetium is measured from the time of injection and diminishes by 50% within five minutes, unless there is reflux into the ventricle. In this case, 20 minutes are allowed before concluding the test. Technetium diffuses freely throughout the body (peritoneum, circulation, chest) and into the space where the distal tubing terminates.

A normal pressure of a shunt system does not exclude or confirm a proximal or a distal obstruction. ICP that does not fall with respiration suggests proximal obstruction. Poor flow through the butterfly tubing and difficulty aspirating CSF also implies proximal obstruction. High opening and closing pressures of the shunt system imply distal obstruction. Wide changes in ICP amplitude with each heartbeat imply a stiff, noncompliant brain. The best available test for adequate shunt function is a normal technetium clearance test.

The two common shuntogram methods combine elements of the shunt tap and technetium clearance tests. In the first method,[37] the reservoir is punctured and pressure is measured. High pressure is defined as greater than 15 cm CSF and implies distal obstruction. Normal pressure implies a normally functioning shunt or proximal obstruction. The proximal catheter is considered to be patent when CSF can be aspirated with ease. CSF is collected for analysis and culture. Technetium 99m pertechnetate (18 megabequerels in 0.5 ml normal saline) is instilled, and clearance of the technetium is monitored. Reflux of technetium into the ipsilateral ventricle can occur if the proximal catheter is open or if there is distal obstruction. When no reflux occurs, 50% of the radioactivity disappears within 5 minutes. When reflux occurs, especially with gross ventriculomegaly, up to 20 minutes is allowed for disappearance of 50% of the radioactivity. The technetium trail is followed to the distal catheter tip. Pooling or failure to disperse freely implies loculation or obstruction (see Fig. 34.5). Normal shunt function is determined by a pressure of lower than 15 cm CSF, easy aspiration of CSF, reflux of technetium into the ipsilateral ventricle, clearance of CSF within the allotted time, and free dispersal throughout the abdominal cavity.

A similar method uses technetium 99m pertechnetate, 100 μCi in 0.1 ml of normal saline.[46] Access

463

to the reservoir is established and pressure measured. The technetium is injected, and the rate of clearance is monitored. Reflux of technetium into the ventricle without spontaneous clearance implies distal obstruction. Typically, 50% of the technetium clears from the injection site within five minutes. The technetium trail is followed distally; extravasation, loculation, or free dispersal is observed. When pumping is required in order to visualize the distal tubing, proximal dysfunction is suspected. Normal function is determined by an ICP of lower than 20 cm CSF, 50% technetium clearance within five minutes, and free dissemination throughout the abdominal cavity.

An advantage of technetium clearance studies is that sites of disconnection and tubing degradation with rupture are easily observed and localized by the leaking and accumulation of technetium along the path of the system.[8,17,37]

After the shunt system is accessed, CSF is collected and sent for culture, Gram stain, and cell count. A "shunt tap" measures pressure, quantifies the drip rate, injects radionuclide, decompresses the system, and offers critical advantages that outweigh the theoretical risks of introducing infection.[48] Infection and mechanical dysfunction induced by a shunt tap are extremely rare. When a technetium study is unavailable, the other elements of this test help rapidly distinguish proximal from distal obstruction. In addition, the shunt tap allows for immediate gradual decompression through the reservoir in case of distal obstruction.[1]

Distal Obstruction

A distal shunt obstruction is easier to diagnose and treat than a proximal obstruction. Causes of distal obstruction include disconnection of the catheter, fibrosis or catheter plugging with cellular debris, kinking, catheter migration, and loculations of CSF. Plain radiographs can locate the cause in most cases. On manual evaluation of the system, the pumping chamber refills promptly in approximately 80% of cases. The CT scan shows enlarged ventricles or subtle signs of increasing ICP such as flattened sulci and gyri, loss of perimesencephalic cisternal volume, and transependymal CSF assimilation. Pressure within a shunt system can be measured by a "shunt tap." High pressure indicates elevated ICP. CSF drip rate is one drop or more every

20 seconds. A technetium study reveals a delayed or absent clearance, and abnormal or absent distal dissemination.

Pending definitive neurosurgical intervention, medical therapy is initiated in the emergency department. *Osmotic agents,* given intravenously, include glycerol (1 g/kg every 6 hours), mannitol (0.25–1 g/kg every 6 hours) and isosorbide (2 g/kg every 6 hours). Osmotic agents are effective primarily by extracting water from brain parenchyma but are relatively ineffective when there is little cortical mantle from which to extract.[49] A 1% increase in serum osmolarity can result in as much as a 6% decrease in CSF production following administration of osmotic agents.[50] The potential dangers of the use of osmotic agents are: (1) osmotic diuresis exacerbates dehydration in a child who is vomiting and has poor oral intake because of increased ICP; (2) when surgical intervention does not take place within 24 hours and osmotic agents are stopped, rebound intracranial hypertension can occur; and (3) water is drawn from the interstitial space of the entire body in the 5–10 minutes immediately following administration of an osmotic agent. This results in a markedly higher cardiac output and transiently elevated cerebral blood flow and blood volume. When osmotic agents are given, an already elevated ICP can increase further before it begins to decrease.

Diuretic agents such as acetazolamide (25 mg/kg per day) and furosemide (1 mg/kg per day) are also used to lower elevated ICP.[49–51] At recommended doses, both agents decrease CSF production by 50–60%. CSF reduction begins within 30 minutes after an intravenous injection and peaks at 90 minutes; duration of effect is up to 2.5 hours. Exacerbation of dehydration is a potential concern with the use of diuretic agents.[50] Furosemide therapy can cause contraction alkalosis, dehydration, and hypokalemia.

Routine use of acetazolamide in the emergency department is not recommended because its use is associated with an immediate increase in ICP due to drug-induced cerebral acidosis. The acidosis causes vasodilation and an increase in cerebral blood volume. In response to this increased intracranial volume, the ICP can increase to 75–150% above baseline, where it can remain for up to three hours. Therefore, acetazolamide is used in less critical situations and after the intracranial space has been mechanically decompressed. Chronic use of acetazolamide causes a hyperchloremic metabolic acidosis, dehydration, diarrhea, and tachypnea.

In cases of life-threatening distal obstruction, mechanical decompression is performed by slowly removing CSF from the ventricular compartment.[1] A 23-gauge butterfly needle is attached to a manometer with a three-way stopcock. The reservoir or pumping chamber (when there is no separate reservoir) is punctured with a needle and the manometer allowed to fill passively. The stopcock is turned, allowing only the CSF in the manometer to be drained and collected. This process is repeated slowly and carefully until the ICP falls to 10–15 cm CSF. The complications of mechanical decompression that occur when the pressure is lowered too rapidly include subdural hemorrhage, subarachnoid hemorrhage, and pneumocranium.[35,52–55]

Proximal Obstruction

Proximal obstruction of the ventricular catheter of the CSF shunt system occurs from cellular debris, fibrosis, infection, envelopment by the choroid plexus, and catheter migration.[33] Symptoms and signs of elevated ICP are present. Radiographic surveys show intact connections of the shunt system. Absent or delayed refill of the pumping chamber can be present. The CT scan can show enlarged ventricles, and migration of the catheter tip outside the ventricular system can confirm the diagnosis. A low CSF drip rate is present 95% of the time when the shunt is "tapped." Combined with low or normal shunt pressure, a technetium study showing delayed or absent clearance helps to confirm the diagnosis of proximal obstruction in a shunt system.

When the ventricular catheter is blocked, intracranial space cannot be decompressed through the reservoir or the pumping chamber. The clinical condition may require the physician to perform a *ventricular puncture* to reduce the elevated ICP gradually.[4] After the scalp site is prepared, a spinal needle appropriate to the age and size of the child is used to perform a ventricular puncture. A 1.5-inch needle is used for newborns, a 2.5-inch needle is used for children up to 4 years of age, and a 3.5-inch needle is used for children over 4 years of age. The intracranial space is entered through the coronal suture approximately 1 cm lateral to the midline or at the farthest lateral margin of an open anterior fontanelle. The needle is directed straight to the base of the skull on a plane parallel to the falx. After the dural "pop" is felt, the needle is redirected toward the base of the skull in line with the inner canthus of the ipsilateral eye. The goal is to remove an amount of CSF sufficient to reduce ICP to 10–15 cm CSF.

Slit Ventricle Syndrome

Small ventricles on the CT scan can be a normal finding after placement of a CSF shunt.[56] In many cases, the small ventricles may appear normal on the CT scans of children who present with intermittent symptoms and signs of shunt dysfunction. This recurrent phenomenon, which commonly resolves by itself, is called the *slit ventricle syndrome.* Conditions responsible for this syndrome include low ICP from overdrainage of CSF, secondary pressure waves from sudden vasodilation (akin to migraine headaches), intermittent high ICP from intermittent proximal catheter obstruction, and intermittent high ICP despite normal shunt function.[20–22,56–63]

Rapid clearance of CSF from the intracranial space results in sudden *intracranial hypotension,* commonly induced by postural change or exercise, and manifested clinically by cold sweats, a sunken fontanelle, a slack encephalocele, or depressed craniotomy sites.[21–23,60] An extreme form of this phenomenon results when there is sudden upward traction on the brainstem from intracranial hypotension causing sudden respiratory arrest, syncope, bradycardia, opisthotonus, or cranial nerve findings. Placing the child in a Trendelenburg position at 15–30 degrees helps to alleviate the symptoms. Definitive treatment requires upgrading the shunt valve and use of an antisiphon device.[52,57,63]

The phenomenon of secondary *vasomotor pressure waves* can result in symptomatic episodes, despite normal shunt function and normal ICP.[19,59,61,62] A child with hydrocephalus who has received a CSF shunt does not tolerate intracranial volume expansion well because the intracranial volume pressure curve is "steeper" than usual. At relatively low volumes and low ICPs, compliance deteriorates markedly. Abrupt clinical deterioration can occur following minor alterations in cerebrovascular tone. When there is a family history of migraine in this group of patients, antimigraine therapy aimed at preventing the episodic vasodilation can be considered after intermittent proximal occlusion is excluded as a possible cause of these symptoms and signs.[56,59,64]

Slit ventricle syndrome can also occur because of intermittent high pressure, secondary to *intermittent proximal catheter occlusion*.[20,56,57,59–62] Especially with small ventricles, coaptation of the ventricular walls can contribute to transient obstruction of the ventricular catheter tip.[23] More commonly, the catheter is partially occluded or "ball-valved" because of cellular debris, fibrotic material, or partial migration. Evaluation during the symptomatic period is most typically consistent with proximal shunt obstruction. Spontaneous resumption of adequate shunt function ameliorates the symptoms, but shunt revision and placement of an antisiphon device are required to prevent recurrence.

Ventriculitis

Shunt infection causing ventriculitis typically results in fever in children with CSF shunts without any other apparent source of infection.[1,4,65] Two to 5% of all shunts become infected.[66] *Staphylococcus aureus* and gram negative infections can cause fulminant life-threatening infections. More than 50% of shunt infections are caused by *Staphylococcus epidermidis* and present in an insidious fashion. Two-thirds of all shunt infections occur within one month of shunt surgery, and 80% occur within six months of the previous shunt operation. Cellulitis, erosion, and purulence over the insertion site are associated with shunt system infection.[25] Fever occurs in two-thirds of cases of shunt infection in which external evidence of wound (skin) infection is present.[67] When there is no external evidence of wound infection, more than 90% of children with shunt infection present with fever. Seeding the peritoneum with infected CSF can result in peritonitis or localized collections of infected CSF.[68,69]

In ventriculoatrial shunt infections, in contrast to ventriculoperitoneal shunt infections, blood cultures are positive more than 80% of the time.[65] Pumping the shunt prior to obtaining the blood cultures increases the yield. Systems that do not terminate in the systemic circulation, such as ventriculoperitoneal shunts, rarely have positive blood culture results. Shunt infection typically results in only mildly elevated CSF white blood cell counts of 50–200 cells/ml, which cannot be distinguished from typical CSF cellularity induced by the presence of the shunt itself.[65] CSF eosinophilia is a sign of ventricular infection; however, some feel that it represents an "allergic reaction" to the siliconized rubber of the shunt system or a reaction to the intraoperative use of intrathecal antibiotics.[70] The CSF Gram stain may not show any organisms; this occurs with slime-producing *Staphylococcus* species, which become tightly adherent to the shunt tubing. However, CSF cultures are positive in 96% of shunt system infections causing ventriculitis.[65]

When CSF cannot be aspirated from the shunt system, lumbar puncture is performed cautiously. An elevated ICP is excluded prior to the lumbar puncture.[71] In noncommunicating hydrocephalus, lumbar CSF is not contiguous with CSF in the lateral ventricles, and routinely has elevated protein levels and monocytosis because of decreased CSF circulation. This presentation can lead to an incorrect diagnosis of infection.[65]

CSF Shunts in Pregnancy

Pregnancy in women with CSF shunts, especially ventriculoperitoneal shunts, increases the likelihood of shunt malfunction.[72,73] Shunt malfunction can complicate pregnancy and can lead to premature delivery. Often, cesarean section is necessary. In addition to the other risks associated with CSF shunts, pregnancy results in decreased free intraperitoneal volume, increased intra-abdominal pressure, increased brain water (decreased cerebral compliance), and increased cerebral venous volume (decreased cerebral compliance). More than 50% of pregnant women with CSF shunts experience symptoms of ICP, and more than 75% experience neurological complications. Up to 25% of women who have been followed through their pregnancy and the subsequent year require shunt revision.[72]

Miscellaneous Complications of CSF Shunt Systems

Almost all non-CNS complications of CSF shunt systems are influenced by the final destination of the distal tubing.[3] For example, in *ventricle-gallbladder* shunts, the most common complication is gallbladder atony. Ascending infection to the CNS from cholecystitis, obstructive jaundice, fistula formation to the small bowel, and reflux biliary ventriculitis have been reported.[74]

With *ventriculopleural shunts,* symptomatic hydrothorax can occur at any time.[75,76] Pneumothorax and pneumocranium can occur secondary to erosion into the bronchiolar system.[77]

Some non-CNS complications associated with the *ventriculoatrial shunts* are life-threatening.[25,78] Descending shunt infection causes endocarditis with potential valve incompetence and heart failure. Pulmonary embolus can result from a migrating thrombus generated at the distal shunt tubing. Cardiac tamponade results when the distal shunt tubing erodes through the right atrium. A disconnected catheter can embolize to the pulmonary artery or cause dysrhythmia. Insidious onset of shortness of breath, decreased exercise tolerance, dry cough, and occasionally frank cor pulmonale in a patient with ventriculoatrial shunt can be due to multiple small pulmonary emboli.[78] Long-standing endocarditis, secondary to ventriculoatrial shunting, causes prolonged deposition of immune complexes on the renal basement membrane.[79] The resulting shunt nephritis is potentially reversible, provided the ventriculoatrial shunt is removed and the endocarditis is treated.

Ventriculoperitoneal systems commonly malfunction due to partial or complete obstruction of the peritoneal end of the catheter.[69,80] This results from kinking or plugging, or from migration of the catheter and CSF loculation. Peritoneal catheters can migrate into the abdominal wall, out of the peritoneal cavity, into the pleural space, into the vagina, into the retroperitoneal space, through the bladder, and into the rectum.[80] Hepatic abscess has occurred after the distal catheter has become insinuated into the liver. Perforation of the gallbladder, small bowel, colon, and stomach has occurred.[80,81] Bowel can be strangulated by peritoneal tubing causing obstruction and necrosis.[82,83] Peritonitis can result from a descending shunt infection or by perforation of the bowel by the distal tubing. Mixed organisms or coliforms found in CSF suggest an ascending infection secondary to bowel perforation.[68] Fewer than 25% of cases of bowel perforation resulting from shunt malfunction are associated with clinical peritonitis. Intestinal perforation can present with protrusion of shunt tubing from the anus.[84,85]

Loculations of CSF known as *pseudocysts* can present with abdominal distension, nausea, and vomiting.[68,86,87] The diagnosis is made by abdominal ultrasound or dye shuntography. A physical clue to the presence of a CSF pseudocyst is swelling around the abdominal insertion site and a palpable mass. Because loculation of CSF prevents its free diffusion of CSF, it can also cause distal obstruction and symptoms of shunt malfunction.

An unusual complication of a CSF ventriculoperitoneal shunt is the opening of the tunica vaginalis, and the creation of a large inguinal hernia or migration of the shunt tubing itself into the scrotum.[88] The ensuing *hydrocele* can prompt evaluation in the emergency department.

When a CSF shunt placement is necessary due to complications of a brain tumor, there is the potential for tumor cells to seed into the peritoneal cavity, creating *brain tumor metastasis* by CSF.[89] A shunt system can be fitted with a filter to prevent this complication. A CSF shunt system with a filter is at increased risk for obstruction due to tumor cells.

Chronic hydrocephalus can cause erosion of the base of the skull, especially at the ethmoid plate. The siphoning effect, inherent in shunt systems, can then cause enough negative pressure to draw air into the cranium, and cause headache and mental status changes. This *pneumocranium* is readily diagnosed on CT imaging.[54]

Although erosion of a blood vessel by the proximal tube is extremely rare, it can be a catastrophic complication of a CSF shunt.[90] The erosion results in either intraventricular or intraparenchymal hemorrhage.

PEARLS AND PITFALLS

- Nonspecific complaints of fever, nausea, and vomiting are more likely to be due to common non-shunt-related illness than to shunt malfunction. However, delaying investigations of possible shunt malfunction can have fatal consequences.

- Pumping the shunt is not an adequate shunt evaluation. "Normal pumping" and refill is accurate only 80% of the time. Further investigations to assess possible shunt malfunction are necessary.

- Life-threatening events from shunt malfunction can occur without evidence of ventricular enlargement on CT imaging.

- Altered sensorium, cranial nerve findings, and autonomic instability (especially breathing pattern) can indicate impending brain herniation.
- A child with a CSF shunt who presents with periodic breathing, declining Glasgow Coma Scale score, hypertension for age, or a low-normal or low heart rate for age cannot wait for neurosurgery to assume care. Immediate measures are undertaken in the emergency department to reduce increased ICP. Depending on the clinical condition, ventricular puncture may be needed when CSF cannot be easily drained from the shunt reservoir.
- In cases of distal shunt obstruction, decompression of the CSF shunt system is easily accomplished and can be life-saving.

REFERENCES

1. Guertin SR. Cerebrospinal fluid shunts; evaluation, complications, and crisis management. *Pediatr Clin North Am.* 1987;34:203.
2. Jordan KT. Cerebrospinal fluid shunts. *Emerg Med Clin North Am.* 1994;12:779.
3. Blount JP, Campbell JA, Haines SJ. Complications in ventricular cerebrospinal fluid shunting. *Neurosurg Clin North Am.* 1993;4:633.
4. Madsen MA. Emergency department management of ventriculoperitoneal cerebrospinal fluid shunts. *Ann of Emerg Med.* 1986;15:1330.
5. Key CG, Rothrock SG, Falk JL. Cerebrospinal fluid shunt complications: an emergency medicine perspective. *Pediatr Emerg Care.* 1995;11:265.
6. Drake JM, Kestle J. Determining the best cerebrospinal fluid shunt valve design: the pediatric valve design trial. *Neurosurgery.* 1996;38:604.
7. Watkins L, Hayward R, Andar U, et al. The diagnosis of blocked cerebrospinal fluid shunts: a prospective study of referral to a pediatric neurosurgical unit. *Childs Nerv Syst.* 1994;10:87.
8. Uvebrant P, Sixt R, Bjure J, et al. Evaluation of cerebrospinal fluid shunt function in hydrocephalic children using ^{99m}Tc-DTPA. *Childs Nerve Syst.* 1992;8:76.
9. Liptak GS, Masiulis BS, McDonald JV. Ventricular shunts, survival in children with neural tube defects. *Acta Neurol Clin.* 1985;74:113.
10. Hobar J. Annual report 1994: Vermont Oxford neonatal network integrating research and clinical practice to improve the quality of medical care.
11. Marro PJ, Downsfield DA, Mott SH, et al. Post-hemorrhagic hydrocephalus; use of an intravenous type catheter for cerebrospinal fluid drainage. *AJDC.* 1991; 145:1141.
12. Dykes FD, Dunbar B, Lazarra A. Posthemorrhagic hydrocephalus in high-risk preterm infants: natural history, management, and long-term outcome. *J Pediatr.* 1989;114:611.
13. Piatt JH Jr, Carlson CV. A search for determinants of cerebrospinal fluid shunt survival: retrospective analysis of a 14-year institutional experience. *Pediatr Neurosurg.* 1993;19:233.
14. Brydon HL, Bayston R, Hayward R, et al. The effect of protein and blood cells on the flow-pressure characteristics of shunts. *Neurosurgery.* 1996;38:498.
15. Post EM. Currently available shunt systems: a review. *Neurosurgery.* 1985;16:257.
16. Aldrich EF, Harmann P. Disconnection as a cause of ventriculoperitoneal shunt malfunction in multicomponent shunt systems. *Pediatr Neurosurg.* 1990–91;16:309.
17. Elisevich K, Mattar AG, Cheeseman F. Biodegradation of distal shunt catheters. *Pediatr Neurosurg.* 1994;21:71.
18. Shapiro K, Fried A, Marmarou A. Biomechanical and hydrodynamic characterization of the hydrocephalic infant. *J Neurosurg.* 1985;63:69.
19. Shapiro K, Fried A. Pressure-volume relationships in shunt-dependent childhood hydrocephalus. *J Neurosurg.* 1986;64:390.
20. Walker ML, Fried A, Petronio J. Diagnosis and treatment of the slit ventricle syndrome. *Neurosurg Clin North Am.* 1993;4:707.
21. Faulhauer K, Schmitz P. Overdrainage phenomena in shunt treated hydrocephalus. *Acta Neurochir.* 1978; 45:89.
22. Kiekens R, Mortier W, Pathmann R, et al. The slit-ventricle syndrome after shunting in hydrocephalic children. *Neuropediatrics.* 1982;13:190.
23. Constantini S, Beni L. Reversible opisthotonus following intracranial pressure changes in Chiari malformation. *Childs Nerv Syst.* 1993;9:350.
24. Tzekov C, Cherninkova S, Gudeva T. Neuroophthalmological symptoms in children treated for internal hydrocephalus. *Pediatr Neurosurg.* 1991–92;17:317.
25. Bell WE, McCormick WF. Hydrocephalus. In: Bell WE, McCormick WF, eds. *Raised Intracranial Pressure in Children: Diagnosis and Treatment.* Philadelphia, Pa: WB Saunders Co; 1978.
26. Arroyo HA, Jan JE, McCormick AQ, et al. Permanent visual loss after shunt malfunction. *Neurology.* 1986; 35:25.
27. Vassilouthis J. The syndrome of normal-pressure hydrocephalus. *J Neurosurg.* 1984;61:501.
28. Carmel PW. Surgical syndromes of the hypothalamus. *Clin Neurosurg.* 1980;27:133.
29. Connolly MB, Jan JE, Cochrane DD. Rapid recovery from cortical visual impairment following correction of prolonged shunt malfunction in congenital hydrocephalus. *Arch Neurol.* 1991;48:956.

30. Hack CH, Enrile BG, Donat JF, et al. Seizures in relation to shunt dysfunction in children with meningomyelocele. *J Pediatr.* 1990;116:57.

31. Saukkonen AL. Electroencephalographic findings in hydrocephalic children prior to initial shunting. *Childs Nerv Syst.* 1988;4:339.

32. Venes JL, Dauser RC. Epilepsy following ventricular shunt placement. *J Neurosurg.* 1987;66:154.

33. Sekhar LN, Moossy J, Guthkelch N. Malfunctioning ventriculoperitoneal shunts. *J Neurosurg.* 1982;56:411.

34. Rekate HL. Shunt revision: complications and their prevention. *Pediatr Neurosurg.* 1991;17:155.

35. Di Rocco C, Caldarelli M. Surveillance of CSF shunt function. In: Di Rocco C, ed. *The Treatment of Infantile Hydrocephalus.* Boca Raton, Fla: CRC Press Inc; 1987;2.

36. Piatt JH Jr. Physical examination of patients with cerebrospinal fluid shunts: is there useful information in pumping the shunt? *Pediatrics.* 1992;89:470.

37. Reilly PL, Savage JP, Doecke L. Isotope transport studies and shunt pressure measurements as a guide to shunt function. *Br J Neurosurg.* 1989;3:681.

38. Neuren A, Ellison PH. Acute hydrocephalus and death following V-P shunt disconnection. *Pediatrics.* 1979;64:90.

39. LeRoux P, Berger M, Benjamin D. Abdominal x-ray and pathological findings in distal unishunt obstruction. *Neurosurgery.* 1988;23:749.

40. El-Gohary MA, Forrest DM, Starer F. The role of the CT scan in the management of blocked ventricular shunt. *Pediatr Surg.* 1988;4:247.

41. Kalsbeck JE, DeSousa AL, Kleiman MB, et al. Compartmentalization of the cerebral ventricles as sequela of neonatal meningitis. *J Neurosurg.* 1980;52:547.

42. Rahman N, Adam KAR. Congenital polycystic disease of the brain: report of an unusual case. *Dev Med Child Neurol.* 1986;28:62.

43. Johnson DL, Fitz L, McCullough DC, et al. Perimesencephalic cistern obliteration: a CT sign of life-threatening shunt failure. *J Neurosurg.* 1986;64:386.

44. Wolpert SM. Radiological investigation of pediatric hydrocephalus. In: Scott RM, ed. *Concepts in Neurosurgery.* Baltimore, Md: Williams & Wilkins; 1990;3.

45. Drake J, Martin A, Henkelman R. Determination of cerebrospinal shunt obstruction with magnetic resonance phase imaging. *J Neurosurg.* 1991;75:535.

46. Hayden PW, Rudd TG, Shurtleff DB. Combined pressure-radionuclide evaluation of suspected cerebrospinal fluid shunt malfunction: a seven-year clinical experience. *Pediatrics.* 1980;66:679.

47. Sood S, Kim S, Ham SD, et al. Useful components of the shunt tap test for evaluation of shunt malfunction. *Childs Nerv System.* 1993;9:157.

48. Noetzel MJ, Baker RP. Shunt fluid examination: risks and benefits in the evaluation of shunt malfunction and infection. *J Neurosurg.* 1984;61:328.

49. Gilmore HE. Medical treatment of hydrocephalus. In: Scott RM, ed. *Concepts in Neurosurgery.* Baltimore, Md: Williams & Wilkins, 1990;3.

50. Di Rocco C. The medical treatment. In: Di Rocco C, ed. *The Treatment of Infantile Hydrocephalus.* Boca Raton, Fla: CRC Press Inc; 1987.

51. Shinnar S, Gammon K, Bergman E Jr, et al. Management of hydrocephalus in infancy: use of acetazolamide and furosemide to avoid cerebrospinal fluid shunts. *J Pediatr.* 1985;107:31.

52. Gruber R, Jenny P, Herzog B. Experiences with the anti-siphone device (ASD) in shunt therapy of pediatric hydrocephalus. *J Neurosurg.* 1984;61:156.

53. Epstein F. How to keep shunts functioning or "The Impossible Dream." *Clin Neurosurg.* 1985;32:608.

54. Ruge JR, Corullo LJ, McLone DG. Pneumocephalus in patients with CSF shunts. *J Neurosurg.* 1985;63:532.

55. Kirkpatrick PJ, Knibb AA, Downing HA. Rapid decompression of chronic hydrocephalus resulting in bilateral extradural hematomas; a general surgical complication. *J Pediatr Surg.* 1993;28:744.

56. Epstein F, Lapras C, Wisoff JF. Slit-ventricle syndrome: etiology and treatment. *Pediatr Neurosci.* 1988;14:5.

57. McLaurin RL, Olivi A. Slit-ventricle syndrome: review of 15 cases. *Pediatr Neurosci.* 1987;13:118.

58. Coker SB. Cyclic vomiting and the slit ventricle syndrome. *Pediatr Neurol.* 1987;3:297.

59. Obana WG, Raskin NH, Cogen PH, et al. Antimigraine treatment of slit ventricle syndrome. *Neurosurgery.* 1990;27:760.

60. Wisoff JR, Epstein FJ. Diagnosis and treatment of the slit ventricle syndrome. In: Scott RM, ed. *Concepts in Neurosurgery.* Baltimore, Md: Williams & Wilkins; 1990;3.

61. Rekate HL. Classification of slit-ventricle syndromes using intracranial pressure monitoring. *Pediatr Neurosurg.* 1993;19:15.

62. Di Rocco C. Is the slit ventricle syndrome always a slit ventricle syndrome? *Childs Nerv Syst.* 1994;10:49.

63. Hyde-Rowan MD, Rekate HL, Nulsen FE. Re-expansion of previously collapsed ventricles: the slit ventricle syndrome. *J Neurosurg.* 1982;56:536.

64. James HE, Nowak TP. Clinical course and diagnosis of migraine headaches in hydrocephalic children. *Pediatr Neurosurg.* 1991–92;17:310.

65. Venus JL. Infections of CSF shunt and intracranial pressure monitoring devices. *Infect Dis Clin North Am.* 1989;3:289.

66. Schoenbaum SC, Gardner P, Shillito J. Infections of cerebrospinal fluid shunts: epidemiology, clinical manifestation and therapy. *J Infect Dis.* 1975;131:543.

67. Odio C, McCracken GH, Nelson JD. CSF shunt infections in pediatrics. *AJDC.* 1984;138:1103.

68. Rush DS, Walsh JW, Belin RP, et al. Ventricular sepsis and abdominally related complications in children

with cerebrospinal fluid shunts. *Surgery*. 1985;97: 420.

69. Bryant MS, Bremer AM, Tepas JJ, et al. Abdominal complications of ventriculoperitoneal shunts. *Am Surg*. 1988;54:50.

70. Duhaime AC. Eosinophilia following shunting. *J Neurosurg*. 1992;76:724.

71. Addy DP. When not to do a lumbar puncture. *Arch Dis Child*. 1987;62:873.

72. Wisoff JH, Kratzert KJ, Handwerker SM, et al. Pregnancy in patients with cerebrospinal fluid shunts: report of a series and review of the literature. *Neurosurgery*. 1991;29:827.

73. Cusimano MD, Meffe FM, Gentili F, et al. Management of pregnant women with cerebrospinal fluid shunts. *Pediatr Neurosurg*. 1991–92;17:10.

74. West KW, Turner MK, Vane DW, et al. Ventricular gall bladder shunts: an alternative procedure in hydrocephalus. *J Pediatr Surg*. 1987;22:609.

75. Piatt JH Jr. How effective are ventriculopleural shunts? *Pediatr Neurosurg*. 1994;21:66.

76. Yellin A, Findler G, Barzilay Z, et al. Fibrothorax associated with a ventriculopleural shunt in a hydrocephalic child. *J Pediatr Surg*. 1992;27:1525.

77. Jones RFC, Currie BG, Kwok BCT. Ventriculopleural shunts for hydrocephalus: a useful alternative. *Neurosurgery*. 1988;23:753.

78. Lundar T, Langmoen IA, Hovind KH. Fatal cardiopulmonary complications in children treated with ventriculoatrial shunts. *Childs Nerv System*. 1991;7: 215.

79. Zamora I, Lurbe A, Alvarez-Garijo A, et al. Shunt nephritis: a report on five children. *Childs Brain*. 1984; 11:183.

80. Agha FP, Amendola MA, Shimzi KK, et al. Abdominal complications of ventriculoperitoneal shunts with emphasis on the role of imaging methods. *Surg Gynecol Obstet*. 1983;156:473.

81. Oshio T, Matsumura C, Kirino A, et al. Recurrent perforations of viscus due to ventriculoperitoneal shunt in a hydrocephalic child. *J Pediatr Surg*. 1991;26: 1404.

82. Hlavin ML, Mapstone TB, Gauderer MWL. Small bowel obstruction secondary to incomplete removal of ventriculoperitoneal shunt: case report. *Neurosurgery*. 1990;26:526.

83. Sanan A, Jaines SJ, Nyberg SL, et al. Knotted bowel: small-bowel obstruction from coiled peritoneal shunt catheters. *J Neurosurg*. 1995;82:1062.

84. Hornig GW, Shillito J. Intestinal perforation by peritoneal shunt tubing: report of two cases. *Surg Neurol*. 1990;33:288.

85. Miserocchi G, Simi VA, Ravagnati L. Anal protrusion as a complication of ventriculo-peritoneal shunt. *J Neurosurg Sci*. 1984;24:43.

86. Gaskill SJ, Marlin AE. Pseudocysts of the abdomen associated with ventriculoperitoneal shunts: a report of twelve cases and a review of the literature. *Pediatr Neurosci*. 1989;15:23.

87. Hahn YS, Engelhard H, McClone DG. Abdominal CSF pseudocyst. *Pediatr Neurosci*. 1985–86;12:75.

88. Moazam R, Glenn JD, Kaplan BJ, et al. Inguinal hernias after ventriculoperitoneal shunt procedures in pediatric patients. *Surg Gynecol Obstet*. 1984;159:570.

89. Hoffman JH, Hendrick EB, Humphreys RP. Metastasis via ventriculoperitoneal shunt in patients with medulloblastoma. *J Neurosurg*. 1976;44:562.

90. Snow RB, Zimmerman RD, Derinsky O. Delayed intracerebral hemorrhage after ventriculoperitoneal shunting. *Neurosurgery*. 1987;19:305.

35
Pediatric Infections of the Central Nervous System

JANE L. TURNER

SUMMARY Infections of the central nervous system (CNS) in children are potentially lethal. Timely recognition and treatment are critical to assure an optimal outcome. The symptoms and signs of CNS infections are frequently nonspecific, especially in the infant or the very young child. Analysis of cerebrospinal fluid can be diagnostic. Treatment often is initiated presumptively while definitive diagnostic information is processed. The emergency physician faces special challenges in diagnosis when a child who has been taking antibiotics presents with symptoms that can be due to CNS infection.

Introduction

Infections of the central nervous system (CNS) in infants and children, as in adults, can be devastating. Timely recognition and appropriate intervention are critical to avoid acute complications, long-term morbidity, or death. Diagnosis is particularly challenging in infants and young children because their presenting symptoms and signs are often nonspecific. The challenge to the emergency physician is to recognize the signs of CNS infections in infants and children, confirm the diagnosis quickly, and treat appropriately.

CNS infections in children include meningitis, encephalitis, meningoencephalitis, and brain abscesses. Meningitis is the most common CNS infection and is primarily a pediatric disease. In the United States, 75% of all instances occur in individuals under 18 years of age; 60% are children under 5 years of age. Most cases of meningitis are aseptic or viral, with seasonal enteroviruses being responsible for more than 75% of all cases of viral meningitis. Bacterial meningitis caused by *Haemophilus in-*

fluenza type B primarily affected children between 2 months and 5 years of age until the recent introduction of conjugated polysaccharide vaccines (Hib) against this pathogen. Since 1991, there has been a dramatic decline in invasive *H. influenza* disease in countries where Hib is given routinely. Use of Hib has resulted in an overall decline in the number of cases of meningitis in children under 5 years of age; however, there has been little change in the numbers of cases of meningitis due to other pathogens. Key points in the recognition, diagnosis, and emergency department management of CNS infections in pediatric patients are discussed in this chapter, with a focus on meningitis.

Prehospital Management

Prehospital management of the infant, toddler, or child with suspected CNS infection is similar to the management of a very ill child. Vital signs are assessed and monitored. Endotracheal intubation and mechanical ventilation are undertaken in any child

Sid M. Shah and Kevin M. Kelly, eds., *Emergency Neurology: Principles and Practice.* Copyright © 1999 Cambridge University Press. All rights reserved.

with an altered level of consciousness, respiratory compromise, unstable vital signs, or decorticate or decerebrate posturing. With evidence of shock, fluid resuscitation is initiated with care not to overhydrate the child. An initial bolus of 20 ml/kg of parenteral normal saline is recommended. Once hypovolemia is corrected, fluids with a low sodium content (i.e. 5% dextrose in 0.18% saline) are administered at a rate approximately 20% of maintenance intake. Fluids are restricted because inappropriate secretion of antidiuretic hormone commonly occurs in children with meningitis.[1]

Emergency Department Evaluation and Differential Diagnosis

The patient's airway, breathing, and circulatory status are assessed on arrival in the emergency department. Endotracheal intubation and mechanical ventilation are undertaken when indicated. Antibiotics are given intravenously after blood cultures have been drawn when sepsis or meningitis is suspected and lumbar puncture (LP) cannot be done in a timely manner. Antibiotics are administered intramuscularly when intravenous access cannot be obtained. In a critically ill child with suspected sepsis or meningitis, antibiotics are administered within 30 minutes of arrival in the emergency department. Cerebrospinal fluid (CSF) obtained after antibiotics have been given may not yield a pathogen on culture, but cell counts, Gram stain, and examination for bacterial antigens can lead to a diagnosis of meningitis. Bacterial antigens can be present in the urine. Encephalitis is suspected in a child presenting with fever and status epilepticus with no apparent cause of the fever.[1] Antiepileptic drugs are administered and an antiviral agent such as acyclovir is begun when herpes simplex encephalitis is suspected.[1]

Infants under 2 Months of Age

Meningitis is considered seriously in the differential diagnosis of any ill infant. Presenting symptoms can be as vague as poor feeding or increased somnolence. Irritability and inconsolable crying can be the only complaints described by the parent. Fever can be absent. Some infants with meningitis and sepsis are hypothermic on presentation.

Encephalitis in the newborn due to herpes simplex virus (HSV) can present with generalized symptoms of lethargy and poor feeding. Many infants with HSV encephalitis do not have characteristic mucocutaneous vesicles, and approximately 33% of infants with HSV infection have encephalitis without disseminated disease.[2] Typically, these infants are brought to the emergency department during the second or third week of life. The presentation can include focal, multifocal, or generalized seizures, apnea, bradycardia, and cranial nerve abnormalities. There may be no history of HSV infection in the mother. CSF findings are nonspecific and variable. Typically, pleocytosis and an increased protein level are found. CSF cultures and antibody studies for HSV can confirm the diagnosis, but results are not available immediately. The polymerase chain reaction procedure holds the potential for expediting diagnosis, but clinical experience is not sufficient to rely on this test currently. Parenteral acyclovir at a dose of 20 mg/kg every 8 hours is recommended when HSV infection of the CNS is suspected clinically.[3]

Because of the lack of specificity in symptoms and signs, the differential diagnosis for CNS infection in infants under 2 months of age is extensive. Metabolic disorders, congenital anomalies of the CNS, sepsis, urinary tract infections, and traumatic brain injury due to child abuse are among the more serious causes of lethargy and poor feeding. Irritability can be due to mild upper respiratory infections, otitis media, overstimulation, or "colic," among many other causes. Evaluation of the newborn presenting with lethargy, poor feeding, somnolence, irritability or fever begins with a thorough history and physical examination. Specific findings on physical examination such as a bulging fontanelle or mucocutaneous vesicles can help the physician make a diagnosis of CNS infection. However, the absence of such findings does exclude the diagnosis. An acute illness such as otitis media does not eliminate the possibility of concurrent CNS infection. LP is performed in an infant suspected of having CNS infection. Urine is obtained for microscopic analysis and culture, because infants with urinary tract infections can present with similar nonspecific symptoms and signs. Bacterial antigen studies can be performed on a urine specimen.

The diagnosis of CNS infection is made on the basis of CSF findings. Normal values for CSF cell

TABLE 35.1. Cerebrospinal Fluid Analysis

	Normal			Bacterial	Viral
	Preterm	Term	>6 mo		
Cell count (WBC/mm³)					
Mean	9	8	0	>500	<500
Range	0–25	0–22	0–4		
Predominant cell type	Lymph	Lymph	Lymph	80% PMN leukocyte	PMN leukocyte initially, lymphocyte later
Glucose (mg/dl)					
Mean	50	52	>40	<40	>40
Range	24–63	34–119			
Protein (mg/dl)					
Mean	115	90	<40	>100	<100
Range	65–150	20–170			
CSF/blood glucose (%)					
Mean	74	81	50	<40	>40
Range	55–150	44–248	40–60		
Gram stain	Negative	Negative	Negative	Positive	Negative
Bacterial culture	Negative	Negative	Negative	Positive	Negative

counts and glucose and protein levels vary according to the age of the infant and gestational maturity. Age-specific values of CSF examination are listed in Table 35.1.

Infants 2–24 Months of Age

As in very young infants, presenting symptoms of CNS infections in infants 2–24 months are typically nonspecific. Fever is often the chief complaint. History of the infant's feeding and responsiveness can be very helpful, because infants with meningitis can be irritable and lethargic. An infant who is feeding well, smiles responsively, and interacts playfully is unlikely to have a serious infection.

Seizures can be the presenting symptom in an infant or toddler with meningitis or encephalitis. CNS infection is considered in the differential diagnosis of an infant or toddler who presents with fever and seizure. However, seizure as the only manifestation of meningitis in children with fever is extremely rare or nonexistent.[4] A child with meningitis who pre-

sents with a seizure is likely to be lethargic, irritable, and vomiting.[5] LP is indicated for the child with fever and seizure, the very young child, the child treated with antibiotics, and the child with a complex seizure.[5,6] The infant or toddler who appears healthy with normal mental status and absence of meningeal signs is not likely to have CNS infection. There is no consensus regarding when a child with fever and seizure does not require an LP. However, there is general agreement that this procedure is not necessary in all febrile children with seizure.[4–6]

Physical examination findings often are nonspecific in infants and toddlers with meningitis. As with younger infants, a bulging fontanelle suggests CNS infection, but a flat or nonpalpable fontanelle does not exclude it. Nuchal rigidity can be present in older infants but is not found consistently in children younger than 2 years of age with meningitis. Twenty-seven percent of infants under 6 months of age with bacterial meningitis have nuchal rigidity; 95% of patients 19 months of age and older with meningitis have nuchal rigidity.[7] The level of consciousness, responsiveness to surroundings, and willingness to interact with the care provider or examiner are the most critical components of the physical examination of a child. As with younger infants, a localizing sign that can account for fever does not eliminate the possibility of CNS infection. Otitis media often is present in infants with meningitis. CNS infection is suspected in any febrile infant or toddler who appears toxic or has an altered mental status.

Laboratory tests including white blood cell (WBC) count, band cell count, and acute phase reactants are obtained to identify infants and toddlers at high risk for serious infections. One study found quantitative C-reactive protein (CRP) to be the most sensitive and specific blood test for identifying infants with bacterial meningitis.[8] A higher sensitivity in identifying meningitis was noted when CRP was combined with physical findings such as meningeal signs or signs of increased intracranial pressure (ICP).

The diagnosis of CNS infection is made on the basis of CSF findings. CSF cell counts, and glucose and protein levels contribute to the diagnosis (see Table 35.1). On a peripheral blood smear, nucleated cell count is the most predictive of a positive bacterial culture.[9] CSF is cultured when the initial values are normal because in rare instances cultures have been positive for a CSF sample without any cells and with normal glucose and protein levels.[9]

The differential diagnosis for CNS infections in infants and toddlers includes the numerous causes of fever in this age group. Respiratory infections, otitis media, pneumonia, gastroenteritis, and urinary tract infections are among the most common causes of fever in this age group. Evaluation in the emergency department is guided by the child's history and findings on physical examination. Urine for microscopic analysis and culture is included in the laboratory evaluation of any infant or toddler who has fever and no historical or physical findings to explain it. Urine is obtained prior to the administration of antibiotics.

Children 24 Months and Older

In children 2 years of age and older, symptoms and physical findings are more specific for meningitis. Headache, fever, lethargy, and stiff neck are likely to be present. Physical examination reveals meningismus in most cases, and fever is virtually always present. The list of differential diagnoses becomes shorter as the findings become more specific. Physical examination in many cases strongly suggests the diagnosis of meningitis, and LP is necessary only for confirmation and identification of a specific pathogen. However, diagnosis is not self-evident in all cases. Neck stiffness can be due to cervical lymphadenitis, trauma to the neck, tumor, muscle injury, or oculogyric crisis from phenothiazine ingestion.[10] A cerebrovascular accident or subarachnoid hemorrhage can cause headache, stiff neck, and altered consciousness.[10] Heatstroke can cause fever, altered consciousness, and meningismus.[10]

As with younger children, examination of the CSF is the definitive diagnostic study. LP is deferred with hemodynamic instability. Computerized tomography (CT) of the brain is performed prior to LP when increased ICP or a mass lesion such as tumor or hematoma is suspected. Prompt administration of antibiotics is important when bacterial infection is suspected.

Patients with viral meningitis can also present with fever, headache, and stiff neck. In contrast to children with bacterial meningitis, children with viral disease rarely appear toxic.[7] CSF results usually confirm the diagnosis. CSF is obtained for viral studies. The presentation of encephalitis and meningoencephalitis is similar to that of meningitis with altered sensorium and fever. Nuchal rigidity may or may not be present.

Microbiology and Pathophysiology

Most pathogens reach the CNS hematogenously. Direct transmission can occur when there is a mechanical disruption of the meninges such as in neurosurgical procedures, a skull fracture with persistent leak of CSF, or in children with a congenital defect that provides communication between skin and meninges such as meningomyelocele. Direct extension of pathogens from infection in a sinus or orbit can occur. Foreign bodies in the CNS, such as a ventriculoperitoneal shunt, are a potential nidus for bacterial infection.

Bacteria that cause meningitis in the newborn belong to the maternal flora or the environment of the infant. Group B streptococci, gram negative bacilli, and *Listeria monocytogenes* are the most common pathogens in the very young infant. *Haemophilus influenza* (type B or nontypable) is occasionally responsible for meningitis in this age group, especially in infants over 1 month of age.

In infants over 2 months of age, the bacteria responsible for meningitis are largely upper respiratory tract flora. These include *H. influenza* type B. *Streptococcus pneumoniae,* and *Neisseria meningitidis.* Meningitis caused by *Pseudomonas aeruginosa, Staphylococcus epidermidis, Salmonella,* or *L. monocytogenes* is uncommon. The likelihood of identifying an uncommon pathogen is increased in children with immune deficits or anatomical defects. *Mycobacterium tuberculosis,* although uncommon, can cause meningitis in all age groups. Enteroviruses, especially echovirus and coxsackievirus, are responsible for most cases of viral meningitis or meningoencephalitis. Other viral agents that cause meningoencephalitis include mumps, herpes simplex, California equine, St. Louis equine, and Western equine viruses. *Mycoplasma pneumoniae* has been implicated in encephalitis and meningoencephalitis in a number of children.[11–15] The pathophysiology of CNS manifestations of *M. pneumonia* infection is not well understood; however, direct invasion of the CNS by the *M. pneumonia* is not likely.[15] Manifestations of *M. pneumonia* CNS infection can be varied, including altered level of consciousness, seizures, ataxia, transverse myelitis, polyradiculitis, and symptoms and signs attributable to disease of the basal ganglia. Diagnosis is based on changes in serum titers.[11–15]

Emergency Department Management and Disposition

As with all critically ill children, careful attention is paid to the oxygenation and cardiovascular status of the patient throughout evaluation in the emergency department. Antibiotics given intravenously are the mainstay of treatment for patients with bacterial meningitis. Treatment with a third-generation cephalosporin, cefotaxime 200 mg/kg per day given every 6 hours, or ceftriaxone, 100 mg/kg per day given every 12 hours, is a currently accepted protocol. Chloramphenicol, 100 mg/kg per day is given every 6 hours, is recommended for children allergic to beta lactam antibiotics. The treatment is adjusted once culture results and sensitivities become available. All children with bacterial meningitis are admitted to the hospital.

The standard therapy for newborns with early-onset disease (i.e., under 7 days old) is ampicillin and an aminoglycoside, usually gentamicin or tobramycin. Infants over 7 days old can be treated with a third-generation cephalosporin (cefotaxime or ceftriaxone) plus ampicillin as an alternative. Ampicillin is included in children under 2 months of age to cover possible infection with *L. monocytogenes.* Ampicillin, 100 mg/kg, is given as the initial dose; the initial dose of aminoglycoside is gentamicin, 2.5 mg/kg, or tobramycin, 2.5 mg/kg. The typical initial dose of cefotaxime is 50–75 mg/kg. Total daily doses per kilogram are adjusted according to the age of the infant and the gestational age (as reflected by the infant's weight). This adjustment is made by altering the dosing interval; the initial dose in the emergency department is not changed.

The recent emergence of penicillin-resistant strains of *Streptococcus pneumoniae* is cause for considerable concern. The incidence of resistance strains varies from community to community, but the problem is growing nationwide.[16,17] Some experts recommend empirical therapy with cefotaxime and vancomycin for all children with meningitis because of emerging resistance to cephalosporins and to penicillin.[17] Others recommend the addition of vancomycin only when gram-positive diplococci are found in the CSF or when there is strong suspicion of pneumococcal disease clinically.[16,17] Antibiotic susceptibility testing is critical in guiding therapeutic decisions later in the course of the illness. A repeat LP at 24–48 hours is recommended in children infected by strains with reduced susceptibility to penicillin.[17]

In some studies, the use of dexamethasone was found to improve outcome from bacterial meningitis in children. Neurological sequelae, specifically hearing impairment, are observed less often in children who receive dexamethasone.[18,19] These studies were done at a time when *H. influenza* was the most common pathogen in meningitis in children. It is not known whether steroid treatment is as effective when other pathogens are involved. There is yet no consensus regarding the appropriateness of the use of dexamethasone in the initial management of meningitis,[17,20,21] and the decision to use corticosteroids is individualized.[20,21] Complications from dexamethasone use include gastrointestinal bleeding,[22] hypertension, hyperglycemia, leukocytosis, and rebound fever following the last dose.[23] The recommended dose of dexamethasone is 0.15 mg/kg given intravenously every 6 hours for 4 days, with the first dose given prior to the first dose of antibiotic.[23,24]

Supportive treatment in the emergency department includes careful fluid management. Hydration is necessary when the child is dehydrated or hypovolemic on arrival. Once normovolemia is established, fluids are restricted to 50–66% maintenance to avoid complications of the syndrome of inappropriate antidiuretic hormone (SIADH) secretion.

Children with septic shock require aggressive fluid resuscitation and vasoactive agents. Endotracheal intubation with mechanical ventilation and controlled hyperventilation is indicated for signs of increased ICP. Administration of furosemide or mannitol may be indicated.

Seizures occur commonly in children with meningitis. Intravenous administration of diazepam or lorazepam is recommended for immediate seizure control. Phenytoin can be administered to reduce the risk of recurrence while avoiding CNS depression.[23]

Special Circumstances

Children treated with antibiotics at the time they present to the emergency department pose a challenge. This is a common occurrence due to the widespread use of oral antibiotics in children, especially in those with common respiratory infections. Children with partially treated meningitis present differently from children who have not received any antibiotics. Children with partially treated meningitis are more likely to have a history of vomiting and to have a longer duration of symptoms.[25] They are less likely to show signs of altered mental status or have a temperature over 38.3°C. They are also more likely to have findings of an ear, nose, or throat infection.[25] The threshold for performing an LP is lower for children taking antibiotics who present with apparently minor illnesses.[25] CSF parameters are also altered by partial treatment with antibiotics, and it can be difficult to distinguish between patients with viral meningitis and those with partially treated bacterial disease.[25]

Another challenge commonly faced by emergency physicians is the blood-contaminated CSF from traumatic LP. The difficulty occurs in the interpretation of the WBC counts in blood-contaminated fluid. CSF WBC counts are expected to be proportional to the peripheral blood WBC when all the cells are introduced from blood. When this occurs, the existence of a CSF pleocytosis is considered to be unlikely. However, it has been demonstrated that CSF WBC counts can be significantly lower than expected from this assumption,[26] and a clinically significant CSF leukocytosis can be missed when this formula is applied. Interpretation remains problematic. Close clinical monitoring is advised when meningitis is suspected and the LP is traumatic, regardless of the WBC count of the specimen.[26]

PEARLS AND PITFALLS

- The younger the child, the less specific the symptoms and signs of meningitis.
- Children on an oral antibiotic with meningitis present differently from children who have not been on an antibiotic.
- There is no reliable way to interpret the cell count of a traumatic LP.
- Seizures often accompany meningitis but are rarely or never the only symptom.
- Most cases of meningitis are due to viral pathogens.
- Once hypovolemia has been corrected, fluids are restricted to avoid overload due to SIADH.
- Recommendations for antibiotics to treat meningitis may change in the near future due to emergence of resistant organisms.

REFERENCES

1. Henning R. Emergency transport of critically ill children: stabilization before departure. *Med J Aust.* 1992;156:117–24
2. Guerina NG. Viral infections in the newborn. In: Cloherty JP, Starkf AR, eds. *Manual of Neonatal Care.* 3rd ed. Boston: Little, Brown and Co; 1991:114–46.
3. Annunziato PW, Gershon A. Herpes simplex virus infections. *Pediatr Review.* 1996;17:415–23.
4. Green SM, Rothrock SG, Clem KJ, Zurcher RF, Mellick L. Can seizures be the sole manifestation of meningitis in febrile children? *Pediatrics.* 1993;92: 527–34.

5. Al-Eissa YA. Lumbar puncture in the clinical evaluation of children with seizures associated with fever. *Pediatr Emerg Care.* 1995;11:347–50.
6. Hirtz DG. Febrile seizures. *Pediatr Review.* 1997;18:3–35.
7. Walsh-Kelly C, Nelson DB, Smith DS, Losek JD, Melzer-Lange M, Hennes HM, et al. Clinical predictors of bacterial versus aseptic meningitis in childhood. *Ann Emerg Med.* 1992;21:910–4.
8. Lembo RM, Marchant CD. Acute phase reactants and risk of bacterial meningitis among febrile infants and children. *Ann Emerg Med.* 1991;20:36–40.
9. Rodewald LE, Woodin KA, Szilagyi PG, Arvan DA, Raubertas RF, Powell KR. Relevance of common tests of cerebrospinal fluid in screening for bacterial meningitis. *J Pediatr.* 1991;119:363–9.
10. Barkin RM, Rosen P, eds. *Emergency Pediatrics.* St. Louis, MO: Mosby–Year Book, Inc; 1994.
11. Thomas NH, Collins JE, Robb SA, Robinson RO. Mycoplasma pneumonia infection and neurological disease. *Arch Dis Child.* 1993;69:573–6.
12. Koskiniemi M. CNS manifestations associated with *Mycoplasma pneumonia* infections: summary of cases at the University of Helsinki and review. *Clin Infect Dis.* 1993;17 (Suppl):S52–7.
13. Lerer RJ, Kalavsky SM. Central nervous system disease associated with *Mycoplasma pneumonia* infection: report of five cases and review of the literature. *Pediatrics.* 1973;52:658–68.
14. Narita M, Matsuzono Y, Togashi T, Kajii N. DNA diagnosis of central nervous system infection by *Mycoplasma pneumonia. Pediatrics.* 1992;90:250–3.
15. Ponka A. Central nervous system manifestations associated with serologically verified *Mycoplasma pneumoniae* infection. *Scand J Infect Dis.* 1980;12:175–84.
16. Orenstein JB. Invasive pneumococcal infection in a community hospital, 1993 to 1995. Characteristics of resistant strains. *Arch Pediatr Adolesc Med.* 1996;150:809–14.
17. Bradley JS, Kaplan SL, Klugman KP, Leggiadro JJ. Consensus: management of infections in children caused by *Streptococcus pneumoniae* with decreased susceptibility to penicillin. *Pediatr Infect Dis.* 1995;14:1037–41.
18. Schaad UB, Lips U, Gnehm HE, Blumber A, Heinzer I, Wedgwood J. Dexamethasone therapy for bacterial meningitis in children. *Lancet.* 1993;342:457–61.
19. Lebel MH, Freij BJ, Syrogiannopoulos GA, et al. Dexamethasone therapy for bacterial meningitis: results of two double-blind, placebo-controlled trials. *N Engl J Med.* 1988;319:964–71.
20. Report of the Committee on Infectious Diseases of the American Academy of Pediatrics. *Dexamethasone Therapy for Bacterial Meningitis in Infants and Children.* 23rd ed. Elk Grove Village, Ill: American Academy of Pediatrics; 1991:558–9.
21. Wald ER, Kaplan SL, Mason EO, et al. Dexamethasone therapy for children with bacterial meningitis. *Pediatrics.* 1995;95:21–8.
22. Prober CG. Infections of the central nervous system. In: Behrman RE, Kliegman RM, Nelson WE, eds. *Nelson: Textbook of Pediatrics.* Philadelphia, Pa: WB Saunders Co; 1996:707–16.
23. Ioannidis JPA, Samarel MD, Lau J, Drapkin MS. Risk of gastrointestinal bleeding from dexamethasone in children with bacterial meningitis. *Lancet.* 1994;343:702.
24. Bonadio WA. Adjunctive dexamethasone therapy for pediatric bacterial meningitis. *J Emerg Med.* 1996;14:165–72.
25. Rothrock SG, Green SM, Wren J, Letai D, Daniel-Underwood L, Pillar E. Pediatric bacterial meningitis: is prior antibiotic therapy associated with an altered clinical presentation? *Ann Intern Med.* 1992;21:146–52.
26. Rubenstein JS, Yogev R. What represents pleocytosis in blood-contaminated ("traumatic tap") cerebrospinal fluid in children? *J Pediatr.* 1985;107:249–51.

36 Pediatric Cerebrovascular Disorders

IMAD JARJOUR

SUMMARY Stroke in children can occur from fetal life to adolescence. A systematic diagnostic approach, modern neuroimaging techniques, and selective laboratory investigation can establish a definitive diagnosis of stroke, and an etiology in two-thirds of the patients. Medical and surgical therapies are available to help. Psychological support to the child with stroke and the family is very important. Recognizing the various disorders that mimic stroke can eliminate the need for extensive testing. New approaches to the treatment of strokes in adults, such as thrombolysis, have not been studied in children.[1]

Introduction

Stroke occurs much less commonly in infants and children than in adults. Pediatric stroke has causes and manifestations that differ according to age group. In the United States, the true incidence of stroke in childhood is likely underestimated, with a reported annual incidence of 2.52 cases per 100,000 children.[2] When estimated over a two-year period in the greater Cincinnati, Ohio, area, there was an incidence of 2.6 cases per 100,000 in white children and 3.1 cases per 100,000 in African American children.[3] The higher incidence of stroke in African American children is likely related to sickle cell disease. Of all incidences of childhood stroke, 20–50% are idiopathic.[4]

As with stroke in adults, stroke in children can be classified either as ischemic or hemorrhagic or, according to pathophysiological mechanisms, as cerebral embolism, arterial thrombosis, venous thrombosis, and intraparenchymal hemorrhage. Stroke in childhood can accompany congenital heart disease, systemic illnesses, dehydration, leukemia, infections, sickle cell disease, bleeding diathesis, and anticoagulant therapy. Stroke can also occur in seemingly healthy children as the first manifestation of cerebrovascular disorders such as moyamoya disease and arteriovascular malformation (AVM).

Children with stroke caused by cerebral embolism or arterial thrombosis typically present with a sudden onset of focal neurological deficits such as hemiparesis or focal seizures, and an impaired level of consciousness. Transient ischemic attacks (TIAs) are a common presentation of cerebrovascular anomalies such as moyamoya disease. Children with intraparenchymal hemorrhage present with sudden neurological deficits, headache, and rapid loss of consciousness. Children with dural sinus thrombosis can have a similar presentation, but the onset usually is subacute and when experienced, occurs late in the course of the disease. In young children, sinus thrombosis can mimic bacterial meningitis clinically as well as by virtue of abnormal CSF findings. Alternatively, bacterial meningitis can cause strokes due to arterial or venous thrombosis.[5] Various potential risk factors for stroke in children are listed in Table 36.1.

Conditions that Mimic Stroke

Sudden focal neurological deficits, seizures, headache, and an impaired level of consciousness are the typical manifestations of childhood strokes.

TABLE 36.1. Etiologies of Stroke in Children

Vascular Disorders

Vasculitis
Meningitis

Vasculitis

Infection-mediated:
Viral and post-viral infections
Bacterial meningitis
Zoster arteritis
Autoimmune-mediated:
Cerebral Lupus
Polyarthritis nodosa
Polymyositis
Wegener's granulomatosis
Takayasu's arthritis
Henoch-Schonlein purpura
Kawasaki disease
Hemolytic-uremic syndrome

Vascular Dysplasias

Moyamoya disease
Neurofibromatosis type I
Fibromuscular dysplasia
Vascular malformations
Ehlers-Danlos syndrome
Sturge-Weber syndrome
Hereditary hemorrhagic telangiectasia

Vasculopathy

Sickle cell disease
Radiation therapy
Trauma
Systemic hypertension
Diabetes mellitus

Vasospasm

Migraine
Cocaine abuse
Glue sniffing
Wasp/scorpion sting
Ergot poisoning

Hematologic Disorders

Sickle cell disease
Polycythemia
Leukemia

Hypercoagulable States

Protein S deficiency
Protein C deficiency
Anti-thrombin III deficiency
Lupus anticoagulant
Oral contraceptives
Thrombocytosis
L-asparaginase
Disseminated intravascular coagulation
Iron deficiency anemia

Metabolic Disorders

Homocystinuria
Mitochondrial disorders
Sulfite oxidase deficiency
Fabry's disease
Urea cycle defects

Cardiac Disorders

Congenital heart defects
Endocarditis
Cardiomyopathy
Atrial myxoma
Arrhythmias
Air and fat emboli

These symptoms can be encountered in children with other conditions, such as migraine, epilepsy, hypoglycemia, and alternating hemiplegia of childhood.

Migraine is common in children and can be associated with unilateral neurological symptoms and signs such as unilateral numbness, aphasia, and hemiparesis.[6] These can occur before or during the course of a vascular headache. Numbness typically occurs in the face and arm, and rarely in the leg. Paresthesias occur in the perioral region and extremities. Symptoms of a vertebrobasilar arterial distribution, such as vertigo, weakness, ataxia, and dysarthria can occur in basilar artery migraine. Hemiplegic migraine is more common in adolescents and can be familial and associated with loss of consciousness.[7,8] A hemibody syndrome occurs during the aura, resolves within 1 hour, and is replaced by a vascular headache that is commonly contralateral but can also be bilateral or diffuse. Aphasia can occur and is usually nonfluent. Some children are confused. The hemibody syndrome rarely persists beyond 24 hours. After 24 hours, a stroke syndrome is considered. Headaches with focal neurological deficits occur in children with AVM and other cerebrovascular anomalies, such as moyamoya disease. Neuroimaging is recommended in these patients. Magnetic resonance imaging (MRI) with magnetic resonance angiography (MRA) of the circle of Willis is preferred over computerized tomography (CT) (Figs. 36.1A and B).

Trauma-triggered migraine can mimic stroke and frequently is unrecognized as the cause of a child's transient neurological deficit following minor closed-head injury.[9,10] These children usually have a brief lucid period between a few minutes and four hours after the injury, and develop a hemibody syndrome, agitation and confusion, loss of consciousness, or cortical blindness. The neurological deficit resolves within minutes to a few hours. The child commonly has a concurrent vascular headache. Typically, a family history of migraines exists and the child has experienced migraine prior to the injury. Electroencephalography obtained when the child is symptomatic typically shows slow electrocerebral activity. Migraine and stroke can be related

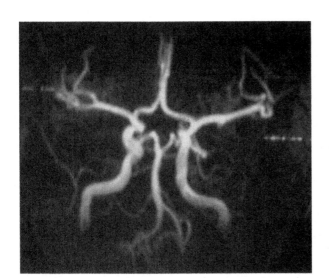
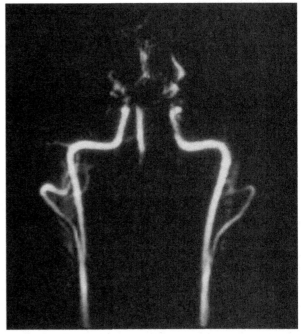

FIGURE 36.1. (A) Normal magnetic resonance angiography of the circle of Willis in a 15-year-old girl. (B) Magnetic resonance angiography of the circle of Willis in a 9-year-old girl with moyamoya disease. Occlusion of both internal carotid arteries is observed.

to one another, especially in young adult women and those with migraine with aura. Migrainous symptoms can be seen in patients with other symptoms of ischemic strokes; alternatively, a hemiplegic aura persists for more than 60 minutes but less than one week and may be associated with ischemic brain infarct on neuroimaging.[11] Prospective studies of migraine as a risk factor for stroke in children are needed.

Epileptic seizures can be followed by a Todd's paralysis that resolves within a few hours. Occasionally, the deficit lasts beyond 24–48 hours, in which case the question of stroke causing the seizure and the hemiparesis is raised. When the seizure is not witnessed but the child has known epilepsy, observation is recommended. Children who have an intracranial pathology such as a neoplasm or AVM can have a history of focal seizures or unilateral headaches, and present to the emergency department with a new focal neurological deficit. In these cases, neuroimaging is indicated. Although rare, hemiparetic seizures that present with acute lateralized weakness and preserved mental state can be a form of partial epilepsy.

Diabetic children can experience unilateral neurological deficits during severe hypoglycemia, which can preferentially affect the left cerebral hemisphere, leading to right-sided weakness or aphasia.[12,13] Measurement of blood glucose concentration and the history of insulin therapy help make the correct diagnosis.

Alternating hemiplegia of childhood can mimic stroke. The first hemiplegic attack typically occurs before the age of 18 months, followed by lateralized hemiplegic episodes that can last for a few minutes to a few days. Bilateral hemiplegia occurs rarely. Patients may have associated dysautonomia, oculomotor dysfunction, and extrapyramidal symptoms. Children with alternating hemiplegia are developmentally delayed or mentally retarded. Flunarizine, a calcium channel blocker, has been used as prophylaxis with limited success.[14]

Neonatal Stroke

Neonatal stroke has been recognized more frequently in recent years due to advanced neuroimaging and to greater survival rates of premature infants and babies with severe cardiorespiratory failure. These strokes are divided into cerebral infarction due to arterial occlusion, intracranial hemorrhage, and cerebral dural sinus thrombosis.

Arterial Occlusion. Incidence of this type of stroke in the neonate is unknown. A review of 592 neonatal autopsies showed an incidence of cerebral infarction of 5.4% due to arterial occlusion, with 17% occurring in term infants. Certain pathological findings suggested intrauterine occurrence of stroke.[15] Other reports from the same institution suggested antenatal occurrence of cerebral infarctions.[16] The incidence of stroke in sick, premature neonates is probably higher and can reach 10%. In these cases, the stroke typically involves hemorrhagic venous infarction. Cerebral infarction was found in 50% of 44 neonates and infants who died after treatment of severe cardiorespiratory failure with extracorporeal membrane oxygenation (ECMO), a temporary life support procedure requiring ligation of the common carotid artery and internal jugular vein.[17] A common presentation of neonatal arterial infarction is that of focal seizure activity.[18] Given that cerebral angiography is invasive and not commonly performed in the neonate, cerebral infarction in the neonate is often labeled idiopathic. An example of such infarction is seen in Figure 36.2. Risk factors for cerebral infarction in the neonate include hypercoagulable states, sepsis, and hypoxic/ischemic injury, which can result in unilateral cerebral artery occlusion and disseminated intravascular coagulation.

Intracranial Hemorrhage. Although rare, subarachnoid hemorrhage from birth trauma does occur. The incidence of SAH in neonates is unknown. It is typically asymptomatic, but occasionally it can result in neonatal seizures in the first 24 hours of life. The hemorrhage resolves spontaneously. However, intraparenchymal and intraventricular hemorrhage in the neonate can have serious consequences such as severe neurological impairment and hydrocephalus. Coagulopathies, either inherited or acquired, such as disseminated intravascular coagulation and idiopathic thrombocytopenia, are risk factors for severe intracranial hemorrhage (Fig. 36.3). Neonates with congenital vascular abnormalities, such as arteriovenous malformation, vascular

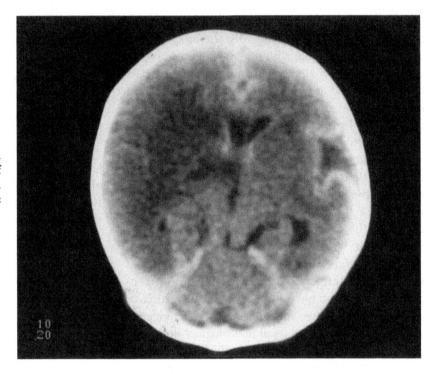

FIGURE 36.2. Brain (CT or MRI) in a neonate with cerebral infarction of undetermined etiology in the MCA territory. The infant had focal clonic seizures.

tumors, and aneurysms, can develop severe neonatal intracranial hemorrhage. Premature birth remains the most common cause of intracranial hemorrhage in the neonate.[19]

Cerebral Dural Sinus Thrombosis. Thrombosis of the cerebral sinuses is detected in neonates by MRI, typically presenting with multifocal seizures, with or without subarachnoid hemorrhage. Hemorrhagic infarctions can also occur. Commonly, the etiology is undefined, but polycythemia, dehydration, congenital heart disease, hypercoagulable state, or infection can be the cause. Treatment is symptomatic.[20]

Stroke in Infants and Children

As stated previously, the etiologies and manifestations of strokes in children are different from those in adults, despite a similar initial pathophysiological process, including thrombi, emboli, and hemorrhages.

Vascular Disorders. Infections of the CNS resulting in angiitis are a common cause of stroke. Either cerebral veins or arteries become occluded due to inflammation of the vessel wall by direct infection. This occurs during bacterial and viral infections.

Meningitis is a common cause. Usually, the subarachnoid arteries are affected. A child with meningitis presents with focal seizures or a focal neurological deficit. There is usually evidence of an ischemic brain lesion on neuroimaging. Patients with bacterial endocarditis can develop septic emboli that can cause direct infection of the cerebral vessels. This often manifests as an intracranial hemorrhage. These children have fever with petechial hemorrhages in the skin and usually have a newly developed heart murmur. Some children have a pre-existing congenital heart disease. Neuroimaging reveals multifocal hemorrhages. Cerebral vasculitis has also been reported in children with human immunodeficiency virus (HIV) infection.[21] This can result in either occlusive cerebral infarction or intracranial hemorrhage. Infection with HIV can also result in cerebral aneurysms.[22] Other viral infections such as herpes zoster can result in vasculitis, which can present with acute hemiplegia. It is controversial whether zoster-related stroke can precede the skin manifestations of herpes zoster and varicella infection. A history of preceding viral infection is commonly elicited in children with stroke where no other etiology is found. Immunological processes may be the cause of a postviral syndrome of acute multifocal necrotizing hemorrhagic

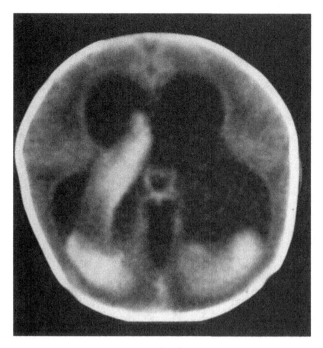

FIGURE 36.3. Intraventricular hemorrhage in a neonate with severe idiopathic thrombocytopenia. Associated hydrocephalus is observed.

leukoencephalopathy in childhood. Systemic lupus erythematosis (SLE) can cause cerebral vasculopathy. Inflammation of the blood vessels has not been documented. The mechanism for cerebral infarction in these children is that of occlusive arterial disease. The infarcts are typically small. When a large cerebral infarction is encountered in a patient with SLE, antilupus anticoagulant-related embolism is considered. Other connective tissue disorders can result in cerebral infarctions. Polyarteritis nodosa can affect the CNS in 20–40% of patients. Stroke can occur in children with polymyositis, mixed connective tissue disease, and progressive systemic sclerosis. Wegner's granulomatosis is a rare cause of stroke in children. Coarctation of the aorta can cause stroke in children. Similarly, involvement of the aorta with Takayasu's arteritis has been associated with thrombotic stroke. Children with Henoch-Schönlein purpura can develop stroke due to arteritis. Hemiplegia and seizures have been reported to occur in children with Kawasaki's disease. Children with hemolytic-uremic syndrome can develop stroke and encephalopathy, which typically involve the basal ganglia. A thorough physical examination and laboratory testing for systemic vasculitis or con-nective tissue disorders usually helps in identifying vasculitis as the cause of stroke in these children.

Drug abuse in children is on the rise. Cerebral infarction and intracerebral hemorrhages can occur with cocaine abuse. The pathophysiological mechanism is likely severe vasoconstriction. Subarachnoid hemorrhage appears to occur more commonly in cocaine users who have occult intracranial aneurysms or arterial venous malformations than among those who have normal cerebral vasculature. Glue-sniffing has been reported to cause cerebral infarction that can be associated with peripheral neuropathy. The use of excessive ergot medications and the abuse of amphetamines can also result in strokes.

Moyamoya disease is observed in children under 15 years of age and presents in this age group with either TIAs or acute focal neurological deficits. In adults, it commonly presents with intracranial hemorrhage. The disorder is related to progressive occlusion of the intracranial supraclinoid internal carotid arteries. There is fibrosis and thickening of the arterial wall. The resultant collateral circulation between the external carotid arteries and the posterior circulation from the vertebral arteries takes the form of a "puff of smoke" on cerebral angiography, which is the meaning of "moyamoya" in Japanese (Fig. 36.4). Moyamoya disease is considered in the differential diagnosis of childhood stroke. A child with TIAs who manifests old cerebral infarction on CT, and exhibits evidence of prominent vasculature in the basal ganglia on MRI, is suspected to have moyamoya disease, which can be confirmed by cerebral angiography (Fig. 36.5). Although MRA can identify the occlusion in the intracranial portion of the internal carotid arteries, it does not easily demonstrate the cortical small arteries and the collateral network (Fig. 36.1A and B). Most incidences of moyamoya disease in children have no apparent etiology, although moyamoya syndrome has been reported in patients with neurofibromatosis, sickle cell disease, tuberculous meningitis, and fibromuscular dysplasia, and following CNS irradiation. The natural history in children with moyamoya syndrome has not been fully defined. Over the past several years, surgical treatment involving bypass anastomosis of the stenotic arteries to increase cerebral blood flow has been performed. Different surgical techniques have been used with variable degrees of success. Medical therapy is limited to the use of antiplatelet agents

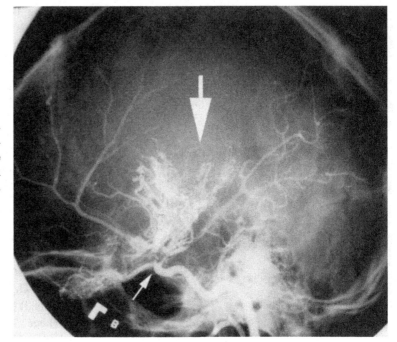

FIGURE 36.4. Moyamoya disease in a 9-year-old girl presenting with TIAs and complicated migraine. There is occlusion of the left internal carotid artery (small arrow) and a network of collateral vessels; "moyamoya, or puff of smoke" (large arrows).

and to prevention of complicated migraine, which occurs frequently in these patients. Anticoagulation with heparin or warfarin is not advocated for these children.

Congenital structural abnormalities of cervical or cerebral vasculature can result in thrombotic stroke in children. Cerebral aneurysms and AVMs can occasionally cause thrombotic stroke. Cerebrovascular and cervical carotid dysplasia can result in stroke in children, either as an idiopathic entity or associated with other disorders such as neurofibromatosis, Ehlers-Danlos syndrome, and Marfan's syndrome. The diagnosis in these cases is made by angiography. Skin manifestations of neurofibromatosis such as café-au-lait spots or the neurofibromas, or fragile skin and hyperextensible joints with poor wound healing, in the case of Ehlers-Danlos syndrome, aid in diagnosis. Some patients with these conditions can develop a dissection of the involved arteries, resulting in cerebral ischemia.

Stroke is a major complication of sickle cell disease in children. Cerebral infarction occurs in approximately 6% of patients with sickle cell disease. There is pathological evidence of large cerebral vessel involvement in patients with this disease, as well as small cerebral vessel obstruction due to the decreased compliance of sickled erythrocytes. Recurrence of stroke usually can be prevented with

chronic transfusion therapy.[23] In addition, children with sickle cell trait can develop stroke.[24,25]

Trauma can cause stroke in children by various mechanisms. Intracerebral hemorrhage, epidural and subdural hematomas, and multifocal hemorrhages are commonly observed in children with severe traumatic brain injuries. However, minor head and neck trauma can result in stroke by injuring either the carotid or the vertebral arteries. The carotid arteries can be injured by intraoral trauma to the tonsillar fossa, such as falling while holding a sharp object in the mouth. In these cases, there is usually dissection of the arterial wall with secondary thrombosis. The vertebral arteries can be injured during aggressive chiropractic manipulations or extreme stretching, torsion, and traction of the neck in other circumstances.[26] Traumatic dissection of the internal carotid artery typically manifests with neck pain and acute hemiplegia. Angiography is the method of choice to diagnose arterial dissection, and MRA may be adequate in some cases.

Hematological Disorders. Besides sickle cell disease, various hematological disorders are associated with stroke in children. Children with leukemia develop stroke as the result of various complications of their treatment or because of direct invasion of the meninges and the cerebral vessels by leukemic

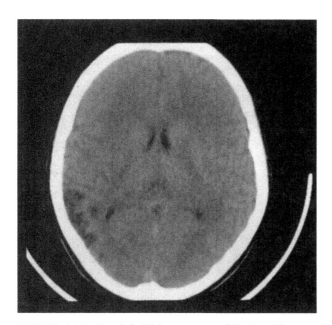

FIGURE 36.5. Cranial CT in a 9-year-old girl with moyamoya disease when presenting first time to the emergency department with transient paresthesias in the left leg.

cells. Stroke can occur as intracerebral hemorrhage due to thrombocytopenia or to disseminated intravascular coagulopathies. Another mechanism is that of cerebral sinus thrombosis associated with treatment with L-asparaginase.[27,28] Cranial irradiation can injure the cerebral vasculature and result in delayed stroke.[29]

Hypercoagulable states can lead to either embolic or thrombotic stroke in children. Deficiencies of protein S and protein C lead to increased spontaneous clotting, which can result in stroke. Antithrombin III deficiency results in strokes that can be arterial or venous in nature. Such deficiencies are typically congenital but can be acquired with liver disease or the nephrotic syndrome. Specific measurement of these proteins leads to the proper diagnosis. Antiphospholipid antibodies are a cause of stroke, in both children and young adults. The lupus anticoagulant and anticardiolipin antibodies are the primary examples. These antibodies are not restricted to patients with SLE. A false positive serological Venereal Disease Research Laboratory test (VDRL) suggests the presence of antiphospholipid antibodies. Cerebral infarction and TIAs have been reported in children with these antibodies. Anticoagulation therapy has been advocated in

adults; however, the risk of a CNS hemorrhage can limit its use in children.[30] In young adolescent women, a hypercoagulable state can be caused by the use of oral contraceptives. This is especially a risk factor in the presence of migraine headache. Chronic smoking in these women also enhances the risk of stroke. Pregnancy and postpartum period are associated with hypercoagulable states, and cerebral vein thrombosis can manifest as severe headache, seizures, and acute hemiparesis or paraparesis. Anticoagulation therapy usually is recommended in these cases. Coagulation factor deficiencies, such as in hemophilia A, hemophilia B, and factor IX deficiency, commonly predisposes the child to intracranial bleeding after seemingly trivial trauma.[31,32] Intracranial hemorrhages are also observed in patients with severe thrombocytopenia. Primary thrombocytosis is very rare in children and has been associated with arterial and cerebral vein thrombosis. Treatment with antiplatelet agents provides some benefit in children with primary thrombocytosis.

Iron deficiency anemia with or without thrombocytosis can cause one of three forms of cerebrovascular accidents. First, patients with severe anemia can present with TIAs.[33,34] Second, iron deficiency anemia can cause cerebral sinus venous thrombosis.[35] Figure 36.6 demonstrates cerebral deep vein thrombosis in a female infant with severe iron deficiency anemia (hemoglobin concentration of 4 g/dl) and thrombocytosis presenting with symptoms and signs of meningitis. Blood transfusions and iron replacement relieved symptoms, and the stroke syndrome resolved. Third, arterial ischemic infarctions occur in adults with iron deficiency anemia.[36,37]

Metabolic Disorders. Homocystinuria is a rare autosomal recessive disorder characterized by the elevation of serum and urine homocystine, skeletal and neurological abnormalities, and thromboembolic disease. Typically, children with homocystinuria are mentally retarded and have seizures. Psychiatric manifestations are relatively common. Myocardial infarcts and pulmonary embolism occur. Endothelial injury due to excessive homocystine leads to platelet aggregation with occlusion of the vessels. Venous thrombosis also occurs. Treat-

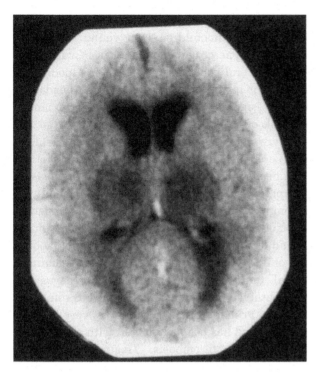 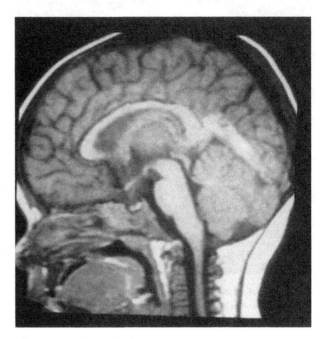

FIGURE 36.6. (A) Unenhanced CT scan of the head in a 14-month-old infant with meningitic signs. Thalamic attenuation and a clot in the deep cerebral vein are observed. (B) Thrombosis of the cerebral veins and straight sinus in a 14-month-old infant with iron deficiency anemia.

ment with folate and vitamin B_{12} can improve symptoms in some patients.[38]

Mitochondrial myopathy, encephalopathy, lactic acidosis, and strokelike episodes (MELAS) is a disorder related to a mutation in mitochondrial deoxyribonucleic acid (DNA). An elevated level of lactate in the serum, or more consistently in the CSF, supports the diagnosis. Molecular analysis of blood specimens confirms the diagnosis. The most common presenting symptom is acute hemiparesis with hemianopia. A maternal family history of migraine and severe headache prior to strokelike episodes is common. Other physical signs include sensorineural hearing loss, dementia, and short stature. Other rare metabolic disorders that cause stroke in childhood include sulfite oxidase deficiency, an autosomal recessive disorder of sulfur amino acid metabolism. These patients have mental retardation, seizures, lens displacement, and acute hemiplegia. The urinary concentrations of sulfites and s-sulfocysteine are high. There is no effective treatment. Fabry's disease, a lipid storage disorder, is due to accumulation of ceramide dihexoside deficiency in various tissues, particularly the kidney, the vascular endothelium, and cornea. Symptoms can become apparent in childhood or adolescence. Painful paresthesias and angiokeratomas typically are the first symptoms and signs, followed by renal failure. Occlusive strokes can also occur. This disorder is X-linked, and there is no effective therapy. Other metabolic causes of stroke include urea cycle defects such as ornithine transcarbamylase deficiency.

Cardiac Disorders. Cardiac causes of stroke in children include both congenital and acquired cardiac conditions. Embolic stroke is common in children with cyanotic congenital heart disease. Conventional echocardiography demonstrates the cardiac defect; however, transesophageal echocardiography conducted with Valsalva bubble studies provides an increased probability of detecting evidence of a right-to-left shunt. Valvular heart disease can result in embolic stroke due to vegetations. Bacterial endocarditis, discussed previously, can result in either embolic stroke or intracerebral hemorrhages. Delayed intracranial hemorrhage due to a mycotic aneurysm remains a risk factor for stroke in patients with bacterial endocarditis. Stroke can also occur in the course of cardiovascular surgery to correct congenital heart disease. ECMO is another cause of stroke in children treated with this temporary heart-lung bypass for severe respiratory or cardiac disease. The mechanism of stroke in these children is either associated with the ligation of internal carotid artery, the internal jugular vein, anticoagulation with heparin, factors related to the bypass equipment itself, or due to disseminated intravascular coagulation in very ill infants.[17]

Cerebrovascular Abnormalities. In addition to moyamoya disease and vascular dysplasia, bleeding from cerebral arterial aneurysms and AVMs is another cause of stroke in children. The most common presentation of AVM is that of intracranial hemorrhage, typically in the form of subarachnoid hemorrhage when an aneurysm ruptures. For this reason, cerebral angiography is performed on children with unexplained intracranial hemorrhage. Intraparenchymal hemorrhage can also occur with symptoms of compression of adjacent brain structures. The aneurysm is typically saccular and can occur in a familial pattern with both dominant and recessive autosomal inheritance. The risk factors for arterial aneurysm in children include polycystic kidney disease, coarctation of the aorta, Ehlers-Danlos syndrome, and pseudoxanthoma elasticum. In the latter condition, the usual clinical manifestations include angioid streaks, laxed joints, and yellowish skin plaques of the flexor creases, neck, axilla, and abdomen.[39] AVMs can present with seizures or intracranial hemorrhage. AVMs are characterized by direct anastomoses of arteries with veins. Cerebral angiography is diagnostic, however the malformation can be occult. In these cases, conventional MRI demonstrates the AVM.[40] Vein of Galen malformations typically present in the neonate with congestive heart failure. A loud cranial bruit can be heard in these patients. In infants and older children, a vein of Galen aneurysm can present with hydrocephalus because of obstruction of the aqueduct of Sylvius. Ruptured aneurysms and AVMs require neurosurgical consultation.[41] Other cerebral vascular malformations include cavernous angiomas, a cluster of vessels without intervening brain

parenchyma, which may bleed. Venous angiomas are a rare source of intracranial hemorrhage. Finally, capillary telangiectasia consists of dilated blood vessels separated by normal intervening brain tissue. Usually they are found incidentally on autopsy. Intracranial aneurysms occur simultaneously with AVMs in about 20% of patients.[42]

Diagnostic Evaluation

The evaluation of a neonate or a child with acute focal neurological deficits and suspected stroke has two primary goals. First, a diagnosis of stroke is established and conditions that mimic stroke are excluded. Second, the etiology of stroke is established, whenever possible. (See Table 36.2.) A comprehensive, problem-oriented medical history, physical and neurological examinations are most important in making a correct diagnosis and appropriately managing a child with an acute lateralizing deficit or suspected stroke. Given the variable presentations of childhood stroke and the various etiologies of stroke among different pediatric age groups, consultation with a pediatric neurologist and a neuroradiologist can increase the probability of correct diagnosis and appropriate treatment.

Following history and neurological examinations, the evaluation proceeds with noninvasive, commonly used tests. In the neonate, cranial ultrasound provides screening information. An arterial occlusion in the term neonate can reveal a wedge-shaped area of increased echogenicity; however, most infarctions appear less well-defined and are patchy in appearance. However, it may not be possible with ultrasound to distinguish between bland and hemorrhagic infarctions.[43] Moreover, an intraparenchymal hemorrhage can mimic infarction, and cortical infarcts can be missed with cranial ultrasound. Usually, cranial CT is readily available in emergency situations. However, in acute ischemic stroke, the CT scan can be negative in the first few hours following the onset of symptoms. Intracranial hemorrhages can be observed readily on CT acutely unless it consists of a microscopic subarachnoid hemorrhage. At times, decreased attenuation on CT in the area of infarction takes days to appear after the acute event.

TABLE 36.2. Diagnostic Evaluation in Childhood Stroke

General Laboratory Tests

1. CBC, differential, and platelet count
2. Erythrocyte sedimentation rate (ESR)
3. PT/PTT
4. Electrolytes and glucose
5. Cholesterol and triglycerides
6. Toxicology screen
7. Brain CT or MRI

Specific Investigations

1. CSF examination: total protein, glucose, cell count, cultures, lactate, and pyruvate levels
2. Coagulation panel (protein S, C, antithrombin III assays)
3. ANA, RF
4. Urinalysis
5. Blood cultures
6. Antiphospholipid antibody and lupus anticoagulant assays
7. Plasma amino acids
8. Urine for organic acids
9. Echocardiogram/transesophageal
10. MR angiography
11. Intra-arterial carotid/vertebral angiography
12. Chest radiograph
13. Blood lactate/pyruvate
14. EKG
15. Hemoglobin electrophoresis
16. VDRL, HIV

Alternatively, MRI provides greater resolution and structural detail than does CT, particularly of the infratentorial structures. Diffusion-weighted MRI can demonstrate cerebral infarction very early after the onset of stroke.[44,45] MRI is also superior in demonstrating cerebral sinus venous thrombosis. In the neonate, heavily T2-weighted images (TR = 3000 ms, TR <120 ms) are necessary to separate the early changes of infarction from the normal high signal of the immature brain.[43] MRA, particularly of the circle of Willis, or magnetic resonance venography (MRV) of the veins can detect major vascular obstruction or demonstrate large vascular anomalies.[46] MRA can be insensitive to peripheral cerebral vascular lesions, and show false positive results of occlusion actually due to turbulent flow in large vessels.

Other laboratory testing can be obtained soon after arrival to the emergency department or after review of neuroimaging studies. These tests include complete blood counts, white blood cell differential counts, platelet count, sedimentation rate, prothrombin time, partial thromboplastin time, glucose concentration, serum electrolyte level, and, in at-risk patients, a hemoglobin electrophoresis. An electrocardiogram and chest radiograph can be obtained. In patients with fever, with or without signs of meningitis, lumbar puncture is performed after increased intracranial pressure (ICP) and risk of brain herniation are assessed by visualizing the optic fundi and reviewing neuroimaging results. Other potential concerns regarding LP are considered, such as severe bleeding diatheses. A review of the results of the initial blood evaluations helps in this regard. Lumbar puncture can be helpful in patients who are afebrile and have an unexplained acute focal deficit, and an inflammatory brain process such as tuberculous meningitis or herpes encephalitis cannot be excluded.

When the etiology of stroke is not identified at this point of evaluation, further testing occurs after E.D. management is complete. It is directed by the individual case, and can include blood specimens for VDRL, HIV, lactate concentration, pyruvate, a hypercoagulability profile with attention to protein S, protein C, anticardiolipin antibodies, and antithrombin III levels, and a lupus anticoagulant. Plasma and urine amino acids can be sent, and urine can be tested for organic acids. A blood lipid profile with triglycerides, cholesterol, and lipoprotein concentrations can be ordered. Rheumatological tests, including antinuclear antibodies, antiDNA antibodies, and rheumatoid factor may be helpful. When a cardiac cause is strongly suspected, conventional or transesophageal echocardiography is considered. Scraping of hemorrhagic skin lesions in the case of suspected bacterial endocarditis and microscopic examination after proper staining can readily demonstrate bacterial agents and guide appropriate antibiotic therapy.

Cerebral angiography is the standard diagnostic procedure for detailed information of extracranial and intracranial vasculature, minor and major. A neuroradiologist experienced with this procedure in the pediatric population can obtain and interpret the results, which can be essential in defining an etiology of the stroke syndrome, and in directing appropriate intervention, particularly in the case of moyamoya syndrome and patients with cerebral aneurysms or AVMs.

Electroencephalography (EEG) is useful in investigating children presenting with an acute neurological deficit although its use in the emergency department is limited. An EEG is particularly relevant when a child has no history of epileptic seizures. The EEG can demonstrate ongoing electrographical seizure activity in the unconscious patient who has used medications prior to arrival in the emergency department. Focal or diffuse slowing of the EEG can correlate to the neuroanatomical location of cerebral infarction. This is valuable information, particularly when neuroimaging is normal. EEG interictal paroxysmal discharges increase the likelihood of epileptic seizure activity as a cause of lateralized weakness. However, focal slowing or focal epileptiform discharges can occur in the postictal state after epileptic seizures, and in migraine.

Treatment

The emergency treatment of childhood stroke depends on the initial manifestations. An acute hemiparesis in a child who is maintaining consciousness and has no associated symptoms requires psychological support, observation for a deteriorating level of consciousness, and a heightened alertness for the potential development of seizures. A rapid increase in ICP with resulting brain herniation can be caused by an intracranial hemorrhage due to a ruptured arterial aneurysm or an AVM. The triad of acute lateralized weakness or neurological deficit, progressive headache, and progressive deterioration of consciousness suggests an evolving and expanding intracranial hemorrhage, until proven otherwise. In these patients, protection of the airway and hyperventilation are important. Sedation and analgesia can mitigate further increases in ICP, which can result in rapid brain herniation and poor clinical outcome. The child with stroke related to an underlying systemic illness, such as dehydration, sickle cell disease, severe anemia, bacterial meningitis, or bacterial endocarditis receives appropriate treatment for the underlying illness.

Although the use of anticoagulation therapy in the adult patient with ischemic cerebral infarction is widely recommended, such therapy in children is not without risk due to the greater probability of subsequent head trauma and intracranial bleeding. However, anticoagulant therapy can be required in children with chronic valvular heart disease or right-to-left shunting. Thrombolytic therapy in the pediatric population is not recommended.

PEARLS AND PITFALLS

- Stroke in children occurs from fetal life to adolescence.
- The etiologies and manifestations of stroke are different in children compared to adults.
- Congenital heart disease is a common underlying cause of stroke in children.
- Stroke occurs in approximately 6% of patients with sickle cell disease.
- Migraine, epilepsy, hypoglycemia, and alternating hemiplegia of childhood can mimic stroke.
- Consider substance abuse and physical abuse in children as a possible cause of stroke.
- Thrombolytic therapy is not used to treat stroke in children.

REFERENCES

1. Becker RC. Thromboneurology and the search for safe and effective stroke therapies. *Editorial Stroke.* 1997;28:1657–9.
2. Schoenberg BS, Mellinger JF, Schoenberg DG. Cerebrovascular disease in infants and children; a study of incidence, clinical features, and survival. *Neurology.* 1978;28:763–8.
3. Broderick J, Talbot GT, Prenger ES, Leach A, Brott T. Stroke in children within a major metropolitan area: the surprising importance of intra-cerebral hemorrhage. *J Child Neurol.* 1993;8:250–5.
4. Druser A, Goutieres F, Aicardi J. Ischemic stroke in children. *J Child Neurol.* 1986;1:131.

5. Snyder RD, Stovring J, Cushing AH, Davis LE, Hardy TL. Cerebral infarction in childhood bacterial meningitis. *J Neurol Neurosurg Psychiatry.* 1981;44:581–5.

6. Barlow CF. Headaches and migraine in childhood. Philadelphia, Pa: JB Lippincott Co; 1984:93–125.

7. Marchioni E, Galimberti CA, Soragna D, et al. Familial hemiplegic migraine versus migraine with prolonged aura: an uncertain diagnosis in a family report. *Neurology.* 1995;45:33–7.

8. Bradshaw P, Parsons M. Hemiplegic migraine, a clinical study. *Q J Med.* 1965;334:65–85.

9. Haas DC, Lourie H. Trauma-triggered migraine: an explanation for common neurological attacks after mild head injury. *J Neurosurg.* 1988;68:181–8.

10. Guthkelch AN. Benign post-traumatic encephalopathy in young people and its reaction to migraine. *Neurosurgery.* 1977;1:101–6.

11. Cephalalgia. Headache Classification Committee of the International Headache Society. Classification and diagnostic criteria for headache disorders, cranial neuralgias, and facial pain. 1988;8(suppl 7):1–96.

12. Foster JW, Hart RG. Hypoglycemic hemiplegia: two cases and a clinical review. *Stroke.* 1987;18:944–6.

13. Jarjour IT, Ryan CM, Becker DJ. Regional cerebral blood flow during hypoglycemia in children with IDDM. *Diabetologia.* 1995;38:1090–5.

14. Caers LI, DeBeukelaas F, Amery WK. Flunarizine, a calcium-entry blocker in childhood migraine, epilepsy and alternating hemiplegia. *Clin Neuropharmacol.* 1987;10:162–8.

15. Baramada MA, Moosy J, Shuman RM. Cerebral infarcts with arterial occlusion in neonates. *Ann Neurol.* 1979;6:495–502.

16. Scher MS, Belfar H, Martin J, Painter MJ. Destructive brain lesions of presumed fetal onset: antepartum causes of cerebral palsy. *Pediatrics.* 1991;88:898–906.

17. Jarjour IT, Ahdab-Barmada M. Cerebrovascular lesions in infants and children dying after extracorporeal membrane oxygenation. *Pediatr Neurol.* 1994;10:13–19.

18. Clancy R, Malin S, Laraque D, Baumgart S, Younkin D. Focal motor seizures heralding stroke in full-term neonates. *Am J Dis Child.* 1984;139:601–6.

19. Volpe JJ. Intracranial hemorrhage: subdural, primary subarachnoid, intracerebellar, intraventricular (term infant), and miscellaneous. *Neurology of the Newborn.* 3rd ed. Philadelphia, Pa: WB Saunders Co, 1995;10:373–402.

20. Rivkin M, Anderson M, Kaye E. Neonatal idiopathic cerebral venous thrombosis. An unrecognized cause of transient seizures or lethargy. *Ann Neurol.* 1992;32:51–7.

21. Park YD, Belman AL, Kim FS, et al. Stroke in pediatric acquired immunodeficiency syndrome. *Ann Neurol.* 1990;28:303–11.

22. Husson RN, Saini R, Lewis LL, Butler KM, Patronas N, Pizzo PA. Cerebral artery aneurysms in children infected with human immunodeficiency virus. *J Pediatr.* 1992;121:927–30.

23. Russell MO, Goldberg HI, Reis L, et al. Transfusion therapy for cerebrovascular abnormalities in sickle cell disease. *J Pediatr.* 1976;88:382–7.

24. Greenberg J, Massey EW. Cerebral infarction in sickel cell trait. *Ann Neurol.* 1985;18:354–5.

25. Williams J, Goff JR, Anderson HR Jr, Langston JW, Thompson E. Efficacy of transfusion therapy for one to two years in patients with sickle cell disease and cerebrovascular accidents. *J Pediatr.* 1980;96:205–8.

26. Garg BP, Ottinger CJ, Smith RR, Fishman MA. Strokes in children due to vertebral artery trauma. *Neurology.* 1993;43:2555–8.

27. Priest JR, Ramsey KC, Steinherz PG, et al. A syndrome of thrombosis and hemorrhage complicating L-asparaginase therapy for childhood acute lymphoblastic leukemia. *J Pediatr.* 1982;100:984–9.

28. Packer RJ, Rorke LB, Lange BJ, et al. Cerebral vascular accidents in children with cancer. *Pediatrics.* 1985;76:194–201.

29. Ball WS Jr, Prenger EC, Ballard ET. Neurotoxicity of radial chemotherapy in children: pathologic and MR correlation. *Am J Neuroradiol.* 1992;13:761.

30. Ravelli A, Martini A, Burgio G. Antiphospholipid antibodies in pediatrics. *Eur J Pediatr.* 1994;153:472–9.

31. Eyster ME, Jill FM, Blatt PM, et al. Central nervous system bleeding in hemophiliacs. *Blood.* 1978;51:1179–88.

32. Andes WA, Wulff K, Smith WB. Head trauma in hemophilia – A prospective study. *Arch Intern Med.* 1984;144:1981–3.

33. Shahar A, Sadeh M. Severe anemia associated with transient neurologic deficits. *Stroke.* 1991;22:1201–2.

34. Young RSK, Rannels DE, Hilmo A, Gerson JM, Goodrich D. Severe anemia in childhood presenting as transient ischemic attacks. *Stroke.* 1983;14:622–3.

35. Belmar AL, Rogue CT, Ancona R, Anand AK, Davis RP. Cerebral venous thrombosis in a child with iron deficiency anemia and thrombocytosis. *Stroke.* 1990;21:488–93.

36. Atkins PT, Glenn S, Nemeth PM, Derdeyn CP. Carotid artery thrombosis associated with severe-iron deficiency, anemia, and thrombocytosis. *Stroke.* 1996;27:1002–5.

37. Alexander MB. Iron deficiency anemia, thrombocytosis, and cerebrovascular accident. *South Med J.* 1983;76:662–3.

38. Boers GHJ, Smalls AGH, Trijbels FJM, et al. Heterozygosity for homocystinemia in premature arterial disease. *N Engl J Med.* 1985;313:709–15.

39. Iqbal A, Alter M, Lee SH. Pseudo-xanthoma elasticum: a review of neurological complications. *Ann Neurol.* 1978;4:18–20.

40. Kelly JJ, Mellinger JF, Sundt TM. Intracranial arterial venous malformations in childhood. *Ann Neurol.* 1978;3:338–43.

41. Hladky J, LeJeune J, Blond S, et al. Cerebral arterial venous malformations in children: a report on 62 cases. *Childs Nerve Cyst.* 1994;10:328–33.

42. Roach ES, Riela AR. Pediatric cerebral vascular disease. Mount Kisco, NY: Futura Publishing Co; 1988.

43. Ball WS Jr. Cerebrovascular occlusive disease in childhood. *Pediatr Neuroradiol.* 1994;4:393–421.

44. Warach S, Schiend Li W, et al. Fast magnetic resonance diffusion-weighted imaging of acute human stroke. *Neurology.* 1992;42:1717–23.

45. Warach S, Boska M, Welch KMA. Editorial pitfalls and potential of clinical diffusion-weighted MR imaging in acute stroke. *Stroke.* 1997;28:481–2.

46. Wiznitzer M, Masaryk T. Cerebral vascular abnormalities in pediatric stroke: assessment using parenchymal and angiographic magnetic resonance imaging. *Ann Neurol.* 1991;29:585–9.

37 Pediatric Seizures

RAE R. HANSON

SUMMARY New-onset febrile and nonfebrile pediatric seizures commonly present to the emergency department. When a previously normal child has a seizure and recovers to a normal baseline, a focused evaluation is indicated. A more extensive evaluation in the emergency department is based on factors other than the occurrence of the seizure. Management of status epilepticus requires aggressive treatment that adheres to a timetable based on a clear understanding of the pharmacokinetics of the antiepileptic drugs used. The treating emergency physician has the responsibility to answer the initial questions of frightened and concerned parents about their child's prognosis.

Introduction

The incidence of seizures and epilepsy is increased at the extremes of age; it is highest in very young children (infants) and in the elderly population. When febrile seizures and status epilepticus (SE) are included in the incidence rate, children outnumber adults in these categories. The age-adjusted prevalence of epilepsy is approximately the same in children and adults.[1]

The causes and therapy of seizures and SE in children are different from those in adults. Effective treatment in the ED requires understanding of the special needs of children and their families. Parents are often highly anxious about the immediate and the long-term treatment. Concerns include the sequelae of seizure, the side effects of anticonvulsants and the social stigmata of a seizure disorder. Issues of prognosis and the need for long-term therapy are frequently raised in the emergency department. These issues are addressed by the emergency physician, who begins the process of parent education, determines immediate disposition, and provides a plan for follow-up. The following sections focus on specific seizures, epileptic syndromes, and treatment considerations unique to childhood.

Status Epilepticus

The *World Health Organization Dictionary of Epilepsy* defines SE as an epileptic seizure that is sufficiently prolonged or repeated at sufficiently brief intervals to produce an unvarying and enduring epileptic condition. In clinical practice, SE is any seizure that lasts 30 minutes or more, or occurs so frequently that the patient does not recover between seizures.

Epidemiology

SE occurs in 50,000–60,000 patients annually in the United States, the majority of whom are children.[2] When febrile seizures are included, more than 50% of these children present with SE as their first or only seizure episode. In a large study, 24% of children with a first nonfebrile seizure presented with SE. Between 1% and 16% of all patients with epilepsy experience SE at some time, with higher percentages occurring in children.[3] SE is most common in young children; the average age is under 3 years.[4]

Sid M. Shah and Kevin M. Kelly, eds., *Emergency Neurology: Principles and Practice.* Copyright © 1999 Cambridge University Press. All rights reserved.

Etiology

Seizures can occur without provocation in a patient with prior central nervous system (CNS) injury. This is referred to as remote symptomatic etiology. In a large prospective series, 13% of children presenting with SE had a remote symptomatic etiology, 5% had a progressive encephalopathy, and the remainder were evenly distributed between febrile, idiopathic, and acute symptomatic causes. Acute symptomatic causes included CNS infection, anoxia, stroke, hemorrhage, trauma, antiepileptic drug (AED) withdrawal, intoxication, and metabolic abnormalities.[5]

Outcome

The outcome of SE in children, as in adults, is related to etiology. Mortality ranges from 3–11%, and was 6% and 3.6% in two recent series, with nearly all deaths due to the underlying cause.[3,4,5] Morbidity varied from 9–28% and was lower in recent accounts.[4] Morbidity was more common in younger children, likely related to a higher incidence of more serious causes of SE. Morbidity was low or nonexistent in previously healthy children with an idiopathic or remote cause of SE when treated quickly and appropriately.[5,6]

Prehospital Management

Intervention for SE begins when contact with the emergency department is made by a parent from home or by a physician in another treatment facility. Information obtained from a parent by the prehospital care providers includes the patient's current health, the presence of any developmental or neurological problems, a history of seizures or epilepsy, and any current medications, including AEDs. When the patient has a known epileptic disorder, the parent is asked if diazepam or lorazepam is used at home rectally. Out-of-hospital use of these medications by parents or paramedics can shorten the duration of SE and decrease the likelihood of persistent seizure activity on arrival in the emergency department.[7] In this regard, lorazepam is preferred to diazepam because it causes less respiratory depression.[8] Dosages for these and subsequent AEDs are provided in Table 37.1, and are discussed in the following section. When a patient is transferred from another facility, his or her airway, breathing, and

circulation are assessed and treated as indicated. An oral or nasal airway is used when tolerated. Patients with hypoventilation, hypoxemia, or significant systemic acidosis are intubated prior to transport.[9] Treatable causes of SE such as hypoglycemia, drug overdose, or electrolyte imbalance are managed prior to transport. Management of the patient's seizures can be as simple as rectal administration of a benzodiazepine, or it can require intravenous administration of AEDs and treatment of systemic problems. When intravenous access cannot be obtained, intramuscular or rectal midazolam can be given. The patient is transported under close observation.

Emergency Department Evaluation and Management

Acute management of the patient consists of a planned treatment schedule that includes a specific time line for each step. The duration of SE is the greatest risk to the patient. It is likely that neuronal death begins within 90–120 minutes following onset of SE.[10] The longer SE lasts, the more difficult it is to treat. There are three goals of treatment: (1) to control seizures; (2) to preserve vital functions; and (3) to diagnose the underlying pathology. An outline of the recommended treatment of SE in children is given in Figure 37.1. This treatment plan details the traditional therapy of SE and includes new AEDs and treatment alternatives. The plan assumes that 80% of patients respond to diazepam in 5 minutes, and is similar to lorazepam.[11–13] In a recent study comparing these two medications, convulsions stopped in less than 60 seconds in all patients who responded to the first dose of medication. Lorazepam had fewer side effects, and fewer patients required a second AED to control SE completely.[8,11,14] Because of these advantages, many clinicians regard lorazepam as the benzodiazepine of choice in treating patients with SE. Recent data suggest that midazolam is superior to either diazepam or lorazepam in efficacy and side effects, and that it may be given intravenously, intramuscularly, or intranasally.[15] Midazolam's onset of action is rapid for all routes, and seizures terminate in less than 5 minutes. Midazolam is an ideal agent for continuous intravenous infusion in those patients who do not respond to bolus infusions. Mild hypotension can occur. Patients recover quickly when midazolam infusion is stopped.[16–24]

THERAPEUTIC OUTLINE FOR MANAGEMENT OF STATUS EPILEPTICUS IN CHILDREN

0 Minutes
- Vital signs, manage airway, breathing and circulation (ABCs) as appropriate
- BUN, glucose, electrolytes, Ca, Mg, drug levels, CBC, ABGs, toxicology screen as indicated
- Begin IV with D10NS to maintain serum glucose at about 150 mg/dl and limit fluids (consider a bolus of D50- one 50 cc ampule if dextrostix glucose is low or unavailable)
- Obtain history of prior seizures, medications, blood levels, compliance, recent illnesses, trauma, medical problems, drug (substance) abuse or exposure
- Observe and re-evaluate patient as needed while doing above

0-10 Minutes

Diazepam: rectal - 0.3 mg - 0.5 mg/kg (max 10 mg)
IV infusion - 0.3 mg/kg at 5 mg/min (max 10 mg)

OR

Midazolam: rectal: 0.5 - 1.0 mg/kg
IM: 0.3 - 0.8 mg/kg
IV: bolus 0.1 mg/kg - 0.3 mg/kg followed by infusion of 0.05 - 0.40 mg/kg/hr

AND

Phenytoin: IV infusion - 50 mg/min or 1 mg/kg/min in children <50 kg, total of 20 mg/kg (30 mg/kg can be used in previously untreated patients) OR
Fosphenytoin: IV infusion - same dose using phenytoin equivalents at 150 mg/kg/min

OR

Lorazepam: IV or rectal - 0.05 - 0.1 mg/kg at 2 mg/kg/min (max 4 mg)

5-10 Minutes

Diazepam: IV infusion - 0.5 mg/kg at a rate of 1.0 mg/min (max 10 mg)

OR

Lorazepam: IV infusion – 0.05 – 0.1 mg/kg and begin IV phenytoin if seizures persist

20 Minutes

If seizures continue:
Phenobarbital: IV infusion - 100 mg/min until seizure stops or a total of 20 mg/kg has been infused. Prepare for assisted ventilation

If seizures persist consider:
Valproic acid: rectal - 250 m/5 ml diluted 1:1, dose of 30 mg/kg. The dose of IV valproate is the same - max rate of 20 mg/min

45- 50 Minutes
- Intractable SE - general anesthesia
- May try in lieu of or while waiting for general anesthesia: Thiopental - IV infusion - bolus with 1.0 - 3.5 mg/kg then 1.0 –2.0 mg/kg/hr

OR

Pentobarbital : IV bolus - 5 mg/kg then 1.0 –3.0 mg/kg/hr

OR

Phenobarbital: IV infusion - continue initial infusion until seizures stop (need assisted ventilation)
OR

Midazolam: IV bolus - 0.1 mg/kg - 0.3 mg/kg followed by infusion of 0.05 - 0.40 mg/kg/hr

FIGURE 37.1. Adapted from Delgado-Escueta, Westerlain, Treiman, and Porter[12]

TABLE 37.1. AEDs Used in the Treatment of Pediatric Status Epilepticus

Drug	Dosage Range (mg/kg)	Route	Rate of Infusion	Recommended Dose (mg/kg)	Maximum Dose (mg)
Diazepam	0.1–0.5	IV	1–2 mg per minute	0.3	20
	0.5–1.0	Rectal		0.5	10–30
Lorazepam	0.05–0.1	IV		0.1	4
	Same	Rectal		0.1	4
Midazolam	0.1–0.3	IV IM	Bolus followed by infusion at 0.05–0.40 mg/kg per hour		
Phenytoin	20–30	IV	50 mg per minute or 1–2 mg/kg per minute	20	
Fosphenytoin	20–30 phenytoin equivalents	IV	150 mg per minute in adults no pediatric dose established	20 phenytoin equivalents	
Phenobarbital		IV	100 mg per minute or 1–2 mg/kg per minute	20	
Valproic acid		Rectal		30	

Phenytoin takes nearly 20 minutes to reach peak brain levels after intravenous infusion. However, phenytoin's peak effect occurs much earlier, with 80% of patients responding by the end of a 20-minute infusion.[25] Fosphenytoin, the prodrug of phenytoin, provides similar bioavailability of phenytoin when infused at rates of 100–150 mg per minute, and is better tolerated. It can be given intramuscularly when no other route is available.[26]

Similar to phenytoin, phenobarbital has an onset of effect before peak brain levels are reached.[27] An alternative approach for treating patients with SE who have failed to respond to benzodiazepines consists of giving repeated boluses of phenobarbital until SE stops. This approach is safe and effective, and usually does not result in significant respiratory depression.[28]

Valproic acid is effective in terminating SE when given rectally. An intravenous preparation of valproic acid is available. Intravenous valproic acid may be used rectally for SE that does not respond to treatment as outlined above. Table 37.1 summarizes the AEDs used in the treatment of pediatric SE.

Nonconvulsive Status Epilepticus

Absence SE, atypical absence SE, or complex partial SE may present as nonconvulsive SE. Typical symptoms include waxing and waning levels of consciousness, and motor activity that varies from multifocal twitching to frank automatisms. Complex partial SE is treated as outlined in Table 37.1. Absence SE and atypical absence SE are treated most effectively with benzodiazepines. When needed, valproic acid can be given in the dosages listed in Table 37.1. Rarely, benzodiazepines can provoke tonic SE in patients with Lennox-Gastaut syndrome (LGS).[29] Tonic SE in these patients can be difficult to treat. Valproic acid, phenytoin, and phenobarbital are used. Consultation with a neurologist is recommended.

Neonatal Status Epilepticus

In cases of unexplained SE in infants 18 months of age or younger, 100 mg of pyridoxine is given intravenously while respirations are monitored.[30,31] Initial treatment is as described in Figure 37.1, or with phenobarbital as the initial AED. Two protocols for administering phenobarbital are suggested. The first protocol begins with phenobarbital, 20 mg/kg given intravenously, followed by repeated boluses of 5–10 mg until the seizures stop or a level of 40 μg/ml is achieved.[32] The second protocol requires phenobarbital, 30 mg/kg given intravenously over 15 minutes.[33] If these measures fail, the infant is loaded with phenytoin, 20 mg/kg given intravenously as above, and the protocol in Figure 37.1 is followed. The high-dose phenobarbital (30 mg/kg) method used for children may also be employed.

Febrile Seizures

A febrile seizure is a seizure occurring with high fever in a child between 3 months and 5 years of age, with no cause identified other than the fever itself.[34] "High fever" is not defined clearly, but commonly it means a temperature greater than 102°F. Most patients with febrile seizure have temperatures of 103°F or higher.[35] Etiology is typically a viral illness. Some experts suggest a lower age limit of 1 month for infants with febrile seizures, based on the end of the neonatal period, and set no upper limit. Most neurologists use the more conservative definition, because most patients are in this age range and it avoids misclassification and possible misdiagnosis of younger and older patients. Children who present with seizures and meningitis virtually always have other abnormal findings that do not mimic those in children with uncomplicated febrile seizures.[36] Risk factors for additional febrile seizures include a lower temperature, a shorter duration of fever (especially less than 1 hour), a family history of febrile seizures, and age less than 18 months.[35] A family history of epilepsy and complex febrile seizures does not correlate with an increased risk for recurrent febrile seizures. Overall, approximately 30% of children will have a recurrent febrile seizure with a risk of 13–50%, depending on the risk factors present.[35] Febrile seizures are typically described as simple or complex. Simple febrile seizures are generalized, brief (less than 15 minutes), do not repeat within 24 hours, and generally do not repeat during the same illness.[37] These types of febrile seizure distinguish patients with a low or high risk of subsequent nonfebrile seizures that

ranges from 1% with simple febrile seizures to 10% with two or more complex features.[38] Treatment of patients with complex febrile seizures has not lowered their risk of experiencing subsequent nonfebrile seizures.

Evaluation

A history is obtained, including duration of illness, prior antibiotic treatment, trauma, medications the child or other persons in the household are taking, potential toxin exposure, recent trauma, and any chronic illnesses. A clear description of the seizure and its circumstances is obtained to determine any focal features. Risk factors for recurrent febrile seizures are reviewed so that initial counseling of the parents can be performed prior to patient discharge.

Management depends greatly on the presentation of the patient. Most patients present with a history of a brief (generally 6 minutes or less), generalized tonic-clonic seizure, which is often the first evidence of fever.[39] The patient is either postictal and improving, or has recovered by the time of arrival in the emergency department and has a temperature of greater than 102°F (generally above 103°F). A source of infection is diagnosed in 73% of patients; 50% have otitis media.[35,39] Examination findings are normal, or nonfocal with mild obtundation. Patients who present with a decreased mental status usually recover quickly during the initial observation period. These patients likely experienced a simple febrile seizure and require virtually no further evaluation. The National Institutes of Health (NIH) consensus conference found that complete blood counts, electrolyte levels, serum glucose levels, and computerized tomography (CT) of the brain are rarely useful, a finding confirmed by subsequent studies.[40]

Patients who have seizures with focal features, focal findings on examination, continued or profound obtundation, meningeal signs, trauma, toxin or medication exposure, or chronic conditions that predispose to seizures are evaluated appropriately for these conditions. The decision to perform a lumbar puncture is based on clinical information and may be unnecessary in the patient with a first uncomplicated seizure or a recurrent febrile seizure.[34,41,42] CT scanning or magnetic resonance imaging (MRI) of the brain is performed on any patient with focal findings, and consideration is given to a possible diagnosis of herpetic encephalitis. This reevaluation may not be necessary when there is a history of a similar presentation that was adequately evaluated, or when no new history or findings are present. An electroencephalography (EEG) is rarely obtained in the emergency department.

Management

An identified cause of a febrile seizure is treated appropriately. Self-limited febrile seizures rarely require acute treatment or initiation of maintenance therapy in the emergency department. The primary physician is contacted and follow-up is arranged. The effectiveness of prophylactic rectal diazepam for the prevention of future seizures is not established. A decision for its use is made by the primary care physician or pediatric neurologist at the time of follow-up for the acute event. Parents are given instructions for the management of fever and simple seizure first aid, and indications for return to the emergency department. The decision not to treat a child with a febrile seizure is outlined below.

Parent Counseling

Parents need to be reassured that the febrile seizure itself is benign whether it is simple, focal, prolonged, or presenting as SE.[5] The probability of recurrence is based on the risk factors previously described and the presence of an underlying neurological condition. A second febrile seizure occurs in 13–50% of patients; 50% of these experience a third seizure.[35] Because febrile seizures are a benign, self-limited disorder of early childhood, the only indication to treat them would be the possibility of decreasing the risk of subsequent epilepsy. Frequently occurring simple febrile seizures slightly increase the risk for the development of nonfebrile seizures.[43] Complex febrile seizures raise this risk by 10%. Regardless of the risk, no treatment for febrile seizures has decreased the risk of subsequent epilepsy. Parents can be advised that the decision to treat or monitor for further febrile seizures should be discussed in detail with the child's primary physician.

Nonfebrile Seizures

In the United States, the reported annual incidence rate of seizures in children through the age of 14 is 0.048–0.134%; the rate is 0.089% in a recent prospective community-based study of children in Sweden through the age of 15. By age 15, 3.5% of children experience a seizure of any type. The cumulative risk for a nonfebrile seizure is 1% by age 14. By age 20, 1% of children are diagnosed with epilepsy, and 0.5% of children have active epilepsy at any one time.[1,43,44] Children presenting to the emergency department with a nonfebrile seizure are divided into those with a first nonfebrile seizure and those with epilepsy. Epilepsy is defined as two or more unprovoked seizures. Pediatric patients are unique in that several characteristic epileptic syndromes have an age-dependent appearance, one or more characteristic seizure types, a natural history, and a prognosis. The presentation and AED treatment of selected syndromes are described.

Infantile Spasms

Infantile spasms are brief seizures characterized by axial flexion, appendicular extension, or a combination of both. In 90% of patients, seizures begin in children between 3 and 12 months of age. Earlier and later onsets can occur. Typically, the seizures start as a cluster of spasms that begin after awakening and last a few minutes. Consciousness is preserved, but the infant can become fretful toward the end of a flurry of seizures. Early recognition and treatment are important to prevent the development of mental retardation in children who are born healthy. Early treatment likely does not affect the outcome of children who are not born healthy or who have an identified cause of infantile spasms. Initial treatment is usually adrenocorticotropin hormone (ACTH) or prednisone. Valproic acid, phenobarbital, or a benzodiazepine is given when initial treatment fails. Vigabatrin may become the treatment of choice in the future; it is not yet approved for use in the United States. Typically, infants begin to regress shortly after seizure onset, and long-term prognosis for intellectual development is grave.

Lennox-Gastaut Syndrome

LGS begins between 1 and 7 years of age. Seizures are myoclonic, tonic or atonic, and atypical absence. Patients are either developmentally delayed at the onset of the syndrome or become so over time. No treatment is fully effective, and many patients with poorly controlled seizures are prescribed numerous AEDs. They can present to the emergency department with increased seizure frequency or with episodes of absence SE. AED toxicity occurs commonly due to drug–drug interactions and the high doses often used in an attempt to control seizures. AED toxicity can mimic, complicate, or exacerbate seizures, and is considered as a potential cause of worsening seizures in the evaluation of these patients.

Benign Rolandic Epilepsy

Benign rolandic epilepsy (BRE) begins between 2 and 13 years of age; peak incidence is between 4 and 10 years of age. BRE is manifested by simple partial seizures involving the face, jaw, and oropharyngeal muscles, with variable and less common involvement of the upper extremity on the same side. Occasional sensory symptoms can be reported. BRE can present with nocturnal grand mal seizures. The patient with BRE is neurologically intact and the EEG shows a prominent, high-amplitude centromidtemporal spike on normal background activity. Typically, seizures are infrequent and resolve spontaneously before age 16 years. BRE has a typical presentation, infrequent seizures, and benign outcome. Many patients do not require treatment, even for repeated seizures.

Other Syndromes

Many other genetic syndromes of infancy, childhood and adolescence are associated with seizures. Treatment is based on the seizure type.[45,46]

The Child with a First Nonfebrile Seizure

Evaluation of Nonfebrile Seizures

A history is obtained, and a detailed neurological examination is performed in the emergency department. Acute symptomatic causes such as toxic ingestions, head trauma, intracerebral hemorrhage, stroke, encephalitis, and metabolic abnormalities are investigated and treated immediately. Hypertension may first present with a seizure in a child. When no cause is determined, possible unrecognized seizures, present neurological problems such as developmental delay, or remote events that can predispose to subsequent seizures and epilepsy (many of these events are those that cause acute symptomatic seizures) are investigated. A family history of genetic, metabolic or neurological disease can be helpful. A detailed description of the seizure is important in order to determine if it was partial or generalized from outset. A parent who witnesses a seizure may need help in considering the sequence of seizure activity, which side of the body it started on and changes in the level of consciousness. A post ictal state may be frightening to parents as well. The neurological examination is directed toward any focal or lateralizing findings that may suggest a focal onset of seizures, or the possibility of a focal structural lesion. A brain CT or MRI is obtained in these cases. In the absence of these findings, emergency imaging is usually not indicated; however, patients with partial seizures should be evaluated with MRI of the brain on an outpatient basis. An EEG usually is arranged as an outpatient study.

Prognosis of Nonfebrile Seizures

Several studies estimate the risk of seizure recurrence after a first non-febrile seizure to be 23–71%.[47] Most of the difference in study results is explained by methodological differences such as inclusion criteria and study design. Factors found to correlate with risk of recurrence are etiology, EEG findings, and type of seizure. Risk of seizure recurrence is as low as 24% in a healthy child with a normal EEG; risk is as high as 65% in a child with two risk factors. Partial seizures are an independent risk factor in children with symptomatic seizures. Patients who present with a nocturnal seizure are more likely to have recurrent seizures, and additional seizures typically occur in the same stage of sleep as the original.[48] The occurrence of SE as the first nonfebrile seizure does not definitely correlate with an increased risk of subsequent seizures or SE in an otherwise healthy child.[5] Recurrence rates are highest immediately after the first seizure and rapidly decrease thereafter, with 80–90% of second seizures occurring in the first year. Patients with a second seizure have a 80–90% probability of having a third seizure.[49] Interestingly, studies do not show a consistent effect of AED treatment on the rate of risk of recurrence of a second seizure, despite the clear efficacy of AEDs in patients with epilepsy.[50]

Treatment of Nonfebrile Seizures

A decision to treat nonfebrile seizures is based on the likelihood of a second or subsequent seizure, and the need to treat those recurrences. Most pediatric neurologists in the United States do not treat the patient until criteria are met for the diagnosis of epilepsy: two or more unprovoked nonfebrile seizures, regardless of the assessed risk of a second seizure. For BRE including repeated seizures, treatment usually is not prescribed, unless they are very frequent or unacceptably disturbing to the patient or the family. Selection of an AED depends on the seizure type, age of the patient, available AED formulations, AED side effects, safety, ease of administration, and the physician's preferences. Phenobarbital, primidone, phenytoin, and carbamazepine are used to treat complex partial or generalized tonic-clonic seizures. Phenobarbital has side effects manifested by decreased concentration, increased motor activity, behavioral problems, and possibly long-term deleterious effects on intelligence level. Primidone is metabolized to phenobarbital and phenylethylmalonamide (PEMA) and has many of the same side effects of other barbiturates. Phenytoin has undesirable cosmetic side effects and nonlinear kinetics that make it difficult to use, particularly in younger children. Carbamazepine has no known long-term effects on appearance or cognition, has linear kinetics, and comes in pediatric formulations. Evidence suggests that except for a shorter half-life, absorption and serum levels are the same in adults, children, and infants. In pediatric trials, carbamazepine is as effective for treatment of these seizure types as it is in adults. It is the drug of choice for children older than 1 year. It can be used in children younger than 1 year in certain instances. For children older than 1 year, phenytoin is the second choice, and barbiturates are the third. For children younger than 1 year, barbiturates are the accepted first-line medication. Phenytoin is not recommended in this age group because of difficulty obtaining and maintaining adequate blood levels. Recently marketed AEDs such as gabapentin, lamotrigine, topirimate, and tiagabine have better kinetics and less toxicity, and may replace the older AEDs in the future. They have not been adequately studied for use as monotherapy in children and should not be used in the emergency department. Pediatric formulations and doses of first-line medications for generalized tonic-clonic and complex partial seizures are given in Table 37.2.

Treatment of Recurrent Seizures

Recurrent or uncontrolled seizures can be due to an underlying condition, medication interactions, decreased AED levels, or a paradoxical effect of the AEDs. When the patient presents to the emergency department, a careful history is obtained that includes current medications and doses, missed doses, or new AEDs. Medications such as major tranquilizers and antihistamines can lower the seizure threshold in susceptible children. Carbamazepine can increase seizures in some patients, even at therapeutic serum levels. Toxic phenytoin serum levels of greater than 40 μg/ml can cause increased seizure activity. Stopping carbamazepine or withholding phenytoin doses may be necessary in such cases. When serum levels are low because patients have missed doses, a loading dose that increases serum levels to a desired concentration is calculated using the formula (weight/kg) $\times$ (volume of distribution, Vd) $\times$ (desired change in concentration). The Vds for the commonly used medications are: phenytoin, 0.75 l/kg; carbamazepine, 1.0 l/kg; phenobarbital, 0.6–0.7 l/kg in infants and older children; valproic acid, 0.25–0.35 l/kg. In patients with refractory seizure disorders such as LGS, none of these conditions may be operative, and benzodiazepines such as lorazepam or a change in AEDs may be required.

AED Toxicity

AED toxicity can occur because of increased blood levels of the parent drug, decreased protein binding in highly bound drugs such as phenytoin, increased metabolites, or as a consequence of polypharmacy with decreased tolerance for high, but still therapeutic, serum levels of individual AEDs. It is important to remember that therapeutic ranges of serum AED levels are only guidelines for treatment. Patients can be toxic in the therapeutic range of an AED or tolerate serum levels well above

TABLE 37.2. Common AEDs for Initial Treatment of Seizures in Children

Medication	Formulation (mg)	Starting dose* (mg/kg per day)	Maintenance Dose* (mg/kg per day)	Schedule	Significant Drug Interactions
Carbamazepine (CBZ)	Liquid, 100 mg/5 ml	3 ×5 days, 6 ×5 days,	10–20	tid–qid	Erythromycin increases levels dangerously
	Chewable tab, 100 mg	10 per day final		bid	
	Tablet, 200 mg			bid	VPA increases 10,11-epoxide
Phenytoin (PHT)	Liquid, 125 mg/5 ml	5	4–7	tid	VPA increases free fraction
	Chewable tab, 50 mg			bid	
	Capsule, 30, 100 mg			bid	
Phenobarbital (PB)	Liquid, 20 mg/5 ml	5	2 mo–1 yr 4–11 1–3 yr 3–7	qd	VPA increases levels
	Tablet, 15, 30, 45 mg		3+ 3–5		
Valproic acid (VPA)	Liquid, 250 mg/5 ml	5 ×5 days, 10 ×5 days,	15–30	tid–qid	PB decreases levels
	Sprinkles, 125 mg	15 per day final		bid	
	125, 250, 500 mg			bid	

*Doses recommended are for children on initial monotherapy who are not taking other medications.

the published maximums. Two AED combinations that are commonly used in pediatrics are valproic acid and phenytoin, or valproic acid and carbamazepine. Valproic acid increases the level of free or unbound phenytoin, causing toxicity with total phenytoin levels that are well within the therapeutic range. When coadministered with carbamazepine, valproic acid inhibits the epoxide hydrolase enzyme responsible for hydrolysis of the initial carbamazepine epoxide metabolite, leading to elevation of the 10,11-carbamazepine epoxide that can reach 50% or higher in the presence of valproic acid and other enzyme-inducing AEDs. Valproic acid significantly decreases the clearance of phenobarbital and the newer AED, lamotrigine, leading to increased serum levels of these AEDs. Valproic acid is associated with many more serious side effects in children age

2 years or younger. It is toxic at normal levels in those with carnitine deficiency.

Events Mimicking Seizures

Many events in childhood can mimic seizure disorders. *Breath holding* may occur from infancy through early childhood but is most common in toddlers. Events are always provoked, begin with crying, and eventually lead to cyanosis and a brief loss of consciousness. Patients can become stiff at the end of the episode and demonstrate a few clonic jerks. Brief confusion afterward may occur. *Benign paroxysmal vertigo* consists of brief episodes of unsteadiness during which patients appear frightened, and may hang onto a parent or wedge themselves in a corner. Nystagmus may be present. In children old enough to express themselves, some sense of movement may be described. Events last one to five minutes and can occur several times per month. These episodes are likely migraine-related and resolve spontaneously with age. *Sandifer's syndrome* occurs in infants and is manifested by postprandial episodic dystonic posturing and head-turning caused by gastroesophageal reflux. *Shuddering attacks* are brief (five seconds or less) episodes of stiffening, fine tremor, and sometimes flexion of the head, trunk, and lower extremities, occurring in infants and children. They can occur hundreds of times per day and can cause falls when the child is standing. These are benign events likely related to essential tremor. *Sleep-related behaviors* are sometimes mistaken for seizures in children and include head or body rocking, and night terrors. The latter are characterized by sudden panicked or frightened awakening from sleep during which the child is inconsolable and only minimally responsive. After several minutes, the child can awaken or simply go back to sleep with no later recall of the event.[51] *Pseudoseizures* are considered in any child presenting with prolonged atypical events, particularly when the child has previously not responded to adequate trials of AEDs.

PEARLS AND PITFALLS

- Treatment of status epilepticus requires a treatment strategy and timetable.
- Healthy children who present with status epilepticus as their first seizure do not need to be started on antiepileptic medication in the emergency department.
- Simple febrile seizures do not require evaluation or treatment in the emergency department; fever and its cause are treated appropriately.
- Complex febrile seizures require evaluation but do not require treatment with chronic antiepileptic medication.
- Children presenting to the emergency department with new-onset seizures who recover to a normal baseline require a focused evaluation. Treatment decisions usually are made with the patient's primary physician or neurologist.

- Not everything that looks or sounds like a seizure is a seizure.

REFERENCES

1. Hauser WA, Hesdorffer DC. *Epilepsy: Frequency, Causes and Consequences.* New York, NY: Demos Publications; 1990.
2. Hauser WA. Status epilepticus: epidemiologic considerations. *Neurology.* 1990;40(suppl 12):9–13.
3. Hauser WA. Status epilepticus: Frequency, etiology, and neurologic sequelae. *Adv Neurol.* 1983;34:3–14.
4. Dunn DW. Status epilepticus in infancy and childhood. *Neurol Clin.* 1990;8:647–57.
5. Maytal J, Shinnar S, Moshe SL, Alvarez LA. Low morbidity and mortality of status epilepticus in children. *Pediatrics.* 1989;83:323–31.
6. Lacroix J, Deal C, Gauthier M, Rousseau E, Farrell CA. Admissions to a pediatric intensive care unit for status epilepticus: a 10-year experience. *Crit Care Med.* 1994;22:827–32.
7. Dieckmann RA. Rectal diazepam therapy for prehospital pediatric status epilepticus. *West J Med.* 1991; 155:287–8.
8. Appleton R, Sweeney A, Choonara I, Robson J, Molyneux E. Lorazepam versus diazepam in the acute treatment of epileptic seizures and status epilepticus. *Dev Med Child Neurol.* 1995;37:682–8.
9. Henning R. Emergency transport of critically ill children: stabilisation before departure. *Med J Aust.* 1992;156:117–24.
10. Treiman DM. General principles of treatment: responsive and intractable status epilepticus in adults. In: Delgado-Escueta AV, *Advances in Neurology.* New York, NY: Raven Press, Ltd; 1983;377–84.
11. Crawford TO, Mitchell WG, Snodgrass SR. Lorazepam in childhood status epilepticus and serial seizures: effectiveness and tachyphylaxis. *Neurology.* 1987;37: 190–5.
12. Delgado-Escueta AV, Wasterlain C, Treiman DM, Porter RJ. Current concepts in neurology: management of status epilepticus. *N Engl J Med.* 1982;306:1337–40.
13. Lacey DJ, Singer WD, Horwitz SJ, Gilmore H. Clinical and laboratory observations: lorazepam therapy of status epilepticus in children and adolescents. *J Pediatr.* 1986;108:771–4.
14. Chiulli DA, Terndrup TE, Kanter RK. The influence of diazepam or lorazepam on the frequency of endotracheal intubation in childhood status epilepticus. *J Emerg Med.* 1991;9:13–17.
15. Kendall JR, Reynolds M, Goldberg R. Intranasal midazolam in patients with status epilepticus. *Ann Emerg Med.* 1997;29:415–17.
16. Galvin GM, Jelinek GA. Midazolam: an effective intravenous agent for seizure control. *Arch Emerg Med.* 1987;4:169–72.

17. Gherpelli JL, Luccas FJ, Roitman I, Troster EJ. Midazolam for treatment of refractory neonatal seizures. A case report. *Arq Neuropsiquiatr.* 1994;52:260–2.

18. Jelinek GA, Galvin GM. Midazolam and status epilepticus in children. *Crit Care Med.* 1994;22:1340–1.

19. Kumar A, Bleck TP. Intravenous midazolam for the treatment of refractory status epilepticus. *Crit Care Med.* 1992;20:483–8.

20. Lahat E, Aladjem M, Eshel G, Bistritzer T, Katz Y. Midazolam in treatment of epileptic seizures. *Pediatr Neurol.* 1992;8:215–16.

21. Orebaugh SL, Bradford SM. Intravenous versus intramuscular midazolam in treatment of chemically induced generalized seizures in swine. *Am J Emerg Med.* 1994;12:284–7.

22. Ramoska EA, Linkenheimer R, Glasgow C. Midazolam use in the emergency department. *J Emerg Med.* 1991;9:247–51.

23. Rivera R, Segnini M, Baltodano A, Perez V. Midazolam in the treatment of status epilepticus in children. *Crit Care Med.* 1993;21:991–4.

24. Wroblewski BA, Joseph AB. Intramuscular midazolam for treatment of acute seizures or behavioral episodes in patients with brain injuries. *J Neurol Neurosurg Psychiatry.* 1992;55:328–9.

25. Wilder BJ, Efficacy of phenytoin in treatment of status epilepticus. *Adv Neurol.* 1983;34:441–6.

26. Ramsay RE, DeToledo J. Intravenous administration of fosphenytoin: option for the management of seizures. *Neurology.* 1996;46(suppl 1):S17–19.

27. Painter MJ, Gaus LM. Phenobarbital: Clinical Use, in *Antiepileptic Drugs,* R.H. Levy, R.H. Mattson, and B.S. Meldrum, Editor. New York, NY: Raven Press, Ltd; 1995.

28. Crawford TO, Mitchell WG. Very-high dose phenobarbital for refractory status epilepticus in children. *Neurology.* 1988;38:1035–40.

29. Tassinari CA, Dravet C, Roger J, Cano JP, Gastaut H. Tonic status epilepticus precipitated by intravenous benzodiazepine in five patients with Lennox-Gastaut syndrome. *Epilepsia.* 1972;13:421–35.

30. Kroll JS. Pyridoxine for neonatal seizures: an unexpected danger. *Dev Med Child Neurol.* 1985;27:377–9.

31. Goutieres F, Aicardi J. Atypical presentations of pyridoxine-dependent seizures: a treatable cause of intractable epilepsy in infants. *Ann Neurol.* 1985;17:117–20.

32. Gilman JT. Rapid sequential phenobarbital treatment of neonatal seizures. *Pediatrics.* 1989;83:674.

33. Donn SM, Grasela TH, Goldstein GW. Safety of a higher loading dose of phenobarbital in the term newborn. *Pediatrics.* 1985;75:1061–4.

34. Consensus-Development-Panel. Febrile seizures: long term management of children with fever associated seizures. *Pediatrics.* 1980;66:1009–12.

35. Berg A, Shinnar S, Hauser WA, et al. A prospective study of recurrent febrile seizures. *N Engl J Med.* 1992;327:1122–7.

36. Green SM, Rothrock SG, Glem KJ, Zurcher RF, Mellick L. Can seizures be the sole manifestation of meningitis in febrile children? *Pediatrics.* 1993;92:527.

37. Nelson KB. Can treatment of febrile seizures prevent subsequent epilepsy? In: Nelso KB, Ellenberrg JH, eds. *Febrile Seizures.* New York; NY: Raven Press, Ltd; 1981.

38. Nelson KB, Ellenberf JH. Prognosis in children with febrile seizures. *Pediatrics.* 1978;61:720–7.

39. Farwell JR, Febrile seizures: recent developments. *Pediatr Ann.* 1991;20:25–28.

40. Nypaver MM, Reynolds SL, Tanz RR, Davis AT. Emergency department laboratory evaluation of children with seizures: dogma or dilemma? *Pediatr Emerg Care.* 1992;8:13.

41. Joint Working Group of the Research Unit of the Royal College of Physicians and the British Pediatric Association. Guidelines for the management of convulsions with fever. *Br Med J.* 1991;303:634–6.

42. Wears RL, Luten RC, Lyons RG. Which laboratory tests should be performed on children with apparent febrile convulsions? An analysis and review of the literature. *Pediatr Emerg Care.* 1986;2:191–6.

43. Annegers JF, Hauser WA, Shirts SB, Kurland LT. Factors prognostic of unprovoked seizures after febrile convulsions. *N Engl J Med.* 1987;316:493–8.

44. Sidenvall R, Forsgren L, Blomquist HK, Heijbel JA. A community-based prospective incidence study of epileptic seizures in children. *Acta Paediatr.* 1993;82:60–5.

45. Luders H, Lesser RP, eds. Epilepsy: electroclinical syndromes. In: Conomy JP, Swash M, eds. *Clinical Medicine and the Nervous System.* New York, NY: Springer-Verlag; 1987.

46. Aicardi J. Epilepsy in children. In: Pocopis PG, Rapin I, eds. *The International Review of Child Neurology.* 2nd ed. New York, NY: Raven Press, Ltd; 1994.

47. Berg AT, Shinnar S, Hauser WA, Leventhal JM. Predictors of recurrent febrile seizures: a metaanalytic review. *J Pediatr.* 1990;116:329–37.

48. Shinnar S, Berg AT, Ptachewish Y, Alemany M. Sleep state and the risk of seizure recurrence following a first unprovoked seizure in childhood. *Neurology.* 1993;43:701–6.

49. Hirtz DG, Ellenberg JH, Nelson KB. The risk of recurrence of nonfebrile seizures in children. *Neurology.* 1984;34:637–41.

50. Berg AT, Shinnar S. The risk of seizure recurrence following a first unprovoked seizure: a quantitative review. *Neurology.* 1991;41:965–72.

51. Evans OB. Episodic disorders in childhood. *Semin Neurol.* 1988;8:42–50.

38 Hypotonic Infant

MARSHA D. RAPPLEY AND SID M. SHAH

SUMMARY The assessment of hypotonia in the infant requires a focused history and a careful physical examination to distinguish hypotonia from weakness. Symptoms and findings on examination can localize the problem neuroanatomically and generate a differential diagnosis. The important role of emergency department management is to treat life-threatening complications of hypotonia and to initiate the diagnostic process with appropriate referrals when hypotonia is not a result of asphyxia, sepsis, trauma, or toxicity.

Introduction

Evaluation of the hyptonic, or "floppy" infant in the emergency department is difficult because the potentially broad differential diagnosis including neurological disorders and life-threatening conditions. The diagnostic evaluation of the hypotonic infant is organized around salient features of the history and physical examination. This leads to the efficient use of diagnostic studies and appropriate disposition of the patient.

It is important to clarify the terminology used in describing hypotonia and muscle weakness in infants. *Hypotonia* refers to decreased muscle tone. This is the least resistance that a quiet, alert infant offers when the examiner passively moves the extremities and head. A healthy baby is not flaccid. Hypertonia is a stiffening or extensor response to stimulation. *Weakness* refers to a decrease in muscle power generated by the infant. Muscle strength can be felt in the active movement of a healthy infant. It can be adequately assessed in a crying infant; a healthy baby is not easily moved from a position of flexion while crying. A weak baby is always hypotonic, but a hypotonic baby may be able to generate muscle strength. Characterizing muscle tone and strength assists in generating a differential diagnosis.

Prehospital Care

A healthy infant who suddenly becomes hypotonic activates the prehospital care system. Acute life-threatening events, sepsis, and trauma are considered in the hypotonic infant. Patency of the airway, and adequate ventilation and circulation are the main objectives of transport to the emergency department, where a focused evaluation begins and management continues.

Neuroanatomy and Physiology

The neurophysiology of the hypotonic infant involves the central nervous system (CNS) and four components of the motor unit: the lower motor neuron, the peripheral nerve, the neuromuscular junction, and the muscle (Fig. 38.1). Muscle tone is a result of the coordinated sequence of events across these elements (Figure 38.1).[1,2] Muscles mature into distinct fibers at 20–24 weeks of gestation in the growing fetus. The motor unit matures with this growth. Fetal movement can be felt at this point in gestation, and increases in intensity and frequency until birth. Concomitant development of the brainstem and spinal cord tracks results in the primitive reflexes. Maturation of cortical function over the first several months of life allows higher functions

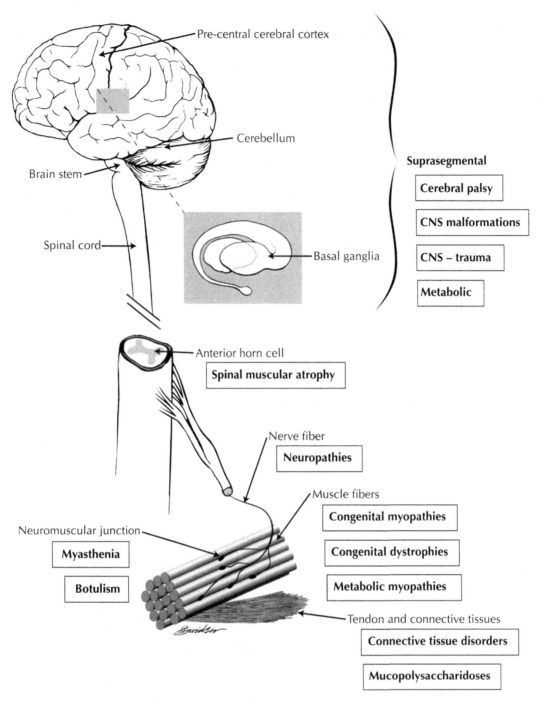

FIGURE 38.1. Anatomical approach to disorders producing hypotonia.

to override these primitive reflexes. CNS lesions that affect the brain diffusely are commonly associated with global cognitive and motor function impairment. Upper motor neuron lesions involve the descending tracts within the brain and spinal cord; lower motor neuron lesions involve the anterior horn cell and the peripheral motor nerve. Disorders of the neuromuscular junction involve chemical neurotransmitters such as acetylcholine. Disorders of the muscle involve muscle fibers, enzyme systems, tendons, and connective tissue.

Emergency Department Evaluation

History

The chief complaint concerning a hypotonic infant can be feeding problems with poor suck and swallow, recurrent respiratory infection, or delay in motor milestones. Parents may express concern that the infant is not active, lies in a passive position, and seems weak. Infants who present with lethargy or a potential acute life-threatening event require assessment for sepsis, apnea, and trauma. For the hypotonic infant who does not appear acutely ill, it is important to identify the onset of apparent symptoms of hypotonia or decreased movement. This history includes details of fetal movement; polyhydramnios; toxic, infectious, or drug exposure in utero; prematurity; and complications of the birth process. The gestational age of the infant is considered in the history and physical examination because premature infants are hypotonic compared to full-term infants. Apgar ratings for tone, irritability, and respiratory effort can suggest problems at birth. Arthrogryposis is a condition of congenital joint contractures that is apparent at birth, results from immobility in utero, and can be of CNS or neuromuscular origin. Onset of hypotonia at 12–24 hours of age is suggestive of a metabolic disorder related to feedings.

The course of hypotonia over time helps to differentiate its cause. Hypotonia might not be apparent to parents until 8–12 weeks after birth, when the baby is expected to have more purposeful movement in interaction with family members. Hypotonia that improves and develops into hypertonia suggests cerebral palsy.

A review of normal developmental milestones of the younger infant includes following a visual stimulus and turning the head toward an auditory stimulus at 4 weeks, smiling socially at 4–8 weeks, lifting of the head in the prone position slightly at 8 weeks and well at 12 weeks, making cooing sounds at 8 weeks, and attempting approximate reaching movements toward objects of interest at 12 weeks. The head can lag when the infant is pulled to a sitting position at 8 weeks, but strength is evident. Early head control with a bobbing motion begins at about 12 weeks. When giving a history of an older infant or toddler, parents are often uncertain of these early milestones. Parents are usually able to describe that the baby sits alone or attempts to sit with a tripod formation using arms for support by the age of 7 months and that the baby attempts to crawl by scooting or pulling by the age of 8 months. In the older infant the most reliable milestone is age at walking; this is usually accomplished by age 14 months.[13] However, the hypotonic infant might not do any of these age-appropriate activities.

The family history is particularly important when investigating neuromuscular disease because many of these disorders have a genetic basis. Consanguinity of parents increases the possibility of recessive disorders. A maternal history of neurological disease or muscle weakness is sought. This can indicate a neonatal manifestation of myasthenia gravis or a hereditary disorder. A positive family history may give evidence of a neuromuscular disorder. A negative family history does not exclude a neuromuscular disorder because many families have too few known members and the expression of many disorders is extremely variable.

Physical Examination

Observation of the infant in various stages of arousal is critical. Hypotonia is suspected in any infant who has bizarre and unusual postures and is relatively immobile.[4] Dubowitz gave the first comprehensive description of the hypotonic infant, which forms the basis for current understanding of the assessment of this disorder.[5] The normal-term infant shows active movement of flexed limbs when placed in a supine position. The way the infant lies in the parent's arms can provide information about the baby's muscle tone and strength. A classic pre-

TABLE 38.1. Common Disorders of the Motor System Causing Hypotonia or Weakness in Infants

Central Nervous System	Motor Neuron	Nerve	Neuromuscular Junction	Muscle
Chromosome disorders	Spinal muscular atrophy	Dejerine-Sottas disease	Myasthenic syndromes	Congenital myopathy
Inborn errors of metabolism	(Werdnig-Hoffmann disease)	Charcot-Marie-tooth disease	Passive transfer from affected mother	Metabolic myopathy
Brain dysgenesis		Congenital neuropathy	Inborn error of neuromuscular junction	Congenital muscular dystrophy
Brain injury			Juvenile myasthenia gravis	Congenital myotonic dystrophy
Benign congenital hypotonia			Infant botulism	
Spinal cord injury				

Source: From Crawford TO. Clinical Evaluation of the Floppy Infant. *Pediatric Annals.* 1992;21(6):349.

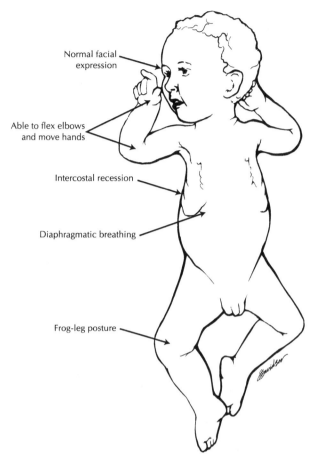

Normal facial
expression

Able to flex elbows
and move hands

Intercostal recession

Diaphragmatic breathing

Frog-leg posture

FIGURE 38.2. Infant with hypotonia.

sentation of hypotonia is the frogleg position, with abduction of hips and extension of limbs when the infant is supine (Fig. 38.2).[6,7] Observation includes assessment of possible dysmorphic features, abnormalities of the skin, and relative proportion of head, trunk, and limbs.

A detailed examination of the respiratory system is indicated in the hypotonic infant. The examination assesses respiratory rate, excursion, diaphragmatic movement, and the use of accessory muscles. The examination notes the condition of the heart, the size of the liver and spleen, status of the genitalia, range of motion of the joints, tendon length or contractures, the quality of muscle mass and subcutaneous fat, and the status of the skin.

The mental status examination of an infant assesses the level of alertness, nature of the cry, degree of irritability, consolability, and interaction.

Primitive reflexes are characteristic of the newborn. Moro's reflex, reflex stepping, and plantar and palmer grasps are examples of primitive reflexes present at birth. These reflexes persist after a few months with CNS dysfunction.

The cranial nerve examination assesses facial symmetry, the ability to suck and swallow, the ability to fixate and follow, eye movements with the oculocephalogyric reflex using gentle rotation of the head, condition of the fundi, and tongue movements or possible fasciculations.

Muscle tone is assessed and hypotonia confirmed by: (1) decreased resistance of limbs through passive range of motion; (2) the frogleg posture in supine position; and (3) abnormal axillary suspension when the infant is held under the axillae and slips through the examiner's hands.

Muscle strength is assessed and weakness confirmed by: (1) decreased ability of the limbs to resist gravity, which can be demonstrated by holding the infant in horizontal suspension causing the limbs to fall loosely; (2) abnormal ventral suspension with curvature of head, trunk, and limbs when the infant is held prone over the examiner's arm and hand; (3) abnormal head lag when the infant is pulled from a supine to a sitting position; (4) decreased trunk and head control with these maneuvers, or with sitting position for older infants. Muscle strength is apparent when the infant is able to keep the extremities in a flexed position, pushes against the examiner or parent, and withdraws extremities or moves against gravity.

The distribution of weakness is important to note (see Table 38.2). Proximal muscle weakness can be associated with muscular dystrophy and progressive spinal atrophy. Distal weakness is characteristic of peripheral neuropathies and myotonic dystrophy. Weakness of the facial muscles may indicate congenital myopathy, myotonic dystrophy, or fascioscapulohumeral muscular dystrophy.

Deep tendon reflexes (DTRs) are most easily elicited in the biceps, knees, and ankles of the normal infant. Increased or absent DTRs can be associated with CNS lesions. Decreased reflexes are associated with weak muscles.

Sensory levels can be determined by a withdrawal response of the infant and are used to differentiate transection of the spinal cord from spinal muscular atrophy. Weakness can make evaluation of sensation difficult because of the dependence of the withdrawal response on adequate muscle strength. Rare disorders of infancy resulting in decreased sen-

TABLE 38.2. General Regions of Weakness Characteristic of Motor Unit Disorders in Infants

Location of Disorder	Region of Weakness
Motorneuron	Diffuse weakness sparing eye movement, diaphragm, and sphincter
Nerve	Intrinsic hand and foot muscles, producing "claw" hand deformity and pes cavus
Neuromuscular junction	Ptosis, extraocular muscles, sucking, and swallowing
Muscle	Weakness of proximal limb muscles, facial diplegia

Source: Crawford TO. Clinical Evaluation of the Floppy Infant. *Pediatric Annals.* 1992;21:349.

sation include Charcot-Marie-Tooth and Dejerine-Sottas syndromes.

Fatigability is typically difficult to demonstrate in an infant but can be apparent from the history. The infant appears hungry and starts feeding with a good suck but tires quickly. This assessment requires that a maximum effort is sustained by the infant. Fatigability is characteristic of myasthenia gravis.

Range of motion of the joints helps to differentiate collagen disorders such as Ehlers-Danlos syndrome, which is associated with laxity but normal strength. Increased laxity is a physical finding that is more helpful than a decreased range of motion because the healthy newborn or crying infant may be flexed tightly.

Differential Diagnosis

The differential diagnosis of infantile hypotonia can be generated by first determining whether hypotonia is associated with weakness (see Figure 38.3). *CNS disorders* are suggested by the loss of developmental milestones or evidence of mental retardation. These disorders can be obscured by severe malnutrition, systemic illness, or weakness that prevents the infant from normal interaction. *Isolated*

connective tissue disorders are suggested by laxity of joint movements; weakness and hypotonia are not prominent features. Examples of CNS disorders that can present with hypotonia but without significant weakness include hypoxic-ischemic encephalopathy and intracranial hemorrhage. Chromosomal disorders associated with hypotonia include Prader-Willi syndrome and Down's syndrome. Osteogenesis imperfecta is an example of a connective tissue disorder that also affects the CNS. It presents with hypotonia, blue sclera, multiple fractures, and retarded development.

The following disorders are associated with significant weakness and secondary hypotonia.

- *Spinal muscular atrophy, Werdnig-Hoffmann syndrome,* is an autosomal recessive disorder with a carrier frequency of 1:60 to 1:80. It involves loss of anterior horn cells and of the hypoglossal nucleus. There is profound symmetrical weakness and loss of spontaneous movement. Muscle atrophy can be obscured by subcutaneous fat. The diaphragm is affected late in the disease process. DTRs are reduced or absent. Infants are alert, and there is no loss of cognitive function. In its most severe form, onset of spinal muscular atrophy is noted at birth or within the first month of life. These infants rarely survive to 1 year of life.[7]
- *Congenital muscular dystrophies* are inherited disorders with slow onset in early life. They are characterized by preferential involvement of proximal muscles, loss of DTRs, and pseudohypertrophy of muscle. This form has onset at birth and is commonly associated with contractures. Other types typically present at age 2–5 years or older, depending on the type. There is no effective treatment for the muscular dystrophies.[4,7]
- *Myasthenia gravis* of infants can be of two types: (1) transient neonatal or (2) congenital type. Transient neonatal disease occurs in approximately one in seven infants born to mothers with myasthenia gravis. There are elevated antibodies against the acetylcholine receptors in mother and baby. Symptoms appear from one to three days of life. There is a weak cry and difficulty in swallowing. The duration of transient neonatal myasthenia gravis is commonly less than five weeks, but symptoms can be severe. With early hospital discharge, close observation is maintained for in-

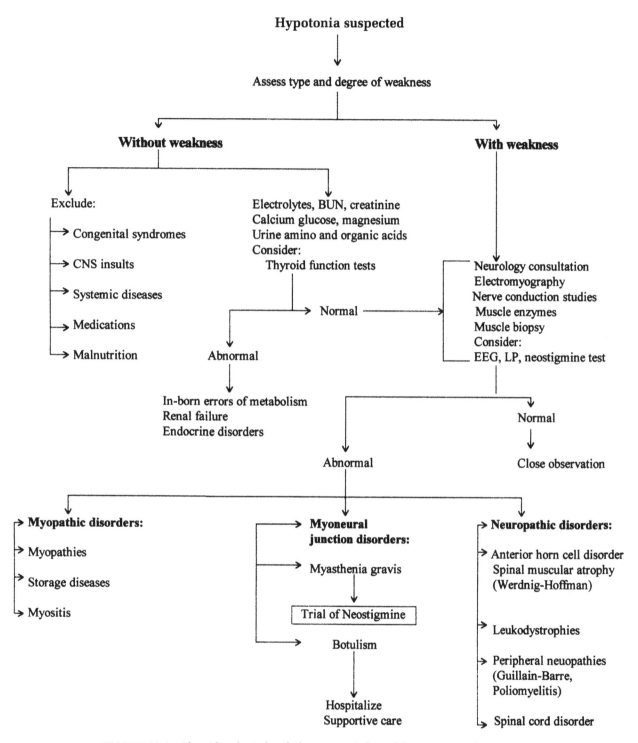

FIGURE 38.3. Algorithm for infantile hypotonia (adapted from Berman[13]).

509

fants born to mothers with myasthenia gravis. Congenital myasthenia gravis occurs in infants born to mothers without myasthenia gravis. The symptoms of congenital disease in infancy usually are not as severe as those of the transient neonatal type, but they persist and are typically refractory to therapy. The hallmark of the history is fatigability. Diagnosis is confirmed by transient improvement in muscle strength with edrophonium or neostigmine. Treatment of infants usually is symptomatic.[7]

- *Congenital myotonic dystrophy* can present with choking, difficulty sucking and swallowing, respiratory problems, arthrogryposis, skeletal deformities, facial diplegia, diminished or absent DTRs, mental retardation, abdominal distension and ileus. These abnormalities are the result of failure of voluntary muscle to relax after contraction. Many genetic and biochemical defects are associated with the various forms of myotonic dystrophy. The congenital form is commonly associated with an affected mother. The clinical course is one of gradual deterioration.[4,7]

- *Guillain-Barré syndrome* is uncommon but described in infants ranging from 1 month to 16 months of age. Presentation is typically that of remarkable respiratory infection with profound hypotonia. Characteristic elevation of the protein level of the cerebrospinal fluid is found.[8,9]

- *Toxic causes of hypotonia* include *Clostridium botulinum, C. tetani,* and venom of the cobra and of the black widow spider, all of which affect the neuromuscular junction. Infantile botulism presents in 95% of cases between 3 weeks and 6 months of age with poor suck and swallow, weak cry, drooling, or obstructive apnea. These symptoms relate to bulbar palsies. A classic presentation of infantile botulism includes internal and external ophthalmoplegia.[7,10]

A list of diagnoses resulting in hypotonia of infancy is listed in Table 38.3.[7,11]

Diagnostic Studies

Results of blood chemistry analysis are compared to age-referenced values that often are not provided on printed sheets of laboratory results. These are available in comprehensive pediatric textbooks or pocket

TABLE 38.3. Diagnosis of 107 Cases of Floppy Infant

Diagnosis	Number of Cases
Infantile muscular atrophy	67
Congenital muscular dystrophy	3
Polymyositis	1
Myasthenia gravis	1
Scurvy	2
Cerebral disease (atonic cerebral palsy)	14
"Benign congenital hypotonia"	17

Source: Menkes JH. Diseases of the Motor Unit. In: Textbook of Child Neurology. Baltimore, MD: Williams and Wilkins, 1995. (page 819).

manuals.[10,12] Creatine phosphokinase (CPK), for example, can be increased tenfold in the first week of life. However, elevations associated with muscular dystrophies range in the thousands. Evaluation of chemistries should include CPK, lactate dehydrogenase (LDH), (ALT), aspartate transaminase (AST), calcium, and electrolytes. Thyroid function tests are obtained because neonatal screens of thyroid disease do not examine all levels of the hypothalamic-pituitary-thyroid axis. When the history suggests a metabolic disorder, glucose level, venous pH, ammonia, complete blood count with differential, serum and urine organic acids, and serum amino acids are considered. Chromosomal analysis with a specific request for karyotyping of suspected Prader-Willi syndrome or Down's syndrome may be indicated. Lumbar puncture is indicated for consideration of an infectious etiology or possible Guillain-Barré syndrome. Neuroimaging can be useful for detecting disorders of the CNS suggested by hypotonia without weakness.

Hypotonia with weakness requires the use of electrophysiology and biopsy studies. Information from these studies on neonates and infants is most useful when appropriately interpreted in the context of the infant's age. Electromyography, nerve conduction studies, and biopsies of muscle and nerve have normal developmental expressions in the neonate and young infant that can mimic pathological findings in an older infant or child. These studies can be useful in differentiating specific disorders or localizing lesions but might require expertise available at centers specializing in neurological electrophysiology and pathology of infants and children.

Ultrasound imaging of muscle can be useful in identifying the characteristic muscle patterns of Werdnig-Hoffmann disease or Duchenne's muscular dystrophy. Additionally, this procedure can be useful for obtaining biopsy specimens.

Management and Disposition

Hospitalization is commonly required to observe a hypotonic infant and to continue with diagnostic evaluation, for example, when a metabolic disorder is suspected and feedings are withheld. Typically, acute management is directed at problems secondary to the hypotonia and weakness such as respiratory compromise, feeding difficulties, aspiration, and recurrent respiratory infections. A pediatric neurologist is consulted in order to determine the need for further diagnostic procedures or to initiate treatment of an underlying neurological disorder.

PEARLS AND PITFALLS

- Decreased muscle tone (hypotonia) is distinct from decreased muscle power (weakness).
- Hypotonia is considered in an infant who has feeding problems with poor suck and swallow, recurrent respiratory infections, or a delay in developmental milestones.
- Hypotonia might not be apparent until 8–12 weeks of age.
- Proximal muscle weakness can be associated with muscular dystrophy and progressive spinal atrophy.
- Distal muscle weakness is characteristic of peripheral neuropathies and myotonic dystrophy.
- Diagnostic evaluation of hypotonia *with* weakness requires electrophysiological studies and a muscle biopsy.

- Transient neonatal myasthenia gravis is considered in an infant born to a mother with myasthenia gravis; this might be associated with severe symptoms.
- In infantile botulism, 95% of cases present between 3 weeks and 6 months of age with poor suck, swallow, weak cry, drooling, or obstructive sleep apnea.
- An infant with hypotonia is hospitalized for observation and evaluation when symptoms or diagnostic procedures place the child at risk for complications secondary to the hypotonia.

REFERENCES

1. Gay CT, Bodensteiner JB. The floppy infant: recent advances in understanding of disorders affecting the neuromuscular junction. *Neurol Clin North Am* 1990; 8:715–25.
2. Crawford TO. Clinical evaluation of the floppy infant. *Pediatr Annals.* 1992;21:348–54.
3. Needleman RD. Growth and development. In: Nelson WE, Behrman RE, Kleigman RM, Arvin AM, eds. *Nelson Textbook of Pediatrics.* 15th ed. Philadelphia, Pa: WB Saunders Co; 1996:41.
4. Cole CH. Hypotonia. In *Primary Pediatric Care,* 3rd ed. Hoekelman RA, Friedman SB, Nelson NM, Seidel HM, Weitzman ML, eds. St. Louis, Mo: CV Mosby; 1997.
5. Dubowitz V. *The Floppy Infant.* Philadelphia, Pa: JB Lippincott Co; 1980.
6. Miller G. Hypotonia and neuromuscular disease. In: Fanaroff AA, Martin RJ, eds. *Neonatal-Perinatal Medicine, Diseases of the Fetus and Infant.* 6th Ed. St Louis, Mo: CV Mosby; 1997; 1.
7. Menkes JH. *Textbook of Child Neurology.* 5th ed. Baltimore, Md: Williams & Wilkins; 1995.
8. Carroll JE, Jedziniak M, Guggenheim MA. Guillain-Barré syndrome: another cause of the "floppy infant." *Am J Dis Child.* 1977;131:699–700.
9. Gilmartin RC, Ch'ien LT. Guillain-Barré syndrome with hydrocephalus in early infancy. *Arch Neurol.* 1977;34:567–9.
10. Nelson WE, Behrman RE, Kliegman RM, Arvin AM. *Nelson Textbook of Pediatrics.* 15th ed. Philadelphia, Pa: WB Saunders Co; 1996.
11. Walton JH. The limp child. *J Neurol Neurosurg Psychiatry.* 1957;20:144–54.
12. Barone MA. *The Harriet Lane Handbook.* 14th ed. St. Louis, Mo: CV Mosby; 1996.
13. Berman S. Infantile hypotonia. In: Berman S, eds. *Pediatric Decision Making.* Philadelphia, Pa: BC Decker and CV Mosby; 1985:137.

SIX Neurological Emergencies of Pregnancy

39 Pregnancy Related Neurological Emergencies

MARY J. HUGHES

SUMMARY The challenging spectrum of neurological disorders in pregnancy extends from life-threatening eclamptic seizures to self-limiting *meralgia paresthetica*. Eclampsia, a disorder specifically related to the pregnant or newly delivered patient, carries a significant morbidity and mortality to the mother and the fetus. The emergency physician is likely to encounter not only the conditions resulting directly from pregnancy but also preexisting conditions changed by the gravid state of the patient. Certain types of neuropathies and movement disorders occur specifically during pregnancy or result from the gravid state. Emergency physicians generally well versed in managing common conditions such as migraine headaches and seizures in the nonpregnant patient can be challenged by the same conditions in the pregnant patient.

Introduction

There are several neurological emergencies that are unique to pregnancy. Some of these are potentially life-threatening to the mother and fetus. This chapter focuses on emergency department evaluation and treatment of neurological problems including eclampsia, seizures, headache, and cerebrovascular disorders.

Prehospital Considerations

The health of the unborn depends on the well-being of the mother. Prehospital care providers focus on the immediate needs of the pregnant patient. Assessment of airway, breathing, and circulation is of fundamental importance. A pregnant patient with hypertension receives supplemental oxygen. Intravenous access is established, and transportation is provided to the nearest hospital capable of delivery and management of this high-risk medical patient. Large amounts of intravenous fluids are avoided unless specifically indicated. Eclamptic seizures are commonly preceded by changes in mental status, vision, or headaches in the prehospital setting. Any of these symptoms require appropriate seizure precautions. Benzodiazepines are the first-line medication for initial management of seizures regardless of cause. A left lateral Sims' position during transport not only allows adequate venous return to the heart but also may prevent aspiration if the patient experiences a seizure. Intractable seizures generally require aggressive airway management such as endotracheal intubation.

Eclampsia

Introduction and Incidence

Eclampsia is a significant cause of maternal and fetal morbidity and mortality. Eclampsia, a condition with an obscure cause, divergent and sometimes controversial treatment protocols can result in significant morbidity for the mother and the fetus.[1] Eclampsia is one of the hypertensive disorders of pregnancy and is defined as the occurrence of generalized seizures during pregnancy, during labor, or within one to two weeks of delivery, not caused by epilepsy or other convulsive disorders. It is the third most common cause of maternal death.[2]

Eclampsia is primarily a disease of young primigravidas and women older than 35 years of age.[3] The incidence varies from 0.2–1.5% of all deliveries, with an increased incidence in twin pregnancies.[4,5] Preeclampsia occurs in approximately 5% of pregnancies, and 1 out of 1150 deliveries develops eclampsia.[6,7]

Preeclampsia has traditionally been defined as pregnancy-induced hypertension (PIH) plus proteinuria and/or generalized edema. It is now believed that edema is such a common finding in pregnant women that its presence or absence does not validate the diagnosis of preeclampsia. Proteinuria, an important sign of preeclampsia, is defined as 300 mg or more of urine protein per 24 hours, or 100 mg/dL or more on at least two random urine samples done at least 6 hours apart. Proteinuria is also a sign of a worsening clinical condition. The combination of proteinuria and PIH markedly increases the risk of perinatal morbidity and mortality. Hypertension is the *sine qua non* of preeclampsia, and once the blood pressure exceeds 140/90, PIH is considered to be present and is managed appropriately.[8]

Emergency Department Evaluation and Differential Diagnosis

When convulsions and altered sensorium occur in the pregnant patient beyond 20 weeks of gestation or in the first 2 weeks postpartum, eclampsia is considered the most likely cause. Other disorders such as epilepsy, endocrine or metabolic disorders, infections, mass lesions, or intracerebral hemorrhages are also possibilities.[9]

Emergency department evaluation begins with close attention to the pregnant patient's vital signs. "Normal" blood pressure readings can be a sign of preeclampsia. Knowledge of the prenatal blood pressure is essential to judge the relevance of the reading. Vital signs are monitored frequently. A thorough history and physical examination is important. A history of any preexisting clinical conditions is sought.

Unrelenting headache, visual disturbances, and, occasionally, right upper quadrant abdominal pain in the preeclamptic patient can precede convulsions.[10] Ocular manifestations of eclampsia can parallel cerebral dysfunction and require serial funduscopic examinations. The initial change in optic fundi is arteriolar narrowing without arteriovenous crossing

compression.[12] Vasospasm can be severe enough to cause central retinal artery occlusion. Retinal edema follows, beginning peripherally, progressing to retinal hemorrhage, exudates, and retinal detachment. Generally the patient's vision improves rapidly after delivery, and retinal reattachment occurs within three days.[11,12] Cortical blindness in eclampsia is thought to be caused by multiple infarcts and microhemorrhages with edema in the occipital gray matter.[10–12] Magnetic resonance imaging (MRI) in patients with cortical blindness supports the theory that reversible arterial vasoconstriction is the etiology of these changes.[13]

Cerebral hemorrhage is a cause of death in patients with eclampsia. Hemorrhagic lesions can be microscopic or detectable on computerized tomography (CT) scanning of the brain. Coma is another expression of neurological impairment; typically, it follows a sudden and severe elevation of blood pressure, resulting in the inability of the brain to autoregulate cerebral flow, causing overt cerebral edema. Another cause of coma in these patients is intracranial hemorrhage from a ruptured aneurysm or arteriovenous malformation (AVM). Fever associated with convulsions can indicate cerebral hemorrhage.[7,14]

Seizures can occur any time before, during, or after labor, and are typically generalized tonic-clonic (grand mal) events. Seizures are most common in the last trimester, increasing in frequency as the patient approaches term. Approximately 25% of eclampsia develops postpartum. Generally, any grand mal seizure that occurs more than 48 hours postpartum may indicate another etiology; however, classic eclampsia, especially in primigravidas, can be encountered up to 10–14 days postpartum.

In patients with antepartum eclampsia, spontaneous labor commonly ensues following the seizure. Often the labor is rapid and intense, and delivery of the fetus is imminent. The fetus can develop bradycardia following a maternal seizure secondary to hypoxia and lactic acidosis generated by convulsions. The emergency department staff must be well equipped and prepared to handle an emergency delivery of a newborn.

Epigastric or right upper quadrant abdominal pain is thought to result from hepatocellular necrosis and edema that stretches the liver capsule. This pain is typically accompanied by elevated serum liver enzyme levels secondary to periportal hemorrhagic necrosis. Most often these enzyme level elevations are accompanied by thrombocytopenia. This is known as the hemolysis, elevated liver enzymes, low platelets (HELLP) syndrome. Bleeding may cause hepatic rupture or may form a subcapsular hematoma. Thrombocytopenia also increases the risk of maternal intracranial hemorrhage and excessive bleeding during parturition.[8]

As preeclampsia develops, renal perfusion and glomerular filtration rates are reduced, leading to elevations in serum creatinine levels and decreases in creatinine clearance.[8]

Laboratory and Radiological Studies

Laboratory findings can be inconsistent in eclampsia, and none are pathognomonic. In more than 50% of patients, abnormal values for uric acid, creatinine, and creatinine clearance are found. Hemoconcentration and increased viscosity are common. In 20–74% of patients, liver enzyme elevation is found.[15]

CT imaging of the brain is obtained in patients with focal deficits or seizures and commonly reveals cerebral edema. Hemorrhage may also be observed.[16–18]

Emergency Department Management

Delivery of the fetus and placenta is the definitive treatment of eclampsia. Typically, delivery is delayed until seizures and hypertension are well controlled, and hypoxia and acidosis have been corrected.[19]

Seizures. Seizures increase the maternal and fetal morbidity. Most obstetricians support the use of magnesium sulfate to *prevent* eclamptic seizures in known high-risk patients. Seizures are treated promptly and aggressively. Benzodiazepines such as diazepam and lorazepam are rapidly effective in the treatment of eclamptic seizures; however, they are used with caution because large doses are known to suppress fetal activity and respirations, and cause maternal hypoventilation.[18,20]

Obstetricians and neurologists differ on the treatment plan of eclamptic seizures. Clinically, and on the electroencephalogram (EEG), eclamptic seizures are indistinguishable from generalized tonic-clonic seizures, and neurologists feel that they should be treated as such.[21,22] Since 1955, Parkland Hospital (Dallas, Texas) has popularized a regimen that in-

TABLE 39.1. Medications for Seizure Control and Prophylaxis in Eclampsia

A Benzodiazepines: intravenous; intramuscular or rectal
B Magnesium Sulfate Dosage Schedule:
1. Give 4 g of magnesium sulfate ($MgSo_4;·7H_2O$, USP) as a 20% solution intravenously at a rate not to exceed 1 g/min.
2. Follow with 10 g of 50% magnesium sulfate solution, one half (5 g) injected deep in each buttock. (Addition of 1.0 ml of 2% lidocaine may be used to decrease discomfort.)
   a. If convulsions persist after 15 minutes, give up to 2 g more intravenously as a 20% solution at a rate not to exceed 1 g/min. If the woman is large, up to 4 g may be given slowly.
3. Every 4 hours thereafter give 5 g of a 50% solution of magnesium sulfate injected deep into alternate buttocks, if:
   a. the patellar reflex is present.
   b. respirations are not depressed.
   c. urine output the previous 4 hours exceeded 100 ml.
4. Magnesium sulfate is discontinued 24 hours after delivery.
C Phenytoin Schedule:
1. Initial dose 10 mg/kg IV (rate not to exceed 25 mg/min).
2. 5 mg/kg IV 2 hours later.
3. 12 hours later begin maintenance dose of 200 mg TID (IV or PO).
4. Check phenytoin and albumin levels at 6 and 12 hours after second bolus and daily thereafter.

Source: Adapted from Cummingham FG, MacDonald PC, Gant NF, Leveno KJ, Gilstrap LC III. Common complications of pregnancy. *Williams Obstetrics.* 19th ed. Norwalk, Conn: Appleton & Lange; 1993:763–803.

corporates the use of magnesium sulfate in the management of eclamptic seizures. In their experience, there is little need for other antiepileptic drugs, although other institutions have not been able to duplicate their results.[21] The main features of this care regimen include: controlling convulsions with magnesium sulfate; intermittent injections of hydralazine to control the blood pressure; avoidance of diuretics and hyperosmotic agents; limiting intravenous fluids unless fluid loss is excessive; prompt delivery of the fetus (Table 39.1).[23]

Magnesium is almost exclusively cleared by the kidneys. Serum magnesium levels are measured frequently, and the maintenance doses of magnesium are decreased in patients with eclampsia-induced renal impairment. Seizures are almost always controlled with plasma magnesium levels between 4 and 7 mEq/l. Early symptoms and signs of magnesium toxicity are nausea, a sensation of warmth and flushing, somnolence, diplopia, dysarthria, and weakness. When serum magnesium levels approach 10 mEq/l (9–12 mg/dl), patellar reflexes are lost. At higher levels, respiratory depression develops. Respiratory paralysis and arrest occur with levels greater than 12 mEq/l (15–17 mg/dl). Cardiac arrest occurs at levels of 30–35 mg/dl.[24,25] At the first signs of toxicity, calcium gluconate, 1 g, is given intravenously and infusion of magnesium sulfate is discontinued.[23]

In patients with myasthenia gravis, magnesium is contraindicated, and phenytoin is used with caution.

Neurologists are much more likely to recommend traditional antiepileptic drug therapy for the treatment of eclamptic seizures. Phenytoin has little effect on the respiratory drive, gastric emptying time, or level of consciousness. Therefore, it is likely a better drug to provide control throughout the peripartum period, when eclamptic women are most at risk for seizures.[21,26] Contraindications for the use of phenytoin include allergy to phenytoin, severe atherosclerotic heart disease, which is rare in this patient population, or marked bradycardia, especially when associated with atrial flutter or fibrillation. Phenytoin is free of tocolytic activity, and neonatal effects are nonexistent.[27] However, in order to prevent bleeding associated with phenytoin-induced coagulopathy, a single dose of vitamin K is given to neonates born to mothers on phenytoin at the time of delivery.[28]

A prospective study evaluated intravenous magnesium sulfate and intravenous phenytoin in patients with PIH requiring seizure prophylaxis. The results demonstrated no statistically significant difference between the two groups in occurrence of seizures and maternal or neonatal complications. The conclusions were that both were effective, had limited side effects, and were well tolerated by patients and neonates.[29] The routine use of magnesium sulfate for this purpose has been recommended by the American College of Obstetricians and Gynecologists, which sets the standards of care for obstetric practice in the United States."[24]

Hypertension. Blood pressure must be controlled in the pregnant patient to prevent maternal intracerebral hemorrhage and other complications of preeclampsia and eclampsia.[30]

Controlling hypertension is essential for normal CNS functioning in these patients. The Parkland formula uses hydralazine intravenously whenever the patient's diastolic blood pressure is greater than 110 mg/Hg. The typical initial dose is 5 mg, titrated in doses of 5–10 mg at intervals of 15–20 minutes until the patient achieves a diastolic blood pressure of 90–100 mmHg. A lower blood pressure is generally avoided because it may compromise placental perfusion.[23]

Antihypertensive medicines that are avoided in the pregnant patient include diazoxide, calcium channel blockers, angiotensin converting enzyme (ACE) inhibitors, diuretics, trimethaphan, reserpine, nitroprusside, and hyperosmotic agents. ACE inhibitors and calcium channel blockers reduce blood pressure in pregnant women; however, ACE inhibitors may cause fetal hypotension, and animal studies have shown calcium channel blockers to cause fetal hypoxemia and acidemia. Therefore, when adequate blood pressure control can be obtained with current regimens, the ACE inhibitors and calcium channel blockers are avoided.[30,31]

Fluids. Expansion of extracellular fluid space is physiologic in pregnancy. Vasospasm caused by eclampsia is responsible for the apparent contraction of the intravascular fluid space. Therefore, the eclamptic patient can be sensitive to the administration of large fluid volumes and also to the rapid blood loss associated with parturition. Fluid therapy is aimed at replacing physiological losses unless excessive fluid loss from diaphoresis, nausea, vomiting, diarrhea, or blood loss from delivery are encountered.[23]

Disposition

All patients with eclampsia and many with preeclampsia are admitted to the hospital. Evaluation for the HELLP syndrome is made in patients with preeclampsia or eclampsia. This syndrome is often misdiagnosed as hepatitis, pyelonephritis, cholelithiasis, or other abdominal disorders.[32]

Seizures in Pregnancy

Seizures are the most common serious neurological problem encountered by obstetricians. Seizures during pregnancy carry an increased risk to the fetus from hypoxia, metabolic acidosis, and hypoglycemia. Status epilepticus carries a maternal and fetal mortality rate of up to 25% and 50% respectively.[33]

The incidence of seizures in pregnancy is 0.3–0.6%.[34] Pregnancy has variable effects on the patient with epilepsy, exacerbating preexisting seizure disorders in 25–50% of patients. In part, this is likely related to the degree of seizure control experienced prior to pregnancy.[20,35,36]

Seizure activity itself may increase fetal anomalies and stillbirths independent of the increased risk for fetal malformations associated with the use of anticonvulsants such as valproic acid and trimethadione. The most common fetal abnormalities include neural tube defects, cardiac anomalies, and dysmorphic facies, including cleft, finger anomalies.[36–40]

Immediate emergency department management of the convulsing pregnant patient is no different from that for the nonpregnant patient. (For details, see Chapter 12, "Seizures.")

Emergency Department Management

Emergency department management of the pregnant patient in the postictal state includes supplemental high-flow oxygen, intravenous access, positioning the patient in the left lateral Sims' position or placing a pillow under the right hip, and stabilization of the maternal acid–base status. Fetal monitoring is undertaken in the emergency department as soon as possible. Anticonvulsant levels are obtained as well as blood tests, to determine whether electrolyte abnormalities or occult infection may have predisposed the patient to seizures. Phenothiazines are known to lower the seizure threshold and are avoided in the pregnant patient with seizures who has hyperemesis. Sleep deprivation, hyperemesis gravidarum, changes in protein binding, hepatic metabolism, volume of distribution of antiepileptic drugs and medication noncompliance can affect antiepileptic drug levels and lower seizure thresholds.[33,41]

Coagulopathy related to the maternal use of antiepileptic drugs, observed primarily in the fetus, is treated by giving the mother oral vitamin K, 20 mg daily for one month, or 10 mg intramuscularly 4 hours before delivery, or 1 mg intramuscularly to the baby at the time of delivery. Internal hemorrhage resulting from the coagulopathy may occur in the fetus or neonate, and fresh frozen plasma may be necessary. This coagulopathy may also lead to stillbirth.[33,41–43]

Status epilepticus occurs in 1% of epileptics during their pregnancy. Management of status epilepticus is discussed in Chapter 12, "Seizures." Continuous fetal monitoring in the emergency department is required.

Of particular note is the infant born to the mother managed on phenobarbital throughout her pregnancy. Approximately seven days postpartum the infant will develop a withdrawal syndrome that may last from two weeks to four months and is manifested by hyperexcitability, tremor, high-pitched cry, and feeding problems despite the child always seeming hungry.[37]

Headache

Headache is one of the most common neurological problems that brings the pregnant patient to the emergency department. Quite common during pregnancy, headache is generally benign but can occasionally herald serious pathology. New-onset headache in the pregnant patient alerts the emergency physician to serious disorders such as preeclampsia, eclampsia, uncontrolled hypertension, pheochromocytoma, subarachnoid hemorrhage, pseudotumor cerebri, a rapidly expanding tumor, and cortical vein thrombosis, as well as infectious etiologies such as encephalitis and meningitis.[44–46]

The incidence of migraine in the general population is 3–5%, with a female preponderance.[47] During pregnancy, the frequency of migraine headaches decreases in two-thirds of patients with a known history of perimenstrual migraine and in one-half of the patients who do not routinely experience a migraine at the time of menstruation.[48,49]

The key to an accurate diagnosis of headache in the pregnant patient is a thorough history and a comprehensive physical examination. Commonly, the diagnosis of tension headache or migraine can be made and further evaluation (such as CT of the brain) can be avoided during this period. However, when intracranial pathology is suspected, the appropriate radiographic tests are performed despite pregnancy.

Management

The goals of headache management in the pregnant patient are: (1) identification of etiology or precipitating factors; (2) relief of pain with medications that are least toxic to the mother and the fetus; and (3) reduction of severity and frequency of headaches.

Foods known to aggravate the patient's migraines are common triggers. Alcohol, aged cheeses, chocolate, chicken livers, pickled herring, canned figs, pods of raw beans, monosodium glutamate, and cured meats are common offenders. Hypoglycemia is avoided by eating three well-balanced meals per day or frequent small meals in the late third trimester as needed and avoiding an overabundance of carbohydrates at any one meal.

The use of ergot alkaloids in the treatment of migraine during pregnancy is avoided because these may increase uterine contractility. The treatment primarily depends on the use of analgesics, antiemetics, and sedatives. Chlorpromazine, 0.1 mg/kg given intravenously, has been shown to be very effective in treating patients with migraines and is a class C drug in pregnancy.[44,50,51] Acetaminophen or acetaminophen with codeine is also acceptable in pregnancy. Occasionally, meperidine and other narcotic derivatives may also be used. Aspirin is avoided, as are nonsteroidal anti-inflammatory drugs during pregnancy. Propranolol is an effective drug for migraine prophylaxis.[37,44,51] However, because propranolol crosses the placenta and causes fetal bradycardia, its use is limited to the pregnant patient with refractory migraine headaches. All medications should be approved by the patient's obstetrician and neurologist.

Movement Disorders

As with other neurological disorders, movement disorders can occur in women of reproductive age and, therefore, may be associated with pregnancy.

Chorea gravidarum is any chorea associated with pregnancy or occurring during pregnancy. Primary chorea is idiopathic or hereditary such as that associated with Huntington's disease, Wilson's disease,

or neuroacanthocytosis. Chorea gravidarum is associated with a wide spectrum of disorders such as infections (group A *Streptococcus*, rheumatic fever), immune disorders (systemic lupus erythematosus, antiphospholipid antibody syndrome), vascular disorders (due to infarction or hemorrhage in the subthalamic or caudate nuclei), and certain endocrine disorders. Drugs are likely one of the more common etiologies for chorea gravidarum. The use of medications such as antiepileptic drugs, amphetamines, dopamine receptor agonists and antagonists, and estrogen preparations are frequently implicated. Drugs of abuse such as cocaine can also be associated with chorea.[52]

The mean age of patients with chorea gravidarum is 22 years, with 80% of the attacks occurring in first pregnancies. Half of affected patients develop chorea in the first trimester, and one-third in the second trimester. Two-thirds of patients have had chorea previously, often Sydenham's chorea associated with rheumatic fever, although this is rare.[53] Chorea gravidarum typically resolves spontaneously in a few months or after parturition. When unrelenting, chorea can lead to hyperthermia, rhabdomyolysis, myoglobinuria and, rarely, death.[54,55]

Chorea gravidarum is generally a diagnosis of exclusion. Inherited and other identifiable causes of choreiform movements are excluded before phenothiazines or haloperidol are prescribed for intractable and disabling choreiform movements.

Restless legs syndrome has an incidence of 11–19% during pregnancy and can be confused with chorea gravidarum. It is characterized by crawling dysesthesias, primarily of the legs, after resting, and usually is relieved by walking. The neurological examination is normal, and symptoms usually resolve after delivery. There is no specific therapy for restless legs syndrome, in the pregnant patient.[52,55] Table 39.2 lists common drugs associated with various movement disorders.[52]

Peripheral Nerve Disorders

Peripheral neuropathies associated with or exacerbated by pregnancy are reviewed in this section.

TABLE 39.2. Common Drug-induced Movement Disorders

Movement Disorder Syndrome	Drugs
Akathisic movements	DDA, DRA, cinnarizine, ethosuximide, flunarizine, levodopa, reserpine, tetrabenazine
Ataxia	Alcohol, lithium carbonate
Chorea	AC, amphetamines, cocaine, DDA, DRA, estrogen (birth control pill and vaginal cream), levodopa, lithium, methylphenidate, TCA, theophylline
Dystonia	DDA, DRA, levodopa
Myoclonus	AC, DRA, levodopa, TCA
Restless legs	None
Rigidity (neuroleptic malignant syndrome)	DRA, withdrawal of antiparkinsonian medication in Parkinson's disease
Tics	Carbamazepine, DDA, DRA, IDA, levodopa
Tremors (postural)	Adrenocorticosteroids, aminophylline, amiodarone, cyclosporin A, DRA, epinephrine, levodopa, levothyroxine, lithium carbonate, oxytocin, terbutaline, valproic acid, withdrawal state (alcohol, sedatives)
Symptomatic parkinsonism	Alpha-methyldopa, DRA, lithium carbonate, reserpine, tetrabenazine, toxins (carbon monoxide, carbon disulfide, cyanide, disulfiram, manganese, methanol, MPTP)

Note: AC, anticonvulsants; DRA, dopamine receptor antagonists; DDA, direct dopamine agonists (apomorphine, bromocriptine, lisuride, pergolide); IDA, indirect dopamine agonists (amantadine and others); TCA, tricyclic antidepressants; MPTP, 1-methyl-4-phenyl-1,2,3,6-tetrahydropyridine.
Source: Adapted from Rogers JD, Fahn S. Movement disorders and pregnancy. In: Devinsky O, Feldman E, Hainline B, eds. *Neurological Complications of Pregnancy.* New York, NY: Raven Press, Ltd; 1994:163–78.

Carpal Tunnel Syndrome

Carpal tunnel syndrome (CTS) is the most common nerve entrapment syndrome associated with pregnancy and is the result of median nerve compression under the transverse carpal ligament of the wrist. It is commonly associated with fluid retention in pregnancy and is more likely to occur as the pregnancy progresses, often resolving in the postpartum period. Because it is self-limiting and generally resolves spontaneously, symptomatic treatment in the form of nocturnal wrist splints, occasional local steroid injections, supplemental oral vitamin B_6, or diuretics usually suffices. In severe cases with disabling pain, surgery can be performed with the patient under local anesthesia with little risk to the fetus.[56–58]

Bell's Palsy

The annual incidence of Bell's palsy is 45.1 per 100,000 births in pregnant females, compared to 17.4 per 100,000 cases in age-matched nonpregnant counterparts. The highest incidence is in the third trimester and early puerperium, calculated to be 118.2 per 100,000 births annually.[59]

Bell's palsy is a condition of facial weakness due to impaired function of the ipsilateral seventh cranial nerve. Generally unilateral, it typically presents in an abrupt fashion and its cause is often not clearly known. Sensation to the face is intact, but occasionally loss of taste on the anterior two-thirds of the ipsilateral tongue may occur. It can be associated with hyperacusis of the ipsilateral ear. Most cases resolve spontaneously and completely. The provision of artificial tears and systemic steroids, particularly when the patient presents early in the course of the disease, is considered.[57–59]

Lateral Femoral Cutaneous Neuropathy

Meralgia paraesthetica is a self-limiting sensory syndrome in which the lateral femoral cutaneous nerve is trapped under the inguinal ligament medial to the anterior superior iliac spine or retroperitoneally where the nerve angulates over the sacroiliac joint. It is manifested by pain, paresthesias, or dysesthesias in the middle one-third of the lateral thigh and may be bilateral. The onset is often during the 30th week of gestation and is thought to be secondary to increased weight gain and exaggeration of the lumbar lordosis during pregnancy. Meralgia paresthetica is exaggerated by hip extension (standing) and is relieved by rest. It tends to resolve within three months of delivery and often recurs in subsequent pregnancies. Management includes reassuring the patient of the transient nature of the syndrome. In severe cases symptoms may be controlled by infiltration of local anesthesia or hydrocortisone at the level of the anterior superior iliac spine.[57–59]

Traumatic Neuropathies

The passage of a large fetal head through the birth canal, the use of forceps, improper leg position in the stirrups, or trauma with hematoma secondary to cesarean section can cause certain peripheral nerves of the mother to be injured during labor and delivery. The most common injury is postpartum foot drop secondary to compression of the lumbosacral plexus by the fetus's head or a midforceps rotation. It may also result from poorly positioned stirrups that cause compression of the lateral peroneal nerve as it crosses the fibular head. The second most common injury is a femoral neuropathy, which occurs secondary to compression of the femoral nerve during vaginal delivery or cesarean section. It manifests as difficulty climbing steps and

anterior thigh paresthesias. Occasionally, the obturator nerve is compressed, causing weakness in hip adduction and rotation, and decreased sensation to the upper medial thigh.[57–59]

Myasthenia Gravis

Myasthenia gravis (MG) is an autoimmune disorder that causes a decrease in the postsynaptic acetylcholine receptor (AChR) activity at the neuromuscular junction. Clinically, MG is characterized by weakness and fatigue due to involvement of ocular, bulbar, or voluntary muscle groups.[60–62]

Pregnancy has a variable effect on MG. Approximately one-third of pregnant patients go into remission, one-third show no change, and one-third experience a relapse. Of all pregnancy-related exacerbations, a recent study showed that approximately 41% occurred during the pregnancy and approximately 30% occurred in the puerperium. MG increases the incidence of spontaneous abortion and has a 3–10% maternal mortality.[63] Anticholinesterase medication (pyridostigmine) is continued during pregnancy when needed. Numerous medications are detrimental to the patient with MG, and each medication is evaluated prior to use in the patient (see Table 39.3). Principles of management of pregnant patients with myasthenic crises are similar to those of nonpregnant patients. See Chapter 18, "Neuromuscular Disorders," for details.

Neonatal myasthenia gravis (NMG) occurs in 12–19% of live-born infants of myasthenic mothers. The onset may occur within hours of birth to four days postpartum and may last 10 days to 15 weeks.[63] Symptoms include feeding difficulties (87%), generalized weakness (69%), respiratory difficulty (65%), feeble cry (60%), and facial weakness (54%).[64] Treatment may include anticholinesterase drugs (see Chapter 18, "Neuromuscular Disorders," on myasthenia gravis for common dosages).

It must be noted that *magnesium is contraindicated in the pregnant patient* with MG because it increases muscle weakness by decreasing acetylcholine release and decreasing the excitability of the postsynaptic membrane.[60] Alternative therapy for patients with preeclampsia or eclampsia is benzodiazepines or phenobarbital. Phenytoin also is used with caution in the patient with MG.

TABLE 39.3. Drugs Potentially Harmful in Patients with Myasthenia Gravis

Antibiotics	Neuromuscular Blocking Agents	Cardiovascular	Antirheumatics	Anticonvulsants	Others	Psychotropics
Aminoglycosides	Pancuronium	Lidocaine	Chloroquine	Phenytoin	Magnesium sulfate	Lithium carbonate
Neomycin	Succinylcholine	Quinidine	D-penicillamine	Trimethadione	Corticosteroids	Chlorpromazine
Streptomycin		Quinine			Thyroid replacement	
Kanamycin		Procainamide			Adrenocorticotropic hormone	
Gentamicin		Beta-blockers			Anticholinesterases	
Tobramycin		Calcium channel blockers				
Amikacin		Trimethaphan				
Polymyxin A						
Polymyxin B						
Colistin						
Lincomycin						
Clindamycin						
Tetracyclines						

Source: Adapted from Gilchrist JM. Muscle disease in the pregnant woman. In: Devinsky O, Feldmann E, Hainline B, eds. *Neurological Complications of Pregnancy.* New York, NY: Raven Press, Ltd; 1994:193–208.

Cerebrovascular Disease

Introduction

Approximately 5–10% of maternal deaths are due to cerebrovascular disease.[65–67] The incidence of cerebrovascular disease in pregnant women varies widely with the population studied, ranging from 1 per 481 deliveries to 0 per 26,099 live births.[68,69]

In the Parkland experience, 20% of patients with acute strokes died, and 40% of the survivors were left with residual neurological deficits.[70] The Maternal Mortality Collaborative Report noted that of 601 maternal deaths from 1980–85, 8.5% were due to stroke.[66] The mortality rate of ischemic stroke is 30% in pregnant patients versus 10% in age-matched nonpregnant women.[35]

Ischemic Cerebrovascular Disease

Acute arterial occlusion accounts for 60–80% of all cerebral infarcts in pregnancy and the postpartum period.[71,72] Arterial distribution infarcts are more common in the second and third trimesters and first week postpartum, whereas venous thrombosis is more likely to occur early postpartum.[71] Risk factors for ischemic stroke include diabetes, hypertension, and hyperlipidemia.[35]

The exact etiology of cerebral infarcts in the pregnant patient is not understood completely, but the hypercoagulability associated with pregnancy and antiphospholipid antibodies are thought to be contributing factors.[73,74]

Acute cerebral arterial occlusions have been associated with arteriopathies, hematological disorders, cardiogenic emboli from noncardiac sources, and miscellaneous conditions such as substance abuse and migraine. Occasionally, the cause is not found.[75–77]

Sudden and severe hypotension can lead to cerebral infarctions in watershed areas of the brain. It can also result in acute pituitary necrosis (Sheehan's syndrome) during labor and delivery.[78]

Cerebral venous thrombosis is more common in the puerperium. Thrombosis of the sagittal sinus with secondary extension into the cortical veins and a primary thrombosis of the cortical vein are the most common sites involved. The clinical syndrome of venous thrombosis typically presents with progressive headache associated with nausea, vom-

iting, visual disturbances, and altered mentation secondary to increased intracranial pressure. Focal and generalized seizures may occur.[75] Venous infarcts are more likely to be hemorrhagic.[71] Diseases that predispose to this condition include polycythemia vera, cancer, leukemia, dehydration, and sickle cell anemia.[71] The overall mortality rate of patients with cerebral venous thrombosis is approximately equal to 25%.[79]

Hemorrhagic Cerebrovascular Disease

Hemorrhagic stroke is classified as either subarachnoid or intracerebral. Subarachnoid hemorrhage has been reported to be the third most common nonobstetrical cause of maternal death. Subarachnoid hemorrhage may be due to or associated with ruptured aneurysms, AVMs, eclampsia, or "crack" cocaine use.[35] Intracerebral hemorrhage may occur as a result of eclampsia, hypertension not related to eclampsia, ruptured vascular malformations, intracranial venous thrombosis, vasculitis, and choriocarcinoma.[77]

Cerebral aneurysms typically arise at the branching points of major arteries traversing the base of the brain. Approximately 1% of females of reproductive age have a cerebral aneurysm. The probability of rupture is related to the size of the aneurysm.[69,80,81] Clinically, the typical presentation of a ruptured cerebral aneurysm is an explosive headache, vomiting, meningismus, photophobia, mental status change, or coma. Coma, regardless of time of occurrence, is a poor prognostic sign. As many as 50% of patients will have had a less severe or "sentinel" bleed in the preceding weeks or months. A careful review of pertinent clinical details and a thorough neurological evaluation of all pregnant patients with headache aids in the diagnosis of a previously ruptured cerebral aneurysm. The risk of rupture of an aneurysm during pregnancy is controversial, with a recent study showing that pregnancy may have little or no effect on the incidence of rupture.[69] Other studies have suggested that the risk of rupture is approximately five times that of a nonpregnant patient.[82] The risk of subarachnoid hemorrhage due to AVM in the pregnant patient is 85% versus 10%, nonpregnant group, and AVM is the cause of subarachnoid hemorrhage 50% of the time in pregnant patients, as opposed to 10% of the time if in nonpregnant patients. The risk of hemorrhage after an

AVM rupture is 27% in the same pregnancy.[83] AVMs tend to rupture between 20 weeks of gestation and 6 weeks postpartum.[84] Hemorrhage from AVMs during pregnancy carries a 20% mortality rate, as opposed to a 10% mortality rate in the nonpregnant population. The overall mortality rate for patients with a ruptured aneurysm is 35%, which is nearly the same rate for a nongravid patient.[85,86] The incidence of intracerebral hemorrhage from aneurysms and AVMs is approximately equal to 0.07–0.05% of all pregnancies, with 77% due to aneurysms and 23% due to AVMs.[85,87]

It is important to differentiate eclampsia with intracerebral hemorrhage from a ruptured aneurysm or AVM because definitive management differs. Because proteinuria and hypertension occur in approximately 11–34% of patients with intracerebral hemorrhage secondary to AVMs and aneurysms, they cannot be used exclusively to differentiate the hemorrhage associated with eclampsia from that associated with AVM or aneurysm.[87]

Management of Cerebrovascular Events

The emergency department management of the pregnant patient with an acute cerebrovascular event focuses on prompt evaluation and identification of any correctable cause. Appropriate radiographic studies are utilized with shielding of the abdomen to limit exposure of the fetus to the radiation.[35,75] Surgery reduces mortality in patients with a ruptured aneurysm or AVM and should not be withheld in the pregnant patient.[85] Mortality rates from an initial AVM hemorrhage are approximately 10%. When the AVM is not surgically corrected, approximately 33–50% of patients will hemorrhage again, with a 50% mortality rate.[35]

Pseudotumor Cerebri

Pseudotumor cerebri (PC) is defined as prolonged elevation of intracranial pressure without focal neurological deficits, or intracranial pathology, and with normal cerebrospinal fluid (CSF).[35,56,88,89] PC is an uncommon condition that commonly presents in young, obese females and is associated with headache and visual disturbances including diplopia, an enlarged blind spot, blurred vision, and papilledema.

The incidence of PC is 1 per 870 to 1 per 5263 in obstetric patients. It is seen most often in the first half of gestation but can occur at any time.[35,56,88–90] When PC is suspected, a CT scan of the brain is performed and, when negative, lumbar puncture follows. When the opening pressure of lumbar puncture is 250 mm CSF or more in a relaxed patient, the intracranial pressure is elevated.[35,89]

Management of PC to prevent visual loss may include carbonic anhydrase inhibitors to decrease CSF production. Analgesics with codeine can be given for headache. Diuretics are used cautiously in pregnant patients due to decreased placental blood flow from decreased circulating blood volume. Monitoring of amniotic fluid levels with ultrasound is suggested when carbonic anhydrase inhibitors or diuretics are used.[35,56,89]

When these measures are unsuccessful, prednisone for two to four weeks or repeated lumbar puncture for CSF evacuation may be used. A lumboperitoneal shunt may be needed in refractory cases. Occasionally, optic nerve decompression is employed to attempt to improve the patient's vision.[35,56,89,91]

Permanent visual damage may occur, and visual fields are monitored closely. The risk of recurrence in patients during a subsequent pregnancy is 10–30%, which necessitates close follow-up for these patients.[35,88]

Multiple Sclerosis

Multiple sclerosis (MS) is a demyelinating disease of the central nervous system that often affects young women and therefore is of concern when these patients become pregnant. Meta-analysis of clinical studies has indicated a significantly lower rate of relapse during the prepartum period than in the nonpregnant period in the same patients, and the gestational relapse rate is lower than in the nonpregnant period in all female patients. Therefore, pregnancy is a period of relatively decreased MS activity. However, there is a high risk of relapse in the first three months postpartum as compared to pregnant or nonpregnant periods. The individual risk is approximately 20–40%.[92,93]

Delivery is no more complicated in the patient with MS, and obstetrical criteria should guide the mode of delivery. Therapy for the patient with gestational relapse is similar to that for the nonpregnant patient. The lowest possible dose of corticosteroids is used, and the patient is counseled about any risks.

Brain Tumors

The incidence of maternal malignant brain tumors is approximately 3.6 per million live births. It is estimated that in the United States, 90 females per year will have a brain tumor and be pregnant at the same time.[94–96] The effects of brain tumors may mimic common complaints in pregnancy such as headache, nausea, and vomiting. A constant daily headache should not be attributed to pregnancy alone, especially in the patient with no history of headache. Hyperemesis gravidarum is generally maximal in the first trimester and improves thereafter. The nausea and vomiting in patients with brain tumors can occur at any time and persists. A thorough neurological examination is imperative in any patient with hyperemesis or pregnancy-induced headache to assess for abnormal findings. MR or CT scan of the brain is obtained to assess for intracranial pathology in patients in whom symptoms are persistent or progressive. New-onset seizures, especially focal seizures, can be the initial presenting sign of a brain tumor. However, an evaluation for possible eclampsia is necessary.[96] Often pregnant patients with brain tumors develop seizures or elevated intracranial pressure that may require emergency treatment. Antiepileptic drugs and steroids can be used but do present some risk to the fetus.[96]

The type of brain tumor and the patient's clinical course determine the need for and type of treatment. Depending on tumor type, a pregnancy can be allowed to go to term followed by definitive treatment. Radiation therapy in the pregnant patient is teratogenic in the first trimester and increases the risk of childhood leukemia in the second and third trimesters. Chemotherapy is dangerous to the fetus but often can be delayed until after delivery.[96]

PEARLS AND PITFALLS

- Preeclampsia may progress rapidly to eclampsia and status epilepticus.

- In eclampsia, the mainstays of therapy are seizure control, blood pressure control, and limiting fluid intake unless there is documented fluid loss. Use of central nervous system depressants, diuretics, and osmotic agents may worsen maternal, and thus fetal, outcome.

- In eclampsia, delivery is the ultimate goal of therapy. When possible, delivery is delayed until the mother is stable.

- Each patient has her own autoregulatory control of cerebral blood flow and blood pressure. Abnormally high blood pressure may begin at 140/90 in a teenager or at 180/110 in a patient with previous hypertension, resulting in a wide range of blood pressures at the onset of eclampsia. Therefore, there is no absolute blood pressure value above which the diagnosis of eclampsia is certain or below which eclampsia can be excluded.

- Management of seizures may include use of diazepam in small doses; it also involves the use of magnesium sulfate or phenytoin when the etiology is eclampsia.

- In the evaluation of the pregnant patient with upper abdominal pain, a diagnosis of the HELLP syndrome is always considered because imminent delivery is indicated regardless of the fetal gestational age.

- Differentiation of generalized convulsive seizures due to epilepsy from those due to eclampsia is important because in the latter, delivery is part of the definitive treatment.

- Magnesium is contraindicated in the eclamptic patient with MG.

REFERENCES

1. Loudon I. Some historical aspects of toxemia of pregnancy. A review. *Br J Obstet Gynaecol.* 1991;98: 853–8.
2. Davey DA, MacGillivray I. The classification and definition of the hypertensive disorders of pregnancy. *Am J Obstet Gynecol.* 1988;158:892–8.
3. Baird D. Epidemiological aspects of hypertensive pregnancy. *Clin Obstet Gynecol.* 1974;4:531.
4. Sibai BM, McCubbin JH, Anderson GD, et al. Eclampsia I. Observations from 67 recent cases. *Obstet Gynecol.* 1981;58:609–13.
5. Lopez-Llera M, Linares GR, Horta JLH. Maternal mortality rates in eclampsia. *Am J Obstet Gynecol.* 1976;124:149–55.

6. Kolawole TM, Patel PJ, Yaqub B, et al. Computed tomographic changes of the brain in toxemia of pregnancy. *European J Radiol.* 1990;11:46–53.

7. Cunningham FG, MacDonald PC, Gant NF. Hypertensive disorders in pregnancy. In: *Williams Obstetrics.* 18th ed. Norwalk, Conn: Appleton and Lange; 1989; 653–94.

8. Cummingham FG, MacDonald PC, Gant NF, Leveno KJ, Gilstrap LC III. Common complications of pregnancy. *Williams Obstetrics.* 19th ed. Norwalk, Conn: Appleton & Lange; 1993:763–803.

9. Eguchi K, Lin YT, Noda K, et al. Differentiation between eclampsia and cerebrovascular disorders by brain CT scan in pregnant patients with convulsive seizures. *Acta Med Okayama.* 1987;41:117–24.

10. Mandelkern D, Burger A. Cortical blindness in postpartum preeclampsia progressing to eclampsia: case report. *Mount Sinai J Med.* 1992;59:72–4.

11. Lau SP, Chan FL, Yu YL, et al. Cortical blindness in toxemia of pregnancy: findings on computed tomography. *Br J Radiol.* 1987;60:347–9.

12. Donaldson JO. Eclampsia. In: Donaldson JO, ed. *Neurology of Pregnancy.* 2nd ed. Philadelphia, Pa: WB Saunders Co; 1989;269–310.

13. Coughlin WF, McMurdo SK, Reeves T. MR imaging of postpartum cortical blindness. *J Comput Assist Tomogr.* 1989;13:572–6.

14. Will AD, Lewis KL, Hinshaw DB, et al. Cerebral vasoconstriction in toxemia. *Neurology.* 1987;37:1555–7.

15. Sibai BM, Anderson GD, McCubbin JH. Eclampsia II. Clinical significance of laboratory findings. *Obstet Gynecol.* 1982;59:153–7.

16. Dunn R, Lee W, Cotton DB. Evaluation by computerized axial tomography of eclamptic women with seizures refractory to magnesium sulfate therapy. *Am J Obstet Gynecol.* 1986;155:267–8.

17. Raroque HG, Orrison WW, Rosenberg GA. Neurologic involvement in toxemia of pregnancy: reversible MRI lesions. *Neurology.* 1990;40:167–9.

18. Brown CE, Purdy P, Cunningham FG. Head computed tomographic scans in women with eclampsia. *Am J Obstet Gynecol.* 1988;159:915–20.

19. Sibai BM, Abdella TN, Spinnato JA, Anderson GD. Eclampsia: V. The incidence of nonpreventable eclampsia. *Am J Obstet Gynecol.* 1986;154:581–6.

20. Dalessio DJ. Seizure disorders and pregnancy. *N Engl J Med.* 1985;312:559–63.

21. Kaplan PW, Lesser RP, Fisher RS, et al. No, magnesium sulfate should not be used in treating eclamptic seizures. *Arch Neurol.* 1988;45:1361–4.

22. Kaplan PW, Lesser RP, Fisher RS, et al. A continuing controversy: magnesium sulfate in the treatment of eclamptic seizures. *Arch Neurol.* 1990;47:1031–2.

23. Pritchard JA, Cunningham FG, Pritchard SA. The Parkland Memorial Hospital protocol for treatment of eclampsia: evaluation of 245 cases. *Am J Obstet Gynecol.* 1984;148:951–63.

24. Sibai BM. Magnesium sulfate is the ideal anticonvulsant in preeclampsia eclampsia. *Am J Obstet Gynecol.* 1990;162:1141–5.

25. McCubbin JH, Sibai BM, Abdella TN, et al. Cardiopulmonary arrest due to acute maternal hypermagnesaemia. *Lancet.* 1981;1058.

26. Moosa SM, Zayat SG. Phenytoin infusion in severe preeclampsia. *Lancet.* 1987:1147–8.

27. Ryan G, Lange IR, Naugler MA. Clinical experience with phenytoin prophylaxis in severe preeclampsia. *Am J Obstet Gynecol.* 1989;161:1297–304.

28. Slater RM, Wilcox FL, Smith WD, et al. Phenytoin infusion in severe preeclampsia. *Lancet.* 1987;1: 1417–21.

29. Appleton MP, Keuhl TJ, Raebel MA, et al. Magnesium sulfate versus phenytoin for seizure prophylaxis in pregnancy-induced hypertension. *Am J Obstet Gynecol.* 1991;165:907–13.

30. Hennessy A, Horvath JS. Newer antihypertensive agents in pregnancy. *Med J Aust.* 1992;156:304–5.

31. Calhoun DA, Oparil S. Treatment of hypertensive crisis. *N Engl J Med.* 1990;323:1177–83.

32. Weinstein L. Syndrome of hemolysis, elevated liver enzymes, and low platelet count: a severe consequence of hypertension in pregnancy. *Am J Obstet Gynecol.* 1982;142:159–67.

33. Krumholz A. Epilepsy and pregnancy. In: Goldstein PJ, ed. *Neurological Disorders of Pregnancy.* Mount Kisco, NY: Futura Publishing Co; 1986;65–88.

34. Collaborative Perinatal Study of the National Institute of Neurological Diseases and Stroke: Neurologic and Psychiatric Conditions. In: Niswander KR, Gordon MJ, Berendes HW, eds. *Women and Their Pregnancies.* Philadelphia, Pa: WB Saunders Co; 1972.

35. Albert JR, Morrison JC. Neurological diseases in pregnancy. *Obstet Gynecol Clin North Am.* 1992;19:765–81.

36. Yerby MS, Devinsky O. Epilepsy and pregnancy. In: Devinsky O, Feldmann E, Hainline B, eds. *Neurological Complications of Pregnancy.* New York, NY: Raven Press, Ltd; 1994:45–64.

37. Donaldson JO. Epilepsy. In: Donaldson JO, ed. *Neurology of Pregnancy.* 2nd ed. Philadelphia, Pa: WB Saunders Co; 1989;228–68.

38. Jones KL, Lacro RV, Johnson KA, et al. Pattern of malformations in the children of women treated with carbamazepine during pregnancy. *N Engl J Med.* 1989; 320:1661–6.

39. Lindhout D, Omtzigt J, Cornel MC. Spectrum of neural-tube defects in 34 infants prenatally exposed to antiepileptic drugs. *Neurology.* 1992;42(suppl 5): 111–18.

40. Friis ML, Hauge M. Congenital heart defects in liveborn children of epileptic parents. *Arch Neurol.* 1985;42:374–6.

41. Cunningham FG, MacDonald PC, Gant NF, Leveno KJ, Gilstrap LC III. *Williams Obstetrics.* 19th ed. Norwalk, Conn: Appleton & Lange; 1993:1243–58.

42. Gimovsky ML, Petrie R. Maternal anticonvulsants and fetal hemorrhage. A report of two cases. *J Reprod Med.* 1986;31:61–2.

43. Jagoda A, Riggio JA. Emergency department approach to managing seizures in pregnancy. *Ann Emerg Med.* 1991;20:80–5.

44. Reik L. Headaches in pregnancy. *Semin Neurol.* 1988; 8:187–92.

45. Rapoport AM. The diagnosis of migraine and tension-type headache, then and now. *Neurology.* 1992;42 (suppl 2):11–15.

46. Gonzalez MD, Rutecki GW, Whittier FC. Headaches in a pregnant woman with a history of preeclampsia. *Hosp Pract.* 1993;28(10A):79–82.

47. Feller CM, Franko-Filipasic KJ. Headaches during pregnancy: diagnosis and management. *J Perinat Neonatal Nurs.* 1993;7:1–10.

48. Epstein MT, Hockaday JM, Hockaday TD. Migraine and reproductive hormones throughout the menstrual cycle. *Lancet.* 1975;1:543–8.

49. Lance JW, Anthony M. Some clinical aspects of migraine. *Arch Neurol.* 1966;15:356–61.

50. Cameron JD, Lane PL, Speechley M. Intravenous chlorpromazine vs intravenous metoclopramide in acute migraine headache. *Acad Emerg Med.* 1995;2: 597–602.

51. Dalessio DJ. Classification and treatment of headache during pregnancy. *Clin Neuropharmacol.* 1986;9:121–31.

52. Rogers JD, Fahn S. Movement disorders and pregnancy. In: Devinsky O, Feldman E, Hainline B, eds. *Neurological Complications of Pregnancy.* New York, NY: Raven Press, Ltd; 1994:163–78.

53. Donaldson JO. Movement disorders. In: Donaldson JO, ed. *Neurology of Pregnancy.* 2nd ed. Philadelphia, Pa: WB Saunders Co; 1989:87–102.

54. Donaldson JO. Neurological emergencies in pregnancy. *Obstet Gynecol Clin North Am.* 1991;18: 199–212.

55. Aminoff MJ. Pregnancy and disorders of the nervous system. In: Aminoff MJ, ed. *Neurology and General Medicine.* 2nd ed. New York, NY: Churchill Livingstone; 1995:567–83.

56. Bray RS, Lynch R, Gossman RG, et al. Management of neurosurgical problems in pregnancy. *Clin Perinatol.* 1987;14:243–57.

57. Donaldson JO. Neuropathy. In: Donaldson JO, ed. *Neurology of Pregnancy.* 2nd ed. Philadelphia, Pa: WB Saunders Co; 1989:23–59.

58. Beric A. Peripheral nerve disorders in pregnancy. In: Devinsky O, Feldmann E, Hainline B, eds. *Neurological Complications of Pregnancy.* New York, NY: Raven Press, Ltd; 1994:179–92.

59. Cohen BS, Felsenthal G. Peripheral nervous system disorders and pregnancy. In: Goldstein PJ, ed. *Neurological Disorders of Pregnancy.* Mount Kisco, NY: Futura Publishing Co; 1986:153–96.

60. Reptke JT, Klein VR. Myasthenia gravis in pregnancy. In: Goldstein PJ, ed. *Neurological Disorders of Pregnancy.* Mount Kisco, NY: Futura Publishing Co; 1986;213–34.

61. Donaldson JO. Muscle disease. In: Donaldson JO, ed. *Neurology of Pregnancy.* 2nd ed. Philadelphia, Pa: WB Saunders Co; 1989;61–85.

62. Gilchrist JM. Muscle disease in the pregnant woman. In: Devinsky O, Feldmann E, Hainline B, eds. *Neurological Complications of Pregnancy.* New York, NY: Raven Press, Ltd; 1994:193–208.

63. Plauché WC. Myasthenia gravis in mothers and their newborns. *Clin Obstet Gynecol.* 1991;34:82–99.

64. Namba T, Brown SB, Grob D. Neonatal myasthenia gravis: report of two cases and review of the literature. *Pediatrics.* 1970;45:488–504.

65. Gibbs CE. Maternal death due to stroke. *Am J Obstet Gynecol.* 1974;199:69–75.

66. Rochat RW, Koonin LM, Atrash HK, Jewett JJ, et al. Maternal mortality in the United States: report from the maternal mortality collaborative. *Obstet Gynecol.* 1988;72:91–7.

67. Kaunitz AM, Hughes JM, Grimes DA, et al. Causes of maternal mortality in the United States. *Obstet Gynecol.* 1985;65:605–12.

68. Srinivasan K. Cerebral venous and arterial thrombosis in pregnancy and puerperium: a study of 135 patients. *Angiology.* 1983;34:731–46.

69. Wiebers DO, Whisnant JP. The incidence of stroke among pregnant women in Rochester, Minn, 1955–1979. *JAMA.* 1985;254:3055–7.

70. Simolke GA, Cox SM, Cunningham FG. Cerebrovascular accidents complicating pregnancy and the puerperium. *Obstet Gynecol.* 1991;78:37–42.

71. Wiebers DO. Ischemic cerebrovascular complications of pregnancy. *Arch Neurol.* 1985;42:1106–13.

72. Cross JN, Castro PO, Jennett WB. Cerebral strokes associated with pregnancy and the puerperium. *Br Med J.* 1968;3:214–21.

73. Levine SR, Welch KMA. Antiphospholipid antibodies. *Ann Neurol.* 1989;26:386–9.

74. Branch DW. Antiphospholipid antibodies and pregnancy: maternal implications. *Semin Perinatol* 1990; 14:139–46.

75. Wilterdink JL, Easten JD. Cerebral Ischemia. In: Devinsky O, Feldmann E, Hainline B, eds. *Neurological Complications of Pregnancy.* New York, NY: Raven Press, Ltd; 1994:1–11.

76. Brick JF. Vanishing cerebrovascular disease of pregnancy. *Neurology.* 1988;38:804–6.

77. Biller J, Adams HP Jr. Cerebrovascular disorders associated with pregnancy. *Am Fam Physician.* 1986;33: 125–32.

78. Wong MCW, Giuliani MJ, Haley EC Jr. Cerebrovascular disease and stroke in women. *Cardiology.* 1990;77 (suppl 2):80–90.

79. Krayenbuhl HA. Cerebral venous and sinus thrombosis. *Clin Neurosurg.* 1967;14:1–24.

80. Holcomb WL Jr, Petrie RH. Cerebrovascular emergencies in pregnancy. *Clin Obstet Gynecol.* 1990;33:467–72.

81. Stehbens WE. Aneurysms and anatomical variation of cerebral arteries. *Arch Pathol.* 1963;7:45.

82. Wiebers DO. Subarachnoid hemorrhage in pregnancy. *Semin Neurol.* 1988;8:226–9.

83. Robinson JL, Hall CJ, Sedzimir CB. Arteriovenous malformations, aneurysms and pregnancy. *J Neurosurg.* 1974;41:63–70.

84. Sadasivan B, Malki GM, Lee C, Ausman JI. Vascular malformations and pregnancy. *Surg Neurol.* 1990;33:305–13.

85. Dias MS, Sekhar LN. Intracranial hemorrhage from aneurysms and arteriovenous malformations during pregnancy and the puerperium. *Neurosurgery.* 1990;27:855–65.

86. Heros RC, Yong-Kwang T. Is surgery necessary for unruptured arteriovenous malformations? *Neurology.* 1987;37:279–86.

87. Dias MS. Neurovascular emergencies in pregnancy. *Clin Obstet Gynecol.* 1994;37:337–54.

88. Digre KB, Varner MW, Corbett JJ. Pseudotumor cerebri and pregnancy. *Neurology.* 1984;34:721–8.

89. Koontz WL, Herbert WNP, Cefalo RC. Pseudotumor cerebri in pregnancy. *Obstet Gynecol.* 1983;62:324–7.

90. Durcan FJ, Corbett JJ, Wall M. The incidence of pseudotumor cerebri, population studies in Iowa and Louisiana. *Arch Neurol.* 1988;45:875–7.

91. Keltner JL, Albert DM, Lubow M, et al. Optic nerve decompression. *Arch Ophthalmol.* 1977;95:97–104.

92. Birk K, Rudick R. Pregnancy and multiple sclerosis. *Arch Neurol.* 1986;43:719–26.

93. Cook SD, Troiano R, Bansil S, et al. Multiple sclerosis and pregnancy. In: Devinsky O, Feldmann E, Hainline B, eds. *Neurological Complications of Pregnancy.* New York, NY: Raven Press, Ltd; 1994:83–95.

94. Haas JF, Janisha W, Staneczek W. Newly diagnosed primary intracranial neoplasms in pregnant women: a population based assessment. *J Neurol.* 1986;49:874–80.

95. Simon RH. Brain tumors in pregnancy. *Semin Neurol.* 1988;8:214–21.

96. DeAngelis LM. Central nervous system neoplasms in pregnancy. In: Devinsky O, Feldmann E, Hainline B, eds. *Neurological Complications of Pregnancy.* New York, NY: Raven Press, Ltd; 1994:139–52.

SEVEN Neurotoxicology and Brain Resuscitation

40 Neurotoxicology

MARY BETH MILLER

SUMMARY Neurological symptoms are common to all toxidromes. The key to successful treatment of the poisoned patient in the emergency department is good supportive care. Airway, breathing, and circulation are stabilized as in any other critically ill patient. A specific antidote may not be available for most poisoned patients. Efforts are focused on basic medical management and decontamination measures. The recognition of toxidromes, or common features associated with specific categories of toxins, helps to narrow the differential diagnosis and aids in medical management.

Introduction

The American Association of Poison Control Centers Toxic Exposures Surveillance System reported over 1,900,000 human exposures in 1994. Eleven percent of these were defined as intentional. Children under 3 years of age accounted for 40% of the poison exposure.[1] Due to inherent flaws in the reporting system, these data underrepresent the true incidence of the problem. Of those patients requiring medical intervention, most seek care in the emergency department.

Any individual with a history of intentional ingestion is taken to the nearest emergency department for evaluation. When the individual is unwilling to be transported, the police are contacted so that the patient can be restrained legally as needed. A person who has attempted to commit suicide is not considered competent to refuse transportation to an emergency department. Those individuals whose ingestion is determined to require no further medical treatment still require psychiatric evaluation.

Prehospital Management

Stabilization of the patient takes priority in prehospital patient care. A set of vital signs is obtained, the level of consciousness is assessed, and appropriate supportive treatment is instituted as warranted. Treatment with oxygen, thiamine, glucose, and naloxone is considered in all unconscious patients. A history is obtained. Useful information regarding known ingestion includes the name of medication taken, and how much, when, and for whom the medication was prescribed. It is useful to have a family member collect all medications to which the patient has had access, including all nonprescription items and herbal/vitamin preparations.

Emergency Department Evaluation

General Approach to the Poisoned Patient

In the emergency department, vital signs including temperature are reassessed. Airway, breathing, and circulation are assessed and stabilized before further treatment is instituted. Endotracheal intubation and assisted ventilation are performed for patients with hypoxia or respiratory compromise. Hypotension is treated initially with a bolus of intravenous fluids when there is no contraindication. External warming or cooling measures are initiated to correct abnormal core body temperatures.

The unconscious patient requires additional stabilization measures. Rapid determination of blood glucose level is done at the bedside and levels of less than 60 mg/dl are treated with 50 ml of 50% dextrose in the adult, 4 ml/kg of 25% dextrose in children, and 5 ml/kg of 10% dextrose in neonates. Thiamine, 100 ml, is given intravenously prior to the administration of glucose in adults to prevent the precipitation of a Wernicke's encephalopathy. The use of naloxone is indicated for patients in coma, or those with respiratory depression, pinpoint pupils, or circumstantial evidence of opioid abuse. The initial dose is 2 mg given intravenously in adults and children (0.01 mg/kg in neonates), although as much as 10 mg may be needed in some cases. Flumazenil is not used routinely in the unconscious patient because it can precipitate withdrawal symptoms in those patients chronically using benzodiazepines[2] and its use has been associated with seizures in the setting of mixed ingestions, particularly tricyclic antidepressants.[3–6]

A comprehensive history and physical examination follow. Family members, friends, or emergency medical services personnel can provide pertinent information for those patients who are unable or unwilling to provide a history. The time, type, and route of exposure, and all substances to which the patient had access, are determined. A list of all nonprescription medications, vitamins, herbal preparations, and household chemicals is helpful. Treatments rendered at home are required. A medical, psychiatric, and alcohol or substance abuse history is sought. A social history including occupation and hobbies can be helpful. A thorough physical and neurological examination are required, especially when the diagnosis is unclear. A careful examination can reveal a clinical pattern consistent with one of the toxidromes described below. It is important to undress the patient fully to allow detailed inspection.

Laboratory evaluation includes analysis of arterial blood gas and serum electrolyte levels to determine the presence of acidosis. A pregnancy test in women of childbearing age is done when applicable. An electrocardiographic tracing helps to determine the presence of drugs such as tricyclic antidepressants that can cause dysrhythmias. Possible aspiration pneumonia or noncardiogenic pulmonary edema is assessed on a chest radiograph. Alcohol and acetaminophen levels are obtained. Toxico-logical screening tests can detect the presence of unexpected substances but rarely alter decisions regarding clinical management.[7] Specific drug levels (such as aspirin, theophylline) are obtained when specific ingestion is suspected.

Decontamination is performed for every patient with suspected poisoning. Inhalation and dermal exposures can be treated by removal from the source of exposure. Dermal exposure requires flushing with water. Care is taken to prevent the emergency department staff from additional exposure. When the substance is known, the regional poison center can provide information regarding the extent of precautions to be taken by the staff.

Gastrointestinal decontamination is an essential part of treatment, but is not performed until after securing stable vital signs, particularly the airway. The best method of decontamination has been the subject of controversy for a long time (see Fig. 40.1). Syrup of ipecac, once favored by many as initial home treatment, can remove only 40% of the ingested material under optimal conditions and has not been shown to change clinical outcome. Its use is contraindicated in the presence of acids or alkalis. In patients with diminished mental status who are unable to protect their airway, vomiting can cause aspiration of gastric contents. Therefore, syrup of ipecac is not used in patients with ingestion of a substance known to cause central nervous system depression or seizures. Additionally, syrup of ipecac can delay the administration of charcoal by as long as 100 minutes.[8] For these reasons, its use is not recommended in the hospital setting.

Gastric lavage is a frequently used means of decontamination. Studies have demonstrated a limited "recovery rate" of approximately 40% of desired material from gastric lavage. Risks associated with its use include perforation of the stomach and aspiration of gastric contents. In comparison to the use of charcoal, lavage offers additional benefit only when performed within one hour of ingestion. When used, gastric lavage is accomplished by oral placement of a large-bore tube (36–40 French in adults, 16–28 French in children) because the diameter of a nasogastric tube is too small to remove most pills. Patients are placed head down on the left side in an attempt to prevent aspiration. With obtundation or no gag reflex, the airway is protected by endotracheal intubation before lavage is undertaken. Aliquots of

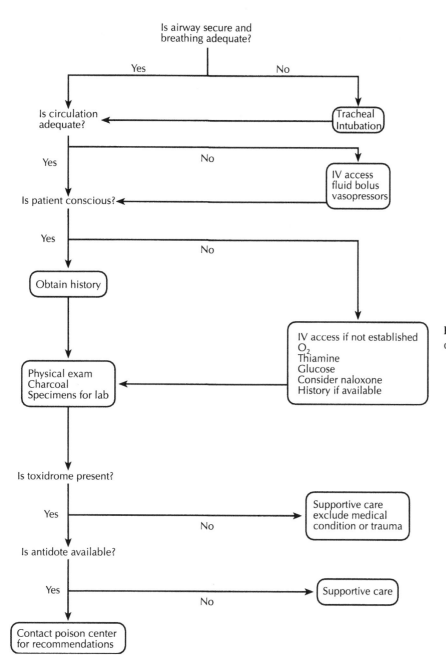

FIGURE 40.1. General management of the poisoned patient.

water no larger than 300 ml are used to avoid pushing gastric contents into the duodenum. Normal saline is used in children to avoid electrolyte imbalance. Gastric lavage is restricted to those patients who present to the emergency department within one hour of a life-threatening ingestion.

Activated charcoal can adsorb most compounds by virtue of its large surface area and thus help prevent the absorption of ingested compounds by the gastrointestinal tract. Activated charcoal can be self-administered by cooperative patients or it can be placed through a small-bore nasogastric tube. The use of activated charcoal as the sole method of decontamination is now advocated by many toxicologists because several studies have confirmed the lack of any additional benefits of gastric emptying (by ipecac or gastric lavage) when charcoal is administered.[8–10] A recent policy statement by the American College of Emergency Physicians supports this approach.[11] The concomitant use of sorbitol to increase transit time through the gut has not been shown to enhance the efficacy of charcoal.[12,13]

TABLE 40.1. Substances Not Significantly Adsorbed by Activated Charcoal

Borates
Bromide
Ethanol
Iron
Lithium
Mineral acids and alkalis
Potassium

The use of sorbitol is not recommended in children because it can cause electrolyte imbalances, and when aspirated, can increase the patient's risk of developing pulmonary edema due to its high osmolarity. The use of multidose activated charcoal can provide good clinical results, but consistent clinical benefits are not proven and its use can lead to bowel obstruction.[14,15] Charcoal is administered in a dose of 1 g/kg to patients suspected of poisoning and to those who have ingested a substance in a potentially toxic dose. Drugs not significantly adsorbed by charcoal are listed in Table 40.1.

When there is a potential diagnosis of poisoning, medical care providers tend to concentrate their efforts on the search for an antidote. The majority of ingested poisons do not have a specific antidote. In fact, most poisoned patients respond to supportive care. Each antidote has its own specific set of indications and contraindications, making indiscrimination use harmful in some cases. Contact with the regional poison control center can aid in the identification and administration of such antidotes.

Recognition and Treatment of Toxidromes

Treatment of a patient with a known ingestion is rarely complicated. Challenging situations include an unknown poison or ingested substance, an unconscious individual with an unknown history, and an alert patient who does not appreciate the relationship between the potentially lethal exposure and benign current symptoms.

The term *toxidrome* was first used in 1970 to describe a constellation of symptoms and signs that indicate poisoning by a particular group of toxins.[16] Recognition of these toxidromes can narrow the diagnostic focus and aid in management. In addition, symptoms not consistent with a toxidrome of a "known" ingestion suggest a coingestant. Many new toxidromes have been added to the list detailed initially; the basic and most frequently encountered toxidromes in the emergency department are reviewed here.

Cholinergic Syndrome

The neurotransmitter acetylcholine is found throughout the nervous system and binds to receptors in the sympathetic and parasympathetic nervous systems, and the neuromuscular junction (Fig. 40.2). Its effects are terminated by the enzyme acetylcholinesterase (AChE), which converts it to acetic acid and choline. Inhibition of AChE by compounds such as organophosphates and carbamate insecticides leads to the accumulation of acetylcholine and overstimulation of its receptors, causing a characteristic set of symptoms and signs commonly known as the cholinergic syndrome.

Organophosphates comprise a group of structurally similar compounds that phosphorylate the active site of AChE, rendering it inactive. The compound becomes irreversibly bound over the next 24–72 hours by a process known as "aging." Once aging has occurred, only renewed synthesis can replenish the supply of AChE, and standard antidotes are ineffective. Carbamate insecticides are N-methyl carbamates, which can bind and inactivate AChE. Unlike organophosphates, their binding is hydrolyzed and thus reversible. Because no aging occurs with N-methyl carbamates, symptoms typically resolve within 24–48 hours after absorption is complete. Because thiocarbamate herbicides and fungicides are not N-methyl carbamates, they do not inhibit AChE and therefore do not produce similar symptoms.

Organophosphate and carbamate insecticides are readily absorbed by dermal, inhalation, and oral routes. Exposure to high concentrations of these agents results in immediate symptoms. Symptoms begin within 12 hours of a significant ingestion; most symptoms manifest within the first 8 hours. The duration of symptoms depends on the lipid solubility of the particular agent. Symptoms are prolonged when

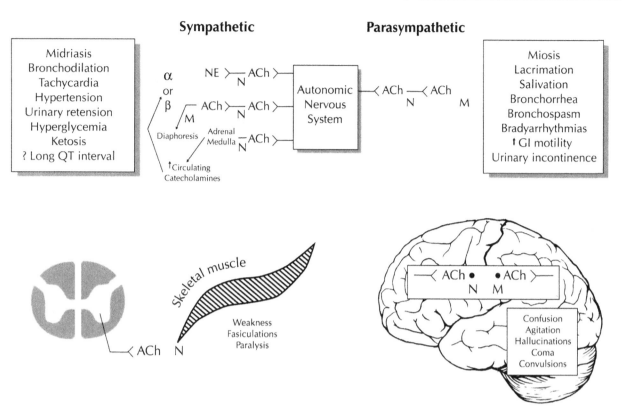

FIGURE 40.2. Pathophysiology of cholinergic poisoning syndrome. ACh = acetylcholine; GI = gastrointestinal; M = muscle; N = nerve; NE = norepinephrine. Adapted from Clark RF, Curry SC. Organophosphates and Carbonates. In Reisdorff EJ, Roberts MR, Wigenstein JC. *Pediatric Emergency Medicine,* Philadelphis, Pa.: WB Saunders Co, 1993: 685. Used with permission

the ingested agent has high lipid solubility. The characteristic findings of excessive muscarinic activity are summarized by the mnemonic SLUDGE (salivation, lacrimation, urination, defecation, gastric emptying) or DUMBELS (defecation, urination, miosis, bronchorrhea, emesis, lacrimation, salivation). Because AChE is not restricted to the parasympathetic nervous system, other findings can be present. Increased sympathetic tone can cause tachycardia or mydriasis, and stimulation of nicotinic receptors can cause fasciculations, weakness, and eventually paralysis (see Fig. 40.2).

The management of the patient with cholinergic syndrome begins with assessment of the airway (Fig. 40.3). Bronchospasm and increased secretions pose an immediate threat to the airway. Endotracheal intubation is performed when appropriate. Atropine is a competitive inhibitor of muscarinic receptors and can be used to control excess parasympathetic findings. Patients receive atropine until bronchospasm is resolved and oral secretions are controlled. Atropine is not to be withheld due to tachycardia or mydriasis. The dosage is higher than usually used (2–5 mg of atropine sulfate, given by intravenous push every two to three minutes for adults, and 0.05 mg/kg, given by intravenous push every two to three minutes in children) and can exhaust the supply of the standard hospital. A continuous intravenous infusion of atropine can be used for refractory or recurring symptoms. Atropine has no effect on nicotinic cholinergic receptors and does not reverse weakness or paralysis.

Pralidoxime (2-PAM) is an antidote for organophosphate poisoning. 2-PAM contains a quaternary nitrogen that is attracted to the anionic site of AChE where 2-PAM is phosphorylated and bound by the organophosphate, thus rejuvenating AChE. Because this reaction occurs only when "aging" has not occurred, 2-PAM is most effective when administered early in the course of therapy. The dose for adults is

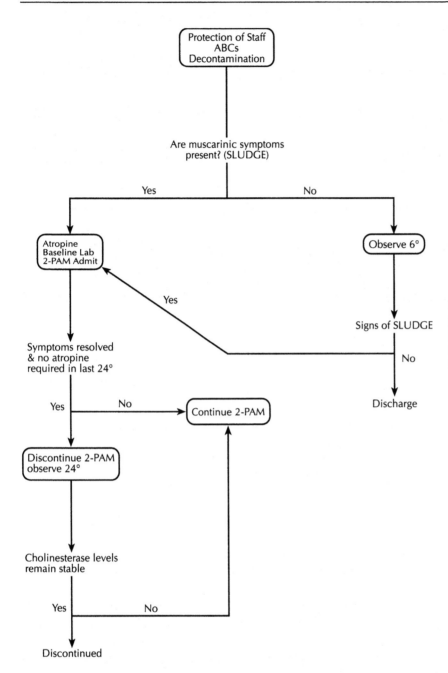

FIGURE 40.3. Management of the patient with cholinergic syndrome. 2-PAM = pralidoxime; SLUDGE = salivation, lacrimation, urination, defecation, gastric emptying.

1–2 gms given intravenously over 10–15 minutes followed by an infusion of 250–500 mg per hour; for children, there is a loading dose of 25 mg/kg and an infusion of 10–20 mg/kg per hour. Although the efficacy of 2-PAM in known carbamate exposures is uncertain, it is best to administer this antidote when the type or name of the compound is unknown.

Decontamination measures are instituted once the patient is stabilized. For oral exposure, lavage may be indicated and charcoal is administered. Dermal exposure requires thorough cleaning measures.

All the patients clothing is removed, and the skin is washed thoroughly with soap and water. Care is taken to clean all skin folds because very small amounts of compound in areas such as the navel can prolong toxicity. Hair is washed repeatedly or shaved. Due to the solubility of these agents, medical staff should be careful to prevent exposure to themselves when treating patients.

Only a nerve biopsy can help to determine synaptic levels of AChE; therefore, red blood cell (RBC) and plasma cholinesterase levels are usually measured. Treatment is not withheld when cholinesterase values are not known. Instead, baseline values are obtained to confirm clinical suspicion, and the rise or fall of these values is used to direct therapy. 2-PAM is continued for 24 hours following resolution of symptoms. RBC and plasma cholinesterase levels are repeated in 24 hours. The stable patient can be discharged to home. A return of symptoms or a fall in RBC and plasma cholinesterase levels to 25–50% of previous levels leads to reinstitution of 2-PAM. Because RBC cholinesterase levels can be decreased long after neuronal levels are adequate, it is not necessary to wait for a "normal" laboratory value before discharging the patient. Most patients with a significant exposure require hospitalization for at least 3 days.

Patients who recover from severe acute toxicity can exhibit confusion, depression, fatigue, and behavioral changes.[17] Most of these effects resolve within a year of exposure.[18] An "intermediate syndrome" that is reported to occur within in 24–96 hours of acute poisoning is most likely explained by residual toxicity of the agent and inadequate treatment.[19] Chronic toxicity results in vague neurological complaints and mild muscarinic symptoms.

Anticholinergic Syndrome

Many medications have anticholinergic properties (Table 40.2). These drugs exert their effects by blocking muscarinic cholinergic receptors throughout the nervous system (Fig. 40.2). Central manifestations include sedation, confusion, agitation, and hallucinations. Patients exhibit a characteristic mumbling speech or repetitive picking at bedsheets and clothing. When exposure is severe, coma and seizures can result. Peripheral effects include fever; flushed, dry skin; anhydrosis (particularly of the axilla); tachycardia; diminished gastrointestinal motility; mydriasis; and urinary retention. Patients can exhibit all, some, or none of the findings described.

Management of an anticholinergic syndrome is supportive. Continuous cardiac monitoring is instituted. Adequate hydration is maintained by intravenous administration of fluids. In expectation of urinary retention, a Foley catheter is placed in the bladder. Tachycardia usually does not require treatment. External cooling methods are used to reduce body temperature when required. Agitation can contribute to fever and lead to rhabdomyolysis, and is

controlled with intravenous benzodiazepines. The use of haloperidol is recommended because of its minimal anticholinergic properties. Profoundly agitated patients may require the use of paralytic agents and mechanical ventilation. Seizures are treated with benzodiazepines or barbiturates. Physostigmine is a cholinesterase inhibitor capable of reversing both central and peripheral anticholinergic effects. Although once commonly used as an antidote, physostigmine has many serious side effects such as bronchospasm, bronchorrhea, bradycardia, heart block, and seizures and is known to increase morbidity.[20–22] The use of physostigmine is reserved for patients whose agitation cannnot be controlled successfully by the use of benzodiazepines or haloperidol.

Adrenergic Syndrome

Both pharmaceutical and illicit compounds can exert adrenergic effects (Table 40.3). Symptoms due to excess catecholamines include tachycardia, hypertension, agitation, tremulousness, mydriasis, hyperreflexia, and metabolic acidosis. Treatment follows the general guidelines reviewed above, and no specific antidote exists. The effects of the adrenergic compound theophylline are reviewed in the section on seizures, below.

Coma and Respiratory Depression

Although many drugs depress the level of consciousness and respiratory drive, the agents most frequently responsible for these effects include narcotics, sedative/hypnotics, and alcohol. The toxicity from any of these agents can cause hypotension, hypothermia, pulmonary edema, and hyporeflexia. Pinpoint pupils suggest narcotic overdose, but this can be masked in drugs such as meperidine (due to its anticholinergic properties) or by the effects of coingestants (see Chapter 41, "Neurotoxicology of Alcohol and Substances of Abuse").

Seizures

A variety of substances cause seizures by lowering seizure threshold, or secondarily from respiratory depression and hypoxia. Poisoning from a select few compounds present with seizure as the initial manifestation of the toxicity.

The most effective way to control seizure activity caused by poisoning is by increased gamma-

TABLE 40.2. Substances with Anticholinergic Effects

Antiarrythmics
Disopyramide
Quinidine
Procainamide

Antihistamines
Astemizole
Azatadine
Brompheniramine
Carbinoxamine
Clemastine
Chlorpheniramine
Cyclizine
Cyproheptadine
Diphenhydramine
Hydroxyzine
Loratadine
Methscopolamine
Phenyltoloxamine
Pyrilamine
Terfenadine
Tripelennamine
Trimeprazine
Tripolindine

**Antinausea drugs/
motion sickness agents**
Dimenhydrinate
Meclizine
Prochlorperazine
Promethazine
Scopolamine
Trimethobenzamide

Antiparkinsonian agents
Amantadine
Benztropine
Biperiden
Ethopropazine
Procyclidine
Trihexyphenidyl

Antipsychotics
Acetophenazine
Chlorprothixene
Chlorpromazine
Clozapine
Fluphenazine
Loxapine
Fluphenazine
Mesoridazine
Molindone
Perphenazine
Promazine
Thioridazine
Thiothixene
Trifluoperazine

Antispasmodics
Cinnamedrine
Clidinium
Dicyclomine
Flavoxate
Hycosamine
Methantheline
Oxybutynin
Propantheline
Tridihexethyl

Cyclic antidepressants
Amitriptyline
Amoxapine
Clomipramine
Desipramine
Doxepin
Imipramine
Maprotiline
Nortriptyline
Protriptyline
Trimipramine

Ophthalmic agents
Atropine
Cyclopentolate
Homatropine
Tropicamide

Plants
Amanita muscaria
Amanita pantherina
Aropa belladonna
Datura stramonium
Mandragora
officinarum

Skeletal muscle relaxants
Cyclobenzaprine
Orphenadrine

Sleep aids
Diphenhydramine
Doxylamine

Miscellaneous
Atropine
Bupropion
Carbamazepine
Glutethimide
Glycopyrolate
Meperidine
Quinine

TABLE 40.3. Substances Causing Adrenergic Syndrome

Albuterol
Amphetamines and derivatives
Caffeine
Cocaine
Dopamine
Dobutamine
Ephedrine/pseudoephedrine
Epinephrine/norepinephrine
Isoproterenol
Methylphenidate
Phenylephrine
Phenylpropanolamine
Theophylline

---

aminobutyric acid (GABA)ergic inhibition of the central nervous system. Both benzodiazepines and barbiturates enhance the activity of GABA and are used in controlling poison-induced seizures. Diazepam and lorazepam are useful for initial seizure control but have relatively short half-lives. Phenobarbitol is used for prolonged control of seizure activity. Typically, phenytoin is ineffective or increases morbidity when used to treat drug- and toxin-induced seizures, particularly seizures induced by ingestion of theophylline or tricyclic antidepressants.[23-25] The use of phenytoin to control seizures is not recommended when the etiology of seizure is suspected to be poisoning. Although most drug-induced seizures respond to standard measures, several compounds require special attention and are discussed below.

Theophylline. Theophylline and other methylxanthines exert their effect by competitive inhibition of adenosine receptors. Presynaptic adenosine receptor activation normally inhibits release of excitatory neurotransmitters. Postsynaptic adenosine receptor activation hyperpolarizes the cell, making it more difficult to reach threshold. The central nervous system symptoms of theophylline toxicity are agitation, tremulousness, and seizures. Similarly, effects of theophylline on the peripheral adrenergic nervous system include tachycardia, cardiac arrhythmias, metabolic acidosis, and rhabdomyolysis.

Adenosine's actions include initiating the interictal phase of seizure. Thus blockade of adenosine receptors can lead to refractory seizures or status epilepticus. Because seizures are the main cause of mortality in theophylline toxicity, prophylactic use of phenobarbital at a dose of 10–20 mg/kg is recommended in severely poisoned patients. The use of phenytoin is avoided. Hemodialysis may be helpful in treating patients with severe theophylline toxicity or when seizures have occurred.

Tricyclic Antidepressants. The most significant properties of tricyclic antidepressants clinically are the anticholinergic effects and the inhibition of sodium channels. It is the latter phenomenon that accounts for the prolongation of the QRS interval of the electrocardiogram. Prolongation of the QRS interval of greater than 100 milliseconds results in an increased probability of developing cardiac arrhythmias and seizures.[26] Sodium bicarbonate is used to increase the serum pH and raise serum sodium concentration, both of which are felt to reverse the effects of sodium channel blockade. Sodium bicarbonate is given until the serum pH is 7.45–7.5, followed by 150 mEq of sodium bicarbonate mixed with one liter of D5W and administered at a rate of 2 ml/kg per hour. Serial measurements of blood pH are used to adjust the infusion rate accordingly. Bicarbonate therapy does not control seizure activity, and other agents such as benzodiazepines and phenobarbital are used.

Isoniazid. Isoniazid (INH) is used in the treatment of tuberculosis, a disease that is currently undergoing resurgence. It is a competitive inhibitor of the enzyme pyridoxine kinase, which is necessary for the synthesis of GABA. Signs of toxicity include vomiting, abdominal pain, coma, metabolic acidosis, and seizures. Seizures usually are refractory to standard treatment, because potentiation of GABA receptor–mediated inhibition by benzodiazepine or barbiturates may not be sufficient when GABA levels are depleted. It is thought that administration of pyridoxine (vitamin B_6) restores this deficiency. For every gram of INH ingested, 1 g of pyroxidine is given intravenously; 5 g are given initially when the amount of ingested INH is unknown.

Lithium. Lithium is a drug used in the treatment of bipolar disorder and has a narrow therapeutic index. Symptoms of chronic toxicity occur despite "therapeutic" serum levels. Clinical findings of toxicity include nausea, vomiting, bradycardia, conduction abnormalities, mental status changes, agitation, fasciculations, hyperreflexia, coma, and seizures. Adequate hydration and restoration of normal sodium levels enhances the renal excretion of lithium. Charcoal does not bind lithium effectively due to its small molecular size. Dialysis is considered for those patients with coma, seizure, cardiovascular toxicity, renal failure, or failure to respond to supportive measures.

Coma and Metabolic Acidosis

An overdose of many compounds can cause metabolic acidosis; examples of commonly ingested agents are reviewed here. Although the finding of metabolic acidosis is the key to diagnosing the ingested compound, the assessment of acid–base status can be complicated by coexisting medical conditions such as dehydration from vomiting or previous seizure.

Salicylates. Salicylates are available in prescription and over-the-counter preparations. They are typically combined with other analgesics to enhance pain relief. A significant overdose of salicylate can result in initial symptoms of vomiting, tinnitus, and respiratory alkalosis and can progress to metabolic acidosis, coma, and seizures. Hypoglycemia can be an additional clue to the diagnosis of salicylate intoxication, especially in children. Glucose levels in cerebrospinal fluid may be low despite normal serum levels, mimicking meningeal irritation. Falling serum levels of salicylate may signal worsening toxicity by indicating movement of the drug from blood into tissue where uncoupling of oxidative phosphorylation occurs. Management of salicylate toxicity includes alkalinization of the urine, which enhances renal elimination. Sodium bicarbonate, 150 mEq, and potassium chloride, 40 mEq, are added to 1 l D5W and administered at two to three times the maintenance rate. Bicarbonate

therapy helps maintain a blood pH of 7.45–7.5, maintain normal blood potassium levels, and maintain urine pH of greater than 7.5. The Dome nomogram has many limitations, and a decision to initiate treatment is best made on clinical grounds. Salicylate levels are drawn and repeated at six hours after ingestion. Asymptomatic patients with low and falling blood salicylate levels can be discharged after psychiatric evaluation. Symptomatic patients are hospitalized and alkalinization is initiated. Hemodialysis is considered for seizures, renal failure, pulmonary edema, or when urinary alkalinization cannot be achieved. The most common presentation of chronic salicylate toxicity is mental status change. Salicylate levels may be within therapeutic range. Treatment is similar to that of acute salicylate toxicity.

Acetaminophen. Acetaminophen is a known hepatotoxin. A patient with significant acetaminophen poisoning can rarely present with coma, renal insufficiency, and metabolic acidosis. Toxicity occurs through the metabolism of acetaminophen to a toxic electrophilic compound that is normally detoxified by glutathione. When the supply of glutathione is depleted, the electrophile is free to bind to macromolecules, causing hepatocellular injury. Acetaminophen levels obtained 4–24 hours postingestion can be plotted on the Rumack-Matthew nomogram to determine the need for treatment (Fig. 40.4). The antidote *N*-acetylcysteine is a precursor to glutathione and likely exerts its antidotal effect by replenishing depleted glutathione stores. Patients with an acetaminophen level on or above the lower line of the Rumack-Matthew nomogram receive a loading dose of *N*-acetylcysteine at 140 mg/kg given orally, followed by 70 mg/kg every 4 hours for an additional 17 doses. No change in dose is necessary when charcoal is administered, and antiemetic medications can be used to control vomiting.

Toxic Gases. Several toxic gases inhibit cytochrome oxidase, resulting in the inhibition of cellular respiration and anaerobic metabolism. Examples of toxic gases include carbon monoxide (CO), cyanide, and hydrogen sulfide. Poisoning by CO may be heralded by nausea, vomiting, and headache.

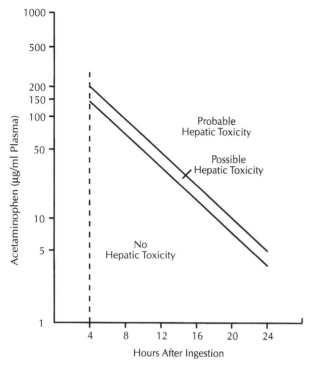

FIGURE 40.4. The Rumack-Matthew nomogram for acetaminophen toxicity (adapted from Rumack and Matthew[29]).

This "nonspecific" presentation is commonly mistaken for influenza ("the flu"). History of exposure to exhaust fumes, gas and coal heaters, house fire, or "sewer gas" alerts the physician to the diagnosis. Treatment of all gases includes removal of the source and supportive measures to assure adequate ventilation. The half-life of CO is reduced by administration of 100% O_2. Hyperbaric oxygen is capable of further reducing the half-life of CO and may not alter the clinical outcome in most patients. Cyanide poisoning is treated by administration of the Lilly Cyanide Antidote Kit which includes instructions for its use. Because the issues surrounding treatment of these gases are complex, contact with a regional poison center is recommended.

Altered Mental Status, Rigidity, and Hyperthermia

Neuroleptic Malignant Syndrome. Neuroleptic malignant syndrome (NMS) is a disorder likely associated with dopamine blockade or depletion in the central nervous system. Symptoms can develop one to seven days after the initiation of the offending agent, typically a neuroleptic and can also occur regardless of the duration of its use. Patients who appear to be ill present with mental status changes, elevated temperature, and autonomic instability. Rigidity can lead to respiratory compromise and rhabdomyolysis. Treatment consists of supportive measures and institution of rapid cooling measures. Although not clearly demonstrated to be effective, dantrolene (0.8–3.0 mg/kg given intravenously every six hours) and bromocriptine (5 mg given orally followed by 2.5–10 mg given orally every eight hours) are commonly used for muscle relaxation and dopamine receptor agonism, respectively. Neuromuscular blocking agents can be used when rhabdomyolysis is severe.

Serotonin Syndrome. Serotonin syndrome is caused by an excess stimulation of serotonin receptors that results from a combination of drugs affecting serotonin receptors, not from an overdose of a single drug. Serotonin syndrome is known to occur with discontinuation of one drug and the initiation of an another before the therapeutic effects of the initial drug have dissipated. A common example is the patient who stops taking monoamine oxidase inhibitor (MAOI) medication and is immediately started on a selective serotonin reuptake inhibitor (SSRI) medication. Symptoms such as head turning, shivering, and leg rigidity may make it possible to distinguish this syndrome from NMS. The patient's medication list may provide important clues (Table 40.4). Treatment includes discontinuation of the offending agent(s) and supportive measures. Cyproheptadine, an antihistamine with nonspecific serotonin antagonist properties, has been used with success in some cases.[27]

PEARLS AND PITFALLS

■ Poisoning is considered in the differential diagnosis of a patient with a "neurological presentation."
■ Coexisting medical illness and occult trauma is considered in a patient with poisoning.
■ Patients with anticholinergic syndrome can be misdiagnosed as having psychiatric illness.

TABLE 40.4. Neuroleptic Malignant Syndrome versus Serotonin Syndrome

	Neuroleptic Malignant Syndrome	Serotonin Syndrome
Commonly Implicated Drugs	Anti-Parkinson agents	Antidepressants (monoamine oxidase inhibitor, selective serotinin reuptake inhibitor, tricyclic antidepressant)
	Butyrophenones	Dextromethorphan
	Phenothiazines	meperidine
Onset after dose	Gradual	Immediate
Altered mental status	Common	Possible
Muscle rigidity	Diffuse	Rare
Hyperthermia	Common	Possible
Autonomic disturbances	Common	Possible
Diaphoresis	Common	Common
Diarrhea	Rare	Common
Head turning	No	Possible
Myoclonus	Rare	Common
Nystagmus	No	Possible
Shivering	Rare	Possible
Elevated creatine phosphokinase	Common	Rare

■ Coingestants are considered in a poisoned patient with a known ingestion.

REFERENCES

1. Litovitz TL, Felberg L, Soloway RA, Ford M, Geller R. 1994 Annual Report of the American Association of Poison Control Centers Toxic Exposure Surveillance System. *Am J Emerg Med*. 1995;13:551–97.
2. Amrein R, Leishman B, Bentzinger C, et al. Flumazenil in benzodiazepine antagonism: actions and clinical use in intoxications and anesthesiology. *Med Toxicol*. 1987;2:411–29.
3. Derlet RW, Albertson TE. Flumazenil induces seizures and death in mixed cocaine-diazepam intoxications. *Ann Emerg Med*. 1994;23:494.
4. Lheureux P, Vranckx M, Leduc D, et al. Flumazenil in mixed benzodiazepine/tricyclic antidepressant overdose: a placebo controlled study in the dog. *Am J Emerg Med*. 1992;10:184–8.
5. Mordel A, Winkler E, Almog S, et al. Seizures after flumazenil administration in a case of combined benzodiazepine and tricyclic antidepressant overdose. *Crit Care Med*. 1992;20:1733–4.
6. Weinbroum A, Halpren P, Geller E. The use of flumazenil in the management of acute drug poisoning: a review. *Crit Care Med*. 1991;17:S32–8.
7. Kellerman AL, Finn SD, LoGerto JP, Copass MK. Impact of drug screening in suspected overdose. *Ann Emerg Med*. 1987;16:1206–16.
8. Kornberg AE, Dolgen J. Pediatric ingestions: charcoal alone versus ipecac and charcoal. *Ann Emerg Med*. 1991;20:648–51.
9. Albertson TE, Derlet RW, Foulke GE, et al. Superiority of activated charcoal alone compared with ipecac and activated charcoal in the treatment of acute toxic ingestions. *Ann Emerg Med*. 1989;18:56–9.

10. Merigan KS, Woodard M, Hedges JR, et al. Prospective evaluation of gastric emptying in the self poisoned patient. *Am J Emerg Med.* 1989;8:479–83.

11. American College of Emergency Physicians. Clinical policy for the initial approach to patients presenting with acute toxic ingestion or dermal or inhalational exposure. *Ann Emerg Med.* 1995;25:570–85.

12. McNamara RM, Aaron CK, Gemborys M, et al. Sorbitol catharsis does not enhance efficacy of charcoal in a simulated acetaminophen overdose. *Ann Emerg Med.* 1988;17:243–6.

13. Neuvonen PJ, Olkkoal KT. Effect of purgatives on antidotal efficacy of oral activated charcoal. *Hum Toxicol.* 1986;5:255–63.

14. Campbell J, Chyka P. Physiochemical characteristics of drugs and response to repeat dose activated charcoal. *Am J Emerg Med.* 1992;10:208–10.

15. Watson WA, Cremes KF, Chapman JA. Gastrointestinal obstruction associated with multiple dose activated charcoal. *J Emerg Med.* 1986;4:401–7.

16. Mofensen HC, Greensher J. The nontoxic ingestion. *Pediatr Clin North Am.* 1970,17:583–90.

17. Tabershaw IR, Cooper C. Sequelae of acute organic phosphate poisoning. *J Occup Med.* 1966;8:5–20.

18. Gershon S, Shaw FH. Psychiatric sequelae of chronic exposure to organophosphate insecticides. *Lancet.* 1961;1:1371–74.

19. Curry SC. Organophosphate-associated "intermediate syndrome": for real? *AACT Clinical Toxicology Update.* 1994;7:1–2.

20. Levy R. Arrhythmias following physostigmine administration in jimsonweed poisoning. *Journal of the American College of Emergency Physicians.* 1977;6:107.

21. Pentel P, Peterson C. Asystole complicating physostigmine treatment of tricyclic overdose. *Ann Emerg Med.* 1980;9:588.

22. Tong TG, Benowitz NC, Becker C. Tricyclic overdose. *Drug Intell Clin Pharm.* 1976;10:711.

23. Goldberg MJ, Spector R, Miller G. Phenobarbital improves survival in theophylline-intoxicated rabbits. *J Toxicol Clin Toxicol.* 1986;24:203–11.

24. Beaubein AR, Carpenter DC, Mathieu LF, et al. Antagonism of imipramine poisoning by anticonvulsants in the rat. *Toxicol Appl Pharmacol.* 1976;38:1–6.

25. Callaham M, Schumaker H, Pentel P. Phenytoin prophylaxis of cardiotoxicity in experimental amitriptyline poisoning. *J Pharmacol Exp Ther.* 1988;245:216–20.

26. Boehnert MT, Lovejoy FH. Value of the QRS duration versus the serum drug level in predicting seizures and ventricular arrhythmias after an acute overdose of tricyclic antidepressants. *N Engl J Med.* 1985;313:474–9.

27. Goldberg RJ, Huk M. Serotonin syndrome from trazodone and buspirone. *Psychosomatics.* 1992;33:235.

28. Clark RF, Curry SC. Organophosphates and carbamates. In: Reisdorff EJ, Roberts MR, Wiegenstein JC, eds. *Pediatric Emergency Medicine.* Philadelphia, Pa: WE Saunders Co; 1993:685.

29. Rumack BH, Matthew H. Acetaminophen poisoning and toxicity. *Pediatrics.* 1975;55:873.

41 Neurotoxicology of Alcohol and Substances of Abuse

SCOTT R. ZITTEL, MARY ELLEN WERMUTH, BRENT FURBEE, AND MARY BETH MILLER

SUMMARY The common neurological complications of alcohol abuse include intoxication syndrome, withdrawal syndrome, alcohol neuropathy, alcohol myopathy, and Wernicke-Korsakoff syndrome. The clinical effects of sedative hypnotic intoxication are similar to those of alcohol intoxication and include ataxia, nystagmus, hypotension, and coma. The hallmarks of narcotic overdose are respiratory depression, coma, and pinpoint pupils. Neurological manifestations of the stimulants, cocaine and amphetamines, include agitation, tremulousness, mydriasis, hyperreflexia, and seizure. Complications of intravenous drug abuse are subacute bacterial endocarditis, meningitis, epidural abscess, mycotic aneurysm, mononeuropathy, and transverse myelitis. Management of these cases is directed at basic stabilization, identification of associated illness, and appropriate pharmacological intervention. Referral for treatment of dependency is made.

Introduction

Approximately 5.5 million people in the United States meet psychiatric criteria for drug abuse disorder. An additional 13 million people meet criteria for alcohol abuse. At least 40% of all hospital admissions and 25% of deaths are related to substance dependence and abuse. Unfortunately, the effects of these addictions reach beyond the lives of these patients. Fifty percent of highway fatalities and cases of domestic violence are associated with drug or alcohol intoxication. At their first prenatal visit, up to 15% of pregnant women have a positive urine screen for drugs of abuse.[1] A high index of suspicion for drug and alcohol abuse in a large segment of the patient population is prudent.

Emergency Department Evaluation

Ethanol

Ethanol is the most commonly used recreational drug in the world. Neurological manifestations of alcohol consumption include neuropathy, myopathy, seizures, stroke, Wernicke-Korsakoff syndrome, metabolic derangement (such as hypoglycemia or acidosis), altered mental status, and coma. Ethanol abuse accounts for about 50% of traffic fatalities and 25% of nontraffic accidental deaths in the United States.

Acute Alcohol Intoxication. Acute ethanol intoxication causes a spectrum of neurological effects ranging from disinhibition and loss of fine motor control

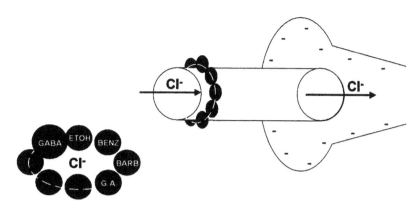

FIGURE 41.1. The GABA receptor on the postsynaptic chloride channel. Stimulation of the GABA receptor leads to an influx of chloride ions (Cl). The resulting hyperpolarization of the postsynaptic neuron produces an inhibitory effect. Indirect stimulation of GABA occurs via ethanol (ETOH), benzodiazepines (BENZ), barbiturates (BARB), general volatile anesthetics (G.A.), and other sedative hypnotics (not pictured).

to nystagmus, dysarthria, ataxia, and coma. Slurred speech, euphoria, disorientation, aggression, and violence are seen in the intoxicated patient with lower blood alcohol levels. As intake increases, impairments of coordination, reaction time, thinking, and judgment occur. These effects are partially produced through gamma-aminobutyric acid (GABA), an inhibitory neurotransmitter of the central nervous system (CNS).[2] Ethanol is an allosteric modulator of the GABA$_A$ receptor and enhances the GABA-mediated influx of chloride ions through the receptor's associated ion channel, and into postsynaptic neurons. The resultant postsynaptic hyperpolarization is responsible for the inhibitory effect of ethanol (see Fig. 41.1).

In alcohol "nontolerant" individuals, blood ethanol levels correlate with neurological impairment to an extent (see Table 41.1).[3] Tolerance of alcohol allows many individuals to survive and maintain

function at much higher levels. Treatment is primarily supportive, and hospital admission is usually not required unless complications such as respiratory compromise occur. Possible traumatic, metabolic, and infectious etiologies are investigated in patients whose mental status does not steadily improve with time. Caffeine, naloxone, and flumazenil are ineffective in counteracting the inebriating effects of ethanol.[4–6] Hemodialysis is used in rare life-threatening conditions caused by profound ethanol intoxication. The CAGE Questionnaire for Alcohol Abuse can help identify those with an alcohol abuse problem. The CAGE Questionnaire for Alcohol Abuse lists four questions. Positive answers to two or more questions indicate a high likelihood of alcoholism.

1. Have you felt you should *cut down* on your drinking?

TABLE 41.1. Clinical Correlation of Blood Alcohol Levels

Blood Ethanol Level (mg/dl)	Clinical Findings
30–120	Fine motor skills less efficient
90–250	Loss of critical judgment, increased reaction time, some muscle incoordination
180–300	Ataxia, muscle incoordination, slurred speech
270–400	Impaired consciousness, incontinence, inability to stand
350–500	Coma, respiratory depression, peripheral vascular collapse
>450	Death from respiratory paralysis

2. Have people *annoyed* you by criticizing your drinking?
3. Have you felt bad or *guilty* about your drinking?
4. Have you ever had a drink first thing in the morning to steady your nerves or get rid of a hangover (*eye-opener*)?

Patients can be safely discharged from the emergency department when alert, oriented, and ambulatory. Information regarding Alcoholics Anonymous or other available substance abuse programs is given at the time of discharge from the emergency department.

Neurological Complications of Chronic Alcohol Abuse

ALCOHOLIC NEUROPATHY. The typical presentation of alcoholic neuropathy is burning pain in the hands and feet, and aching pain in the calves. This pain can be so severe that even light touch can cause discomfort. Typically, symptoms begin in the legs and progress proximally in a symmetrical distribution. Neurological examination may reveal loss of light touch and vibratory sensation, and decreased or absent Achilles and patellar deep tendon reflexes. Muscle wasting and weakness are prominent in the distal extremities. On a neuropathological level, axonal degeneration and demyelination are related to nutritional deficiency or the direct neurotoxic effects of alcohol. A specific vitamin deficiency is yet to be determined. However, treatment is targeted toward resuming a balanced diet with supplementation of B vitamins. Recovery is typically slow and incomplete.

"Saturday night palsy" is characterized by acute onset of wrist drop secondary to radial nerve compression from an arm drooped over the back of a chair or bench, indirectly related to alcohol use at times. Treatment includes use of a cock-up wrist splint. Most episodes resolve spontaneously.

ALCOHOLIC MYOPATHY. Acute alcoholic myopathy is an uncommon but potentially life-threatening complication of chronic alcohol consumption. It is characterized by an elevated creatinine phosphokinase (CPK) level and rhabdomyolysis. Symptoms include acute onset of pain, cramps, tenderness, weakness, and swelling of the legs during a period of prolonged heavy drinking. Myoglobinuria can lead to renal failure and death. Treatment consists of intravenous fluids and alkaline- (sodium bicarbonate) induced diuresis.

WERNICKE-KORSAKOFF SYNDROME. Wernicke's encephalopathy (WE) is characterized by nystagmus, abducens and conjugate gaze palsies, ataxia of gait, and disturbances of consciousness.[7] The onset of these symptoms is either acute or insidious, and the symptoms occur either singly or in various combinations. Wernicke's disease is due to nutritional deficiency of thiamine. Encountered primarily in alcoholic patients, WE is also seen in conditions associated with nutritional deficiencies.

Pathological studies demonstrate bilateral CNS lesions that almost always involve the mamillary bodies. Periventricular structures, especially the tissue around ventricles III and IV and the aqueduct, are commonly involved. Studies utilizing magnetic resonance imaging (MRI) have shown periventricular lesions in up to 80% of patients.[7]

Chronic alcohol abuse leads to thiamine deficiency due to dietary deficiency, decreased gastrointestinal absorption, and depleted hepatic stores. The selective loss of neurons associated with thiamine deficiency may be due to impaired cellular energy metabolism, focal accumulation of lactate and ensuing acidosis, or excitotoxic damage due to the effects of N-methyl-D-aspartate (NMDA) receptor activation by glutamate.[11] Particularly vulnerable areas of the CNS demonstrate a marked increase in metabolic activity and lactate production shortly before the development of WE lesions. This appears to represent a shift from aerobic metabolism to rapid glycolysis associated with a reduction of pyruvate dehydrogenase activity.[12,13] Studies in rat have shown that in thiamine-deficient states, glutamate induces excitotoxic injury in the CNS. This injury is mitigated by thiamine replacement in the early stages of thiamine deficiency.[14] Ethanol has been shown to inhibit glutamate receptors (specifically, NMDA). This chronic inhibition leads to an increase in the number of NMDA receptors and may explain the greater severity of CNS damage observed in alcoholics with WE than in nonalcoholics.[15,16]

WE rarely progresses to Korsakoff's psychosis; however, the continued use of alcohol appears to contribute to that development. Korsakoff's psychosis, observed primarily but not exclusively in alcoholic patients, is characterized by a severe loss of retentive memory, and confabulation. Confabulation is an important feature of Korsakoff's psychosis, in which the patient fills gaps in memory with "made-up stories." Memory impairment, apathy, visuoperceptive abnormalities, and difficulties with problem solving, planning, and abstract thinking are common. Personality changes are also noted.[10] Korsakoff's psychosis is considered to be the psychiatric manifestation of WE. The term *Wernicke's encephalopathy* refers to the symptom complex comprising ophthalmoparesis, nystagmus, ataxia, and an acute global confusional state. When features of Korsakoff's psychosis such as memory and learning loss and confabulation are observed in combination with WE, the symptom complex is called Wernicke-Korsakoff syndrome.

Oculomotor abnormalities such as nystagmus and lateral rectus palsy with dysconjugate gaze are common manifestations of WE and were reported to occur in 96% patients with WE in one study.[8] Nystagmus can be either horizontal or vertical. Weakness of external rectus muscle is observed in combination with weakness or paralysis of conjugate gaze. The palsy of conjugate gaze varies from rapidly extinguishing nystagmus on extreme gaze to a complete loss of ocular movement in that direction. This reflects involvement of vestibular nuclei and oculomotor and abducens nerve involvement.

Gait disturbances are present in the vast majority of patients with WE. These vary from ataxia characterized by abnormal tandem gait, to a severe degree of ataxia where sitting or standing requires assistance. Upper extremity ataxia and dysarthria are observed in 20% of patients.

Mental status changes in patients with Wernicke-Korsakoff syndrome commonly manifest as "global confusional states." Patients appear apathetic, inattentive, and indifferent to their surroundings. Stupor and coma are rare initial manifestations of WE. When Wernicke-Korsakoff syndrome is not diagnosed in its early stages, progressive deterioration of mental status can lead to stupor, coma, and death.

The body stores of thiamine are exhausted in 7–8 weeks in the chronic alcoholic or a patient with persistent vomiting. Administration of glucose when thiamine stores are depleted can cause either precipitation of WE or an early form of the disease to progress rapidly. A single dose of 100 mg of thiamine has been reported to have resolved symptoms in about 3 hours.[17] The exact amount of thiamine re-

quired to treat WE is not known. Blood pyruvate levels are elevated in patients with untreated WE; a more accurate index of thiamine deficiency is blood transketolase. The recommended practice for treating thiamine deficiency is to titrate the amount of administered thiamine to clinical response. Both oral and intravenous regimens are used, and doses range from 50–500 mg of thiamine per day. One recommendation is infusion of 500 mg of thiamine over 10 minutes every 8 hours for 2 days, then 500 mg per day until oral thiamine is tolerated, at which time 100 mg per day is administered.[18] Complete recovery from ataxia occurs in less than 50% of affected patients. Recovery begins within a week of starting thiamine and is maximal by 7 months.[19]

ALCOHOL WITHDRAWAL SYNDROME. Alcohol withdrawal is characterized by a constellation of signs and symptoms that occur after abrupt cessation or reduction of alcohol consumption. Alcohol stimulates GABA receptors, leading to inhibition of neuronal activity. In addition, alcohol inhibits the excitatory effects of NMDA receptor activation. After cessation or reduction of alcohol consumption, the chronic inhibitory effect on neuronal excitability, impulse conduction, and transmitter release is removed. Rebound excitability is clinically manifested as "withdrawal."[20] The biochemical basis of withdrawal seizures is not clearly understood. However, chronic alcohol consumption increases the concentration of calcium channels in neuronal preparations, fostering catecholamine release and lowering seizure threshold.[21] Chronic exposure to ethanol reduces adenosine receptor-stimulated cyclic adenosine monophosphate(cAMP) levels. Adenosine is known to have "endogenous anticonvulsant" properties; hence, decreased cAMP may explain generation of alcohol withdrawal seizures.[22]

Symptoms of alcohol withdrawal develop 6–48 hours after the patient's last drink and may occur before the blood alcohol level has returned to zero. The severity of withdrawal is related to the dose of alcohol consumed and the duration of consumption. Symptoms generally peak by 48–72 hours and subside within 4–5 days.[23] After abstinence from alcohol the patient may first complain of an intense craving for alcohol and "the shakes." Other symptoms of early withdrawal can include autonomic hyperactivity, nausea, anorexia, tremor, diaphoresis, tachycardia, hypertension, insomnia, and anxi-

TABLE 41.2. Symptoms of Ethanol Withdrawal

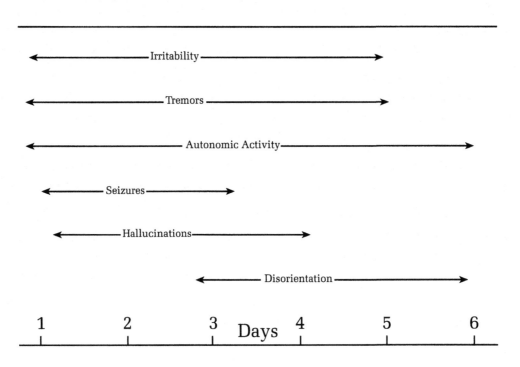

ety. Late alcohol withdrawal is distinguished from early withdrawal by delirium and confusion. The mental status changes of late withdrawal generally begin approximately 48 hours after alcohol cessation are accompanied by profound autonomic hyperactivity and volume depletion (see Table 41.2).

Alcohol withdrawal seizures develop in about a third of untreated patients experiencing alcohol withdrawal. Arising 24–48 hours from the last drink, alcohol withdrawal seizures are generalized and typically single or paired, but can also be multiple.[24] Status epilepticus is uncommon in alcohol withdrawal seizures; it occurs in 3–4% of patients with withdrawal seizures.[25] Focal or multiple seizures should prompt the search for an intracranial lesion.

A comprehensive history and physical examination is necessary for the alcoholic patient. The possibility of alcohol–drug combination, head injury, and cervical spine trauma is considered in patients with altered mental status. Coexisting medical problems, which may have caused the patient to discontinue drinking, are sought and treated. A history of seizures during withdrawal is elicited, because similar patterns tend to occur with each episode. A quiet, supportive environment is essential in caring

for an alcoholic patient. Intravenous fluid therapy is begun as needed. Parenteral administration of thiamine and folic acid is considered.

Acute alcohol withdrawal and alcohol withdrawal seizure are best treated with intravenous diazepam or lorazepam. Lorazepam is principally metabolized in the kidney and is therefore well suited for patients with hepatic disease. Barbiturates, like benzodiazepines, have cross-tolerance with ethanol and are effective in treating seizures and withdrawal symptoms. An advantage of phenobarbital for treatment of alcohol withdrawal seizure is its long duration of action (half-life is approximately 90 hours).

Although beta-adrenergic receptor blockers and clonidine are used to suppress the peripheral manifestations of alcohol withdrawal, they do not prevent seizures: They are used in combination with benzodiazepines for the treatment of alcohol withdrawal symptoms. When hallucination or delirium is unresponsive to benzodiazepines, the neuroleptic agent haloperidol can be given. Antipsychotic agents such as haloperidol are ineffective in treating the underlying withdrawal state and have the potential to lower seizure threshold.

The routine use of magnesium sulfate in alcohol withdrawal is not recommended unless the serum

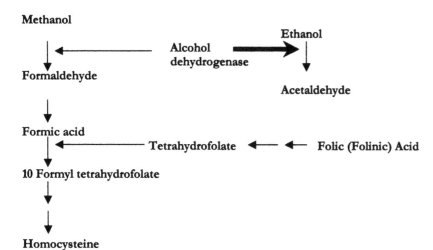

Methanol

Formaldehyde

Formic acid

10 Formyl tetrahydrofolate

Homocysteine

Ethanol

Alcohol dehydrogenase

Acetaldehyde

Tetrahydrofolate ← ← Folic (Folinic) Acid

FIGURE 41.2. Metabolism of methanol. Methanol is metabolized by alcohol dehydrogenase to formaldehyde. Formic acid is the major toxic metabolite. The administration of folate increases conversion of formic acid to 10-formyl tetrahydrofolate, ultimately forming the nontoxic compound homocysteine. The administration of ethanol competes with alcohol dehydrogenase to inhibit the production of formic acid.

magnesium level is low.[26,27] The antiepileptic drug phenytoin does not have a beneficial effect in controlling alcohol withdrawal seizures and is not administered except in the treatment of underlying idiopathic epilepsy.[28] Neither carbamazepine nor valproate is effective in treating withdrawal seizures.[29]

STROKE. The incidence of hemorrhagic and ischemic stroke among heavy drinkers is disproportionately high. Comorbid conditions such as coagulation defects from hepatic disease, hypertension, and smoking contribute to the increased incidence of stroke in alcoholic patients.

Toxic Alcohols

Methanol and ethylene glycol are alcohols found in numerous industrial and household products. Methanol, used as an industrial solvent, is also found in products such as "Sterno." Methanol is used as a gasoline antiknock additive, in antifreeze agents, and in windshield wiper fluid. Ethylene glycol is used in antifreeze agents, deicing agents, fire extinguishers, and refrigerator coolants. Because of their widespread commercial use and easy availability, often they are ingested as "cheap" ethanol substitutes. However, unlike acute ethanol intoxication, acute methanol and ethylene glycol ingestion can lead to permanent neurological damage.

Metabolism and Relevant Pathophysiology

The toxic alcohols methanol and ethylene glycol are both metabolized through the same hepatic enzyme system to toxic intermediaries. Methanol is initially metabolized to formaldehyde by the en-

zyme alcohol dehydrogenase, which is then converted to formic acid (see Fig. 41.2). Typically, formate is metabolized to a nontoxic metabolite homocysteine, a process that requires folic acid (see Fig. 41.2). Formic acid impedes aerobic cellular respiration by inhibiting cytochrome-c and -aa_3 oxidases, leading to metabolic acidosis.[30–32] The presence of acidosis further inhibits cellular respiration and leads to the accumulation of formic acid by inhibiting its metabolism. In optic nerve tissue, inhibition of cytochrome oxidase by formic acid results in the lack of adenosine triphosphate (ATP) formation and subsequent loss of axonal conduction.[33,34] This leads to demyelination of the optic nerve, which helps explain the ocular toxicity of methanol.

Ethylene glycol is initially metabolized to glycolaldehyde via alcohol dehydrogenase; following a series of metabolic reactions, glyoxylic acid and eventually oxalic acid are formed. Glycolic acid appears to be the primary contributor to the development of metabolic acidosis. Oxalic acid forms a complex with calcium to form calcium oxalate. The precipitation of calcium oxalate crystals in the kidneys is responsible for the development of renal failure. Crystal depositions are found in renal, myocardial, pulmonary, and cerebral tissues.[31]

Clinical Manifestations

Symptoms of methanol poisoning typically take 12–24 hours to develop after ingestion, secondary to the slow metabolism of methanol to formic acid. Initially, CNS depression is fairly mild; however, as the metabolic acidosis develops, somnolence, coma, and seizures develop. Nausea, vomiting, abdominal pain, and pancreatitis also occur. Visual disturbances and blindness are the hallmark of methanol poisoning. Eye pain, blurry vision, or blindness can be unilateral or bilateral.[31] Physical examination reveals impaired visual acuity, dilated pupils with a poor pupillary light reflex, and papilledema.[31,35] Visual impairment can be permanent; however, recovery from blindness has been reported.[31] Putamenal hemorrhage and necrosis with corresponding motor impairment is observed in patients with methanol poisoning. Symptoms are similar to those of Parkinson's disease, with predominant findings of dystonias and hypokinesis. Although improvement in motor impairment is observed in some patients when given levodopa, others have little response.[36,37] It is unknown why the basal ganglia and, specifically, the putamen are preferentially affected in methanol poisoning. Various hypotheses include the pattern of venous drainage for the putamen, a greater susceptibility of the putamen to hypoxic and ischemic damage, or a direct cellular toxin affecting the putamen.[37]

Ethylene glycol poisoning is divided into three clinical stages. Stage 1 develops within 30 minutes of ingestion and lasts for approximately 12 hours. Patients appear inebriated. Progressive CNS depression can lead to coma. Stage 2 occurs 12–24 hours postingestion. Findings in this stage are secondary to the development of a metabolic acidosis and include tachypnea, acute respiratory distress syndrome, and cardiovascular collapse. Stage 3 is characterized by acute renal tubular necrosis with anuria, oliguria, and flank pain. This stage develops between 48 and 72 hours after ingestion.[31,38] Hypocalcemia from precipitation of calcium oxalate crystals can manifest as arrhythmias, tetany, or seizures.[30] Multiple cranial nerve deficits can occur, typically 1–2 weeks after the ingestion of ethylene glycol. Cranial nerve VII is consistently affected by ethyl glycol poisoning, which can result in facial diplegia. Dysarthria, dysphagia, and hearing loss can also occur.[38–43] The effects can be permanent despite aggressive treatment of this poisoning. Computerized tomography (CT) of the brain in the patients with cranial nerve deficits from toxic alcohol poisoning is usually normal; however, cerebrospinal fluid (CSF) protein levels can be elevated. Proposed etiologies include calcium oxalate crystal deposition around the cranial nerves, direct toxic effect of ethylene glycol or its metabolites on

the CNS, Guillain Barré syndrome with ethylene glycol triggering an immune system response, or pyridoxine deficiency.[38,40,44]

Laboratory Studies

Confirmation of ethylene glycol or methanol poisoning is obtained through specific measurement of the alcohol in blood or urine by gas chromatography. Serum electrolytes are measured. Low or falling serum bicarbonate levels indicate ethylene glycol or methanol intoxication. Because alcohol levels may not be readily available in the emergency department, and treatment delay can lead to serious sequelae, calculations of anion and osmolar gaps aid in the early diagnosis of poisoning.

If an anion gap acidosis is present, measurement of serum osmolality helps make the diagnosis of toxic alcohol poisoning. Serum osmolality is calculated by the following formula and expressed as mOsm/kg H_2O:

$$2(Na^+) + glucose/18 + blood\ urea\ nitrogen/2.8 + ethanol\ (mg/dl)/4.3$$

Low-molecular-weight alcohols such as ethylene glycol and methanol are osmotically active and increase serum osmolality. An osmolar gap is determined by subtracting the calculated serum osmolality (derived from the above formula) from the serum osmolality as measured by freezing point depression.[45] A normal osmolar gap is considered less than 10 mOsm/kg; however, there is a wide range of values. Therefore, the presence of an osmolar gap may support the diagnosis of toxic alcohol poisoning, but its absence does not exclude this possibility.[46]

Urine calcium oxalate crystals, hypocalcemia, and the presence of fluorescent urine when viewed under a Wood's lamp can be observed with ethylene glycol poisoning. Elevated serum amylase levels may be present with methanol poisoning.[30,31]

Treatment

Initial treatment consists of clinical stabilization with attention to airway, breathing, and circulation. Because the alcohols are rapidly absorbed from the gastrointestinal tract, gastrointestinal decontamination can be done with gastric lavage when the ingestion is recent. The efficacy of adsorbing toxic alcohols to activated charcoal in the gastrointestinal tract is not clearly known;[31] however, activated charcoal is fairly safe and can be given at 1 g/kg, especially when a mixed ingestion is suspected.

Ethanol has a much higher affinity for alcohol dehydrogenase than does methanol or ethylene glycol. Administration of ethanol, by either oral or intravenous routes, successfully blocks further metabolism of these toxic alcohols. Ethanol is given empirically when poisoning with toxic alcohol is suspected, even before laboratory confirmation. Typically, a 10% ethanol solution mixed in D5W is used. Therapy is initiated with a 6.0–10.0 ml/kg loading dose of ethanol over one hour, followed by a maintenance drip of 1.0–2.0 ml/kg. Ethanol levels are checked every one to two hours and the rate adjusted to maintain a serum ethanol level of 100–150 mg/dl.[31] Therapy can be discontinued when the serum ethylene glycol or methanol level is less than 10 mg/dl. Another alcohol dehydrogenase inhibitor, 4-methylpyrazole (4MP), is currently under clinical investigation. The advantages of 4MP include the lack of CNS depression, less frequent dosing, and safe oral or intravenous administration.

Hemodialysis is the definitive treatment for toxic alcohol poisoning. Current indications include methanol and ethylene glycol levels above 25 mg/dl, significant metabolic acidosis, and renal dysfunction. The intravenous ethanol infusion is continued during hemodialysis. Asethanol is also readily dialyzable; the intravenous administration is increased to 1.5–2.0 times its original maintenance rate. Hemodialysis is discontinued when levels are less than 10 mg/dl and metabolic acidosis has resolved.

Adjunctive therapy includes administration of sodium bicarbonate and vitamins. Folic acid, a cofactor in the metabolism of formic acid, is given intravenously, 50 mg every four hours, in methanol poisoning. Thiamine and pyridoxine are cofactors in the metabolism of glyoxilic acid. Thiamine, 100 mg, and pyridoxine, 50 mg, are given intravenously every six hours.

Neurological Complications of Commonly Used Drugs of Abuse

Sedative Hypnotics

Since their introduction at the turn of the twentieth century, sedative hypnotics have become popu-

TABLE 41.3. Sedative-Hypnotic Agents

Barbiturates
Benzodiazepines
Chloral hydrate
Ethanol
Ethchlorvynol (Placidyl)
Glutethimide (Doriden)
Meprobamate (Miltown, Equanil)
Methylqualone
Zolpidem (Ambien)

lar drugs for both legitimate use and frequent abuse. A variety of drugs are classified as sedative hypnotics, for their ability both to reduce anxiety and to induce sleep (see Table 41.3.)

Clinical effects of sedative hypnotic toxicity include ataxia, nystagmus, hypotonia, coma, apnea, bradycardia, hypotension, and hypothermia. Although bulbous skin lesions are attributed to barbiturate overdose, they are not specific and can be due to pressure necrosis. Prolonged and cyclical coma is characteristic of glutethimide and meprobamate.[47–49] Coma produced by ethchlorvynol has been reported to last almost two weeks.[47] Effects of toxicity are rarely fatal unless combined with other substances.[50]

Treatment consists of aggressive airway management and supportive measures. Due to its unique pharmacokinetics, the elimination of phenobarbital is enhanced by alkalinizing the urine. A bolus of 1 mEq/kg of sodium bicarbonate is administered intravenously. A maintenance infusion is prepared by adding 100 mEq sodium bicarbonate to 1 l D5W and administered at 2.5 ml per minute to attain a urine pH of 7.5–8.0.46. Flumazenil (Romazicon) is a competitive inhibitor specific to the benzodiazepine binding site of the $GABA_A$ receptor and does not reverse the effects of barbiturates or other sedative hypnotics (with the exception of zolpidem). The use of flumazenil is restricted to patients with a benzodiazepine overdose, absence of seizure disorder, or benzodiazepine dependence. Its use is not recommended in routine treatment of the comatose patient, and in those suspected of having multiple drug overdose.

Sedative-Hypnotic-Withdrawal. Sedative-hypnotic withdrawal occurs in a time course consistent with the half-life of that particular agent. Clinical manifestations are indistinguishable from those of alcohol withdrawal. Treatment is supportive. Lorazepam is widely used to control agitation and other withdrawal symptoms.

Narcotic Agents

Narcotic agents act on the various opiate receptors to mediate the body's natural response to pain. The classic presentation of narcotic overdose is coma, respiratory depression, and pinpoint pupils. Although the presence of this triad and evidence of drug abuse at the scene are sensitive indicators, the classic features are commonly absent. Meperidine (Demerol) and diphenoxylate (Lomotil) in particular may present with mydriasis. Propoxyphene (Darvon) shares the sodium channel blocking properties commonly associated with the tricyclic antidepressants and may therefore prolong ventricular conduction.[51] Noncardiogenic pulmonary edema is also reported in cases of narcotic toxicity.

Transverse myelitis is a unique neurological complications of heroin use that leads to vascular insufficiency of the thoracic spinal cord and resultant paraplegia. This can occur with intravenous use of heroin following several months of drug abstinence. Heroin also causes a variety of peripheral nerve lesions. Brachial and lumbosacral plexitis are not associated with needle trauma and are characterized by intense neuritic pain, weakness, and sensory deficits. Mononeuropathy can occur as painless weakness of an extremity hours after intravenous injection of heroin. The mononeuropathy is also known to occur at a remote location from the site of injection. Acute and subacute polyneuropathies that resemble Guillain-Barré syndrome can occur with the use of heroin. Heroin use can affect muscle, resulting in acute rhabdomyolysis with myoglobinuria, localized myopathy at recurrent injection sites, and localized crush syndromes.[52]

Treatment is supportive. Naloxone (Narcan) is an opiate receptor antagonist used for both the diagnosis and the treatment of opiate ingestion. It can be administered orally, endotracheally, intramuscularly, intravenously, or sublingually. Dosage is based on incremental administration titrated to the desired effect. The use of physical restraints is appropriate prior to administering naloxone, because combativeness and agitation may accompany arousal. Some compounds are relatively resistant to the effects of naloxone (propoxyphene, methadone, etc.); therefore, doses of up to 10 mg may be needed. Although the use of naloxone potentiates narcotic withdrawal, there are no absolute contraindications for its use. Because the half-life of naloxone is shorter than that of most narcotics, repeat doses or intravenous infusions may be used to maintain the desired levels of arousal. Typically, infusion of two-thirds of the initially required dose per hour achieves the desired effect.[53] In the setting of propoxyphene toxicity, QRS complex duration of greater than 100 milliseconds on electrocardiogram (EKG) is treated with bicarbonate therapy (see Chapter 40, "Neurotoxicology," for discussion of tricyclic antidepressants).[51]

Narcotic Withdrawal. Narcotic withdrawal is the result of abrupt cessation of the chronic stimulatory effects at the opiate receptors. In the case of heroin, withdrawal symptoms develop within four to eight hours after the last dose and last approximately two to three days. In contrast, withdrawal from methadone begins after two to three days after the last dose and lasts approximately two weeks. Symptoms include lacrimation, rhinorrhea, yawning, and anxiety. Tachycardia and hypertension are less severe than that observed in patients with sedative-hypnotic withdrawal. Symptoms may progress to vomiting, diarrhea, and abdominal pain. Piloerection is characteristic (hence the phrase "cold turkey"). Mental status changes, hyperthermia, and seizures are not common in patients undergoing narcotic withdrawal, unlike those undergoing sedative-hypnotic withdrawal. Treatment is supportive. The use of clonidine or methadone is best reserved for inpatient rehabilitation.

Cocaine, Amphetamines, and Other Stimulants

Cocaine, amphetamines, and chemically related drugs are commonly referred to as *sympathomimetics* (see Table 41.4). The use of these compounds results in excessive stimulation of adrenergic receptors. Toxicity causes tachycardia, hypertension, hyperthermia, and metabolic acidosis. Neurological manifestations of acute ingestion include agitation,

TABLE 41.4. Commonly Available Sympathomimetic Agents

Illicit	Over-the-Counter	Prescription
Amphetamine	Desoxyephedrine (Vicks inhaler)	Dextroamphetamine (Dexedrine)
Methamphetamine	Ephedra (Ma Huang)	Fenfluramine (Pondimin)
3,4-methylenedioxymethamphetamine	Ephedrine (Bronkaid, Tedral)	Methylphenidate (Ritalin)
(MDMA, Adam, Ecstasy)		
3,4-methylenedioxyethamphetamine	phenylpropanolamine (Contac,	
(MDEA, Eve)	Dexatrim, Dimetapp, Triaminic)	
	pseudoephedrine (Actifed, Comtrex,	
	Drixoral, Novahistine, Sudafed)	

tremulousness, mydriasis, hyperreflexia, clonus, and seizure. In addition, paranoia and psychosis can occur. Complications associated with toxicity include cerebral vascular accidents, cardiac arrhythmias, and myocardial infarction.

Treatment is supportive. Benzodiazepines used to control agitation and seizures are also useful for initial treatment of hypertension. When hypertension cannot be controlled, the use of nitroprusside (0.5–5 μg/kg per minute) is recommended. The use of beta blockers and labetelol is no longer advocated due to the deleterious effects of relatively unopposed alpha-adrenergic receptor agonism.[54–56] Haloperidol can be used for agitation and psychiatric symptoms such as paranoia and psychosis. Haloperidol is known to lower the seizure threshold. Cocaine can block sodium channel activity, an action commonly associated with tricyclic antidepressants, and malignant cardiac arrhythmias can be treated with sodium bicarbonate.[57] Norepinephrine is the preferred agent for the treatment of cardiovascular collapse.

Phencyclidine

Developed in the 1950s as a dissociative-anesthetic-analgesic agent, phencyclidine (PCP) arrived on the streets as an agent of abuse in the 1960s. A few of the many street names of PCP include angel dust, crystal, rocket fuel, THC, super weed, hog, and hog dust. PCP is sold on the street in capsules, tablets, powder, as a solution (in water or alcohol), or in "rock salt" crystal form. It can be sniffed, smoked, or injected.

PCP interacts with all neurotransmitter systems studied to date. PCP inhibits GABAergic systems. It also produces both an anticholinergic effect and a sympathomimetic effect. PCP causes vasospasm, which has been prevented and reversed with verapamil in animal studies. The high lipid solubility of PCP accounts for its affinity for, and storage within, adipose tissue and the brain. It becomes concentrated in the slightly more acidic CSF. CSF concentrations of PCP are known to be four times higher than that in serum. This explains the long-lasting CNS effect of the drug. The duration of action can be 7–16 hours to as long as a week.

The clinical effects of PCP are highly unpredictable. Intoxication, ataxia, slurred speech, extremity hypesthesia, varying degree of mental status change, sweating, and muscle rigidity accompany ingestion of a "lower" dose of PCP, frequently from snorting PCP. Anesthesia becomes more pronounced at higher doses of PCP. Coma can follow. (For CNS effects of PCP see Table 41.5.)

Treatment is supportive. Seizures are controlled with benzodiazepines. Haloperidol is used to treat agitation and PCP psychosis. Urinary excretion of PCP is increased by as much as 100-fold by acidification of urine.

Neurological Complications of Intravenous Drug Abuse

Besides the chemical effects of the drugs, the lifestyles and habits of intravenous drug users contribute to many neurological complications (see

TABLE 41.5. CNS Findings of PCP Intoxication

Mental Status Changes	Sensory-Motor	Ophthalmologic	Miscellaneous
Calm	Sensory anesthesia	Blurred vision	Seizures
Violent, agitated behavior	Hyperactivity	Miosis (more common) or mydriasis (less common)	Status epilepticus (rare)
Bizarre behavior	Myoclonus	Dysconjugate gaze	Variable deep tendon reflexes
Hallucinations (auditory and visual) are less common than with hallucinogenics	Dystonia (facial grimacing, opisthotonus, torticollis)	Nystagmus: horizontal or vertical	Muscle rigidity causing rhabdomyolysis
Disorientation	Abnormal stereognosis		Hypertension
Paranoia			Tachycardia
Dysphoria			
Unresponsive to comatose			

Table 41.6). Spinal pain, fever, leukocytosis, and progressive weakness suggest spinal or epidural abscess. Altered mental status, low-grade fever, or focal neurological findings can indicate meningitis, abscess, mycotic aneurysm, or subarachnoid hemorrhage. Wound botulism, though rare, has been reported and can occur from innocuous-looking wounds. Although patients with botulism can present with ocular palsies and progressive neurological impairment, the most common prominent initial symptom of botulism is dysphagia.[58] Tetanus is more common among patients with a long history of intravenous abuse. Common findings in tetanus are muscle rigidity and trismus.

The peripheral nervous system is also affected in the intravenous drug abuser. Nontraumatic mononeuropathy is the most common complaint and presents with painless weakness occurring several hours after an injection. A history of compression necrosis usually is lacking. In contrast, traumatic mononeuritis presents with immediate postinjection pain. Paresthesias and loss of motor function in-

TABLE 41.6. Complications of Intravenous Drug Abuse

Peripheral Nervous System	Central Nervous System
Compression injuries	Abscess (cerebral, epidural, spinal)
Nontraumatic mononeuropathy	Meningitis
Plexitis/plexopathy	Mucormycosis
Transverse myelitis	Mycotic aneurysm
Traumatic mononeuritis	Stroke
	Tetanus
	Transient ischemic attack
	Wound botulism

volve a definitive neuronal distribution. These effects of intravenous drug use are frequently permanent; treatment is supportive.

PEARLS AND PITFALLS

- Alcohol-intoxicated patients require a comprehensive evaluation. Failure to recognize and treat coexisting medical problems or associated trauma is a major pitfall in caring for such patients.
- Intravenous ethanol therapy is begun in suspected cases of ethylene glycol or methanol poisoning, even before the results of serum levels are available.
- Nontraumatic mononeuropathy is common in intravenous drug abusers.
- Transverse myelitis can occur in heroin abusers who inject the drug after several months of abstinence.

REFERENCES

1. American Psychiatric Association. Practice Guidelines for the Treatment of Patients with Substance Abuse Disorders: Alcohol, Cocaine, Opioids. *Am J Psychiatry.* 1995;152:11.
2. Suzdak PD, Schwartz RD, Shelwick P, et al. Ethanol stimulates the GABA receptor mediated chloride transport in rat brain synaptoneurosomes. *Proc Natl Acad Sci USA.* 1986;83:4071–83.
3. Dubowski KM. Alcohol determination in the clinical laboratory. *Am J Clin Pathol.* 1980;74:747–50.
4. Nuotto E. Coffee and caffeine and alcohol effects on psychomotor function. *Clin Pharmacol Ther.* 1982;31:68–72.
5. Nuotto E, Pala ES. Naloxone fails to counteract heavy alcohol intoxication. *Lancet.* 1983;2:167–79.
6. Fluckiger A, Hartmann D, Leishman B, Zeigler WH. Lack of effect of the benzodiazepine antagonist flumazenil and the performance of healthy subjects during experimentally induced ethanol intoxication. *Eur J Clin Pharmacol.* 1988;34:273–6.
7. Heye N, Terstegge K, Sirtl C, et al. Wernicke's encephalopathy – causes to consider. *Intensive Care Med.* 1994;20:282–6.
8. Harper CG, Giles M, Finlay-Jones R. Clinical signs in the Wernicke Korsakoff complex: a retrospective analysis of 131 cases diagnosed at autopsy. *J Neurol Neurosurg Psychiatry.* 1986;49:341–5.
9. De Wardener HE, Lenox B. Cerebral beri-beri (Wernicke's encephalopathy). Review of 52 cases in a Sin-

gapore prisoner-of-war hospital. *Lancet.* 1947;1:11–17.
10. Joyce EM, Rio DE, Ruttimann UE, et al. Decreased cingulate and precuneate glucose utilization in alcoholic Korsakoff's syndrome. *Psychiatry Res.* 1994;54:225–39.
11. Butterworth RF. Pathophysiology of cerebellar dysfunction in the Wernicke-Korsakoff syndrome. *Can J Neurol Sci.* 1993;20(suppl 3):S123–6.
12. Hakim AM. The induction and reversibility of cerebral acidosis in thiamine deficiency. *Ann Neurol.* 1984;16:673–9.
13. Hakim AM, Pappius HM. Sequence of metabolic, clinical and histological events in experimental thiamine deficiency. *Ann Neurol.* 1983;13:365–75.
14. Zhang SX, Weilerbacher GS, Henderson SW, et al. Excitotoxic cytopathology, progression, and reversibility of thiamine deficiency-induced diencephalic lesions. *J Neuropathol Exp Neurol.* 1995;54:255–67.
15. Grant KA, Valverius P, Hudspith M, Tabakoff B. Ethanol withdrawal seizures and the NMDA receptor complex. *Eur J Pharmacol.* 1990;6:289–96.
16. Gulya K, Grant KA, Valverius P, et al. Brain regional specificity and time-course of changes in the NMDA recepto-ionophore complex during ethanol withdrawal. *Brain Res.* 1991;547:129–34.
17. Guido ME, Brady W, DeBehnke D. Reversible neurological deficits in a chronic alcohol abuser: a case report of Wernicke's encephalopathy. *Am J Emerg Med.* 1994;12:238–40.
18. Chataway J, Hardman E. Thiamine in Wernicke's syndrome – how much and how long? *Postgrad Med J.* 1995;71:249.
19. Butterworth RF. Effects of thiamine deficiency on brain metabolism: implications for the pathogenesis of Wernicke Korsakoff syndrome. *Alcohol Alcohol.* 1989;24:274–9.
20. Lohr R. Treatment of alcohol withdrawal in hospitalized patients. *Mayo Clin Proc.* 1995;70:777–82.
21. Greenberg DA, Messing RO, Marks SS, Carpenter CL. Calcium channel changes during alcohol withdrawal. In: Porter RA, Mattson RH, Cramer JA, et al., eds. *Alcohol and Seizures: Basic Concepts and Clinical Management.* Philadelphia, Pa: FA Davis Co; 1990:60–7.
22. Diamond I, Mochly-Rosen D, Gordon AS. Reduced adenosine receptor activism in alcoholism: implications for alcohol withdrawal seizures. In: Porter RA, Mattson RH, Cramer JA, et al., eds. *Alcohol and Seizures: Basic Concepts and Clinical Management.* Philadelphia, Pa: FA Davis Co; 1990:79–86.
23. Shuckit MA. *Alcoholism: drug and alcohol abuse: A Clinical Guide to Diagnosis and Treatment.* Shuckit MA ed, New York, NY: Plenum Medical Book Company; 1989:77–95.
24. Victor M, Brausch C. The role of abstinence in the genesis of alcoholic epilepsy. *Epilepsia.* 1967;8:1.

25. Turner RC, Lichstein PR, Peden JG, et al. Alcohol withdrawal syndromes. *J Gen Intern Med.* 1989;4:432–444.

26. Embry CK, Lippman S. Use of magnesium sulfate in alcohol withdrawal. *Am Fam Physician.* 1987;35:167–70.

27. Wilson A, Vulcano B. A double-blind, placebo-controlled trial of magnesium sulfate in the ethanol withdrawal syndrome. *Alcoholism* (NY) 1984;8:542–5.

28. Rathlev NK, D'Odofrio G, Fish SS, et al. The lack of efficacy of phenytoin in the prevention of recurrent alcohol withdrawal seizures. *Ann Emerg Med.* 1994;23:513–18.

29. Sternebring B. Treatment of alcohol withdrawal seizures with carbamazepine and valproate. In Porter RA, Mattson RH, Cramer JA, et al., eds. *Alcohol and Seizures: Basic Concepts and Clinical Management.* Philadelphia, Pa: FA Davis Co; 1990;315–20.

30. Jacobsen D, McMartin K. Methanol and ethylene glycol poisonings. Mechanism of toxicity, clinical course, diagnosis, and treatment. *Med Toxicol.* 1986;1:309–34.

31. Burkhart KK, Kulig KW. The other alcohols. Methanol, ethylene glycol, and isopropanol. *Emerg Med Clin North Am.* 1990;8:913–28.

32. Suit P, Estes M. Methanol intoxication: clinical features and differential diagnosis. *Cleve Clin J Med.* 1990;57:464–71.

33. Sharpe JA, Hostovsky M, Bilbao JM, Rewcastle NB. Methanol optic neuropathy: a histopathological study. *Neurology.* 1982;32:1093–100.

34. Baumbach GL. Methyl alcohol poisoning. Alterations in the morphological findings of the retina and optic nerve. *Arch Ophthalmol.* 1977;95:1859–65.

35. Hayreh MS, Haryeh SS, Baumbach GL, et al. Methyl alcohol poisoning, III: Ocular toxicity. *Arch Ophthalmol.* 1977;95:1851–8.

36. Guggenheim MA, Couch JR, Weinberg WW. Motor dysfunction as a permanent complication of methanol ingestion. *Arch Neurol.* 1971;24:550–4.

37. LeWitt P, Martin S. Dystonia and hypokinesis with putaminal necrosis after methanol intoxication. *Clin Neuropharmacol.* 1988;11:161–7.

38. Spillane L, Roberts J, Meyer A. Multiple cranial nerve deficits after ethylene glycol poisoning. *Ann Emerg Med.* 1991;20:208–10.

39. Berger J, Ayyar D. Neurological complications of ethylene glycol intoxication. *Arch Neurol.* 1981;38:724–6.

40. Factor S, Lava N. Ethylene glycol intoxication: a new stage in the clinical syndrome. *NY State J Med.* 1987;87:179–80.

41. Fellman D. Facial diplegia following ethylene glycol ingestion. *Arch Neurol.* 1982;39:739–40.

42. Mallya K, Mendis T, Guberman A. Bilateral facial paralysis following ethylene glycol ingestion. *Can J Neurol Sci.* 1986;13:340–41.

43. Palmer B, Eigenbrodt E, Henrich W. Cranial nerve deficit: a clue to the diagnosis of ethylene glycol poisoning. *Am J Med.* 1989;87:91–2.

44. Anderson B. Facial-auditory nerve oxalosis. *Am J Med.* 1990;88:87–8.

45. Eisen TF, Lacouture PG, Woolf A. Serum osmolality in alcohol ingestions: differences in availability among laboratories of teaching hospital, nonteaching hospital, and commercial facilities. *Am J Emerg Med.* 1989;7:256–9.

46. Hoffman R, Smilkstein MJ, Howland MA, Goldfrank LR. Osmol gaps revisited: normal values and limitations. *Clin Toxicol.* 1993;31:81–93.

47. Teehan BP, Maher JF, Carey JJH, et al. Acute ethchlorvynol (Placidyl) intoxication. *Ann Intern Med.* 1970;72:875–82.

48. Maher JF, Schreiner GE, Westervelt FB Jr. Acute glutethimide intoxication: clinical experience (22 patients) compared to acute barbiturate intoxication (63 patients). *Am J Med.* 1962;33:70–81.

49. Dennison J, Edwards JN, Volans GN. Meprobamate overdosage. *Hum Toxicol.* 1985;4:215–17.

50. Greenblatt DJ, Shader RI, Abernethy DR. Current status of benzodiazepines, 1: *N Engl J Med.* 1983;309:354–8.

51. Stork CM, Redd JT, Fine K, Hoffman RS. Propoxyphene-induced wide QRS complex dysrhythmia responsive to sodium bicarbonate – a case report. *Clin Toxicol.* 1995;33:179–83.

52. Richter R, Pearson J, Bruun B. Neurological complications of addiction to heroin. *Bull NY Acad Med.* 1973;49:4–21.

53. Goldfrank L, Weisman RS, Errich JK, Lo MW. A dosing nomogram for continuous infusion intravenous naloxone. *Ann Emerg Med.* 1986;15:566–70

54. Ramoska E, Sacchetti A. Propranolol-induced hypertension in the treatment of cocaine intoxication. *Ann Emerg Med.* 1985;14:112–13

55. Sybertz EJ, Sabin CS, Pula KK, et al. Alpha and beta adrenoreceptor blocking properties of labetalol and its R,R-isomer, SCH 19927. *J Pharmacol Exp Ther.* 1981;218:435–43.

56. Briggs RSJ, Birtwell AJ, Pohl JEF. Hypertensive response to labetalol in pheochromocytoma. *Lancet.* 1978;1:1045–6.

57. Parker RP, Beckman KJ, Bauman JL, et al. Sodium bicarbonate reverses cocaine-induced conduction defects. *Circulation.* 1989;80(4 suppl 2):15.

58. MacDonald KL, Rutherford GW, Friedman SM, et al. Botulism and botulism-like illness in chronic drug users. *Ann Intern Med.* 1985;102:616–18.

42 Neurotoxicology of Envenomations

JANET G. H. ENG, ROBERT J. PRODINGER, AND
DAVID J. CASTLE

SUMMARY   The venom of certain species of snake, scorpions, and marine animals produces most of the "neurotoxic" envenomations in humans. In addition to the effects of venom on the nervous system, most of the venoms affect the cardiovascular and hematological systems. The severity of symptoms depends largely on the type of venom and the degree of envenomation. The availability of prompt and effective medical care determines clinical outcome. This chapter reviews the mechanism of toxicity, clinical findings, and key aspects of treatment of common envenomations from snakes, scorpions, and some marine animals.

Snake Envenomations

Neurotoxicity from snake envenomation, attributable primarily to coral snakes in the United States, is rare. However, in other areas of the world, such as Australia, neurotoxicity from snake envenomation is common. Many snake venoms contain more than one neurotoxin in addition to many different toxins affecting other organ systems.[1] Neurotoxicity from a snake bite is produced mostly by snakes of the family Elapidae, which includes coral snakes, cobras (*Naja*), kraits (*Bungarus*), mambas (*Dendroapsis*), and all terrestrial poisonous snakes of Australia.[2] Other snakes that possess neurotoxins include sea snakes of the family Hydrophiidae, the Mojave rattlesnake, the Brazilian rattlesnake (*Durissus teriffi-cus*), and the Russell's viper (*Vipera russeli*).[1]

Elapids have a distinctive appearance. The bullet-shaped heads of the elapids contrast with the more triangular heads of the crotalids (rattlesnakes). Elapids lack a facial pit and have round pupils, whereas the crotalid pupil is slit-like.[3,4] The oral anatomy of elapids that causes neurotoxicity is distinctive. The fangs of the Australian elapids are small and have limited rotation; the coral snake's fangs are fixed to the maxillae and are short.[4,5] These characteristics of venomous snakes produce a bite that can appear either as fang marks or more often as scratch marks on the skin.[5]

The coral snake can be recognized by its characteristic markings. The coral snakes have a black snout, along with red and black bands separated by yellow bands.[3,4] This is in contrast to the scarlet king snake, which has a red snout and red and yellow rings separated by black rings.[4] A description of the offending snake's characteristics is very helpful in establishing the risk of neurotoxicity from envenomation.

Pathophysiology

Snakes use venom as a means of obtaining food, not as a defense mechanism. The venom is used to immobilize the prey and aids in digestion. Snake venoms range from colorless to a dark amber liquid; 90% of the nonaqueous portion is protein.[1] The heat-stable toxins in the venom consist of polypeptide toxins, glycoproteins, low-molecular-weight compounds,[1] and a variety of enzymes such as protease, cholinesterase, hyaluronidase, ribonuclease, desoxyribonuclease, and ophio-oxidase.[6] Some of these enzymes have remained active after 25–50 years of storage.

Snake venom has a curare- and myasthenia gravis like effect. In the past, toxins from the krait and cobra were used to help identify the acetylcholine receptor (AChR) abnormality of myasthenia gravis.[7] The two major sites of action for the neurotoxins are the pre- and postsynaptic AChRs (see Fig. 42.1). Beta-bungarotoxin and γ-bungarotoxin are found in the Formosan krait (*Bungarus multicinictus*). These toxins bind presynaptically to cause depletion of acetylcholine[2,8] and cannot be reversed by a cholinesterase inhibitor or antivenom globulin.[2] Structurally similar to phospholipase A_2, toxins from *B. multicinictus* are similar in action to botulinum toxin. Other toxins with phospholipase A_2 activity include notexin (tiger snake – *Notechis scutatus*), taipotoxin (taipan – *O. scutellatus*), crotoxin (Brazilian rattlesnake – *C. durrissus terrifficus*), and some sea snakes.

The cobra neurotoxin and the α-bungarotoxin from the Formosan krait (*B. multicinictus*) bind hydrophobically to the postsynaptic nicotinic AChRs to cause nondepolarizing neuromuscular blockade.[1,2] This blockade is reversed by cholinesterase inhibitors and antivenom globulin.[2] Clinically, these toxins produce a curare-like neuromuscular blockade[5] and muscle paralysis.[6]

Other neurotoxins with unclear significance include K-neurotoxins found in some kraits. These toxins have little effect on the nicotinic AChRs in muscles but bind selectively to neuronal nicotinic AChRs.[1] Vipotoxin is found in Russell's viper (*V. russelli*) and blocks biogenic amine receptors. Dendrotoxin found in the mamba *Dendroaspis angusticeps* blocks potassium channels and facilitates acetylcholine release at the neuromuscular junction.[1]

Clinical Presentation

The neurological findings are relatively similar in different snake envenomations. The onset of neurotoxic symptoms is typically delayed. Mild local paresthesias occur within 15 minutes; subsequent weakness progresses to paralysis 12 hours or later.[10,11] This delayed onset of symptoms is characteristic of the presynaptic neurotoxins and is commonly observed in coral snake and krait envenomations.[1,11] These bites do not typically present with the marked local reaction that is common with crotalid bites. Frequently there is only minimal local

reaction. The presenting symptoms include headache, nausea, vomiting, and abdominal pain.[8]

Neurotoxic signs manifest as weakness and do not affect the sensorium.[8,11] The initial signs of toxicity are of the "bulbar type" that include ptosis, blurred vision, and difficulty swallowing.[1,11] A sixth cranial nerve palsy or ophthalmoplegia may be followed by progression of paralysis leading to respiratory paralysis.[8,11] Excessive salivation is common from an inability to swallow, not from the increase in secretions. Progression of clinical findings can be rapid.[11] Because aspiration pneumonia can occur in patients who cannot swallow, the airway must be protected.[10] Signs of apprehension, lethargy, and convulsions result from hypoxia; neurotoxins do not cross the blood–brain barrier.[2]

Symptoms of the Mojave rattlesnake envenomation are similar to those of Elapid envenomations. Victims of rattlesnake envenomation develop respiratory distress, muscle fasciculations, spasm and weakness, ptosis, dysphagia, and paralysis. Victims of the Brazilian rattlesnake bite present with cranial nerve palsies, weakness, and convulsions. Respiratory failure is rare in these victims.[1]

Reports of clinical findings following elapid envenomations include a case of Guillain-Barré syndrome[12] and chemical conjunctivitis from the venom of African and Asian spitting cobras.[13]

Prehospital Care

Prehospital treatment for snake envenomations includes rapid patient transport to a health care facility.[9] Delayed absorption of cobra toxin can occur from the use of tourniquets; however, the use of tourniquets can lead to severe and rapid neurotoxicity when removed too quickly.[9] When a tourniquet is used, it is removed in the hospital under controlled conditions. The use of a tourniquet is controversial and is generally not recommended. Incision and suction techniques are not recommended as part of the treatment of snake envenomations.

Emergency Department Evaluation and Management

The bite area is evaluated carefully. Tetanus prophylaxis and general supportive care including wound care and respiratory support are provided. Prophylactic antibiotics are not recommended. Blood tests such as complete blood cell (CBC)

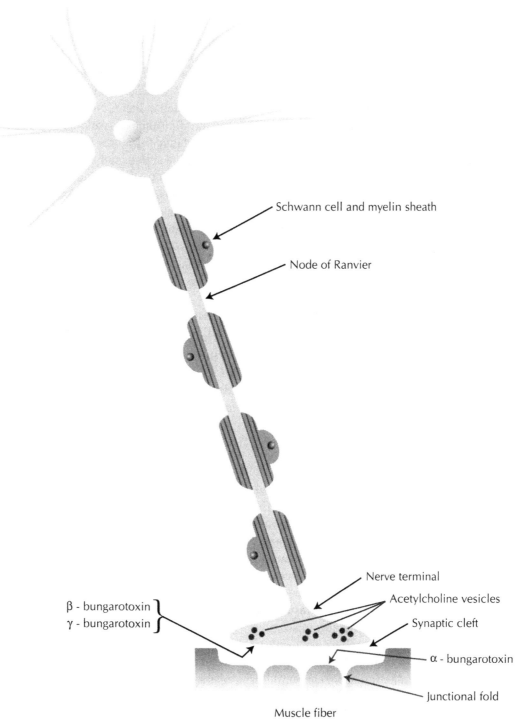

Schwann cell and myelin sheath

Node of Ranvier

Nerve terminal

Acetylcholine vesicles

Synaptic cleft

β - bungarotoxin

γ - bungarotoxin

α - bungarotoxin

Junctional fold

Muscle fiber

FIGURE 42.1. Schematic representation of a neuromuscular junction and sites of action of different snake neurotoxins.

count, electrolyte level, coagulation studies, and urine analysis are not essential for emergency management, because hematological or renal complications do not occur acutely following snake envenomations.[4,5] When the patient appears intoxicated, a blood alcohol level and a urine drug screen can be helpful. Measurement of respiratory peak flow and tidal volume, pulse oximetry, and arterial blood gases helps to monitor respiratory function.[4]

A snake identification kit available in Australia utilizes an enzyme-linked immunosorbent assay (ELISA). Aspirate from the bite site or venom from skin or clothing can help to identify the species of snake.[1,5] Because venom is concentrated and excreted in the urine,[5] a severe envenomation is assumed when the venom is identified in the urine. The vitreous humor of the eye can be analyzed postmortem for presence of venom, especially in bodies undergoing decomposition.

Different antivenins are available worldwide. A polyvalent antivenin against all venomous species would be ideal but is not yet available. In the United States, an antivenin that neutralizes venom from the eastern North American and Texas coral snake is available. This antivenin does not neutralize venoms of Arizona or Sonoran coral snakes or those found in Mexico, Central, or South America.[14] One vial of coral snake antivenin neutralizes approximately 2 mg of venom.[10] Typically, 3–4 vials are administered to a patient with no signs of envenomation. In symptomatic patients with severe pain, numbness, or presence of other neurological findings, 5–6 vials are administered. Envenomation from a large coral snake, capable of injecting greater than 20 mg of venom, can require the use of at least 10 vials of antivenin.[15]

In the United States, all patients are tested for horse serum sensitivity prior to the administration of antivenin. A negative skin test does not exclude the possibility of anaphylaxis during treatment. Antivenin is administered in an intensive care unit, as anaphylactic reactions can be a major complication of this therapy. Patients receiving more than 5 vials of antivenin are at risk for delayed serum sickness.

Indications for antivenin use in Australia includes neurotoxic paralysis, coagulopathy, myolysis, renal impairment, venom detection in urine, seizures, headache, nausea, vomiting, and abdominal pain. Skin testing for antivenin is not recommended because it can be hazardous and it does not reliably predict allergic reaction to the antivenin.[8] A monospecific antivenin is available in Thailand.[13]

The use of anticholinesterase inhibitors is effective in the treatment of certain snake envenomations and should be considered in countries where antivenin is not readily available. A case of snake bite was effectively treated in Papua New Guinea with neostigmine and atropine after a tourniquet and pressure immobilization failed to halt the progression of symptoms.[16]

Atropine sulfate and edrophonium chloride have been used to treat cobra envenomations (*Naja Naja Philippinensis*) in India, Sri Lanka, and Southeast Asia. When clinical improvement is noted, a longer-acting agent such as neostigmine methylsulfate can be used subsequently.[7] However, the efficacy of anticholinesterase inhibitors in treating snakebite victims has not been definitively demonstrated.

Disposition

Hospitalization for observation of patients with suspected coral snakebites is recommended because of the potential for delayed onset of neurotoxicity.[3] Administration of antivenin is recommended by some toxicologists to those patients who present with acute snake envenomations. A delay in definitive treatment until the onset of neurological symptoms can prolong disability.[10] Although administration of antivenin to all victims of a potentially neurotoxic snake envenomation leads to "unnecessary" use of antivenin, the benefits of antivenin appear to outweigh the risks of administration.

Scorpion Envenomation

Introduction

Scorpions are found worldwide, are exothermic, and similar to many invertebrates, possess a hard exoskeleton. Using pedipalps to grasp prey, the segmented tail directs a stinger into the victim and injects venom. Six families of scorpions include approximately 1000 species.

In 1991, 75 poison control centers in the United States reported 6765 scorpion envenomations. Of these, 2968 were from Arizona.[17] The last confirmed death from a scorpion sting in Arizona was that of a 5-month-old child in 1968.[18] Of the nearly 200,000 scorpion stings reported annually in Mexico, approximately 1000 are fatal.[19]

Of the eight species of scorpions found in North America, *Centruroides exilicanda* is the most common and potentially the most lethal. *Centruroides* is found in Arizona, parts of California, Texas, Nevada, and New Mexico.[20] *Centruroides* envenomation primarily affects the central nervous system (CNS) and the cardiovascular system. The clinical findings of *Centruroides* envenomation include local pain, restlessness, roving eye movements, and cranial nerve dysfunction. Generalized seizures are not a prominent manifestation of neurotoxicity from *Centruroides* envenomation. Involuntary tonic and clonic activity may be caused by neuromuscular dysfunction, not seizure activity.

Several other scorpions found throughout the world are potentially lethal. The yellow scorpion, *Leiurus quinquestriatus,* is found throughout the Middle East and northern Africa. Envenomation from *Leiurus* results in indirect neurotoxicity secondary to the profound release of catecholamines. Hypertensive encephalopathy can ensue.[21] Other toxic and potentially lethal species include *Mesobuthus tamulus* of India and Iran, *Hemiscorpion lepturus* of southwestern Iran, the *Paraguthus* and *Buthotus* scorpions of South Africa, and *Tityus* species found throughout South America, the Caribbean, and Brazil.

Pathophysiology

Scorpion venom is water-soluble and antigenic, and contains mucopolysaccharides, small amounts of hyaluronidase and phospholipase, serotonin or histamine-like structures, protease inhibitors, histamine releasers, and "neurotoxins." Toxins of many species of scorpion have been purified and characterized. Each species of scorpion has a unique combination of toxins that produce varying degrees of cholinergic, adrenergic, and other neurotoxic effects.

The severity of the envenomation is related to the amount and composition of the venom. Variables such as the species, age, nutritional status of the scorpion, season, and geographical area determine the potency of the venom.[22] The depth and the site of penetration of the stinger, and the integrity of the stinger are important factors contributing to the severity of scorpion envenomation. The size and the age of the victim are also important, because the severity of the envenomation is dose-dependent.

Prehospital Care

Early interventions such as airway control and early intensive care management contribute to improving patient outcomes and decreasing the morbidity and mortality of scorpion envenomations.[20,23] Rapid transport to a facility for definitive treatment is essential. There is no need for incision and suction of the bite site. Immobilization of the involved extremity provides comfort while ice is applied locally to the bite area. Extensive cooling does not provide additional benefit.

Initial field interventions include appropriate airway management for hypoxia, which can result from heart failure, pulmonary hypertension, or CNS depression. Hemodynamic monitoring with frequent neurological evaluations is important. Close observation for symptoms or signs of hypertensive encephalopathy or cardiovascular instability is crucial. Profound hypotension, hypertension, or cardiac dysrhythmias are treated aggressively.

Emergency Department Evaluation

Symptoms generally begin within minutes following scorpion envenomation but can be delayed up to an hour. Pain at the site of the sting varies in intensity from mild superficial burning to deep or diffuse pain. The site of envenomation and localized erythema or edema are not always obvious. Pain and paresthesias can be elicited by tapping over the envenomed area (tap test). The diagnosis of scorpion envenomation in a child should be suspected clinically when the child is unable to provide an accurate history of a scorpion bite.

CNS symptoms include paresthesias, irritability, tremor, muscle rigidity, extraocular muscle dysfunction, decreased level of consciousness, coma, and seizures. Scorpion envenomation in young children can result in apneic episodes or centrally mediated respiratory compromise caused by acute hypertensive encephalopathy.[24] Allergic (atopic) subglottic narrowing with stridor or expiratory wheeze progressing to airway closure can occur.[24] Heart failure and cardiogenic shock can occur from abnormal left ventricular hemodynamics.[21,25] Abdominal pain, nausea, and vomiting are common manifestations of scorpion envenomation and can be caused by the development of pancreatitis.[26] Hyperthermia, rhabdomyolysis, excessive secretions,

TABLE 42.1. Grades of Severity of Envenomation by *Centruroides sculpturatus*

Grade	Description
I	Local pain and/or paresthesias at the site of envenomation
II	Local pain and/or paresthesias at the site of envenomation, accompanied by pain or paresthesias remote from the site
III	Either cranial nerve or somatic skeletal neuromuscular dysfunction: 1. Cranial nerve dysfunction such as blurred vision, irregular eye movements, difficulty swallowing, tongue fasciculations, slurred speech, occasional upper airway incoordination 2. Somatic skeletal neuromuscular dysfunction such as jerking of extremities, restlessness, severe involuntary shaking, and jerking that may be mistaken for seizures
IV	Both cranial nerve and somatic skeletal neuromuscular dysfunction

Source: Curry, Vance, Ryan, Kunkel, and Northey.[20]

bradycardia, hypotension, miosis, and priapism can also be present.[26]

Management

Aggressive symptomatic management is the mainstay of therapy for the victims of scorpion envenomation. Appropriate wound care and tetanus immunization, when required, are provided. Pain or paresthesias surrounding the site of envenomation are common and are treated with oral analgesics and local application of ice. Intravenous agents such as phenobarbital, benzodiazepines, and narcotics can be used to treat severe pain and restlessness. Pain and paresthesias are present for approximately 24–48 hours but can persist for up to 2 weeks.

A scale grading the severity of symptoms associated with acute *Centruroides* envenomations has been developed (Table 42.1).[20] This grading scale is used as a guide for treatment and is based on the acceleration and severity of symptoms. Rapid onset of

neurological symptoms (within 6 hours) associated with grade III and IV envenomations requires aggressive management. Infants can develop grade III and IV symptoms within 15–30 minutes. Management includes stabilization of the airway and maintaining hemodynamic stability. Fluid balance is assessed and monitored closely. Hypertension that does not respond to sedation and analgesia is treated with antihypertensive agents.[27] The use of vasodilators and diuretics is recommended when signs of acute left ventricular failure, pulmonary edema, and elevated pulmonary capillary wedge pressure are present.[28] Management of left ventricular heart failure with a normal systemic vascular resistance includes use of vasopressors such as dobutamine.[29] Adequate hydration for optimum renal perfusion is important when signs of rhabdomyolysis are present. Alkalinization of the urine to expedite myoglobin excretion may be required. Hyperthermia requires techniques such as evaporative cooling.

Specific antivenins for scorpion venoms have been developed; however, prompt intensive care and symptomatic management have been shown to be more effective in reducing mortality than administration of scorpion antivenin. Despite over 40 years of use, there is no convincing evidence that antivenin is consistently effective in the treatment of scorpion envenomations. Children treated with and without scorpion antivenin had similar cardiovascular complications, and children treated with antivenin had more complications during therapy than did the children who were not treated with antivenin.[30] Despite these findings, antivenin is often used in children presenting with tongue fasciculations or airway compromise. Adult patients usually do not require antivenin unless severe symptoms develop early. Patients with grade III or IV symptoms require hospitalization and intensive care management whether or not antivenin is used. Recipients of antivenin are monitored for symptoms and signs of anaphylaxis.

Disposition

Patients with grade I or II symptoms of scorpion envenomation can be discharged from the emergency department when the symptoms resolve. Patients with even minor progression of symptoms are hospitalized for close observation. Rarely, paresthesias can persist for weeks. Antivenin therapy can be complicated by immediate and delayed serum sickness.

Marine Envenomations

The marine animals are broadly classified into vertebrates and invertebrates.

Marine Vertebrates

There are three classes of marine vertebrates with neurotoxic envenomations: Chondrichthyes, Osteichthyes, and Reptilia. The Chondrichthyes include stingrays, mantas, and rays. Osteichthyes are bony fishes such as scorpionfish and stonefish. Reptilia include sea snakes. Depending on the marine vertebrate, envenomation can cause lacerations, punctures, abrasions, or bites. The toxicity and the amount of tissue damage vary according to the species. The sea snake can cause a painless, essentially inapparent bite that can be lethal; a stingray can cause a painful laceration without any lethal effect.

Stingrays. Stingrays reside in moderate to shallow depths of temperate and tropical waters and strike only in self-defense. They often lie submerged under the sand with only their eyes visible. They vary in size from several inches to 20 feet. An estimated 1500 injuries due to stingrays are reported each year in the United States.[31] Stingrays derive their name from the spine at the end of their whip-like tail, which can be driven into an aggressor, producing deep puncture wounds and long lacerations. The venom glands encased inside grooves on the side of these spines are covered with a membrane. When the integumentary membrane covering the spine is ruptured, venom runs down the grooves and into the victim.[32] The spine can break and becomes embedded in the victim, intensifying the injury. Stingray venom is composed of heat-labile, water-soluble proteins including serotonin, 5'-nucleotidase, and phosphodiesterase.[33,34] Exposure to low concentration of the venom produces cardiac conduction disturbances with mild hypotension; larger doses cause vasoconstriction and cardiac ischemia. A centrally mediated neurotoxic effect of the stingray venom is respiratory depression. In addition to the neurotoxicity, a stingray wound can cause significant physical trauma. Deaths have been reported from penetration of body cavities from stingray spines.[33] The venom does not have a paralytic neuromuscular component, although paralysis of the involved extremity can occur. Seizure activity can also occur.

Stingray envenomations cause immediate pain that increases over the next 1–2 hours and peaks at 2–3 days. Bleeding can be severe. The site appears pale and blanched with dusky wound margins. A mucoid secretion or membranous material may be found in the wound. Systemic symptoms and signs include diaphoresis, nausea, vomiting, vertigo, headache, fasciculations and muscle cramps, tachycardia, hypotension, and death.[35]

Treatment begins with wound cleaning. Wound irrigation with nonscalding hot water (40.5°C/ 105°F) is applied for at least 30–90 minutes as tolerated by the patient. Hot water or local heat is believed to denature the venom. There is no specific antivenin for stingray venom. The patient can be safely discharged from the emergency department after 3–4 hours of observation following stingray envenomation in the absence of systemic symptoms.[31]

Venomous Fish. Species of the family Scorpaenidae, or scorpionfish, have approximately 11–17 venom-containing spines that are used primarily for protection. Out of approximately 330 members of this family, the best known although not the most toxic, is the ornate lionfish or butterfly cod. Found in tropical and subtropical regions, the lionfish is brightly and colorfully striped, with radiating spines extending from its head, fins, dorsum, and pelvis. It is an expensive and prized specimen in many home aquariums. The stonefish, probably the most venomous fish in the world, belongs to the same family as the lionfish. Residing in the Indian and Pacific oceans, the stonefish lives in shallow water, bays, and coral reefs often half-buried in the sand. Their spines are capable of piercing through a lightly soled shoe as well as the skin.

The weeverfish, a member of the Trachinidae family, has dorsal spines containing deadly toxins similar to the stonefish. As a more aggressive creature, the weeverfish is feared among fishermen who work in shallow areas. It is found primarily in the North Atlantic Ocean and Mediterranean Sea.

The venomous spines of the scorpionfish and weeverfish can easily penetrate skin and envenomate the victim. The effects of the potent venom of the stonefish are compared to those of the cobra snake venom.[36] Stonefish toxin is both antigenic and heat-labile.[37] The venom causes paralysis of cardiac and skeletal muscle by acting on the presynaptic and postsynaptic membranes of the neuromuscular junction, depleting neurotransmitter stores and causing irreversible depolarization.[38,39] Lionfish toxin has effects similar to those of the stonefish but is less potent. Weeverfish venom contains a hemotoxin that causes hemolysis.[40]

Envenomation by the scorpionfish or weeverfish is usually nondescript, painful, and not suspected on initial presentation. Radiation of the pain occurs quickly and can be sufficiently severe to cause unconsciousness. Peak intensity of the pain occurs within 60–90 minutes and resolves in 6–12 hours. Severity of toxicity is dependent on the species, the amount of venom, and the age and health of the victim. Local blanching of the extremity can occur, which can progress to cyanosis. Swelling, fasciculations, and paralysis can develop rapidly in the involved extremity. Systemic symptoms include anxiety, headache, tremors, nausea, vomiting, diaphoresis, delirium, seizures, abdominal pain, dysrhythmias, and death. Signs of mild heart failure are common. Respiratory compromise can occur because of pulmonary edema or paralysis of the chest muscles. When the victim survives, convalescence can take months.

Management of scorpionfish and weeverfish envenomation is similar to that for stingrays. Because of the heat lability of the toxins, immediate irrigation of the wound with nonscalding water is initiated and continued for up to 90 minutes. When symptoms recur, irrigation is reinstated. A stonefish antivenin is available in the United States through the Health Services Department, Sea World, San Diego, California. It is manufactured in Australia from horse serum. As with other antivenin, anaphylaxis and serum sickness are potential complications of its use. The use of antivenin is reserved for envenomations that do not respond to supportive care or those with progression of symptoms. Antivenin for weeverfish envenomation is not yet available.

Sea Snakes. There are 52 known species of sea snakes distributed in the tropic and temperate Pacific and Indian oceans. Sea snakes are not found in the Atlantic Ocean, but there are anecdotal reports of sea snake sightings in Caribbean waters. All are venomous and potentially lethal.[32] Sea snakes are inquisitive and can be aggressive. Characteristic markings include a palmated or flattened tail seen in all species. Sea snakes can be up to 3 meters long, and some species can swim to depths of 100 meters. Their fangs are short, are easily dislodged, and usually cannot penetrate a wet suit. Most bites do not result in significant toxicity from the small amount of venom injected; however, sea snake venom is considered to be approximately 20 times more toxic than cobra venom. Venom injected by an adult sea snake of a given species is sufficiently potent to kill 3 individuals.[33] The venom is a mixture of proteins that include cardiotoxins, myotoxins, coagulants and anticoagulants, and hemolytic enzymes. Twenty-nine toxins have been isolated from 9 species.[33]

A sea snake bite may be unrecognized. Minimal swelling or inflammation is present at the site of the bite. Small fang marks number from 1 to 20 and are usually seen in groups of 2 to 4. Victims of sea snake envenomation who remain asymptomatic 8 hours after the bite generally do not develop systemic symptoms. Anxiety and restlessness herald impending toxicity. Rhabdomyolysis with myoglobinuria can develop within 3–4 hours. Muscle fasciculations, trismus, and an ascending paralysis originating from the envenomation site can occur. Respiratory distress, bulbar paralysis, aspiration-related hypoxia, acute renal failure, and coma can complicate sea snake envenomation. Symptoms begin within 1 hour but may not progress for up to 8 hours.

The treatment of sea snake envenomation is rapid administration of antivenin. The use of tourniquets or incision and suction of the wound are generally not recommended. Optimal supportive care is important, but it cannot replace antivenin therapy. Polyvalent sea snake antivenin from Commonwealth Serum Laboratories in Melbourne, Australia, is effective against three different species of sea snakes. If this is not available, a monovalent antivenin can be used. Identification of the sea snake can help guide the choice of antivenin. Antivenin should be administered in an intensive care setting due to the possibility of anaphylactic shock and serum sickness. Careful management of renal function is important. Hemodialysis has resulted in dramatic improvements in electrolyte abnormalities and paralysis.

Marine Invertebrates

Jellyfish. Of approximately 10,000 species of Coelenterates (jellyfish), 100 types are venomous. Most of these are hydrozoa, such as the Portuguese man-of-war, scyphozoa, such as the box jellyfish, and anthozoa, anemones, which are found on soft and stony corals. *Chironex fleckeri,* the box jellyfish, is reported to be the most venomous sea creature and can cause death within 30–60 seconds of envenomation.[32,41] It is found primarily in the waters off the coast of Australia. Rarely seen prior to contact, it is nearly invisible in the water because of its pale blue and transparent, membranous body. The box-shaped body can measure 20 centimeters on a side. Its tentacles are covered with nematocysts (small coiled cystic structures that uncoil, releasing the toxin) and can measure up to 3 meters in length. The tentacles adhere to objects by a sticky jelly-like substance.

Three biochemical properties of box jellyfish venom are a hemolytic component that is not clinically significant, a dermatonecrotic factor that causes rapid skin death, and a lethal component that is cardiotoxic and neurotoxic. Myocardial paralysis occurs during the contraction phase, resulting in cardiac arrest. Envenomation can cause apnea by paralyzing the respiratory muscles. Central respiratory depression can also result in apnea. The overall mortality of a box jellyfish sting is estimated at 15–20%.[31,32]

In order to prevent further discharge of venom from nematocysts, the affected region is covered with acetic acid 5% (vinegar). Local application of vinegar helps prevent further envenomation. Health care providers should wear gloves while removing the tentacles. Rapid administration of box jellyfish antivenin ensures the best possible patient outcome. Analgesics, local anesthetic sprays, or steroid preparations provide relief from local discomfort and pain.

Mollusks. Three of the five main classes of mollusks are hazardous to humans: cephalopods, which include squid, octopus, and cuddlefish; gastropods, which include snails and slugs; and pelecypods, which include oysters, scallops, mussels, and clams.

The latter cause hypersensivity reactions when ingested by people who are allergic to "shellfish."

Octopuses are passive creatures unless provoked. The blue-ringed or Australian ringed octopus, *Hapalochlena lunulata,* is colored yellow brown with rings on its tentacles, is found in tidal pools and seaweed, and is the most common offending species. When the octopus is agitated, the rings on the tentacles become a bright, iridescent blue. This species of octopus can grasp tightly with its tentacles, allowing it to bite down on its prey. Initially, the bite is nondescript and may remain unnoticed. Edema and blister formation develop in a few hours, followed by localized paresthesias. The venom includes hyaluronidase, which assists in the spread of a toxin called maculotoxin. This toxin interferes with sodium conductance in excitable membranes.[42] Rapid neuromuscular blockade occurs primarily at the phrenic nerve.[43] Oral and facial paresthesias develop within 10–15 minutes. Systemic symptoms include visual disturbances, ptosis, mydriasis, dysphagia, dysphonia, generalized weakness, and difficulty in coordination. These symptoms persist for approximately 4–12 hours; weakness can persist longer. Both peripheral and respiratory paralysis are potential complications. Treatment is supportive care.

Cone Shells. Only a small number of more than 400 species of these snails, which are carnivorous, are dangerous to humans. They are found in the Indo-Pacific oceans, the Red Sea, the coastal waters of Florida, and the Caribbean. Some are valued highly by shell collectors. A proboscis extends from the shell and contains a detachable dart-like tooth. When a prey is within striking distance, the snail thrusts one of these teeth into it, impregnating it with a potent neurotoxin. Presynaptic conotoxins inhibit physiological receptors in neuromuscular pathways. Postsynaptic conotoxins inhibit AChRs. Muscle conotoxins inhibit sodium channels and directly block muscle contraction.

Pain can be immediate or delayed. Edema and paresthesias begin at the site of envenomation and are followed by ascending paresthesias and weakness of the involved extremity. Visual disturbances, dysphagia, and dysphonia follow. Rapid, shallow breathing precedes respiratory paralysis, a potential complication. No antivenin is available. Rapid supportive care is important. Paralysis usually begins to reverse within the first 24 hours, but complete recovery may take several weeks.

Differential Diagnosis

The differential diagnosis of marine envenomations includes decompression sickness and infection or cellulitis secondary to laceration or abrasion by a contaminated foreign object. It can be especially difficult to distinguish the neurological symptoms of decompression sickness from the effects of a marine neurotoxin envenomation. Bacterial infection of a wound usually does not involve neurological symptoms until endotoxins or exotoxins of the bacteria induce a state of shock. A careful history of wound occurrence and symptom progression is important to make the correct diagnosis.

PEARLS AND PITFALLS

- The mainstay of therapy for snake and scorpion envenomations is rapid patient transport to a health care facility where aggressive symptomatic care can be delivered.

- Incision and suction at the site of envenomation and routine application of a tourniquet in the field are not recommended. However, when a tourniquet is placed, it should be removed gradually in the emergency department under controlled conditions.

- The use of antivenin for snake envenomation is considered especially when signs of neurotoxicity are present. The antivenin is administered in an intensive care unit where signs of anaphylaxis can be monitored and treated.

- The risk of delayed serum sickness from the antivenin is reviewed with the patient.

- Specific antivenin is available for the stonefish, box jellyfish, and sea snakes.

- Decompression sickness (parasthesias, abdominal cramping, muscular spasms, and seizures) can mimic symptoms produced by certain neurotoxins. A careful history can help to differentiate the two.

- When patient transport times are prolonged in an area where marine envenomation occurs, access to a first aid kit containing vinegar, latex gloves, oral

analgesics, steroids (oral and topical), antihistamines, and bandaging material is crucial.

REFERENCES

1. Minton SA. Neurotoxic snake envenoming. *Semin Neurol.* 1990;10:52–61.
2. Pettigrew LC, Glass JP. Neurologic complications of a coral snake bite. *Neurology.* 1985;35:589–92.
3. Parrish HM, Khan MS. Bites by coral snakes: report of 11 representative cases. *Am J Med Sci.* 1967:561–8.
4. Gaar GG. Assessment and management of coral and other exotic snake envenomations. *J Fla Med Assoc.* 1996;83:178–82.
5. White J, Pounder DJ. Fatal snakebite in Australia. *Am J Forensic Med Pathol.* 1984;5:137–43.
6. Naphade RW, Shetti RN. Use of neostigmine after snake bite. *Br J Anaesth.* 1977;49:1065–8.
7. Watt G, Theakston RDG, Hayes CG, et al. Positive response to edrophonium in patients with neurotoxic envenoming by cobras (*Naja Naja Philippinensis*): a placebo-controlled study. *N Engl J Med.* 1986;315:1444–8.
8. White J. Snakebite: an Australian perspective. *J Wildl Med.* 1991;2:219–44.
9. Watt G, Padre L, Tuazon L, et al. Tourniquet application after cobra bite: delay in the onset of neurotoxicity and the dangers of sudden release. *Am J Trop Med Hyg.* 1988;38:618–22.
10. Kitchens CS, Van Mierop LHS. Envenomation by the eastern coral snake (*Micrurus fulvius fulvius*): a study of 39 victims. *JAMA.* 1987;258:522–5.
11. McCollough NC, Gennaro JF. Coral snake bites in the United States. *J Fla Med Assoc.* 1963;49:968–72.
12. Chuang TY, Lin SW, Chan RC. Guillain-Barré Syndrome: an unusual complication after a snake bite. *Arch Phys Med Rehabil.* 1996;77:729–31.
13. Warrell DA. Venomous bites and stings in the tropical world. *Med J Aust.* 1993;159:773–9.
14. Otten EJ. Antivenin therapy in the emergency department. *Am J Emerg Med.* 1983;1:83–93.
15. Fix JD. Venom yield of the North American coral snake and its clinical significance. *South Med J.* 1980;73:737–41.
16. Currie B, Fitzmaurice M, Oakley J. Resolution of neurotoxicity with anticholineresterase therapy in death-adder envenomation. *Med J Aust.* 1988;148:522–5.
17. Litovitz TL, Holm KC, Bailey KM, Schmitz BF. 1991 annual report of the American Association of Poison Control Centers National Data Collection System. *Am J Emerg Med.* 1992;10:452–505.
18. Likes K, Banner W, Chavez M. Centruroides exilicauda envenomation in Arizona. *West J Med.* 1984;141:634.
19. Dehesa-Davila M, Possani LD. Scorpionism and serotherapy in Mexico. *Toxicon.* 1994;32:1015–18.

20. Curry SC, Vance MV, Ryan PJ, Kunkel DB, Northey WT. Envenomation by the scorpion *Centruroides sculpturatus. J Toxicol Clin Toxicol.* 1983–4;21:417–49.

21. Gueron M, Yarom R. Cardiovascular manifestations of severe scorpion sting. *Chest.* 1970;57:156–62.

22. Yarum R. Scorpion venom: a tutorial review of its effects in man and experimental animals. *Clin Toxicol.* 1970;3:561.

23. Rachesky IJ, Banner W, Dansky J, Tong T. Treatment for *Centruroides exilicanda* envenomation. *Am J Dis Child.* 1984;138:1136–9.

24. Sofer S, Gueron M. Respiratory failure in children following envenomation by the scorpion *Leiurus quinquestriatus:* hemodynamics and neurological aspects. *Toxicon.* 1988;26:931–9.

25. Gueron M, Adolph RJ, Grupp IL, Gabel M, Grupp G, Fowler NO. Hemodynamic and myocardial consequences of scorpion venom. *Am J Cardiol.* 1980;45:979–86.

26. Sofer S, Shalev H, Weizman Z, Shahak E, Gueron M. Acute pancreatitis in children following envenomation by the yellow scorpion *Leiurus quinquestriatus. Toxicon.* 1991;29:125–8.

27. Sofer S, Gueron M. Vasodilators and hypertensive encephalopathy following scorpion envenomation in children. *Chest.* 1990;97:118–20.

28. Sofer S. Scorpion envenomation. *Intensive Care Med.* 1995;21:626–8.

29. Abroug F, Ayari M, Novira S, et al. Assessment of left ventricular function in severe scorpion envenomation: combined hemodynamic and echo-doppler study. *Intensive Care Med.* 1985;21:629–35.

30. Sofer S, Shahak E, Gueron M. Scorpion envenomation and antivenin therapy. *J Pediatr.* 1994;124:973–8.

31. Auerbach PS. Marine envenomations. In Auerbach PS, ed. *Management of Wilderness and Environmental Emergencies.* 3rd ed. St. Louis, Mo: CV Mosby;1995;1327–74.

32. Halstead BW. *Poisonous and venomous marine animals of the world.* Princeton, NJ: Darwin Press; 1978.

33. Edmonds C. *Dangerous Marine Creatures, Field Guide for Medical Treatment.* Flagstaff, AZ. Best Publishing Co; 1995.

34. Halstead BW. *Current Status of Marine Biotoxicology – An Overview.* Colton, Calif: International Biotoxicological Center, World Life Research Institute; 1980.

35. Grainger CR. Occupational injuries due to sting rays. *Trans R Soc Trop Med Hyg.* 1980;74:408.

36. Fisher AA. *Atlas of aquatic dermatology.* New York; NY: Grune & Stratton; 1978.

37. Williamson JA, Exton D. *The Marine Stinger Book.* Queensland, Australia: The Surf Life Saving Association of Australia; 1985.

38. Kreger AS, Molgo J, Comella JX, Hansson B, Thesleff S. Effects of stonefish (*Synanceia trachynis*) venom on murine and frog neuromuscular junctions. *Toxicon.* 1993;31:307.

39. Cohen AS, Olek AJ. An extract of lionfish (*pterois volitans*) spine tissue contains acetylcholine and a toxin that affects neuromuscular transmission. *Toxicon.* 1989;27:1367.

40. Chatwal I, Dreyer F. Isolation and characterization of dracotoxin from the venom of the greater weever fish *Trachinus draco. Toxicon.* 1992;30:87.

41. Sutherland SK. *Venomous Creatures of Australia.* Melbourne, Australia: Oxford University Press; 1981.

42. Sheumack DD, Howden ME, Spence I, Quinn RJ. Maculotoxin: a neurotoxin from the venom glands of the octopus *Hapalochlaena maculosa* identified as tetrodotoxin. *Science.* 1978;199:188.

43. Trewethie ER. Tetrodotoxin in the blue-ringed octopus. *Med J Aust.* 1978;1:506.

43 Brain Resuscitation

W. LEE WARREN AND JAMES E. WILBERGER, JR.

SUMMARY Head injury causes approximately 50% of all trauma-related deaths in the United States, and results in serious morbidity for hundreds of thousands of survivors each year. In the past 20 years, the overall mortality rate for patients with head injuries has declined significantly. This reduction is a result of vigilant attention to the details of patient management and an improved understanding of the significance of secondary brain injury. The appreciation of head injury as a dynamic and evolving process has produced new approaches to therapy aimed at reducing the effects of secondary neurological injury. Clinical trials that have tested the use of different classes of pharmacological agents or hypothermia in patients with traumatic brain injury are reviewed.

Introduction

Extensive clinical and basic science research in the past several decades has significantly increased the understanding of the pathophysiology of traumatic brain injury (TBI). This information has resulted in major improvements in treatment and better patient outcomes. In the 1970s, the mortality rate for patients with severe TBI was nearly 40%;[1] current studies report a mortality rate of less than 20%.[2] This chapter reviews recent developments and trends in brain resuscitation that seek to improve further the patient outcome following TBI.

Primary Neural Injury

Primary neural injury of the brain occurs at the time of impact, resulting in the shearing or destruction of neurons, glia, and vascular structures by the mechanical forces imposed by the impact. This injury is irreversible, and the neurological deficits created by the primary injury have little potential for recovery. When epidural hematoma, subdural hematoma, or brain contusion occurs, the signifi-cance of primary neural injury may be unclear. Typically, prompt and appropriate surgical and medical therapy can improve the patient's condition in these settings. Primary neural injury rarely results in immediate mortality, thus providing the opportunity for affecting survival through postinjury management.

The degree and extent of primary neural injury is fixed at the time of the accident, and depends partially on the mechanism of injury. The only defense against the occurrence of primary neural injury is prevention. Extensive efforts at injury prevention have occurred in recent years; however, the success of programs such as decreased speed limits, mandatory seat belt laws, and passive restraints (air bags) is not confirmed. In Pennsylvania, which has an extensive trauma registry program, there was a 30% decrease in the incidence of severe TBI in 1996 as compared to 1995 (unpublished data). The reasons for this significant decrease are not yet analyzed. Ongoing educational programs, such as Think First®, are aimed at increasing the awareness of the association of risk-taking behaviors, and the potential occurrence of TBI and its consequences.

Secondary Neural Injury

Several clinical and biochemical events occur following primary neural injury. These events cause secondary neural injury that converts a potentially recoverable TBI into one resulting in either mortality or significant long-term disability. Hypotension and hypoxia are the most consistent predictors of poor outcome in head injury, presumably because of their role in facilitating the processes that lead to secondary neural injury. More than 30% of patients with severe TBI present to the emergency department with significant hypotension (systolic blood pressure less than 90 mm Hg) or hypoxia (PaO$_2$ less than 60 mm Hg). The occurrence of hypotension or hypoxia alone increases morbidity of and mortality from TBI by up to 50%.[3] When hypoxia and hypotension occur together, the risk of a poor outcome increases to more than 60%. Adequate prehospital and emergency department resuscitation is of critical importance. The concern of the effects of hypotension underlies one of the cornerstones of head injury management: adequate volume resuscitation and maintenance of euvolemia. Because of the concern that currently used intravenous fluids can potentially exacerbate cerebral edema, especially in areas of blood–brain barrier breakdown, other resuscitative and maintenance fluids are under active investigation. Because of the small volumes required (approximately 8 cc/kg) to maintain an adequate blood pressure, 3% saline has been used as a resuscitative fluid in experimental studies.[4] Hypotensive animals treated with 3% saline had excellent blood pressure maintenance and less brain water content postmortem. Although several clinical studies have used 3% saline as a resuscitative fluid, there has been limited use of 3% saline in the treatment of head injury.[5]

The concept of maintaining an adequate systolic blood pressure in the patient with severe TBI has been refined recently, with the goal of establishing and maintaining adequate cerebral perfusion pressure (CPP). CPP represents the perfusion of cerebral tissue, and is defined as the difference between mean arterial pressure (MAP) and intracranial pressure (ICP): (CPP = MAP − ICP). Current studies indicate a significant improvement in outcome following TBI when CPP is maintained at greater than 70 mm Hg. When an adequate CPP cannot be maintained by volume replacement and control of ICP, pressor agents such as dopamine or neosynephrine are used to elevate the systolic blood pressure to the level that yields a CPP above 70 mm Hg.[6]

A sensitive feedback mechanism normally exists that matches cerebral blood flow (CBF) to the regional and global metabolic needs of the brain. In the first 24 hours after TBI, there is a significant decrease in CBF and cerebral metabolism. Following this, an uncoupling phenomenon can occur between CBF and metabolic demand. CBF returns to normal or elevated levels within 36–48 hours after injury, irrespective of metabolic needs.[7] Uncoupling of CBF and metabolism can result in elevated ICP, adversely affecting CPP and subsequent outcome. Currently, the only clinical methods for detecting this problem are monitoring CBF and indirectly monitoring cerebral metabolism utilizing jugular venous oxygen sampling. CBF can be quantified by a number of methods including xenon-CBF computerized tomography. Alternatively, a catheter placed in the internal jugular vein can sample the amount of oxygen being utilized by the brain. Typically, the brain is ischemic when the oxygen extraction is less than 50%, regardless of the CBF. Therapeutic interventions that attempt to regulate CBF and/or metabolism are limited. Preliminary data suggest that mannitol increases CBF through its ability to alter the rheostatic properties of red blood cell membranes. Elevation of systolic blood pressure can possibly increase CBF, and barbiturates can significantly decrease cerebral metabolic demands.[8] It remains to be proven if these types of interventions significantly affect recovery.

For many years, it was considered standard therapy to hyperventilate patients with TBI. Although hyperventilation-induced hypocapnia lowers ICP acutely, recent investigations have discovered problems with its use. For each mm Hg drop in PaCO$_2$, there is a 3% decrease in CBF. Shortly after injury, when CBF may be quite low, keeping the PaCO$_2$ below 30 mm Hg can result in significant ischemia. Several studies have shown that prolonged prophylactic hyperventilation results in poor outcomes. Therefore, it is recommended that the PaCO$_2$ is maintained at 32–35 mm Hg unless hyperventilation is required to treat otherwise uncontrollable ICP.[6,9]

ICP has been considered a primary determinant of clinical outcome. The longer the ICP is over

20mm Hg, the poorer the outcome.[10] However, there is considerable controversy over whether ICP elevations are either a primary treatable event after severe TBI or an epiphenomenon. Although the treatment of ICP improves survival rates, it has not been shown conclusively to improve other outcomes, such as quality of life.

Recent improved understanding of the biochemical events underlying severe TBI have led to pharmacological interventions designed to attenuate or prevent the deleterious effects of TBI. Following TBI, a cascade of biochemical events occur that are interrelated, are time-linked, and lead to secondary neural injury. These events are potentially amenable to attenuation or reversal by a variety of drug treatments. However, clinical trials of several promising agents have resulted in significant disappointment to date.

Different investigators favor different mechanisms as the primary modulators of secondary neural injury. Recent studies have focused on free radical scavengers, calcium channel blockers, and glutamate receptor antagonists as potential therapeutic agents in treating TBI.

Free Radical Scavengers

Free radicals are normally generated as a byproduct of cellular metabolism. They rarely accumulate in sufficient amounts to be harmful because of endogenous free radical scavengers such as vitamin E or superoxide dismutase (SOD). Following trauma, the production of free radicals increases by several orders of magnitude, rapidly overcoming mechanisms that regulate their concentration. The action of free radicals results in lipid peroxidation, damage to cell membranes, and ultimately, cell death. Thus following TBI, neurons that do not sustain primary injury are susceptible to subsequent injury by free radicals.[11] Clinical studies using free radical scavengers and lipid peroxidation inhibitors have not shown improved outcomes following severe TBI.[12]

Although steroids are the prototypical lipid peroxidation inhibitors, no clinical study has demonstrated improved patient outcome with their use following TBI.[13] Tirilazad, a 21-aminosteroid, demonstrated promising results in laboratory studies of TBI.[14] However, a large-scale clinical trial was terminated prematurely because of excess mortality in tirilazad-treated patients compared with placebo-treated patients. Data analysis indicated that the findings were primarily due to inadequate randomization of patients. When the results were corrected for this variable, there remained no statistically significant improvement in patient outcome with the use of tirilazad (anecdotal data).

The most promising results of studies of free radical scavengers are those using SOD. SOD is a naturally occurring free radical scavenger that is active in experimental models of TBI. Improved recovery has been shown when SOD is used as a primary treatment in experimental models. For clinical use, SOD is conjugated with polyethylene glycol (PEG-SOD) to decrease potential immunogenicity and to prolong its half-life. Several studies have shown beneficial effects on ICP, CBF, and cerebral edema.

A randomized, double-blind, placebo-controlled phase II trial of PEG-SOD was reported in 1993.[15] Random assignment of patients with severe TBI was done between placebo and an escalating dose of PEG-SOD given as a single intravenous bolus within 12 hours of injury. No complications attributable to the drug were described. Patients receiving the higher doses of PEG-SOD required less intensive therapy for ICP control and had fewer ICP elevations above 20 mm Hg. At three months post-TBI, the placebo group had a 43% incidence of death or vegetative outcome, compared with 20% in the cohort treated with PEG-SOD ($p = 0.03$). At six months, the differences, 36% versus 21%, respectively, remained significant ($p = 0.04$). The results of a larger multicenter phase III trial comparing placebo with two different PEG-SOD doses were reported in 1996.[16] In more than 800 patients studied, there was a 9% increase in favorable outcomes for those receiving PEG-SOD, but this difference did not reach statistical significance. Thus, no free radical scavenger has demonstrated improved patient outcome following TBI.

Calcium Channel Antagonists

Several calcium channel antagonists have been studied intensively for their potential effects on brain ischemia and trauma. Trauma causes extensive membrane depolarization, resulting in the opening of voltage-gated calcium channels and subsequent abnormal accumulation of calcium inside neurons and glia. These ionic shifts are associated with a cascade of events, including activation of lipolytic enzymes, proteolytic enzymes, protein kinases and protein phosphatases, and dissolution of microtubules and altered gene expression. These pathophysiologic events can disrupt cellular cytoskeletal architecture, arrest axoplasmic transport, and destroy cellular membranes.[17]

The European Head Injury I and II Trials (HIT-I and-II) recently reported results using the calcium channel blocker nimodipine in more than 1000 patients.[18,19] The HIT-I trial recruited 352 patients in a placebo-controlled study of patients enrolled within 24 hours of injury and treated for 7 days. There were no deleterious effects on blood pressure and no positive benefits to ICP control. No statistically significant difference was observed in favorable patient outcomes between the nimodipine (53%) and the placebo (49%) groups.

The HIT-II trial enrolled 852 patients with similar outcome results: Of the nimodipine-treated patients, 61% had a favorable outcome, compared with 59% of the placebo-treated group. However, a post hoc analysis of the 33% of patients who had posttraumatic subarachnoid hemorrhage on initial CT scanning found a significant reduction in unfavorable outcomes in the nimodipine-treated patients (61%) compared with the placebo-treated patients (41%; $p < 0.025$). Thus it appears that nimodipine does not alter overall outcome in patients with severe TBI, although there may be at least one subset of patients who could benefit from its utilization. Currently, a clinical trial is being initiated with the neuron-specific calcium channel blocker SNXIII. Results will not be available for several years.

Glutamate Receptor Antagonists

Antagonists to N-methyl-D-aspartate (NMDA) and other glutamate receptor subtypes have had substantial preclinical use and are presently in phase II and phase III clinical trials. Binding of excitatory amino acid receptors by glutamate can open the associated receptor-operated ion channel; some of these receptors allow for calcium influx into the neuron. In injury models, an abnormal influx of calcium may occur, initiating the pathophysiological sequences previously described. Most of the available preclinical data were obtained using stroke-ischemia models.[20] The combined results of these studies suggest the ability to provide neuronal protection for greater than 50% of the tissue at risk for ischemia using a variety of NMDA receptor antagonists. Because injury due to ischemia often plays a significant role in many patients with TBI, any agent that provides protection in this situation is attractive.

Several studies have demonstrated improved recovery using NMDA receptor antagonists after experimental TBI. In a rat fluid percussion model, pretreatment with the NMDA receptor antagonist MK-801 produced a dose-dependent decrease in mortality with a concomitant similar improvement in memory and motor function.[21] In a rat subdural hematoma model, an excellent correlation was shown between injury and excess glutamate levels, altered metabolism, and improvement with NMDA receptor antagonist treatment.[22] There was a sevenfold increase in glutamate levels in the cortex directly below the subdural hematoma. The increased glutamate levels and a marked increase in glucose metabolism were both abolished by pretreatment with the NMDA receptor antagonist d-CPP-ene. Additionally, treatment with d-CPP-ene reduced the zone of infarction under the hematoma by 54%.

Several years ago, a phase III clinical trial was initiated in both the United States and Europe based on data concerning the NMDA receptor antagonist CGS19755. Its effects on stroke and TBI were studied. After entry of more than 1000 patients, the study was stopped because of disproportionate mortality rates in patients with stroke treated with CGS19755. Although there were no similar deleterious effects in TBI, the study was not reinitiated and the number of patients with TBI treated to the termination point was too small to draw any valid conclusions about the effectiveness of this agent. More recently, d-CPP-ene was tested in clinical trials in Europe. The trial has recently concluded, but no outcome data are yet available. A more selective NMDA receptor antagonist has recently begun clinical trial in the United States.

Future Directions

Despite many unfavorable results of clinical trials described above, there continues to be optimism that pharmacological intervention following severe

TBI will ultimately limit or prevent secondary injury, and improve patient outcome. Improved patient outcome occurred in two studies that used methylprednisolone following acute spinal cord injury.[23,24] Several compounds of varying types and actions continue to be under active preclinical investigation, and phase I and II clinical trials for severe TBI. Additionally, investigations into the genetic response of neurons to injury and recovery are opening a new avenue of study. Several injury-specific genes such as c-*fos* and c-*jun* have been identified and may be responsible for the abnormal biochemical responses, cellular apoptosis, or cellular repair and recovery.[25]

In addition to attempting cerebral protection by pharmacological agents, other techniques have been developed to protect the injured or ischemic brain from the deleterious effects of secondary injury. Cerebrovascular surgery researchers and clinicians have generated a large body of literature suggesting better subject outcomes when using hypothermia during periods of iatrogenic brain ischemia. Moderate hypothermia has received much attention as a treatment for severe head injury. Studies using hypothermia were first reported in 1943, and have suggested improved outcome in patients with head injury treated with cooling compared with patients treated in normothermia.[26] In a prospective and randomized trial, a significant improvement in neurological outcome was noted at three and six months in a patient group treated with hypothermia.[27] This improved outcome occurred in the patient group who had initial Glasgow Coma Scale scores of 5–7, but no difference was seen in the group with scores less than 5. Although some studies have indicated a higher incidence of medical complications (especially pulmonary) with hypothermia, this study noted no significant difference.

There are a number of documented effects of hypothermia on the brain. Reducing the core body temperature reduces cerebral ischemia, edema, and tissue injury, and preserves the blood–brain barrier during low blood flow conditions. The mechanisms by which these protective effects occur are not fully known. In animal models, one definite effect of hypothermia is lowering of the cerebral metabolic rate, thereby lowering the oxygen demand, and decreasing CBF and ICP. Additionally, hypothermia lowers the extracellular concentrations of some excitatory neurotransmitters (e.g., glutamate) and inflammatory mediators (e.g., IL-1).[28–31]

These experimental findings are potentially important in the prevention or lessening of secondary neural injury; however, they are not established as being applicable in patients with TBI. Moderate hypothermia treatment protocols have not been determined conclusively to be beneficial in patients with TBI and Glasgow Coma Scale scores of lower than 8. Further investigation is required before hypothermia can be recommended as a standard therapy for patients with TBI.

Conclusion

Recent years have brought potential breakthroughs in TBI management. Research into better resuscitation techniques, improved monitoring and treatment systems, and biochemical and genetic therapies has provided new avenues of investigation that seek to improve patient outcome following TBI. It is hoped that severe TBI will be considered not a hopeless situation, but rather one in which a positive impact can be made with aggressive and appropriate therapy.

PEARLS AND PITFALLS

- Brain injury that occurs at the time of impact (primary injury) is relatively fixed.
- Following TBI, several biochemical processes are initiated that lead to further neurological injury (secondary injury). Appropriate management of patients with TBI can ameliorate some or all of the effects of secondary injury.
- Hypotension and hypoxia significantly increase the chance of a poor outcome in patients with TBI.
- Hyperventilation provides an initial benefit in ICP control, but should be avoided because hypocapnia contributes to decreased CBF and ultimately to brain ischemia.
- Maintenance of adequate CPP (>70 mm/Hg) optimizes cerebral perfusion and improves outcome in many cases.

- Mannitol is useful in reducing ICP and possibly improves CBF by affecting red blood cell membranes.
- Several neural protection agents are being tested to establish new avenues of therapy for TBI.
- Moderate hypothermia may be of some benefit to patients with TBI.

REFERENCES

1. Becker DP, Miller JD, Ward JD, Greenberg RP, Young HF, Sakalas R. The outcome from severe head injury with early diagnosis and intensive management. *J Neurosurg.* 1977;47:491–502.
2. Vollmer DG. Prognosis and outcome of severe head injury. In: Cooper PR, ed. *Head Injury.* 3rd ed. Baltimore, Md: Williams & Wilkins; 1993;553–81.
3. Chesnut RM, Marshall LF, Marshall SB. Medical management of intracranial pressure. In: Cooper PR, ed. *Head Injury.* 3rd ed. Baltimore, Md: Williams & Wilkins; 1993:225–46.
4. Gunnar WD, Merlotti GJ, Jonasson O, et al. Resuscitation from hemorrhagic shock: alterations of the intracranial pressure after normal saline, 3% saline and dextran-40. *Ann Surg.* 1986;204:686–92.
5. Shackford SR, Bourguignon PR, Wald SL, et al. Hypertonic saline resuscitation of patients with head injury: a prospective, randomized clinical trial. *J Trauma.* 1998;44:50–8.
6. *Guidelines for the Management of Severe Head Injury.* Philadelphia, Pa: Brain Trauma Foundation and American Association of Neurological Surgeons; 1995.
7. Sioutos PJ, Orozco JA, Carter LP, et al. Continuous regional cerebral cortical blood flow monitoring in head-injured patients. *Neurosurgery.* 1995;36:943–50.
8. Wilberger JE, Cantella D. Barbiturates in intractable intracranial pressure. *New Horizons.* 1995;3:469–73.
9. Muizelaar JP, Marmarou A, Ward JD, et al. Adverse effects of prolonged hyperventilation in patients with severe head injury: a randomized clinical trial. *J Neurosurg.* 1991;75:54–9.
10. Narayan RK, Greenberg RP, Miller JD, et al. Improved confidence of outcome prediction in severe head injury: a comparative analysis of the clinical examination, multimodality evoked potentials, CT scanning and intracranial pressure. *J Neurosurg.* 1981;54:751–62.
11. Hall ED. Free radicals and lipid peroxidation. In: Narayan RK, Wilberger JE, Povlishock JT, eds. *Neurotrauma.* New York, NY: McGraw-Hill Book Co; 1996:1405–19.
12. Wilberger JE. Pharmacologic strategies in head injury. In: Salcsman M, 2nd ed. *Current Techniques in Neurosurgery.* Philadelphia, Pa: Morrison Communications; 1995.
13. Giannotta SL, Weiss MH, Apuzzo MLJ, Martin E. High dose glucocorticoids in the management of severe head injury. *Neurosurgery.* 1984;15:497–501.
14. Dimlich RVW, Tornheim PA, Kindel RM, et al. Effects of a 21-amino acid steroid (U-74006F) on cerebral metabolism and edema after severe experimental head trauma. In: Long DA, ed. *Advances in Neurology.* New York, NY: Raven Press, Ltd; 1990;52:365–75.
15. Muizelaar JP, Marmarou A, Young HF, et al. Improving the outcome of severe head injury with the oxygen radical scavenger polyethylene glycol-conjugated superoxide dismutase: a phase-II trial. *J Neurosurg.* 1993;78:375–82.
16. Young B, Runge JW, Wilberger JE, et al. A multicenter phase-III trial of the oxygen radical scavenger polyethylene glycol-conjugated superoxide dismutase in patients with severe head injury. *JAMA.* 1996;276:538–42.
17. Young W. Death by calcium: a way of life. In: Narayan RK, Wilberger JE, Povlishock JT, eds. *Neurotrauma.* New York, NY: McGraw-Hill Book Co; 1996:1421–31.
18. Bailey I, Bell A, Gray J, et al. A trial of the effect of Nimodipine on outcome after head injury. *Acta Neurochir.* 1991;110:97–105.
19. Karieica A, Braakman R, Schakel EH. Traumatic subarachnoid hemorrhage. Importance in treatment perspective with nimodipine. *J Neurotrauma.* 1993;10 (suppl 1):193.
20. Ozyurt E, Graham DI, Woodruff GN, McCullough J. Protective effect of the glutamate antagonist MK-801 in focal cerebral ischemia in the cat. *J Cereb Blood Flow Metab.* 1988;8:138–43.
21. Hayes RL, Jenkins LW, Lyeth BG. Neurotransmitter mediated mechanisms of traumatic brain injury: acetylcholine and excitatory amino acids. *J Neurotrauma.* 1992;9(suppl 1):S173–88.
22. Chen MH, Bullock R, Graham DI, et al. Ischemic neuronal damage after subdural hematoma in the rat. Effects of pretreatment with a glutamate antagonist. *J Neurosurg.* 1991;79:944–50.
23. Bracken MB, Shepard MJ, Collins WF Jr., et al. Methylprednisolone or Naloxone in the treatment of acute spinal cord injury: one year follow-up results of the National Acute Spinal Cord Injury Study. *J Neurosurg.* 1992;76:23–32.
24. Bracken MB, Shepard MJ, Holford TR, et al. Administration of Methylprednisolone for 24 or 48 hours or Tirilizad Mesylate for 48 hours in the treatment of acute spinal cord injury. *JAMA.* 1997;227:1597–1604.
25. Sheng M, Greenberg ME. The regulation and function of *c-fos* and other immediate early genes in the nervous system. *Neuron.* 1990;4:477–85.

26. Fay T. Observation on generalized refrigeration in cases of severe cerebral trauma. *Assoc Red Nerv Ment Dis Proc.* 1943;24:611–19.

27. Marion DW, Penrod LE, Kelsey SF, et al. Treatment of traumatic brain injury with moderate hypothermia. *N Engl J Med.* 1997;336:540–6.

28. Pomeranz S, Safar P, Radovsky A, et al. The effect of resuscitative moderate hypothermia following epidural brain compression on cerebral damage in a canine outcome model. *J Neurosurg.* 1993;79:241–51.

29. Smith SL, Hall ED. Mild pre- and post-traumatic hypothermia attenuates blood-brain barrier damage following controlled cortical impact injury in the rat. *J Neurotrauma.* 1996;13:1–9.

30. Clasen RA, Pandolfi S, Russel J, et al. Hypothermia and hypotension in experimental cerebral edema. *Arch Neurol.* 1968;19:472–86.

31. Bering EA Jr. Effect of body temperature change on cerebral oxygen consumption of the intact monkey. *Am J Physiol.* 1961;200:417–19.

Index

Printed in the United States
By Bookmasters